WOMEN'S HEALTH AND DISEASE
Gynecologic, Endocrine, and Reproductive Issues

ANNALS OF THE NEW YORK ACADEMY OF SCIENCES

Volume 1092

WOMEN'S HEALTH AND DISEASE
Gynecologic, Endocrine, and
Reproductive Issues

*Edited by George Creatsas, George Mastorakos, and
George P. Chrousos*

Published by Blackwell Publishing on behalf of the New York Academy of Sciences
Boston, Massachusetts
2006

Library of Congress Cataloging-in-Publication Data

Women's health and disease : gynecologic and reproductive issues /
edited by George Creatsas, George Mastorakos, and
George P. Chrousos.
    p. ; cm. – (Annals of the New York Academy of Sciences, ISSN
0077-8923 ; v. 1092)
    This volume is the latest proceedings of a series of meetings that
has been held in Athens for over a decade.
  Includes bibliographical references and index.
  ISBN-13: 978-1-57331-621-7 (alk. paper)
  ISBN-10: 1-57331-621-0 (alk. paper)
  1. Women–Health and hygiene–Congresses.
2. Women–Diseases–Congresses. 3. Gynecology–Congresses.
4. Endocrinology–Congresses. 5. Reproductive health–Congresses.
I. Creatsas, G. II. Mastorakos, George. III. Chrousos, George P.
IV. Series.
  [DNLM: 1. Genital Diseases, Female–Congresses. 2. Reproductive
Medicine–Congresses. 3. Women's Health–Congresses.
4. Neurodegenerative Diseases–drug therapy–Congresses.
W1 AN626YL v.1092 2006 / WP 140 W8723 2006]

  Q11.N5 vol. 1092
  [RA778]
  613'.04244–dc22

                            2006033075

The *Annals of the New York Academy of Sciences* (ISSN: 0077-8923 [print]; ISSN: 1749-6632 [online]) is published 28 times a year on behalf of the New York Academy of Sciences by Blackwell Publishing, with offices located at 350 Main Street, Malden, Massachusetts 02148 USA, PO Box 1354, Garsington Road, Oxford OX4 2DQ UK, and PO Box 378 Carlton South, 3053 Victoria Australia.

Information for subscribers: Subscription prices for 2006 are: Premium Institutional: $3850.00 (US) and £2139.00 (Europe and Rest of World).
Customers in the UK should add VAT at 5%. Customers in the EU should also add VAT at 5% or provide a VAT registration number or evidence of entitlement to exemption. Customers in Canada should add 7% GST or provide evidence of entitlement to exemption. The Premium Institutional price also includes online access to full-text articles from 1997 to present, where available. For other pricing options or more information about online access to Blackwell Publishing journals, including access information and terms and conditions, please visit www.blackwellpublishing.com/nyas.

Membership information: Members may order copies of the *Annals* volumes directly from the Academy by visiting www.nyas.org/annals, emailing membership@nyas.org, faxing 212-298-3650, or calling 800-843-6927 (US only), or +1 212-298-8640 (International). For more information on becoming a member of the New York Academy of Sciences, please visit www.nyas.org/membership.

Journal Customer Services: For ordering information, claims, and any inquiry concerning your institutional subscription, please contact your nearest office:
UK: Email: customerservices@blackwellpublishing.com; Tel: +44 (0) 1865 778315; Fax +44 (0) 1865 471775
US: Email: customerservices@blackwellpublishing.com; Tel: +1 781 388 8599 or 1 800 835 6770 (Toll free in the USA); Fax: +1 781 388 8232
Asia: Email: customerservices@blackwellpublishing.com; Tel: +65 6511 8000; Fax: +61 3 8359 1120
Members: Claims and inquiries on member orders should be directed to the Academy at email: membership@nyas.org or Tel: +1 212 838 0230 (International) or 800-843-6927 (US only).

Printed in the USA.
Printed on acid-free paper.

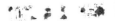

ANNALS OF THE NEW YORK ACADEMY OF SCIENCES

Volume 1092
December 2006

WOMEN'S HEALTH AND DISEASE
Gynecologic, Endocrine, and Reproductive Issues

Editors
GEORGE CREATSAS, GEORGE MASTORAKOS, AND GEORGE P. CHROUSOS

This volume is a result of a meeting entitled **the 6th Athens Congress on Women's Health and Disease: Gynecologic and Reproductive Issues**, held on September 23–25, 2005 in Athens, Greece.

CONTENTS

Part VII. Fetal–Maternal Medicine

Part VIII. Treating Menopausal Women under the WHI Shadow

Part IX. Menopause–Osteoporosis

Part X. Selected Research Papers

Financial assistance was received from:

- Medical School of Athens University
- International Menopause Society (IMS)
- European Menopause and Andropause Society (EMAS)
- International Federation of Gynecology and Obstetrics (IFGO)

Foreword

Women's Health: The World's Safeguard

"The soul suffers when the body is diseased or traumatized, while the body suffers when the soul is ailing."

Aristotle

The new millennium has begun with major social, cultural, ethical, philosophical, and practical questions regarding women, reproduction, and society. In the Western world, women have asserted their rights but still live in a mostly male-run environment, constantly trying to balance their professional and family responsibilities. Major efforts continue to be initiated by international and national organizations to accelerate the process of women's empowerment and attainment of equal rights everywhere on the planet. Day by day, momentum is being gained, with women achieving social autonomy and financial independence, and reaching leadership positions in all aspects of human life.

This marked improvement of status, however, has placed women in highly demanding, stressful conditions, and Western societies at a reproductive disadvantage, resulting in major negative repercussions. Women start families and/or bear children late, frequently requiring expensive and burdensome assisted reproduction medications and procedures. They have at most one or two children, a proportion of them born prematurely or small, with an increased risk of later suffering from developmental disabilities. As a consequence, Western nations now have shrinking and aging populations and face a difficult future with unsustainable resources for continuing to maintain effective social security systems. We progressively realize as a modern society that we must assist women reconcile their unique social and biologic roles, which are linked to the continuance of our very existence in the future.

Recently, an increasing interest has developed within the biomedical community in understanding the dynamic physiologic and psychological changes that occur during a woman's life span and in exploring their major psychological and biologic differences from men. Indeed, women's health departments and centers that target women as subjects and patients have been developed and research funding has been allocated specifically for the study of women. Thus, even for seemingly simple applications, for example, determining gender-specific drug dosology, no extrapolations from male studies should be used, but, rather, the appropriate doses should be determined in women for use by women.

Ann. N.Y. Acad. Sci. 1092: xiii–xv (2006). © 2006 New York Academy of Sciences.
doi: 10.1196/annals.1365.001

This volume represents the edited proceedings of an international congress entitled The 6th Athens Congress on Women's Health and Disease: Gynecologic and Reproductive Issues that was held in Athens, Greece, in the fall of 2005. The meeting took place under the auspices of the Athens University School of Medicine, the International Federation of Gynecology and Obstetrics, and the European Society of Contraception. The program included a well-balanced combination of basic and clinical subjects, without neglecting important psychological aspects of a woman's life.

This volume contains useful information that covers broad aspects of obstetrics, gynecology, endocrinology, and the reproductive sciences, as well as recent progress in molecular biology and genetics pertinent to reproductive health. The papers are clustered by content into ten parts.

In the introductory section, attention is drawn to current methods of contraception favored in everyday practice and the major influence that the metabolic syndrome exerts on a woman's life. The second part covers the topic of the first menstruation, while the third covers adolescent medicine issues, including contraception, anorexia nervosa, and hypothalamic amenorrhea at this critical period of life. In the fourth section, the female metabolic syndrome and its relationship to chronic inflammation are presented, with articles on ovarian and adrenal hyperandrogenism, intrauterine growth restriction, and postnatal development of the metabolic syndrome, premature adrenarche, and polycystic ovary syndrome (PCOS), as well as the recently described low-grade systemic inflammation in PCOS.

The fifth section deals with subjects related to minimally invasive surgery, such as the retroperitoneal approach, the laparoscopic management of hydrosalpinx and adnexal masses, and the safety of hysteroscopic surgery. The sixth and seventh parts draw the attention of the reader to one of the main issues of Western societies today, subfertility. Over the past three decades, assisted reproduction has markedly evolved from a set of procedures that were first faced with skepticism into widely used technologies that help many infertile couples have children. These technologies now offer a higher pregnancy rate than that previously attained by the surgical management of infertility in cases of endometriosis and tubal damage. The section covers assisted reproduction issues, such as oocyte maturation, prevention and management of the ovarian hyperstimulation syndrome, the relationship between fertility drugs and gynecologic cancer, as well as prenatal genetic diagnosis.

We inevitably needed to include issues of maternal–fetal medicine regarding the outcome of pregnancy. Thus, the recent developments in the detection of fetal single-gene disorders in maternal blood, routine ultrasound evaluations in low-risk obstetric populations, the assessment of intrauterine growth restriction by Doppler, the brain-sparing effect of neurotrophins, the symmetric small-for-gestational-age fetus, the roles of reproductive corticotropin-releasing hormone, and the postnatal development of fetal growth-restricted infants are presented and discussed.

As life expectancy has remarkably increased in the Western world, the life of women after menopause has become a long, productive period of major importance to women and to society. Thus, the eighth and ninth sections of the book deal with the treatment of menopausal women in the post-Women's Health Initiative (WHI) study era; hormone replacement therapy for cardioprotection in women with premature menopause, and the importance of this therapy in breast cancer survivors; the expanding estrogen functions emerging from the recently described different types of estrogen receptors; the cardiovascular effects of Selective Estrogen Receptor Modulators (SERMs); and the recent advances in the treatment of postmenopausal osteoporosis. Finally, the last section of the volume was dedicated to selected research papers that enriched The 6th Athens Congress on Women's Health and Disease with novel hypotheses and promising data.

In the ensuing decades, the biomedical community will increasingly broaden and deepen the study of women, facilitating their important and unique roles and achievements, and improving their quality of life, to the benefit of humankind.

GEORGE CREATSAS
GEORGE MASTORAKOS
GEORGE P. CHROUSOS
University of Athens Medical
School, Athens, Greece

Contraception Today

GIUSEPPE BENAGIANO, CARLO BASTIANELLI,
AND MANUELA FARRIS

Department of Gynecological Sciences, Perinatology and Child Care, University
"La Sapienza," Rome, Italy

ABSTRACT: Modern contraceptive methods represent more than a technical advance: they are the instrument of a true social revolution—the "first reproductive revolution" in the history of humanity, an achievement of the second part of the 20th century, when modern, effective methods became available. Today a great diversity of techniques have been made available and—thanks to them, fertility rates have decreased from 5.1 in 1950 to 3.7 in 1990. As a consequence, the growth of human population that had more than tripled, from 1.8 to more than 6 billion in just one century, is today being brought under control. At the turn of the millennium, all over the world, more than 600 million married women are using contraception, with nearly 500 million in developing countries. Among married women, contraceptive use rose in all but two developing countries surveyed more than once since 1990. Among unmarried, sexually active women, it grew in 21 of 25 countries recently surveyed. Hormonal contraception, the best known method, first made available as a daily pill, can today be administered through seven different routes: intramuscularly, intranasally, intrauterus, intravaginally, orally, subcutaneously, and transdermally. In the field of oral contraception, new strategies include further dose reduction, the synthesis of new active molecules, and new administration schedules. A new mini-pill (progestin-only preparation) containing desogestrel has been recently marketed in a number of countries and is capable of consistently inhibiting ovulation in most women. New contraceptive rings to be inserted in the vagina offer a novel approach by providing a sustained release of steroids and low failure rates. The transdermal route for delivering contraceptive steroids is now established via a contraceptive patch, a spray, or a gel. The intramuscular route has also seen new products with the marketing of improved monthly injectable preparations containing an estrogen and a progestin. After the first device capable of delivering progesterone directly into the uterus was withdrawn, a new system releasing locally 20 µg evonorgestrel is today marketed in a majority of countries with excellent contraceptive and therapeutic performance. Finally, several subcutaneously implanted systems have been developed: contraceptive "rods,"

Address for correspondence: Giuseppe Benagiano, 28, Chemin Des Massettes, 1218 Le Grand, Saconnex, Genève, Switzerland. Voice: +3906-490-398; fax: +3906-4997-2544.
e-mail: giuseppe.benagiano@uniroma1.it

Ann. N.Y. Acad. Sci. 1092: 1–32 (2006). © 2006 New York Academy of Sciences.
doi: 10.1196/annals.1365.002

where the polymeric matrix is mixed with the steroid and "capsules" made of a hollow polymer tube filled with free steroid crystals. New advances have also been made in nonhormonal intrauterine contraception with the development of "frameless" devices. The HIV/AIDS pandemic forced policy makers to look for ways to protect young people from sexually transmitted diseases as well as from untimely pregnancies. This led to the development of the so-called dual protection method, involving the use of a physical barrier (condom) as well as that of a second, highly effective contraceptive method. More complex is the situation with antifertility vaccines, still at a preliminary stage of development and unlikely to be in widespread use for years to come. Last, but not least, work is in progress to provide effective emergency contraception after an unprotected intercourse. Very promising in this area is the use of selective progesterone receptor modulators (antiprogestins).

KEYWORDS: contraception; sexual behavior; hormonal contraceptives; intrauterine devices; emergency contraceptives

INTRODUCTION

Discussing contraception usually means discussing technology: old versus new methods; short-acting versus long-acting methods; reversible versus irreversible methods. Yet, modern contraceptive methods represent more than a technical advance: they are the instruments of a true social revolution, or—in more concrete terms—of the "first reproductive revolution" in the history of humanity.

This is because since *homo sapiens* started dwelling in the lands of East Africa, the strategy that characterized human male reproductive behavior remained basically unchanged until the middle of the 20th century. It was a strategy based on two simple mechanisms: ensure continuity of an individual male through the passage of his genes to the largest feasible number of females, and select those females who would provide the highest possible quality of oocytes. The latter was usually achieved by selecting a young female with the best physical characteristics. Female strategies, on the other hand, have always focused around the need for protection and support. A human female, like the females of big apes, has throughout most of the life span of the gender *homo* sought a male capable of providing the best means for her survival and that of their offspring.[1]

Basically, this common strategy, according to which sexual activity is fundamentally justified for reproductive purposes, has remained unchanged throughout human history because conceptive sexuality makes sense since sexual behavior is costly to both sexes.[2] Saving energies to be dedicated to food gathering, hunting, and defense was—in the early days—an imperative and a winning strategy.

Modern anthropology, however, has now delineated a more complex picture since infecund copulations have today been well documented among primates, particularly a species of chimpanzees little known until the second part of the 20th century, called *bonobos*, living on the northern shore of the Congo river.[3] In apes, nonconceptive copulations are of two distinct types: *exchange sex,* in which a female obtains direct nonreproductive benefits, like food, in exchange for sex; and *communication sex,* sexual activity, not necessarily copulative, to develop social relationship or to diffuse tension and avoid aggression.[4] This indicates that, already in the great apes, a more complex sexual behavior began to emerge as a characteristic that can be learned and used for purposes other than reproduction.

In humans, therefore, sexual activity must have started to lose its exclusive reproductive meaning early in the evolution of the species. Indeed, humans must have begun nonconceptive sex since time immemorial if we look at the unique features developed by our females. As nonconceptive sexual activity began to take predominance, external manifestations of an impending ovulation so prevalent in primates (e.g., genital swelling) began to disappear. Under those circumstances nonconceptive sexual activity must have conditioned human evolution, including creating the basis for the trend toward monogamy. Indeed, with a female who is accessible every day of the year, there is less impetus to "look around" for other receptive females.[1] Yet, nonreproductive sexual behavior and the consequent changes that "hid" the appearance of the fertile period created a new necessity, that of *avoiding*, rather than *seeking* conception during intercourse.

In this respect, we know that humans have tried to practice contraception since they began to leave written records. FIGURE 1 shows an Egyptian papyrus describing how to avoid conception during intercourse.

Although contraception has been practiced since ancient times, the contraceptive revolution is an achievement of the second part of the 20th century, when modern, effective methods became available. FIGURE 2, taken from a review by Baird and Glasier, [5] summarizes known potential targets for contraception in men and women, giving an idea of the great diversity of techniques already developed and of possible future developments.

THE POPULATION EXPLOSION

Research on fertility-regulating methods has been prompted by many imperatives; however, at the global level, there is no doubt that the most powerful engine has been the unique feature that characterized the 20th century: population explosion. When we realize that during the last 100 years human population more than tripled from 1.8 to more than 6 billion, we can easily accept that the problem reached such a magnitude that it had to be aggressively addressed and resolved. And this is precisely what happened, since, whenever

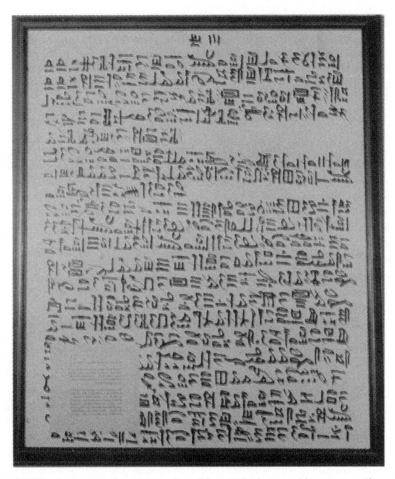

FIGURE 1. An Egyptian papyrus describing methods to avoid pregnancy (from the Ortho museum of contraception).

in human history a global problem reached such a magnitude that its solution could not be delayed, humanity has invariably found the strength and the way to successfully resolve it.

Fertility Rate Decline

Remarkable results have already been achieved, although clearly much remains to be done. Looking at the latest projections made by the United Nations [6] and shown in FIGURE 3, we see space for optimism because of the five different projections made then, today only the lower two seem realistic in view of the results achieved in most countries of the world.

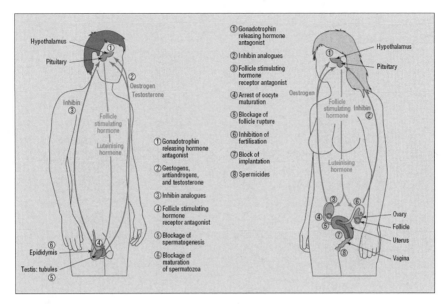

FIGURE 2. Present and possible future targets for contraceptive action (from Baird & Glasier, 1999).[5]

Indeed, as indicated in FIGURE 4A, total fertility rates decreased between 1950 and 2000 from 5.1 to 3.7. This decrease involved most of the countries of the planet including almost all developing countries surveyed since 1990 thanks to an increase in the use of modern contraceptives as shown in FIGURE 4B.

These trends continue according to the findings from more than 100 surveys conducted since 1990. In this connection, the World Fertility Report 2003[7] states that worldwide, contraceptive utilization grew from 38% in the 1970s to 52% in the 1990s. In developing countries the increase has been from 27% to 40%; in one-fourth of them this increase reached 62%.

Distribution of Contraceptive Use

Around the world, more than 600 million married women are using contraception with nearly 500 million in developing countries. Among married women, contraceptive use rose in all but two developing countries surveyed more than once since 1990. Among unmarried, sexually active women, contraceptive use rose in 21 of 25 countries.[7]

There is general agreement that as family planning programs have become widespread, more and more people want smaller families and more succeed in having the size of family that they want. This trend started during the second

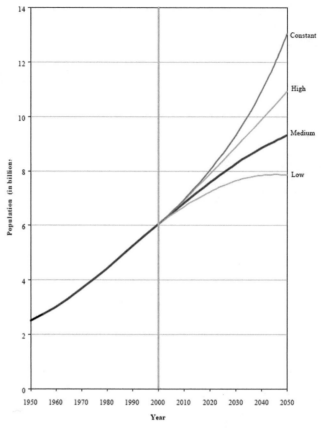

FIGURE 3. Estimated and projected population to the year 2150 (from UN Population Division 2000).[6]

part of the 20th century although, from the beginning, utilization of modern contraception has been higher in the industrialized world than in developing countries: for instance, a recent survey of the distribution of contraceptive methods in five European countries (France, Germany, Italy, Spain, and the UK) showed that 77% of all women of fertile age were regularly using a method. In terms of popularity, 30% used an oral contraceptive (OC); 20% relied on the partner's use of a condom; 11% used a reversible long-term contraception; 11% either partner was sterilized; and 6% of the women relied on "traditional methods." When we look at country-specific differences, OCs are more widely used in France, Germany, and the UK than in Italy and Spain. The proportion of women in each country having experienced the use of an OC (current and former users) was: 89% in Germany, 85% in France, 85% in UK, 55% in Spain, and 50% in Italy.[8]

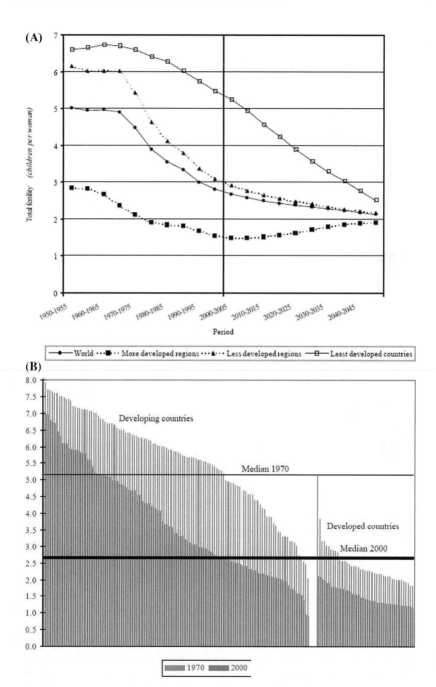

FIGURE 4. (A) Expected trends in world population from 1950 to 2050 (from UN Population Division 2000). **(B)** Fertility levels between 1970 and 2000 (from World Fertility Survey 2003).[6]

Contraceptive use varies substantially among developing countries. In a few countries of Asia and Latin America, at least three-fourths of married women use a contraceptive method with use levels equal to those of developed countries. In contrast, in some sub-Saharan African countries fewer than 10% of married women use contraception. Fertility rates range from just 2.3 children per woman in Vietnam to 7.2 in Niger.[7]

Although fertility is higher and contraceptive use less common in sub-Saharan Africa than elsewhere, surveys suggest that parts of Africa have started down the path already taken in other regions. Fertility fell by more than 1% per year in 9 of 16 sub-Saharan countries where more than one survey was carried out since 1990.[7] An African country that has shown excellent recent progress in family planning is Ethiopia, where modern method contraceptive prevalence increased from 6% in 2000 to 14% in 2005.[9]

It is noteworthy that, in spite of the vast array of methods available today, four of them account for almost three-quarters of all contraceptive use: female sterilization, OCs, injectables, and intrauterine devices (IUDs).

NEW DEVELOPMENTS IN HORMONAL CONTRACEPTION

Oral hormonal contraception, universally known as "the pill," is in fact represented today by a variety of methods using either estrogen-progestin combinations or progestins alone. A number of new routes of administration have also been researched and several of these new modalities have reached the market.

Combined Oral Contraception

In spite of all the new routes of administration available today for the delivery of contraceptive hormones, OCs remain the most important and most widely accepted modality. New strategies for improving OCs include: dose reduction and the synthesis of new active molecules.

Estrogen Dose Reduction

Since the first "pill scare" caused by the finding of an increased risk of venous thromboembolism in women using OCs containing high doses of ethinyl estradiol (EE) 35 years ago, safety has become the main issue in hormonal contraception[10] and the pharmaceutical industry was engaged in efforts to reduce the estrogen content of combined pills. This led in the 1980s and 1990s to the marketing of OCs containing as little as 20 μg of EE. Yet, this massive dose reduction (the first OC ever marketed, Anovlar®, contained 150 μg of mestranol, biologically equivalent to 120 μg of EE) continued even in the 21st century. A newly marketed combination contains as little as 15 μg EE in association with 60 μg gestodene (GSD). Since pharmacodynamic studies have shown that with this very low dosage inhibition of follicular growth and ovarian hormone production cannot be assured with the standard 21-day regimen, a daily administration schedule of 24 days has been implemented. FIGURES 5A and B show in a comparative fashion, circulating levels of estradiol and the mean diameter of the largest "follicle-like structure" with the 21- and 24-day administration of this regimen.[11]

Further dose reduction has also taken place in triphasic formulations; in two of them, recently approved by the FDA, the estrogen content has been reduced to minimize estrogen-related side effects such as breast tenderness, bloating, and nausea. The two formulations contain both 25 μg EE for a better cycle control, and respectively, 180, 215, and 250 μg nomegestrol (NMG) [12] and 100, 125, and 150 g desogestrel (DSG).[13]

A multicenter, randomized, blind study comparing the 25 μg EE-NMG triphasic formulation with a 20 μg EE-norethisterone acetate monophasic one, showed over 13 cycles a better cycle control with the new triphasic, although compliance was similar in the two treatment groups. Interestingly, only 0.4% discontinuation in either treatment regimen was due to nausea.[12]

The triphasic formulation containing DSG has been recently compared in two multicenter, randomized, open-label trials run concurrently to another triphasic formulation containing 30 μg EE and 500, 750, and 1μg norethisterone. In each of the six treatment cycles, rates of amenhorrea, breakthrough bleeding, and spotting were significantly lower among women using the 25 μg/tri-DSG formulation.[13]

Progestin Dose Reduction

In 1981 a pharmacodynamic study by Hirvonen *et al.*[14] found that certain 19-nor progestins, because of their androgenic properties, acted negatively on lipid metabolism. These findings had a profound influence on oral contraception because they started the search for new molecules with high progestational activity, but devoid of metabolic effects. The process led to the development—over the past two decades—of five new progestins: desogestrel, gestodene, norgestimate, drospirenone, and dienogest. It also led to studies aimed at decreasing the dosage of existing progestins; for instance, with levonorgestrel (LNG), the daily content in OCs went from the 500 μg of the racemic form used in 1969 to 250 μg in the 1970s, 150–125 μg in the 1980s, and 100 μg in the 1990s.

Even with the latest generation progestins a dose reduction has recently taken place: as already mentioned, whereas the original OC using gestodene as the progestin contained 75 μg daily, the latest pill contains only 60 μg.

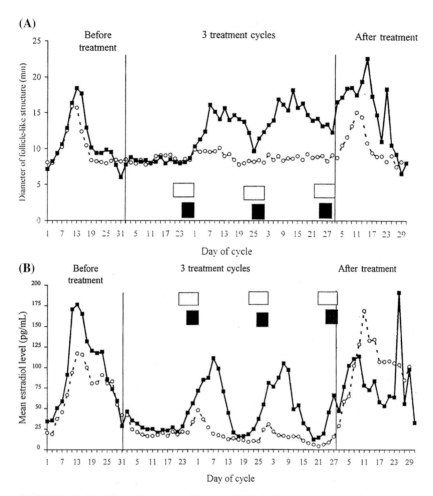

FIGURE 5. (A) Mean diameter of largest "follicle-like structure" with 21- and 24-day administration of a combined OC containing gestodene 60 μg and EE 15μg (Sullivan *et al.*[11]). White rectangles: 7-day pill-free intervals; black squares: 4-day placebo pill interval; diameters with 21-day regimen, square black dots; and with 24-day regimen, white dots. **(B)** Estradiol plasma levels with 21- and 24-day administration of a combined OC containing gestodene 60 μg and EE 15 μg (Sullivan *et al.*[11]). White rectangles: 7-day pill-free intervals; black squares: 4-day placebo pill interval; mean estradiol levels with 21-day regimen, square black dots; and with 24-day regimen, white dots.

Synthesis of New Molecules with Contraceptive Properties

When hormonal contraception was first introduced, only two orally active synthetic estrogens (mestranol and EE) and two progestins (norethisterone and norethynodrel) were available. Today, whereas only EE is used, a variety of progestins are being used in OCs as indicated in FIGURE 6.

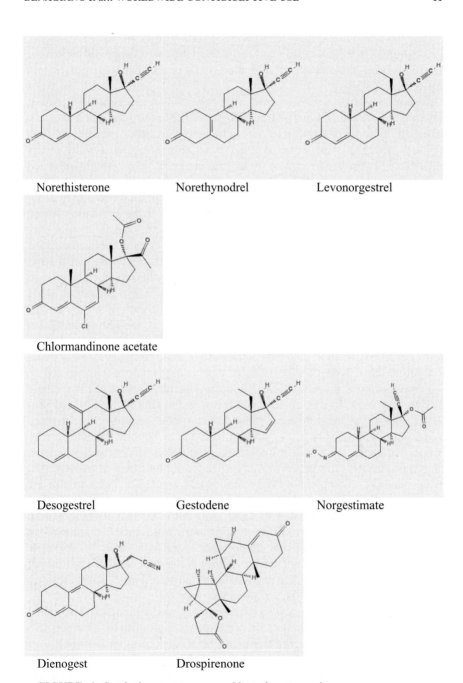

Norethisterone   Norethynodrel   Levonorgestrel

Chlormandinone acetate

Desogestrel   Gestodene   Norgestimate

Dienogest   Drospirenone

FIGURE 6. Synthetic progestogens used in oral contraception.

Progress continues and, for the first time in many years, the natural estrogen, 17β-estradiol, is being reevaluated for use in OCs. New progestin molecules have also been made available over the last 10 years: dienogest (DNG) and drospirenone (DRS).

Dienogest is a 19-nor testosterone derivative with a cyanomethyl group in position C17. It has a unique pharmacologic profile to the point that it has been labeled a "hybrid progestin:" it has no androgenic, estrogenic, mineralcorticoid, or glucocorticoid properties, and it exerts an antiandrogenic activity nearly 30% that of cyproterone acetate. After oral intake, DNG is rapidly adsorbed with a bioavailability of almost 95%. In spite of the high serum concentrations observed after administration of the combined formulation containing 2 mg DNG and 30 μg EE, there is no accumulation of DNG in the circulation during daily intake. When circulating, 90% of the dienogest is bound to albumin. The ovulation-inhibiting dose is 1 mg/day, in the range of that of cyproterone and chlormandinone acetates, while the endometrial transformation dose is similar to that observed with levonorgestrel. This may be explained by its high serum concentration (50 μg/L on average) and the 10% free-circulating DNG fraction.[15] Phase III trials are now examining the feasibility of a "step-down" combination containing DNG and the natural estrogen, estradiol. Estradiol is administered at the dose of 3 mg for the first 2 days, 2 mg from day 3 to 24 and 1 mg from day 25 to 26; DNG at the dose of 2 mg from day 2 to day 5 and 3 mg from day 6 to day 25.[16]

Drospirenone is a derivative of 17α-spironolactone with a pharmacologic profile very close to that of progesterone; it is the first clinically used progestin with antiandrogenic and antimineralocorticoid activities at contraceptive doses. Its peculiarity among progestins is due to the mild antialdosteronic action that characterizes all spiroolactone derivatives thanks to the lactonic ring in position 17; this action makes it specifically indicated in women who, when using OCs, complain of fluid retention or weight gain. Two randomized, open-label, clinical trials have been recently carried out to compare the efficacy, tolerability, and cycle control of 30 μg EE/2mg DRS with that of a monophasic 30 μg EE/150 μg DSG formulation: cycle control with the two combinations was similar, while reported side effects were lower with DRS.[17,18] Two new OC combinations containing DRS are shortly going to be available in Europe; both will contain 20 μg EE, but one will be administered for 21 days, the other for periods from 24 to 120 days without interruption.

Selective progesterone receptors modulators. These compounds, also called SPRMs or antiprogestins, so far have not shown real promise for contraceptive purposes, although a number of trials have been carried out under the aegis of WHO. In this respect, the 1998 WHO's Annual Technical Report of the UNDP-UNFPA-WHO-World Bank Special Programme of Research, Development and Research Training in Human Reproduction [19] stated them under "Planned studies during 1999": "In view of the disappointing interim results obtained in the contraceptive efficacy study involving a daily dose of 0.5 mg mifepristone, no further studies involving the daily administration of this compound are planned. The study to investigate the effect of daily doses of 2 mg and 5 mg of mifepristone on the endometrium and other parameters will be completed in 1999." The subsequent year, however, the section on mifepristone as a contraceptive was omitted altogether.

A suggestion has been made for SPRM to be used as "once a month" pills. In an article discussing the future of contraception, Baird and Glasier [5] argued that "a once a month pill that prevented ovulation or implantation would be welcomed by many women from various countries and cultures, whereas only a minority would be prepared to use a pill taken around the time of expected menses, when implantation of the embryo would already have occurred." They concluded that "current evidence suggests that mifepristone alone or in combination with misoprostol would result in too high an incidence of pregnancy to be useful as a regular method of inducing early menses."

New Administration Modalities

Several international guidelines state that women can safely and effectively use many of the monophasic OCs continuously for some cycles, skipping the pill-free interval or inactive pills.[20,21] This allows women to reduce the number of bleeding days and also side effects related to hormone withdrawal such as migraine, headache, mood changes, and painful monthly withdrawal bleedings.

A new formulation specifically packed for continuous use is being marketed in Europe under the trade name of Seasonale®; it contains 30 µg EE and 150 µg LNG. The package comes in a 3-monthly supply. Women take one active pill per day for 84 days (12 weeks) and then take an inactive pill for 7 days.

This regimen allows a reduction from 13 to 4 bleeding episodes per year; however, during the first 8 or 9 months of use, women taking OCs continuously are about twice as likely as those using conventional regimens to experience breakthrough bleedings.[22]

Progestin-Only Contraception

Progestin-only oral contraception (POP, the so-called "minipill") has been for many years a neglected modality because traditional POPs are associated with higher pregnancy rates than combined OCs, with a 1-year method failure of some 0.5% and a 5% failure in typical use.[23] Recently, however, a new, desogestrel-containing minipill (Cerazette®) has been marketed in a number of countries. It contains 75 µg of the hormone and is based on studies showing that the daily administration of 60 µg desogestrel consistently inhibits ovulation in all women treated. [24,25] A further randomized, double-blind comparative study using daily doses of 30, 50, or 75 µg indicates that the highest dose

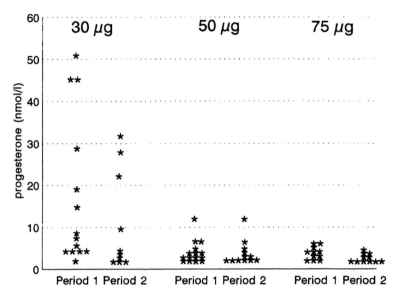

FIGURE 7. Maximum progesterone concentrations per subject per assessment period by dosage group (from Rice et al., 1996).[24]

preparation shows satisfactory suppression of ovarian function with consistent inhibition of ovulation: serum progesterone concentrations never exceed levels of 10 nmol/L,[26] as shown in FIGURE 7.

When the progestin-only OC containing 75 μg of DSG was compared to that containing 30 μg of LNG, Cerazette® inhibited ovulation in 58 out of the 59 cycles studied, while in the LNG group, 16 out of the 57 cycles studied were shown to be ovulatory.[27] It is noteworthy that in this study ovulation was defined as follicular rupture on ultrasound scanning followed by a rise in serum progesterone values. A higher suppression of ovarian function in women treated with the DSG minipill when compared to women treated with LNG can also be inferred both from significantly lower estradiol serum concentrations and from the number of follicles exceeding 30 mm in diameter in spite of similar FSH suppression.[27,28]

The clinical profile and biological effects of Cerazette® have been recently reviewed;[29] available evidence indicates that the more pronounced suppression of the hypothalamic-pituitary-ovarian axis and the consistent inhibition of ovulation are the prerequisites for the better Pearl index for the DSG minipill, close to that reported for OCs. Indeed, with traditional progestin-only pills, compliance with the timing of administration has a major impact on contraceptive use-effectiveness, whereas with Cerazette® a tolerance of 12 h for missed tablets over the regular 24-h intervals is allowed since restoration of the fully suppressed hypothalamic-pituitary-ovarian axis takes as long as with low-dose combined formulations.

The single most important adverse effect of progestin-only contraceptives is represented by bleeding irregularities because a continuous administration does not allow regular withdrawal bleedings, thus giving rise to unpredictable bleeding patterns. These negatively affect both acceptability and compliance by a majority of women, and, as a consequence, the diffusion of the method.

New Administration Routes

When hormonal contraception was first made available as a daily pill, few could have imagined that 50 years later seven different routes of administration would have been investigated. Indeed, today contraceptive hormones can be administered intramuscularly, intranasally (a modality no longer being pursued), intrauterus, intravaginally, orally, subcutaneously, transdermally.

Vaginal delivery. Contraceptive rings to be inserted in the vagina offer a novel approach to the delivery of hormones into the blood stream and use the well-known ability of the vaginal epithelium to absorb a large variety of different substances.[30] Pharmacokinetically, they provide a sustained release of steroids, are user-controlled, can be easily inserted and removed, do not require daily attention, and do not interfere with intercourse.[31]

Although rings delivering only progestins have been researched,[32] only vaginal rings containing both an estrogen and a progestogen (EP-VR) have reached widespread marketing; they are to be inserted before day 5 of the cycle irrespective of the presence of menstrual flow and withdrawn after 21 days, thereby allowing a proper cycle control.

Vaginal rings releasing an estrogen and a progestin. The first EP-VR marketed (Nuvaring®) releases 15 μg EE and 120 μg etonogestrel (ENG, or 3 ketodesogestrel), the active metabolite of DSG.

In a recent study where women using the EP-VR have been followed for 1 year, the overall failure rate was 0.65 pregnancies per 100 woman-years. The majority of women in the study considered insertion and removal of the vaginal ring to be easy and 90% used the device correctly. Adverse effects that led to discontinuation of the ring were mostly related to foreign body sensation, coital problems, and expulsion of the device. However, only 3.6% of women in the study stopped using the device for these reasons. In terms of cycle control, the vaginal ring is associated with a lower incidence of breakthrough bleeding than an OC containing 30 μg EE with a higher rate of normal withdrawal bleeding.[33]

Another EP-VR, releasing 15 mg EE and 150 mg of the progestin nestorone (NSR), is still in clinical trials. NSR is a potent progestin when given in a sustained release formulation, exhibiting a progestational activity stronger than that of DSG or LNG, lacking androgenic, estrogenic, and glucocorticoid activity. The NSR-containing ring is used in the same fashion as the

Nuvaring, its action lasts more than 12 months, and it seems to be more cost-effective.[31,34]

Vaginal rings releasing only a progestin. At present, two progestin-only vaginal rings (P-VR) have been developed: the Progering® containing the natural hormone progesterone and a ring filled with NSR. The Progering® ring releases 10 mg progesterone daily and lasts for 3 months. The method is highly effective among lactating women in whom it provides a level of contraceptive protection not significantly different from an IUD.[35] NSR-releasing rings rely on a potent synthetic progestin and therefore show great potential. This ring is under investigation at different daily release rates: 50, 75, or 100 μg.[36] Progestin-only rings exert their action in much the same way as minipills; thus, they are less effective than combined rings although they are recommended for breast-feeding women in whom they are highly effective and do not interfere with lactation.

Transdermal Delivery

Following the successful introduction of transdermal delivery systems for hormonal replacement therapy, the transdermal route has been investigated also for contraceptive purposes via a contraceptive patch, spray, or gel. This is an innovative and potentially useful approach to hormonal contraception, although at present only one patch has been marketed while gels and sprays are still in development.

Contraceptive patches. The only combined contraceptive patch already in the market (Evra®) releases daily 20 μg EE and 150 μg norelgestromin (NGN), the active metabolite of norgestimate. Each square patch has a 20 cm² surface (4.45 cm each side) and provides steady serum levels of EE and NGN as observed in a pharmacokinetic study lasting 3 months.[37] The absorption of NGN and EE is similar whether the contraceptive patch is applied to the upper outer arm, upper torso (excluding breast), buttock, or lower abdomen.

Patches are user-controlled and require change only once a week, although pharmakokinetic data suggest that there is sufficient absorption of NGN and EE to maintain serum levels within the reference range up to 10 days.[38] For this reason, effectiveness does not depend on reapplying a new patch at exactly the same time every week and if a woman forgets to remove the patch on day 7, there is good evidence that contraceptive protection is provided for a further 2 days. Naturally, if a woman wishes to delay menses, the patch-free week can be delayed, although it is recommended that after six consecutive patches have been used, there should be a patch-free week.

Contraceptive efficacy has been investigated in a comparative study where women were randomized to a triphasic LNG-containing OC or to the patch. The *overall* Pearl index for the contraceptive patch was 1.24 per 100 woman-years (95% CI 0.19–2.33) and for the OC 2.18 (95% CI 0.57–3.8). When *method* failure was considered, the Pearl index for the contraceptive patch was 0.99 (95% CI 0.02–1.96) and for the OC 1.25 (95% CI 0.02–2.47).[39,40]

Compliance with the contraceptive patch was studied in a comparative fashion using an OC; in this open-label, randomized-controlled trial, compliance was measured *subjectively* in well-motivated women and "perfect use" was reported for 88.2% of the subjects using the patch and for 77.7% of those using the OC.[39] Commonly reported side effects associated with the contraceptive patch include: headache (21.9%), nausea (20.4%), site reactions (20.2%), and breast tenderness (18.7%).[40] Worth mention is the fact that breast discomfort seems significantly less common with OC use than with the patch. Some form of local reaction was observed in 20.2% of women using the patch, although this led to discontinuation in only 2.6% of the cases. The mean alteration in body weight during the trial was an average increase of 0.4 kg for both patch and pill users.[39] Breakthrough bleeding and spotting with the contraceptive patch appeared similar to that for a triphasic OC in a randomized, comparative trial. Jointly these side effects were reported by 17.5% of the users in the first cycle, falling to 9.2% by cycle 13.

A second contraceptive patch is in phase III clinical trials. It is a round, transparent patch with a diameter of 3.16 cm and releases 18 μg EE and 50 μg gestodene. In a recent published trial the patch showed to be highly effective in reversibly inhibiting ovulation and it was well tolerated. Ovulation inhibition was achieved in all participants and resumption of ovulation occurred in 85.7% of them, already during the first posttreatment cycle.[41]

Contraceptive sprays. Clinical trials were started in 2004 for a "metered dose transdermal system;" it is a spray-on progestin-only contraceptive using nestorone and relying on a new technique for transferring a preset dose of fast-drying hormone onto the skin. The spray is absorbed almost instantaneously so that there is no risk of washing off. The hormone is collected as a reservoir under the skin from which it diffuses into the bloodstream.[42]

Contraceptive gels. In a preliminary clinical trial, a Nestorone gel applied to the skin daily for 3 months was capable of inhibiting ovulation in 83% of the cases when 1.2 mg per day were applied.[43]

Intrauterine Delivery

The intrauterine administration of progesterone (first introduced in the 1970s with a device named Progestasert®) is capable of exerting good contraceptive activity without inhibiting ovulation [44] since, after its insertion to volunteers, levels of estradiol and progesterone remain within the normal range of their clinical phases.[45] With time, locally released progesterone produces a suppression of the proliferative activity of the endometrium, a diffuse predecidual reaction in the stroma, and changes leading to poorly developed glands.[46–48] Locally delivered progesterone also causes a decrease in vascularity with an increase in the percentage of small vessels with defects.[49] Although these facts point to a mechanism of action at the level of the endometrium, epidemiological data highlighted a different, although still peripheral, mechanism: it was calculated that in women bearing a Progestasert®, failure caused a disproportionate percentage of extrauterine pregnancies.[50] This phenomenon would of course involve an alteration in the progress of the ovum and/or of the zygote in the fallopian tubes.

These findings led to the withdrawal of the device from the market; fortunately, a new LNG-releasing intrauterine system (LNG-IUS) was also being developed [51] and it becomes possible for intrauterine hormonal contraception to see a new season. The system, called Mirena®, releases locally 20 μg of LNG and thereby has a strong direct action on the endometrium. It has a T-shaped polyethylene body with a steroid reservoir on the vertical stem. The recommended duration of use is 5 years, after which the release of LNG is reduced to some 14 μg/day; however, data from randomized trials of contraceptive efficacy show that this dose is effective for up to 7 years.[52]

Mirena® represents both a very effective contraceptive[53,55] and a specific treatment for menorrhagia.[51,56,57] The release of LNG has a marked antiproliferative effect on the endometrium that becomes suppressed and insensitive to the stimulus of endogenous estrogens.[58] Meanwhile, there is no reduction in estradiol levels [53] and ovulatory cycles occur in 85% of women.[56] Indeed, the incidence of anovulatory cycles in users of the LNG system does not differ from that observed in women bearing a copper device.[59]

It must be pointed out that when released directly *in utero*, progestins exert major peripheral effects: they thicken the cervical mucus, inhibit sperm mobility, and prevent endometrial proliferation.[60] In women with an LNG-IUS, the effect on cervical mucus is correlated to the action on ovarian function: in women with ovulatory-like ovarian activity, cervical mucus characteristics are seemingly normal; however, in women with cyclic follicular activity but inadequate luteal activity, mucus production is scanty and viscous and there is a reduction in the mucus penetration test score. Analysis of mucus properties shows that water content in relation to mucin concentration is substantially lower than in women bearing a copper-releasing device.[61]

The LNG-IUS is a system that combines the advantages of oral and intrauterine contraception, being very effective and reversible. Large clinical studies indicate a Pearl index of 0.1 per 100 woman-years.[23] Given what happened with the Progestasert®, a possible increased risk of ectopic pregnancy has been carefully investigated; recent data from randomized trials reported no ectopic pregnancy over a total of 334,944 woman-months of LNG-IUS use. When compared to copper IUDs or to a normal population, ectopic pregnancy rates per 100 woman-years are: 0.02 for LNG; 0.25 for the copper IUD (Nova T); and 12–16 when no contraceptive method is used.

Follow-up studies of women recruited to randomized trials who requested removal of the LNG-IUS to seek pregnancy have documented a rapid return of fertility: the pregnancy rate is 90% in the first year after removal and the mean time to pregnancy is 4 months.[62] Finally, in a systematic review no significant difference has been identified in overall side effects (acne, breast tenderness, headaches, nausea) between women using a LNG-IUD or a copper IUD.[61]

The most striking effect observed with the LNG-IUS is a marked reduction in menstrual blood loss that can lead to hypomenorrhea or amenorrhea and has been used for the treatment of women who experience heavy menstrual bleeding or menorrhagia.[51,56,57,63,64]

Intramuscular Delivery

New activities in this area focus around the marketing of new monthly injectable preparations containing an estrogen and a progestin (MEPI). A number of monthly preparations have been developed and marketed locally since the 1970s and some of them are still in use (the Chinese "Injectable No. 1," also known as Gravibinon and Deladroxate, available in Latin American countries under various trade names, such as Perlutal, Patectro, and Topasel).

Real development, however, did not take place until much later when WHO entered the field and helped provide the necessary safety and effectiveness data.[63] The two MEPIs for which satisfactory data are now available are:

- The combination of 25 mg medroxyprogesterone acetate (MPA) and 5 mg estradiol cypionate (EC), marketed under the names Cyclofem, Cycloprovera, Lunelle, Novafem; today Cyclofem is available in 18 countries, mostly in Latin America and Asia.[64]
- The combination of 50 mg norethisterone enanthate and 5 mg estradiol valerate (Mesigyna, Norigynon).

The primary mode of action of MEPIs is the suppression of ovulation by inhibition of pituitary FSH and LH. In addition, they produce thickening of cervical mucus (mainly due to progestin component), which becomes an obstacle to sperm penetration. Although histologically the endometrium appears decidualized, these changes probably do not contribute to the contraceptive effect. Because MEPIs act very much like OCs, they represent a very effective modality with failure rates between 0.1% and 0.5%; with typical use that does not exceed 0.3%.[23]

Epidemiological evidence of MEPIs' safety is scanty since they have not been in widespread use and for a long enough period. However, it can be assumed that on the basis of theoretical considerations and existing data, both side effects and health benefits of MEPIs will be similar to those of OCs. Both formulations seem well tolerated by most women, although in a minority adverse reactions can lead to discontinuation. Breakthrough bleeding or spotting may occur, especially during the first 3 months of use, when they are more likely to produce prolonged, irregular, or heavy bleeding and amenorrhea than OCs. Also, they may be associated with a longer delay in the return of fertility, although not as prolonged as that associated with the use of progestin-only injectables.[65,66]

Because MEPIs are mostly used in developing countries, an important reason for discontinuation is lack of availability. Many women are unable to go to a clinic or a pharmacy every month for another injection, while clinics sometimes are unable to supply them with the necessary regularity.[67] This situation has been addressed by the Program for Applied Technology in Health (PATH), which is promoting a single-use, prefilled, nonreusable syringe called "Uniject" that would allow health workers to provide the injections at a community level or even self-injection by properly trained women. A study recently conducted in Brazil found that about two-thirds of those participating agreed to receive training to self-administer a MEPI. Of these, 93% correctly self-administered the injectable and 57% preferred self-injection at home over going to a clinic each month.[68]

A woman can have the first MEPI injection within 7 days from the start of her menstrual bleeding and from the onset no additional contraceptive protection is needed. As a matter of fact, the first injection can be given at any other time when the woman is reasonably certain not to be pregnant.

Subcutaneous Delivery

Subcutaneously implanted contraceptives have been made available by the Population Council for decades under the name Norplant®.

Modern research in this field focused on reducing the number of implants by using more potent progestins; on minimizing side effects, particularly bleeding disturbances; and in gathering evidence that implants are safe for use while breastfeeding.

Two types of implants have been developed: contraceptive "rods," where the polymeric matrix (dimethyl–polysiloxane or DPS) is mixed with the steroid, and contraceptive "capsules," made of a hollow polymer tube filled with free steroid crystals.

Norplant-2 (Jadelle®) was designed to deliver the same daily dose of LNG of Norplant-1 using only two rods instead of six capsules. Initially, the system was approved for 3 years, but after studies documented a longer duration of action, many countries have now labeled it for a 5-year use. Indeed, in a clinical trial involving 1,198 women, none became pregnant in the first 4 years of use; the failure rate rose to 1 per 100 woman-years in the fifth year of use.[69] The Chinese "implant system no. 2," also called Sinoplant or Sinoimplant, is nearly identical to Jadelle but contains more levonorgestrel (150 mg instead of 140 mg).

Implanon®. This new single implant with a duration of action of 3 years has already been marketed in a number of countries. It contains a total of 68 mg etonogestrel, delivers daily between 60 and 30 μg of the steroid, and is easier and faster to insert than the Norplant-2. In most cases, Implanon is capable of blocking ovulation, a fact that can explain its very high effectiveness: in a multicenter clinical trial including 1,416 women followed for more than 53,530 cycles not a single pregnancy was observed.[70]

*Uniplant.*This is a single rod system containing 38 mg nomegestrol acetate (NMGA) with a 1-year duration. A recent study evaluated the endocrine status, endometrial histology, and ovarian function (through vaginal ultrasound profiling) of NMGA subdermal implant users at varying times after insertion and found that 75% of all cycles evaluated across the 1 year of implant effect were anovulatory, with 63% showing the development of a persistent nonluteinized follicle. Anovulatory cycles devoid of appreciable follicular development were seen mostly in the first months after Uniplant® insertion. Although ovulatory cycles represented one-quarter of all cycles tested, inadequate luteal phase or dysregulation of follicular growth was a common feature in these cycles, suggesting that the contraceptive effect of Uniplant® involves at least three different endocrine mechanisms: prevention of follicular growth, development of a persistent nonluteinized follicle, and inadequate luteal phase. In addition, there is also disruption of the endometrial architecture.[71]

New Implants. A new implant releasing nestorone is under development by the Population Council. Effective for 2 years, it is a single rod system designed specifically for breastfeeding women since infants of breastfeeding mothers who are using the nestorone implant have no detectable progestin in their blood. Whereas lactating women have found the nesterone implant perfectly acceptable since they had significantly less irregular bleeding, nonlactating ones were not enthusiastic because of prolonged and irregular bleeding even compared to the Copper-T-380A IUD.[72] When effectiveness was tested in a clinical trial (including 200 breastfeeding women followed for 2,000 woman-months of use), no pregnancy occurred in either group.[73]

Implants work primarily by thickening cervical mucus so that it becomes impenetrable to sperm; they also prevent ovulation in many cycles and suppress endometrial growth and maturation. Typical failure rates are between 0.3 and 1.1 pregnancies per 100 woman-years in the first year of use.[23]

Development of new contraceptive implants has been particularly slow because they are expensive to develop and market, their cost is overall too high for many family planning programs, and they require provider training in techniques of insertion and removal.

NEW DEVELOPMENTS IN INTRAUTERINE CONTRACEPTION

Recent research in nonhormonal IUDs focused on the so-called "frameless" IUDs, simple devices without plastic frame.

GyneFix. It is the only frameless IUD available today. It is made without any plastic frame and consists of six copper sleeves threaded on a surgical nylon thread anchored 1 cm deep into the uterine fundus. Insertion or removal of the device requires training and competence in the technique, which is entirely different than that of framed IUDs.[74,75] The simple design is intended to cause less pain and bleeding than framed devices. In spite of this, a recent Cochrane review of framed and frameless devices was unable to identify whether frameless devices were less likely to cause pain in nulliparous women because only parous women were included in the randomized trials reviewed.[76] Nevertheless, it showed to be an effective reversible method of contraception with a net cumulative pregnancy rate of 88% at 12 months and 99% after 2 years of observation.[77]

Moreover, the design characteristics of the frameless IUD (fixed, frameless, and flexible) are responsible for the low expulsion, high effectiveness, and high continuation rates.[78,79]

Frameless systems under development. A new frameless IUD being developed, called FibroPlant-LNG, releases the progestin levonorgestrel, thereby combining the advantages of hormonal contraception to those of IUS. Based on the design of the GyneFix IUD, it too is anchored into the fundus of the uterus. FibroPlant-LNG delivers 14 μg of levonorgestrel daily and prevents pregnancy for at least 3 years.[80] Initial studies suggest that FibroPlant-LNG would be highly acceptable and may reduce bleeding. A pilot study of 109 women approaching menopause found that few women experienced hormonal side effects, such as irregular bleeding or spotting even during the first 3 months after insertion; these features contributed to a 98% continuation rate after 1 year of use.[81]

Another T-shaped levonogestrel-releasing IUS, called Femilis™, with a small version for nulligravidae (who generally have smaller uteri), called Femilis-Slim™, is under development. The aim of this new IUS is to simplify the insertion procedure by using a "push-in technique" that does not require a plunger, as most other IUSs.[82]

FERTILITY-REGULATING VACCINES

For decades it has been hoped that fertility-regulating vaccines (FRV) may provide a valuable addition to the array of methods used today. Over the years, a number of "target molecules" have been identified, such as gonadotropin hormone-releasing hormone (GnRH); sperm and oocyte zona pellucida antigens; and substances produced by the early embryo (such as hCG). Unfortunately, so far, vaccines targeting gamete production have not shown promise since they either affect sex steroid production causing impotence and/or show only a partial rather than a complete effect in inhibiting gametogenesis.[83]

Vaccines based on targeting GnRH on the other hand, are being developed by several pharmaceutical companies as substitutes for castration of domestic pets, farm and wild animals,[84] and for therapeutic anticancer purposes such as ovarian carcinoma.[85] Although to date no application to humans for contraceptive purposes is envisaged, anti-GnRH vaccines may find applications in clinical situations where a blockage of ovarian steroid production may be beneficial (such as uterine fibroids, polycystic ovary syndrome, endometriosis, and precocious puberty).

More promise is offered by FRV-targeting molecules involved in gamete function. Theoretically, sperm constitute the most obvious target for a contraceptive vaccine and infertility caused by antisperm antibodies provides a naturally occurring model to indicate how a vaccine might work in humans. Over the years, several sperm-specific antigens have been identified and are now being actively explored for use in a vaccine. At present, research is focused on identifying appropriate sperm-specific epitopes, and on increasing the immunogenicity (specifically in the local genital tract) and efficacy of the vaccines.[86] Vaccines based on Zona Pellucida proteins are quite efficacious in producing contraceptive effects and are being successfully tested to control populations of domestic (dogs) as well as wild (deer, horses, and elephants) populations of several species of zoo animals and studies are ongoing to test a possible application to humans, although there is concern that they may induce oophoritis, affecting sex steroid production. Current research deals with an attempt at distinguishing between infertility-related epitopes (B cell epitopes) from oophoritis-inducing epitopes (T cell epitopes).[87,88]

Notwithstanding all these promising leads, the development of antifertility vaccines focused for years around the possibility to raise homologous antibodies against hCG, [89,90] amid controversy and unexpected complications.

Two types of controversies arose over the development of an anti-hCG vaccine. The first, purely technical, dealt with the type of antigen to be used: the whole β-hCG molecule or only its specific 37 amino acid carboxy-terminal region. The "whole-β-hCG" approach was pioneered by the Indian group led by Talwar,[91] whereas the "specific-peptide" route was promoted by Stevens and supported by WHO.[92] The second controversy revolved around the acknowledged mechanism of action of this type of vaccine: blocking the effect of hCG; as such, they are by definition "anti-implantation agents" and therefore act exclusively after fertilization.

Two quotes, taken by the WHO's Annual Technical Reports of 1990 and 1999, will give an idea of the problems encountered. In 1991 the report stated ". . . large batches of the vaccine components were prepared, under GLP/GMP conditions for pre-Phase II teratology and a Phase II clinical trial of the prototype vaccine."[93] In 2000 the situation was described as follows: ". . . a Phase II trial with an improved version of this [*the vaccine prototype*] preparation was initiated in early 1994, but was interrupted when unexpectedly high levels of injection-site pain and tissue reaction were encountered in the first few volunteers to receive the preparation."[94] Since then, the situation has not improved and lack of funding has now forced WHO to stop this line of research.

The Indian anti-hCG vaccine moved further and phase II studies were successfully completed [95]; unfortunately, a major shortcoming soon appeared: effective antibody titers (>50 ng/mL) could be raised in only 60–80% of women. Therefore, at least in its present form the Indian version cannot be considered satisfactory.[87]

DUAL METHOD PROTECTION

The resurgence of sexually transmitted diseases and the HIV/AIDS pandemic have given new impetus to attempts aimed at preventing this vast category of infections, now totaling more than 30, bearing in mind the well-established fact that unprotected and casual sex carries two types of distinct, but equally important and inextricably linked consequences: unintended pregnancy and sexually transmitted infections (STIs).

To cope with the new reality, a strategy called "Dual protection" has been designed to concurrently offer a safeguard against unintended pregnancy and HIV/STIs. The need for such a strategy is a direct consequence of the fact that whereas male condoms represent a valid protection against HIV/STIs, they are not the most effective method for preventing unintended pregnancy. There is therefore a need to couple the use of condoms with a highly effective contraceptive modality such as an OC, an IUD, or an injectable.

Since little is known about how to promote dual use, a recent study examined associations of dual method use with women's background characteristics, intrapersonal factors, and relationship characteristics. The study identified three mutually exclusive method use groups: "effective contraceptive only" (users of hormonal methods, IUD, surgical sterilization) (59%), "condom only" (24%), and "dual use" (18%). Findings indicate that women who were younger, reported more than one sexual partner in the past year, and were highly motivated to avoid HIV/STDs, were more likely to use the dual method system. In addition, women confident about using condoms without feeling embarrassed or breaking the sexual mood were more likely to use dual methods rather than a single effective method. Finally, women with confidence in their ability to use condoms correctly are more likely to rely solely on condoms.[96]

It has been argued that—to offer young women full protection—a third variable must be brought into the picture: the safeguard of future fertility. This new vision has been labeled "triple protection" and is intended to explicitly draw out the connection between infertility and STIs.[97] According to the promoters, "understanding differences in perception and weighting of protection concerns by young women and men, whether they wish to start, postpone or avoid pregnancy, is essential for the creation of effective programmes. Building on efforts to promote dual protection, a strategic opportunity exists to include prevention of infertility into safer sex messages and to address the fragmentation of reproductive health and HIV/AIDS programmes."

EMERGENCY CONTRACEPTION

Although a controversial modality, emergency contraception has seen its utilization grow exponentially after the first trials by Yuzpe and his group [98] who, in 1974, began to evaluate the potential postcoital activity of two pills each containing 50 μg EE/ 250 μg levonorgestrel, taken twice at a 12-h interval, as soon as possible within 72 h after unprotected intercourse. Ten years later a new modality was introduced, based on the administration of twice 600 μg levonorgestrel.[99] The dose was subsequently adjusted to 750 μg (taken twice 12 h apart).[100] In a subsequent large, prospective, randomized trial comparing the levonorgestrel with the Yuzpe regimen, the progestin-only method not only showed to be more effective, but also to produce significantly lower side effects.[101] The present status of EC has been recently summarized[102]; for this reason here only recent developments will be reported and these revolve around the use of the selective progesterone receptor modulator (antiprogestin) mifepristone (also known as RU-486).

Mifespristone, best known for its ability to interrupt, in association with a prostaglandin, an early gestation,[103] is highly effective for true emergency contraception. The WHO has contributed in a substantial way to the development of RU-486 for EC[104–107] showing that the dose of 10 mg had the same effectiveness (1.2% failure rate) as 50 or 600 mg in the prevention of pregnancy when administered up to 120 h after unprotected intercourse. It also showed that effectiveness of a single dose of 10 mg of mifepristone was not different from that observed with the two levonorgestrel regimens.[104]

In general, EC acts through several distinct mechanisms, the main one being *inhibition* or *delay* of the ovulation process caused by an interference with the luteinizing hormone (LH) midcycle peak release. There are also cases in which all measured parameters seem to be normal, together with instances in which the LH peak is partially or totally suppressed with a partial or total failure in follicular luteinization, depending on the time in the menstrual cycle in which EC has been administered.[108–111] Additional mechanisms involve impairment of sperm and ovum migration in the genital tract. Kesseru *et al.*[112] reported that following LNG administration there is a reduction in the number of sperm recovered from the uterine cavity beginning 3 h after treatment, a pronounced alkalization (capable of immobilizing sperm) of the uterine fluid starting at 5 h, and an increased viscosity of the cervical mucus beginning at 9 h, blocking further sperm passage. Endometrial functional alterations have also been reported in some studies,[111,113–115] although they seem to be the reflection of an impaired ovarian function rather than a direct effect of EC on the endometrium.

Mifepristone effects on the human menstrual cycle also depend on the stage of the cycle in which it is administered. During the mid-to-late follicular phase RU-486 blocks the further growth of the dominant follicle and counteracts the positive feedback of estradiol, preventing the midcycle LH surge, thereby delaying ovulation.[116]

It is because of this mechanism of action that use of RU-486 is associated with a high incidence rate of cycle disturbances (in 9–18% of all women there is more than a 5-day delay of menses). Other side effects such as nausea and vomiting are less likely with mifepristone when compared to the Yuzpe regimen.[117]

One important ethical objection that has been brought against EC is the fact that it may act as an anti-implantation agent. For sure, there is no final proof that EC acts always before fertilization. However, given that EC is administered as soon as possible after coitus and that the existing experimental and clinical evidence seem to exclude that it could dislodge the embryo after implantation, the balance of evidence seems to indicate that—in a majority of cases—EC acts a true contraceptive.

REFERENCES

1. BENAGIANO, G. 2002. Male and female reproductive strategies. Edwards symposium, Reprod. BioMed. Online, **4**(Suppl. 1): 72–76.
2. WRANGHAM, R. & D. PETERSON. 1996. Demonic males: apes and the origin of human violence. Mariner Books. London.
3. NISHIDA, T. & M. HIRAIWA-HASEGAWA. 1987. Chimpanzees and bonobos; cooperative relationship among males. *In* Primate Societies. B.B. Smuts, D.L. Cheney, R.M. Seyfart, *et al.* Eds.: 165–177. Chicago University Press, Chicago.
4. DE WAAL, F.M.B. 1987. Tension regulation and non reproductive functions of sex in captive bonobos (Pan panicus). Nat. Geo. Res. **3**: 318–335.
5. BAIRD, D. & A.F. GLASIER. Science, medicine and the future: contraception. Brit. Med. J. **319**: 969–972.
6. UN POPULATION DIVISION. 2001. World Population Prospects: The 2000 Revision. United Nations, Department of Economic and Social Affairs (New York) ESA/P/WP.165.
7. UN POPULATION DIVISION. 2004. World Fertility Report 2003. United Nations, Department of Economic and Social Affairs. New York.
8. SKOUBY, S.O. 2004. Contraceptive use and behavior in the 21st century: a comprehensive study across five European countries. Eur. J. Contrac. Reprod. Health Care **9**: 57–68.
9. ETHIOPIA DEMOGRAPHIC AND HEALTH SURVEY. 2005. Preliminary Report. Ethiopia Central Statistical Agency and ORC Macro. Calverton, UK.
10. BENAGIANO, G. & F.M. PRIMIERO. 1998. Safety of modern oral contraception: the options for women. Hum. Reprod. Update **5**: 633–638.
11. SULLIVAN, H. *et al.* 1999. Effect of 21-day and 24-day oral contraceptive regimens containing gestodene (60 μg) and ethinyl estradiol (15 μg) on ovarian activity. Fertil. Steril. **72**: 115–120.
12. HAMPTON, R.M. *et al.* 2001. Comparison of a novel norgestimate/ethinyl estradiol oral contraceptive (Ortho Tri-Ciclen Lo) with the oral contraceptive Fe 1/20. Contraception **63**: 289–295.

13. KAUNITZ, A.M. 2000. Efficacy, cycle control, and safety of two triphasic oral contraceptives: Cyclessa (desogestrel/ethinyl estradiol) and Ortho Novum 7/7/7 (norethindrone/ethinyl estradiol): a randomised clinical trial. Contraception **61:** 25–302.

14. HIRVONEN, E., M. MALKONEN & V. MANNINEN. 1981. Effects of different progestogens on lipoproteins during post-menopausal replacement therapy. N. Engl. J. Med. **304:** 560–563.

15. JUNCHEN, M. *et al.* 1995. Dienogest: Bindungs-studien an veschienden Rezeptor- und Serumprotein. *In* Dienogest- Praklink und Klinik eines neuen Gestagenes. Walter de Gruyter Verlag. A.T. Teichman. Ed.: Berlin. 119–133.

16. HABENICHT, U.-F. 2005. Personal communication.

17. FOIDART, J. M. *et al.* 2000. A comparative investigation of contraceptive reliability, cycle control and tolerance of two monophasic oral contraceptives containing either drospirenone or desogestrel. Eur. J. Contracept. Reprod. Health Care **5:** 124–134.

18. HUBER, H.J. *et al.* 2000. Efficacy tolerability of a monophasic oral contraceptive containing ethinil estradiol and drospirenone. Eur. J. Contracept. Reprod. Health Care **5:** 25–35.

19. SPECIAL PROGRAMME OF RESEARCH, DEVELOPMENT AND RESEARCH TRAINING IN HUMAN REPRODUCTION. UNDP/UNFPA/WHO/WORLD BANK. 1999. Annual Technical Report 1998.WHO/RHR/00/9, World Health Organization, Geneva. 92.

20. FFPRHC, CLINICAL EFFECTIVENESS UNIT. 2003. FFPRHC guidance: first prescription of combined oral contraception. J. Fam. Plann. Reprod. Health Care **29:** 209–223.

21. WORLD HEALTH ORGANIZATION. 2005. Selected Practice Recommendations for Contraceptive Use. Second edition. World Health Organisation. Geneva.

22. KAUNITZ, A.M. 2005. Beyond the pill: new data and options in hormonal and intrauterine contraception. Am. J. Obstet. Gynecol. **192:** 998–1004.

23. TRUSSELL, J. 2004. Contraceptive efficacy. *In* Contraceptive technology. R.A. Hatcher, J. Trussell, F. Stewart *et al.*, Eds.: 18th edition. New York, Ardent Media.

24. RICE, C. *et al.* 1996. Ovarian activity and vaginal bleeding patterns with a desogestrel-only preparation at three different doses. Hum. Reprod. **11:** 737–740.

25. SKOUBY, S.O. 1982. Laboratory and clinical assessment of a new progestational compound desogestrel. Acta Obstet. Gynaecol. Scand. Suppl. **111:** 7–11.

26. VIINIKKA, L. *et al.* 1979. Metabolism of a new synthetic progestogen, Org 2969, in female volunteers. Investigations into the pharmacokinetics after a single dose. Eur. J. Clin. Pharmacol. **15:** 349–355.

27. RICE, C.F. *et al.* 1999. A comparison of the inhibition of ovulation, achieved by desogestrel 75µg and levonorgestrel 30µg daily. Hum. Reprod. **14:** 982–985.

28. RICE, C.F. *et al.* 1998. The effect of desogestrel 75µg and levonorgestrel 30µg on the endometrium and bleeding patterns over one year. Br. J. Obstet. Gynaecol. **105** (Suppl. 17): 114.

29. BENAGIANO, G. & F.M. PRIMIERO. 2003. The new minipill with 75 g of desogestrel. *In* Challenges on Women's Health and Diseases: Gynecologic and Reproductive Issues. Ann. N. Y. Acad. Sci. **997:** 163–173.

30. HUSSAIN, A. & F. AHSAN. 2005. The vagina as a route for systemic drug delivery. J. Control Release **103:** 301–313.

31. UPADHYAY, U.D. 2005. New contraceptive choices. Population Reports. Series M, No.19. Johns Hopkins Bloomberg School of Public Health. Baltimore, MD.
32. DIAZ, S. 1999. Contraceptive vaginal rings. International Planned Parenthood Federation Medical Bulletin. **33:** 3–4.
33. BJARNADOTTIR, R.I., M. TUPPURAINEN & S.R. KILLICK. 2002. Comparison of cycle control with a combined contraceptive vaginal ring and oral levonorgestrel /ethinyl estradiol. Am. J. Obstet. Gynecol. **186:** 389–395.
34. JOHANSSON, E.D. & R. SITRUK-WARE. 2004. New delivery systems in contraception: vaginal rings. Am. J. Obstet. Gynecol. **190** (Suppl 4): S54–S59.
35. MASSAI, R. et al. 2000. Vaginal rings for contraception in lactating women. Steroids **65:** 703–707.
36. SITRUK-WARE, R. 2004. Contraceptive development at the Population Council. Quoted by: Population Reports (31).
37. SMALLWOOD, G.H. et al. 2001. Efficacy and safety of a transdermal contraceptive system. Obstet. Gynecol. **98:** 799–805.
38. STEWART, F.H. et al. 2005. Extended use of transdermal norelgestromin/ethinyl estradiol: a randomized trial. Obstet. Gynecol. **105:** 1389–1396.
39. AUDET, M.C. et al. 2001. Evaluation of contraceptive efficacy and cycle control of a transdermal contraceptive patch vs an oral contraceptive: a randomized controlled trial. J. Am. Med. Assn. **285:** 2347–2354.
40. ZIEMAN, M. et al. 2002. Contraceptive efficacy and cycle control with the Ortho Evra/Evra transdermal system: the analysis of pooled data. Fertil. Steril. **77**(Suppl 2): S13–S18.
41. HEGER-MAHN, D. et al. 2004. Combined ethinyl estradiol/ gestodene contraceptive patch: two-center, open label study of ovulation inhibition, acceptability and safety over two cycles in female volunteers. Eur. J. Contracept. Reprod. Health Care **9:** 173–181.
42. YOUNG, E. 2003. Spray-on female contraceptive to start trial. New Scientist. Nov. 27, 2003.
43. SITRUK-WARE, R. et al. 2003. Nestorone: clinical applications for contraception and HRT. Steroids **68:** 907–913.
44. ERMINI, M. et al. 1976. Effetto dei dispositivi intrauterine liberanti progesterone sull'asse ipotalamo-ipofiso-ovarico nella donna. Patol. Clin. Ostet. Ginec. **4:** 109–115.
45. WAN, L.S. et al. 1977. Effects of the progestasert on the menstrual pattern, ovarian steroid and endometrium. Contraception **16:** 417–434.
46. HAGENFELDT, K. & B.M. LANDGREN. 1975. Contraception by intrauterine release of progesterone-effects on endometrial trace elements enzymes and steroids. J. Steroid Biochem. **6:** 895–898.
47. HAGENFELDT, K. et al. 1977. Biochemical and morphological changes in the human endometrium induced by the progestasert device. Contraception **16:** 183–197.
48. ERMINI, M., F. CARPINO, V. PETROZZA & G. BENAGIANO. 1989. Distribution and effect on the endometrium of progesterone release from a progestasert device. Hum. Reprod. **4:** 221–228.
49. SHAW, S.T. et al. 1981. Effect of progesterone-releasing intrauterine contraceptive device on endometrial blood vessels: a morphometric study. Am. J. Obstet. Gynecol. **141:** 829–839.
50. SNOWDEN, R. 1977. The progestasert and ectopic pregnancy. Br. Med. J. **2:** 1600–1601.

51. NILSSON, C.-G., E.D.B. JOHANSSON & T. A. LUUKKAINEN. 1976. d-norgestrel-releasing IUD. Contraception **13:** 503–514.
52. FACULTY OF FAMILY PLANNING AND REPRODUCTIVE HEALTH CARE. FFPRHC GUIDANCE. 2004. The levonorgestel releasing system (LNG-IUS) in contraception and reproductive health. J. Fam. Plann. Reprod. Health Care **30:** 99–109.
53. BARBOSA, I. *et al.* 1990. Ovarian function during use of a levonorgestrel-releasing IUD. Contraception **42:** 51–66.
54. NILSSON, C.G., P.L.A. LAHTEEMAKI & T. LUUKKAINEN. 1984. Ovarian function in amenorrheic and menstruating users of a levonorgestrel-releasing intrauterine device. Fertil. Steril. **41:** 52–55.
55. FRENCH, R.S. *et al.* 2000. Levonorgestrel-releasing (20 g/day) intrauterine system (Mirena) compared with other method of reversible contraception. Br. J. Obstet. Gynecol. **107:** 1218–1225.
56. LUKKAINEN, T. 2000. The levonorgestrel intrauterine system: therapeutic aspects. Steroids **65:** 699–702.
57. IRVINE, G.A. *et al.* 1998. Randomised comparative trial of levonorgestrel intrauterine system and norethisterone for treatment of idiopathic menorrhagia. Br. J. Obstet. Gynecol. **105:** 592–598.
58. LUUKKAINEN, T., P.L.A. LAHTEENMAKI & J. TOIVONEN. 1990. Levonorgestrel-releasing intrauterine device. Ann. Med. **22:** 85–90.
59. ANDERSSON, K., V. ODLIND & G. RYBO. 1994. Levonorgestrel releasing and copper releasing (Nova T) IUDs during five years of use: a randomised trial. Contraception **49:** 56–72.
60. RIVERA, R., I. YACOBSON & D. GRIMES. 1999. The mechanism of action of hormonal contraceptives and intrauterine contraceptive devices. Am. J. Obstet. Gynecol. 1999 **181:** 1263–1269.
61. JONSSON, B., B.-M. LANDGREN & P. ENEROTH. 1991. Effects of various IUDs on the composition of cervical mucus. Contraception **43:** 447–458.
62. ANDERSSON, K., I. BATAR & G. RYBO. 1992. Return to fertility after removal of a levonorgestrel releasing intrauterine device and Nova T. Contraception **46:** 575–584.
63. FRENCH, R.S. *et al.* 2000. Implantable contraceptives (subdermal implants and hormonally impregnated intrauterine systems) versus other forms of reversible contraception: two systematic reviews to assess relative effectiveness, acceptability, tolerability and cost-effectiveness. Health Technol. Assess. **4:** 1–107.
64. STEWART, A. *et al.* 2001. Effectiveness of the levonorgestrel releasing intrauterine system in menorrhagia: a systematic review. Br. J. Obstet. Gynecol. **108:** 74–86.
65. NEWTON, J.R., C. D'ARCANGUES & P.E. HALL. 1994. A review of "once-a-month" combined injectable contraceptives. J. Obstet. Gynecol. **4** (Suppl 1): S1–S34.
66. RAHIMY, M.H. & K.K. RYAN. 1999. Lunelle monthly contraceptive injection (medroxyprogesterone acetate and estradiol cypionate injectable suspension): assessment of return of ovulation after three monthly injections in surgically sterile women. Contraception **60:** 189–200.
67. INTERNATIONAL PLANNED PARENTHOOD FEDERATION. 2003. Directory of hormonal contraceptives.http://contraceptive.ippf.org/(rlyna245m2v-hrjfqdj304v45)/Default.aspx International Planned Parenthood Federation, London.

68. BAHAMONDES, L. *et al*. 1997. Self-administration with UniJect of the once-a-month injectable contraceptive Cyclofem. Contraception **56:** 301–304.
69. SIVIN, I. *et al*. 1998. The performance of levonorgestrel rod and Norplant contraceptive implants: a 5 year randomized study. Hum. Reprod. **13:** 3371–3378.
70. CROXATTO, H.B. & N. MAKARAINEN. 1998. Pharmacodinamics and efficacy of Implanon. Contraception **58:** 91S–97S.
71. DEVOTO, L. *et al*. 1997. Hormonal profile, endometrial histology and ovarian ultrasound assessment during 1 year of nomegestrol acetate implant (Uniplant). Hum. Reprod. **12:** 708–713.
72. SIVIN, I. *et al*. 2004. Two-year performance of a Nestorone-releasing contraceptive implant: a three-center study of 300 women. Contraception **69:** 137–144.
73. MASSAI, M.R. *et al*. 2001. Contraceptive efficacy and clinical performance of nestorone implants in postpartum women. Contraception **64:** 369–376.
74. WILDEMEERSCH, D. 2001. Further information and recommendations to prevent perforation with the frameless GyneFix IUD. J. Fam. Plann. Reprod. Health Care **27:** 241.
75. BROCKMEYER, A., M. KISHEN & A. WEBB. 2004. New GyneFix introducer. J. Fam. Plann. Reprod. Health Care **30:** 65.
76. O'BRIEN, P.A. & C. MARFLEET. 2005. Frameless versus classical intrauterine device for contraception. Cochrane Database Syst. Rev. **25:** CD 003282.
77. DELBARGE, W. *et al*. 2002. Return to fertility in nulliparous and parous women after removal of the GyneFix intrauterine contraceptive system. Eur. J. Contracept. Reprod. Health Care **7:** 24–30.
78. CAO, X *et al*. 2004. Three-year efficacy and acceptability of the GyneFix 200 intrauterine system. Contraception **69:** 207–211.
79. WU, S., J. HU & D. WILDEMEERSCH. 2000. Performance of the frameless GyneFix and the TCu380A IUDs in a 3-year multicenter, randomized, comparative trial in parous women. Contraception **61:** 91–98.
80. WILDEMEERSCH, D. *et al*. 2002. Development of a miniature, low-dose, frameless intrauterine levonorgestrel-releasing system for contraception and treatment: a review of initial clinical experience. Reprod. Biomed. Online **4:** 71–82.
81. WILDEMEERSCH, D., E. SCHACHT & P. WILDEMEERSCH. 2002. Contraception and treatment in the perimenopause with a novel "frameless" intrauterine levonorgestrel-releasing drug delivery system: an extended pilot study. Contraception **66:** 93–99.
82. WILDEMEERSCH, D. *et al*. 2004. Ease of insertion, contraceptive efficacy and safety of new T-shaped levonorgestrel-releasing intrauterine systems. Proceedings 8th Congress of the European Society of Contraception, Edinburgh, Scotland. June 23–36.
83. NAZ, K.R. *et al*. 2005. Recent advances in contraceptive vaccine development: a mini-review. Hum. Reprod. **20:** 3271–3283.
84. MILLER, L.A., B.E. JOHNSON & G.J. KILLIAN. 2000. Immunocontraception of white tailed deer with nRH vaccine. Am. J. Reprod. Immunol. **44:** 266–274.
85. HSU, C.T. *et al*. 2000. Vaccination against gonadotropin-releasing hormone (GnRH) using toxin receptor binding domain-conjugated GnRH repeats. Cancer Res. **60:** 3701–3705.
86. SURI, A. 2005. Sperm-based contraceptive vaccines: current status, merits and development. Expert Rev. Mol. Med. **7:** 1–16.
87. NAZ, R.K. 2005. Contraceptive vaccines. Drugs **65:** 593–603.

88. GUPTA, S.K. *et al.* 2004. Update on zona pellucida glycoproteins based contraceptive vaccines. J. Reprod. Immunol. **62:** 79–89.
89. STEVENS, V.G. 1973. Immunization of female baboons with hapten-coupled gonadotropins. Obstet. Gynecol. **42:** 496–504.
90. PALA, A., M. ERMINI, L. CARENZA & G. BENAGIANO. 1976. Immunization with hapten-coupled HCG-beta subunit and its effect on the menstrual cycle. Contraception **14:** 579–593.
91. STEVENS, V.C. 1974. Fertility control through active immunization using placenta proteins: Karolinska Symposia on Research Methods in Reproductive Biology. 7th Symposium: *In* Immunological Approaches to Fertility Control. E. Diczfalusy, Ed.: 357–369. Bogtrykkeriet Forum. Copenhagen.
92. TALWAR, G.P. 1974. Fertility control through active immunization using placenta proteins: Karolinska Symposia on Research Methods in Reproductive Biology. 7th Symposium: *In* Immunological Approaches to Fertility Control. E. Diczfalusy Ed.: 370–386. Bogtrykkeriet Forum. Copenhagen.
93. SPECIAL PROGRAMME OF RESEARCH, DEVELOPMENT AND RESEARCH TRAINING IN HUMAN REPRODUCTION. WORLD HEALTH ORGANIZATION. 1991. Annual Technical Report 1990. WHO/HRP/90/91, World Health Organization. Geneva. 99.
94. SPECIAL PROGRAMME OF RESEARCH, DEVELOPMENT AND RESEARCH TRAINING IN HUMAN REPRODUCTION. UNDP/UNFPA/WHO/World Bank. 2000. Annual Technical Report 1999. WHO/RHR/00/9, World Health Organization, Geneva. 127.
95. TALWAR, G.P. *et al.* 1994. A vaccine that prevents pregnancy in women. Proc. Natl. Acad. Sci. USA **91:** 8532–8536.
96. HARVEY, S.M. *et al.* 2004. Protecting against both pregnancy and disease: predictors of dual method use among a sample of women. Women Health **39:** 25–43.
97. BRADY, M. 2003. Preventing sexually transmitted infections and unintended pregnancy, and safeguarding fertility: triple protection needs of young women. Reprod. Health Matters **11:** 134–141.
98. YUZPE, A.A. 1974. Post-coital contraception—A pilot study. J. Reprod. Med. **30:** 12–18.
99. HOFFMAN, K.O. 1984. Postcoital contraception: experiences with ethynil estradiol/norgestrel and levonorgestrel only. *In* Proceedings of the XIth Congress on Fertility and Sterility. R.F. Harrison, J. Bonnar & W. Thompson. Eds.: 311–316. MTP Press. Lancaster.
100. WORLD HEALTH ORGANIZATION. TASK FORCE ON POST-OVULATORY METHODS FOR FERTILITY REGULATION. (SPECIAL PROGRAMME FOR RESEARCH TRAINING IN HUMAN REPRODUCTION.) TASK FORCE ON POSTOVULATORY METHODS OF FERTILITY REGULATION. 1998. Randomized controlled trial of levonorgestrel versus the Yuzpe regimen of combined oral contraceptives for emergency contraception. Lancet **352:** 428–433.
101. TASK FORCE ON POST-OVULATORY METHODS FOR FERTILITY REGULATION. 1987. Post coital contraception with levonorgestrel during the peri-ovulatory phase of the menstrual cycle. Contraception **36:** 257–286.
102. BENAGIANO, G., M. FARRIS & C. BASTIANELLI. 2005. Emergency contraception. *In* Human Reproduction. A.R. Genazzani, J. Schenker, P.G. Artini, T. Simoncini, Eds.: 40–47. CIC Edizioni Internazionali. Roma. 2005.
103. LAHTEEMAKI, P. *et al.* 1987. Pharmacokinetics and metabolism of RU-486. J. Steroid. Biochem. **27:** 859–865.

104. VON HERTZEN, H. *et al.* 2000. Low dose mifepristone and two regimens of levonorgestrel for emergency contraception: a WHO multicentre randomized trial. Lancet **360:** 1803–1810.
105. WORLD HEALTH ORGANIZATION. TASK FORCE ON POST-OVULATORY METHODS FOR FERTILITY REGULATION. 1999. Comparison of three single doses of mifepristone as emergency contraception: a randomized trial. Lancet **353:** 697–702.
106. VON HERTZEN, H. & P.F.A. VAN LOOK. 1996. Research on new methods of emergency contraception. Int. Fam. Plann. Perspect. **22:** 62–68.
107. VON HERTZEN, H. & G. PIAGGIO. 2003. Levonorgestrel and mifepristone in emergency contraception. Steroids **68:** 1107–1113.
108. CROXATTO, H.B. *et al.* 2002. Effects of the Yuzpe regimen, given during the follicular phase on ovarian function. Contraception **65:** 121–128.
109. HAPANGAMA, D., A.F. GLASIER & D.T. BAIRD. 2001. The effects of peri-ovulatory administration of levonorgestrel on the menstrual cycle. Contraception **63:** 123–129.
110. LANDGREN, B.M. *et al.* 1989 The effect of levonorgestrel administered in large doses at different stages of the cycles on ovarian function and endometrial morphology. Contraception **39:** 275–289.
111. DURAND, M. *et al.* 2001. On the mechanism of action of short-term levonorgestrel administration in emergency contraception. Contraception **64:** 227–234.
112. KESSERU, E. *et al.* 1974. The hormonal peripheral effects of dl-norgestrel in post-coital contraception. Contraception **10:** 411–424.
113. CROXATTO, H.B. *et al.* 2001. Mechanism of action of hormonal preparations used for emergency contraception: a review of the literature. Contraception **63:** 111–121.
114. SWAHN, M.L. *et al.* 1996. Effect of post-coital contraceptive methods on the endometrium and the menstrual cycle. Acta Obstet. Gynecol. Scand. **75:** 738–744.
115. MARIONS, L. *et al.* 2002. Emergency contraception with mifepristone and levonorgestrel: mechanism of action. Obstet. Gynecol. **100:** 65–71.
116. CROXATTO, H.B. 2002. Pillules contraceptives d'urgence: comment fonctionnent-elles? IPPF Med. Bull. **36:** 1–2.
117. ASHOK, P.W. *et al.* 2002. A randomized study comparing a low dose of mifepristone and the Yuzpe regimen for emergency contraception. Br. J. Obstet. Ginec. **109:** 553–560.

Women's Health and the Metabolic Syndrome

ASIMINA MITRAKOU

Department of Internal Medicine, Henry Dunant Hospital, Athens, Greece

ABSTRACT: The metabolic syndrome is a cluster of cardiovascular risk factors that identifies individuals at a relatively high, long-term risk for atherosclerosis, cardiovascular disease, and type 2 diabetes. Insulin resistance and central obesity are the main risk conditions underlying the metabolic syndrome. As obesity rates increase worldwide especially in women, accompanying rising frequency of insulin resistance, dyslipidemia, diabetes, and hypertension contribute to increasing rates of cardiovascular morbidity and mortality. According to the latest NCEP/ATPIII definition of the metabolic syndrome almost 25% (from 6.7 up to 43.5% according to age) of the United States and European adult population appear to have the syndrome and in the recent years it has been more prevalent in men than in women. Prevalence is increasing and the increase seems to be steeper in women. The contribution of the different components of the syndrome differs between genders. Age, endocrine dysfunction (especially loss of ovarian estrogens) as well as genetic factors modify the response to underlying factors. Physical inactivity, which diminishes by age, is more prevalent in women than in men. Treatment goals are to prevent cardiovascular disease by both altering the risk factors that are components of the syndrome and more importantly applying lifestyle modifications with caloric restriction and exercise.

KEYWORDS: obesity; cardiovascular disease (CVD); dyslipidemia; hypertension; metabolic syndrome

THE METABOLIC SYNDROME: DEFINITION—EPIDEMIOLOGY

The metabolic syndrome is a cluster of cardiovascular risk factors as abdominal obesity, dyslipidemia, hyperglycemia, and hypertension. The metabolic syndrome definition helps to identify individuals at a relatively high, long-term risk for atherosclerosis, cardiovascular disease, and type 2 diabetes. The risk for

Address for correspondence: Asimina Mitrakou, M.D., Department of Internal Medicine, Henry Dunant Hospital, 77 Mavromichali St., GR 10680, Athens, Greece. Voice: +30-210-7249561; fax: +30-210-7249562.
e-mail: amitrakou@otenet.gr

Ann. N.Y. Acad. Sci. 1092: 33–48 (2006). © 2006 New York Academy of Sciences.
doi: 10.1196/annals.1365.003

major cardiovascular events resulting from the presence of the metabolic syndrome is approximately twice as high as for those without the syndrome[1] and the risk for type 2 diabetes is approximately fivefold greater for those who have it. Type 2 diabetes, although accompanied by increased risk for cardiovascular disease (CVD), carries much more risk for CVD when the metabolic syndrome is concomitantly present especially in women.[2] Although the association has been known for more than 80 years, the clustering received recognition in 1988 when Reaven described the syndrome X as the association of insulin resistance, hyperglycemia, hypertension, low high-density lipoprotein (HDL) cholesterol, and increased very low-density lipoprotein (VLDL) triglycerides.[3] Obesity was omitted in the definition of the syndrome, but is now recognized as an essential component, especially central obesity.[1,4] The syndrome has gone through numerous changes over the past few years to become more clinically useful. Obesity, and in particular central obesity, became the core of diagnostic criteria and it is related to insulin resistance as evaluated by increased circulating insulin levels. Insulin sensitivity declines linearly with body mass index (BMI) independently of gender[5] and adipose tissue. Adipose tissue plays a primary role in the pathogenesis of atherosclerosis through various metabolic and hormonal pathways. The WHO definition puts more emphasis on insulin resistance.[6] The European Group for the study of Insulin Resistance (EGIR) has proposed some changes to the WHO definition of the metabolic syndrome. The EGIR definition excludes microalbuminuria as a core characteristic, since its association with cardiovascular disease is yet to be proven. EGIR also considers that the most appropriate measure of abdominal obesity is in dispute and that the role of insulin resistance, although a consistent early abnormality in the type 2 diabetes pathogenesis, is to be proven in the cardiovascular disease pathogenesis. Thus the EGIR definition of the metabolic syndrome excludes patients with type 2 diabetes; defines central obesity as waist girth ≥ 80 cm for women and ≥ 94 cm for men; and recommends use of fasting insulin levels to estimate insulin resistance (instead of the euglycemic clamp) and impaired fasting glycemia as a substitute for impaired glucose tolerance in epidemiologic studies.[7,8]

The latest definition is the one proposed by International Diabetes Federation (IDF) in 2005[4] where central obesity defined as a waist circumference > 94 cm in men and > 80 cm in women plus any two of the following parameters: TG > 150 mg/dL or treatment for hypertriglyceremia; HDL < 40 mg/dL in men and < 50 in women; BP systolic > 130, diastoloic > 85 mmHg; or fasting plasma glucose ≥ 110 mg/dL or previously diagnosed type 2 diabetes.

For large-scale screening purposes, the NCEP/ATP III[9] classification has been used and the data mentioned in this review refer to this classification of the metabolic syndrome (≥ 3 criteria: central obesity waist ≥ 88 cm in women or ≥ 102 cm in men; HDL < 50 mg/dL in women or < 40 mg/dL in men; triglycerides ≥ 194 mg/dL; hypertension $\geq 135/85$; fasting plasma glucose ≥ 110 mg/dL).

In 2000, 47 million Americans were identified as having the metabolic syndrome, corresponding to about 40% of the adult population.[10] This correlates with the 61% increase in the incidence of obesity between the years 1991 and 2000. The prevalence of the metabolic syndrome increases with age (ranging from 6.7% among people in the age group of 20–29 years to 43.5% for ages 60–69 years, and 42% for those 70 years and older) and there is also a trend toward younger subjects being affected.[10] The increase in prevalence of the metabolic syndrome in later studies seems to be higher in women than in men, especially in the age group of 20–29 years and over the age of 60 years.[11] Young women (20–39 years) had a 76% relative increase of prevalence of the metabolic syndrome compared to a nonsignificant increase of 5% in men in these ages. This difference in increase of the prevalence of the metabolic syndrome is in accordance with the constant rise in obesity in women. There are 2 million more women in the United States categorized as being obese[12] with the trend of obesity and diabetes increasing. In the past decade we have seen a 74% increase in obesity mostly in women.[13] This epidemic needs to be understood and managed to prevent further morbidity and mortality attributed to diabetes and cardiovascular disease. Studies have tried to determine the contribution of the different factors to the metabolic syndrome. Elevated body weight, waist girth, and low HDL cholesterol show a significantly higher effect in women than in men in the French Monica study.[14] In contrast, systolic and diastolic blood pressures were more important factors in men.[14] This difference is due to the different body fat distribution in men compared to women. Men have a higher abdominal fat tissue favoring the early development of insulin resistance dyslipidemia and high blood pressure. Women need a higher degree of adiposity to achieve the same metabolic disturbances.[15]

In Europe there are only sporadic data on the prevalence of the metabolic syndrome. The metabolic syndrome has been found to be more frequent in men than in women. Classification according to WHO criteria generally leads to a 50% higher estimation of prevalence compared with the EGIR criteria in men.[8] This can be explained by the different cutoff points for central obesity employed in the WHO definition. For women the difference is smaller.[7] Two-hour glucose values are a WHO criterion for metabolic syndrome and this may indicate that a number of women will be identified only by this criterion. Baseline measurements of the components of the metabolic syndrome in 1,325 European males (44%) and females (55%) aged 30–60 years, during the RISC study conducted by the EGIR,[16] revealed a 7.9% in men and 5.9% in women prevalence of the metabolic syndrome in the selected healthy population (unpublished data). Similar results have been obtained in a Greek population where 1,128 men and 1,154 women have been studied. The prevalence of the metabolic syndrome was 25.2% in men and 14.6% in women. Men had a higher prevalence until the age of 65 years where the rate was equal for both genders.[17] The prevalence of the metabolic syndrome is three times higher in women with prior diet-treated gestational diabetes than in the general population.[18]

COMPONENTS OF THE METABOLIC SYNDROME IN WOMEN

Abdominal Obesity

Abdominal or central obesity, defined as increased waist circumference, is the form of obesity that is most commonly associated with the metabolic syndrome.[19] This is because abdominal adipose tissue has been shown over the recent years to play a central role in the pathogenesis of atherosclerosis through various metabolic and hormonal pathways.[15]

The pattern of lipid accumulation differs in women and men. Women more often develop peripheral obesity with gluteal fat accumulation whereas men are more prone to central or android obesity. Lower body subcutaneous fat accumulation is associated with a lower likelihood of insulin resistance or diabetes mellitus.[20] The amount of visceral fat increases with age in both genders, and this increase is present in normal weight as well as in overweight and obese subjects but more so in men than in women.[21] However, both types can be found in both sexes. Enzi *et al.* have found that 7.3% of females in their study had an android type of fat topography and 6.5% of the males had a gynoid type of fat distribution.[21] In young women and middle-aged females up to about 60 years of age subcutaneous abdominal fat area is predominant over abdominal visceral fat. Later on, in age, especially after menopause, there is a change to android type of fat distribution and visceral fat increases in a steeper way, almost the same as in men.[22]

Adipose tissue plays an essential role in lipolysis releasing free fatty acids and glycerol into the circulation. The capacity for lipogenesis and lipolysis varies according to body region and sex.[15] It has been shown that the contribution of visceral fat lipolysis to FFA delivery, mainly to the liver, increases with increasing visceral fat and this effect is greater in women than in men.[23] A tendency toward an increase in central obesity is observed in both sexes in advanced age or after gonadectomy.[24] Sex hormone receptors distribution is different in visceral and subcutaneous fat. Estrogen receptor-β is mainly expressed in subcutaneous fat tissue of females whereas androgen receptors are more prominent in visceral fat both in men and women. Higher rates of lipolysis in men are regulated by α or β adrenergic receptors in the abdominal adipocytes.[25] Estrogens decrease noradrenalin-stimulated lipolysis in women by upregulating the number of α-2 adrenergic antilipolytic receptors in adipose tissue.[26] Thus abdominal adipocytes are a main source of free fatty acids, high concentrations of which induce insulin resistance.[27]

Android obesity is particularly linked to increased cardiovascular mortality and the risk of type 2 diabetes.[28] Male obese subjects exhibit altered cortisol secretion, reduced plasma testosterone, and growth hormone levels.[28]

Apart from being a source of fatty acids, visceral fat is an important source of several bioactive compounds, such as inflammatory mediators (TNF-α, interleukins [more importantly IL-6], adipokines, and proteins related to co-agulation [PA-1]) affecting glucose and fat metabolism and contributing to the development of hepatic insulin resistance.[29] The finding that adipose tissue secretes leptin has established adipose tissue as an endocrine organ that communicates with the central nervous system regulating food intake and energy expenditure.[30] In vitro and in vivo studies have revealed that leptin also has angiogenic activity.[31] In fact, prospective studies including only male subjects have shown that leptin may be an independent risk factor for coronary heart disease.[32] Leptin is mainly secreted by the subcutaneous adipose tissue. This is why serum leptin levels are higher in women because they have higher fat mass than men.[33] It has also been speculated that leptin secretion from abdominal fat contributes to the development of visceral adiposity in men.[33] Lower amounts of visceral fat might explain the reduced tendency to develop metabolic syndrome in obese women.[34] Although a correlation between leptin and estrogen has been described there has been no difference in leptin levels between pre- and postmenopausal women.[35]

Adiponectin, another adipose tissue-derived protein with antiatherogenic properties, seems to be higher in women than in men,[36] whereas resistin, an adipose tissue-derived cytokine related to the development of type 2 diabetes, shows a trend of increase in women with polycystic ovary syndrome.[37]

The cytokines secreted by the adipose tissue play multiple roles in the inflammatory process that accelerates atherosclerosis. In particular, Il-6 stimulates the release of CRP by the liver. CRP plays a proatherogenic role acting on the endothelial cells and it is considered a biologic marker of systemic inflammation.[38] CRP has been shown to be a better predictor of future cardiovascular events than LDL cholesterol in women.[39] The potential interrelationships between CRP, the metabolic syndrome, and cardiovascular events were examined in the participants of the Women's Ischemia Syndrome Evaluation (WISE), which enrolled apparently healthy women aged 45 years and older with no prior history of cardiovascular disease or cancer.[40] CRP levels increased linearly with the number of criteria of the metabolic syndrome as defined according to the ATP III guidelines, from 0.68 mg/L for women who met no criteria of the syndrome to 5.57 mg/L for women who met all five criteria. Analysis of the women with metabolic syndrome ($n = 3,597$) indicated that cardiovascular disease risk rose with increasing levels of CRP. However, the WISE study enrolled postmenopausal women aged ≥45 years. The National Health and Nutrition Examination Survey (NHANES) study included women aged ≥20 years with most of the women in the fifth decade of life meeting ≥3 criteria for the metabolic syndrome. The data in this analysis confirm other studies, which show that all the components for the metabolic syndrome are associated with increased levels of hsCRP.[10] A strict relationship of CRP to the metabolic syndrome in women more accurately than in men has been confirmed in the Framingham Offspring Study.[41]

Hypertension

Hypertension is an essential component of the metabolic syndrome. Women show a lower incidence of hypertension than men before menopause. The effect of menopause on hypertension is not clear but studies have shown a higher incidence of hypertension among postmenopausal women even after correcting for age and BMI.[42] Estrogens definitely play a role either by affecting fat accumulation or the renin-angiotensin system (RAS). Estrogen prevents the conversion of angiotensin I to angiotensin II and decreases the sensitivity of angiotensin receptors.[43] Pressure natriuresis, renal hemodynamics, and tubular response to salt are influenced by sex hormones and the RAS.[44] Sex differences have also been found in the association of gene polymorphisms for the proactivator of PPAR γ (PPARGC1) and the angiotensin receptor type 2 (AT_2).[45]

Insulin Resistance

The metabolic syndrome derived from the insulin resistance syndrome means that previous definitions of the syndrome were based on the critical role of insulin resistance in the pathogenesis of atherosclerosis.[3,6] Although such a pathophysiological link has not yet been clarified there is enough evidence from prospective studies that there is an association between insulin resistance measured only by fasting insulin levels and the incidence of cardiovascular disease.[46] Hyperinsulinemia is the result of insulin resistance, enhanced insulin secretion, and reduced insulin clearance.[47]

Hyperinsulinemia and insulin resistance show different frequencies in men and women. Women at their child-bearing age exhibit a greater sensitivity to insulin at the level of the whole body compared to men matched for age, relative body weight, and physical activity fitness (VO2 max measurements) of similar age.[48] This inherent gender difference in insulin sensitivity may explain why many of the associates of hyperinsulinemia, such as hypertriglyceridemia, low HDL cholesterol concentration, hyperuricemia, and impaired glucose tolerance are more commonly observed in men. Heart muscle insulin sensitivity is comparable in both sexes and glucose uptake by the heart expressed per muscle weight correlates with increasing BMI.[49] It is conceivable that some of the cardioprotective effects of estrogens could be mediated via enhanced insulin sensitivity.

In a large series of Caucasian subjects of all ages living in Europe selected with normal glucose tolerance test and normal arterial blood pressure, insulin sensitivity has been measured under euglycemic clamp conditions.[50] Obesity was found to be related to insulin resistance as evaluated by increased circulating insulin levels. Insulin sensitivity declines linearly with BMI independently of gender (1.2 μmoL/kg/FFM/min per unit of BMI). Although obese subjects were more insulin resistant, obesity was found to be associated with a statistically high reduction in insulin sensitivity when insulin-mediated glucose uptake was normalized by lean mass, the metabolically active mass in the body. The obese group was only 15–25% less sensitive to insulin than the lean group with no difference between men and women. This is because most total glucose uptake occurs in skeletal muscle; fat tissue, being mainly a triglyceride mass, contributes much to body weight but little to total glucose uptake. In other studies normalizing insulin-mediated glucose uptake for body weight rather than for lean body mass and using plasma insulin concentrations as a surrogate measure of insulin sensitivity may have contributed to overestimation of insulin resistance. Furthermore, this population studied by the EGIR has been selected to be of normal glucose tolerance and blood pressure. In these normotensive and nondiabetic obese individuals, insulin resistance being relatively low was exceeded by the prevalence of insulin hypersecretion particularly in women with central obesity. Fat distribution had little to do with insulin sensitivity when simultaneously accounting for BMI since an increase in BMI is associated with an increase in subcutaneous fat and not with the topography of fat accumulation.[51] Other investigators, in small study groups, have suggested that in nonobese women, total body fat mass appears to be a primary determinant of tissue sensitivity to insulin, whereas in obese women, body fat topography exerts a more dominant effect.[52] In the EGIR database in pure obesity without other confounding abnormalities, insulin resistance is not as prevalent as previously thought, and is less frequent than insulin hypersecretion. The hyperinsulinemia of obesity is the result of both the compensation to insulin resistance and the primary (central) insulin hypersecretion. The clinical implication of these findings is that the risk for diabetes and/or CVD associated with the predominantly insulin resistant or insulin–hypersecreting obese phenotype may be different. In a subsequent report of the EGIR database,[53] fasting hyperinsulinemia and insulin resistance, although they coexist, also seem to identify with partially different groups of individuals. Subjects with pure insulin resistance seem to have a different phenotype with more central fat distribution, excessive lipolysis, and endogenous glucose production predisposing them to type 2 diabetes, whereas subjects with pure hyperinsulinemia seem to have higher values of systolic blood pressure, lower values of HDL cholesterol concentrations, suppressed lipolysis, and endogenous glucose production making them more prone to advance to cardiovascular abnormalities. These results suggest that total body fat content and body fat topography are associated differently with insulin-mediated glucose metabolism in nonobese and obese women.

Dyslipidemia

Circulating lipids are different and have different significance in women and men.[54] Total cholesterol measurements are higher in men until the fifth decade of life but beyond this age women have greater values.[55,56] High-density lipoprotein values are generally higher in women at all ages. Gender differences in HDL cholesterol levels diminish with advancing age because women experience a relatively mild decline in HDL cholesterol at the time of menopause.[57,58] Women seem to have a less atherogenic lipoprotein subclass profile.[59] The Framingham Offspring Study, however, reported that women have a twofold higher concentration of large HDL particles as compared to men.[59] Elevated triglycerides levels are a more potent independent risk factor for ischemic heart disease in women than in men, and non-HDL cholesterol is a stronger predictor than LDL cholesterol of cardiovascular mortality in women than in men in the Lipid Research Clinics Program Follow-up Study.[60] A recent meta-analysis of 17 studies showed that hypertriglyceridemia increases the relative risk for coronary heart disease by 32% in men compared to 76% in women.[61]

Cardiovascular Events

The metabolic syndrome is associated with an increased number of cardio-vascular events and actually is a better predictor of future cardiovascular events than diabetes.[2,62] Clinical manifestations of cardiovascular disease are coronary artery disease (CAD), myocardial infarction, stroke, and heart failure. Each one of these exhibits gender-specific differences in their pathogenesis progression and severity. The appearance of the syndrome increases the risk for coronary artery disease and stroke about threefold in a mixed population.[62]

Since the release of the previous National Cholesterol Education Program (NCEP) guidelines, the decline in cardiovascular mortality in the United States that predated these guidelines has slowed. In women, there has actually been an increase in the incidence of cardiovascular mortality.[57] This could be contributed to the increasing prevalence of the metabolic syndrome, the metabolic alterations associated with obesity and its increasing prevalence, the increased physical inactivity in women, and gender-specific differences in symptoms and diagnostic approaches of ischemic heart disease in women.

CAD is the predominant cause of morbidity and mortality of women in the Western Hemisphere.[1] It has been convincingly demonstrated that the incidence of CAD is lower in women than in men for all age groups except the very elderly.[38] The risk of CVS increases after menopause, which explains why the onset of atherosclerotic disease begins approximately 10 years later in women than men.[1] Almost 50% of women undergoing coronary angiography because of chest pain suggestive of angina have normal or insignificant CAD as compared to 17% of men.[63] In the WISE II careful follow-up even women who were found not to have significant coronary luminal narrowing but suffered persistent or worsening symptoms often demonstrated test abnormalities that implicated ischemic etiology for these symptoms and experienced adverse cardiovascular events during medium-term follow-up extended 4 to 5 years.[64–66] This has been attributed to microvascular disease or dysfunction whereas the misleading chest pain suggests that women have a lowered pain threshold.[67] The importance of family history in the development of CAD and its adverse events indicates the influence of an individual's genotype to vascular disease susceptibility. The WISE study has begun exploring the genetic predisposition in women and cardiovascular disease.[68]

Women with the metabolic syndrome are at intermediate cardiovascular disease mortality risk when compared to those with normal glucose tolerance or diabetes.[40,62,69,70] The 4-year relative risk of cardiac events increased almost twofold in women with the metabolic syndrome in the WISE study.[71] Central fat distribution as measured by waist circumference accompanied by decreased physical activity were considered the best contributors to these results.

The age differences in cardiovascular risk in women compared to men could be attributed to the loss of ovarian estrogen during menopause that is associated with an android shape and deposition of abdominal fat as well as the greater decrease in physical activity in older women.[72]

In several studies the appearance of metabolic syndrome increased the risk for coronary artery disease and stroke up to threefold and its appearance is a better predictor of future cardiovascular disease compared to diabetes.[9,62,71] The prevalence of cardiovascular disease was the highest in patients with diabetes and the metabolic syndrome (19.2%), lower in patients with the metabolic syndrome (13.9%), and even lower in patients without the metabolic syndrome (8.7%).

In the Framingham Offspring Study, where the metabolic syndrome was also associated with increased risk of cardiovascular events, this increase was associated with the increase in the CRP levels. Increased CRP and metabolic syndrome were independent predictors of cardiovascular disease[73] and the relationship of elevated CRP to CVD was stronger in women than in men.[73]

Treatment

Lifestyle management and behavior modification have a definite role in the treatment of the metabolic syndrome. Ultimately, treatment goals are to prevent cardiovascular disease by altering the risk factors that are components of the syndrome. All individuals with the metabolic syndrome should undergo absolute risk assessment to determine whether they are candidates for preventing drug therapies. The proposition by Kahn *et al.* to just treat the independent risk factors of the metabolic syndrome does not ensure the degree of risk reduction that is implied.[74] At the moment we do not have a drug available to target the syndrome as a whole entity. Future research may reveal such a therapeutic agent. Patients suffering from the metabolic syndrome deserve more intensive intervention with lifestyle approaches. The initial goal is weight loss and reduction of the adipose mass by lowering caloric intake along with exercise. Visceral fat is more sensitive to weight reduction than subcutaneous adipose tissue because omental and mesenteric adipocytes, the major components of visceral abdominal fat, have been shown to be more metabolically active and sensitive to lipolysis.[28] Regarding the effects of exercise *per se* on visceral fat, there appears to be a relative resistance to visceral adipose tissue reduction in obese women, whereas exercise-induced weight loss is associated with significant reductions in visceral fat in men.[75] Reducing adipose tissue mass through lifestyle modification lowers TNF-α and IL-6 and prevents the metabolic syndrome and the development of atherosclerosis and type 2 diabetes. Exercise and weight loss are likely to be fundamental mechanisms by which we can reduce the impact of the inflammatory process.[76] It has been speculated that weight loss is a safe method for downregulating the inflammatory state and counteracting endothelial dysfunction in obese women.[77]

Physical inactivity expressed as the reported no leisure time physical activity is higher in women than in men (35.8% in men and 41% in women).[78] This gender difference is reported even in youth where a higher BMI is associated with greater decline in activity among girls.[79] The relative risk for CVD associated with physical inactivity ranges from 1.5–2.4, an increase in risk comparable to that observed for high cholesterol, high blood pressure, or cigarette smoking.[80] On the other hand, prolonged time of sitting predicts increased risk for cardiovascular risk. In an analysis from the Framingham Heart Study, BMI was directly associated with total cholesterol, blood pressure, and blood glucose levels. These risk factors decreased with weight loss and increased with weight gain. Obesity was also associated with increased relative risks for total mortality, coronary heart disease, and cerebrovascular disease.[81]

Brisk walking for at least 2.5 h per week is associated with 30% reduction in the risk of coronary events in postmenopausal women.[82] These findings are important for women's health because walking is an activity preferred by many women. Even a 3-year lifestyle change in cohorts of free-living populations have shown that 3-year increases in sporting activity were associated with a lowering of waist circumference while increases in physical activity at home had beneficial effects on waist circumference, BMI, triglycerides, and HDL in men.[83] Intensive lifestyle intervention with diet and exercise reduced the incidence of type 2 diabetes by 58% in high-risk population[84] and this effect was superior to the intervention with pharmaceutical agent.[85]

The majority of risk factors for CAD can be improved by lifestyle modification. The ultimate goal in treating women with the metabolic syndrome is to focus on adipose tissue mass reduction by encouraging increased physical activity in any way and by setting realistic goals. A heart healthy lifestyle that will continue into adulthood should be encouraged from youth, but even changes later in life lead to important benefits.

REFERENCES

1. ECKEL, R.H., S.M. BRUNDY & P.Z. ZIMMET. 2005. The metabolic syndrome. Lancet **365:** 1415–1428.
2. ALEXANDER, C.M., P.B. LANDSMAN, S.M. TEUTSCH & S.M. HAFFNER. 2003. Third National Health and Nutrition Examination Survey (NHANES III)I; National Cholesterol Education Program (NCEP). NCEP-defined metabolic syndrome, diabetes, and prevalence of coronary heart disease among NHANES III participants age 50 years and older. Diabetes **52:** 1210–1214.
3. REAVEN, G.M. 1988. Banting Lecture 1988 Role of insulin resistance in human disease. Diabetes **37:** 1595–1607.
4. INTERNATIONAL DIABETES FEDERATION. The IDF consensus worldwide definition of the metabolic syndrome. Available at: htpp://www.idf.org/webdata/docs/IDF_Metasyndrome_definition.pdf.
5. FERRANNINI, E., S. VICHI, H. BECK-NIELSEN, et al. 1996. Insulin action and age. European Group for the Study of Insulin Resistance (EGIR). Diabetes **45:** 947–953.
6. ALBERTI, K.G. & P.Z. ZIMMET. 1998. Definition, diagnosis and classification of diabetes mellitus and its complications Part 1: diagnosis and classification of diabetes mellitus provisional report of a WHO consultation. Diabet. Med. **15:** 539–553.
7. BALKAU, B. & M.A. CHARLES. 1999. Comment on the provisional report from the WHO consultation European Group for the Study of Insulin Resistance (EGIR). Diabet. Med. **16:** 442–443.
8. BALKAU, B., M.A. CHARLES, T. DRIVSSHOLM, et al. 2002. Frequency of the WHO metabolic syndrome in European cohorts, and an alternative definition of an insulin resistance syndrome. Diabetes Metab. **28:** 364–376.
9. EXECUTIVE SUMMARY OF THE THIRD REPORT OF THE NATIONAL CHOLESTEROL EDUCATION PROGRAM (NCEP) EXPERT PANEL ON DETECTION, EVALUATION AND TREATMENT OF HIGH BLOOD CHOLESTEROL IN ADULTS (ADULT TREATMENT PANEL III). 2001. JAMA **285:** 2486–2497.
10. FORD, E.S., W.H. GILES & W.H. DIETZ. 2002. Prevalence of the metabolic syndrome among US adults: Findings from the Third National Health and Nutrition Examination Survey. JAMA **287:** 356–359.
11. FORD, E.S., W.H. GILES & A.H. MOKDAD. 2004. Increasing prevalence of the metabolic syndrome among U.S. adults. Diabetes Care **27:** 2444–2449.
12. HEDLEY, A.A., C.L. JOHNSON, M.D. CARROLL, et al. 2004. Prevalence of overweight and obesity among US children, adolescents and adults 1999–2002. JAMA **291:** 2847–2850.
13. MOKDAD, A.H., E.S. FORD, B.A. BOWMAN, et al. 2003. Prevalence of obesity, diabetes, and obesity-related health risk factors, 2001. JAMA **289:** 76–79.

14. DALLONGEVILLE, J., D. COTTEL, D. ARVEILLER, *et al.* 2004. The association of the metabolic disorders with the metabolic syndrome is different in men and women. Ann. Nutr. Metab. **48:** 43–50.

15. WAJCHENBERG, B.L. 2000. Subcutaneous and visceral adipose tissue their relation to the metabolic syndrome. Endocr. Rev. **21:** 697–738.

16. HILLS, S., B. BALKAU, S. COPPACK, *et al.* 2004. The EGIR-RISC STUDY (The European group for the study of insulin resistance: relationship between insulin sensitivity and cardiovascular disease risk): I. Methodol. Object. Diabetol. **47:** 566–570.

17. PANAGIOTAKOS, D., C. PITSAVOS, C. CHRYSOHOOU, *et al.* 2004. Impact of lifestyle habits on the prevalence of the metabolic syndrome among Greek adults from the Attica Study. Am. Heart J. **147:** 106–112.

18. LAUENBORG, J., E. MATHIESEN, T. HANSEN, *et al.* 2005. The prevalence of the metabolic syndrome in a Danish Population of women with previous gestational diabetes mellitus is three-fold higher than in the general population. J. Clin. Endocr. Metab. **90:** 4004–4010.

19. GRUNDY, S., H. BREWER, H.B. CLEEMAN, JR., *et al.* 2004. Definition of metabolic syndrome: report of the National Heart, Lung, and Blood Institute/American Heart Association conference on scientific issues related to definition. Circulation **105:** 433–438.

20. LIVINGSTON, E.H. 2006. Lower body subcutaneous fat accumulation and diabetes mellitus risk. Surg. Obes. Relat. Dis. **2:** 362–368.

21. ENZI, G., M. GASPARO, P.R. BIONDETTI, *et al.* 1986. Subcutaneous and visceral fat distribution according to sex, age, and overweight evaluated by computed tomography. Am. J. Clin. Nutr. **44:** 739–746.

22. MATSUZAUA, Y., T. NAKAMURA, I. SHIMOMURA, *et al.* 1996. Visceral fat accumulation and cardiovascular disease. *In* Progress in Obesity Research Proceedings of the Seventh International Congress on Obesity (Toronto, Canada, August 20–25, 1994). A. Angel, H. Anderson, C. Bouchard, D. Lau, L. Leitter, R. Mendelson, Eds.: 569–572. John Libbey and Company. London.

23. NIELSEN, S., Z. GUO, C.M. JOHNSON, *et al.* 2004. Splachnic lipolysis in humans. J. Clin. Invest. **113:** 1582–1588.

24. MAYES, J.S. & G.H. WATSON. 2004. Direct effect of sex steroid hormones on adipose tissues and obesity. Obes. Rev. **5:** 197–216.

25. LONNQVIST, F., A. THORNE, V. LARGE & P. ARNER. 1997. Sex differences in visceral fat lipolysis and metabolic complications of obesity. Arterioscler. Thromb. Vac. Biol. **17:** 1472–1480.

26. PEDERSEN, S.B., K. KRISTENSEN, P.A. HERMANN, *et al.* 2004. Estrogen controls lipolysis by up regulating alpha 2 adrenergic receptors directly in human adipose tissue through the estrogen receptor alpha. Implications for the female fat distribution. J. Clin. Endocrinol. Metab. **89:** 1869–1876.

27. BODEN, G. & G.I. SHULMAN. 2002. Free fatty acids in obesity and type 2 diabetes: defining their role in the development of insulin resistance and beta cell dysfunction. Diabetes Care **25:** 1135–1141.

28. BJONTROP, P. 2000. Metabolic difference between visceral fat and subcutaneous abdominal fat. Diabetes Metab. **26**(Suppl. 3): 10–12.

29. RONTI, T., G. LUPATELLI & E. MANNARINO. 2006. The Endocrine function of adipose tissue: an update. Clin. Endocrinol. **64:** 355–365.

30. CARO, J.F., M.K. SINHA & J.W. KOLACZYNSKI, *et al.* 1996. Leptin: the tale of an obesity gene. Diabetes **45:** 1455–1462.

31. SIERRA-HONIGMANN, M.R., A.K. NATH & C. MURAKAMI, *et al.* 1998. Biological action of leptin as an angiogenic factor. Science **281:** 1683–1686.
32. WALLACE, A.M., A.D. MCMAHON, C.J. PACKARD, *et al.*2001. Plasma leptin and the risk of cardiovascular disease in the West of Scotland Coronary Prevention Study (WOSCOPS). Circulation **104:** 3052–3056.
33. MONTAGUE, C.T., J.B. PRINS, L. SANDERS, *et al.* 1997. Depot- and sex-specific differences in human leptin mRNA expression: implications for the control of regional fat distribution. Diabetes **46:** 342–347.
34. KROTKIEWSKI, M., P. BJONTROP, I. SJOSTROM & U. SMITH. 1983. Impact of obesity on metabolism in men and women. Importance of regional adipose tissue distribution. J. Clin. Invest. **72:** 1150–1162.
35. VAN HARMELEN, V., S. REYNISDOTTIR, P. ERIKSSON, *et al.* 1998. Leptin secretion from subcutaneous and visceral adipose tissue in women. Diabetes **47:** 913–917.
36. COSTACOU, T., J.C. ZGIBOR & R.W. EVANS, *et al.* 2005. The prospective association between adiponectin and coronary artery disease among individuals with type 1 diabetes.The Pittsburgh Epidemiology of Diabetes Complications Study. Diabetologia **48:** 41–48.
37. YANNAKOULIA, M., N. YIANNAKOURIS, S. BLUHER, *et al.* 2003. Body fat mass and macronutrient intake in relation to circulating soluble leptin receptor, free leptin index, adiponectin, and resistin concentrations in healthy humans. J. Endocrinol. Metab. **85:** 61–69.
38. RIDKER, F.M. & D.A. MORROW. 2003. C-reactive protein, inflammation and coronary risk. Cardiol. Clin. **21:** 315–325.
39. RIDKER, PM., N. RIFAI, L. ROSE, *et al.* 2002. Comparison of C-reactive protein and low density lipoprotein cholesterol levels in the prediction of first cardiovascular events. N. Engl. J. Med **347:** 1557–1565.
40. RIDKER, P.M., J.E. BURING, N.R. COOK & N. RIFAI. 2003. C-reactive protein, the metabolic syndrome and risk of incident cardiovascular events: an 8-year follow-up of 14719 initially healthy American women. Circulation **107:** 391–397.
41. RUTTER, M.K., J.B. MEIGS, L.M. SULLIVAN, *et al.* 2004. C-reactive protein, the metabolic syndrome and prediction of cardiovascular events in the Framingham Offspring Study. Circulation **110:** 380–385.
42. GOHLKE-BARWOLF, C. 2000. Coronary artery disease is menopause a risk factor. Basic Res. Cardiol. **95**(Suppl 1): 171–183.
43. NICKENING, G. 2004. Should angiotensin II receptor blockers be combined? Circulation **110:** 1013–1020.
44. PESCHERE-BERTSCHI, A. & M. BURNIER. 2004. Female sex hormones, salt and blood pressure regulation. Am. J. Hypertens. **17:** 994–1001.
45. CHEURFA, N., A.F. REIS, D. DUBOIS LAFORGUE, *et al.* 2004. The Gly482Ser polymorphism in the peroxisome proliferator-activated receptor-gamma coactivator-1 gene is associated with hypertension in type 2 diabetic men. Diabetologia **47:** 1980–1983.
46. HAFFNER, S.M., R.A. VALDEZ, H.P. HAZUDA, *et al.* 1992. Prospective analysis of the insulin resistance syndrome (syndrome X). Diabetes **41:** 715–722.
47. LAASKO, M. 1993. How good a marker is insulin level for insulin resistance? Am. J. Epidemiol. **137:** 959–965.
48. YKI-JARVINEN, H. 1984. Sex and insulin sensitivity. Metabolism **33:** 1011–1015.
49. NUUTILA, P., J. KNUUTI, M. MAKI, *et al.* 1995. Gender and insulin sensitivity in the heart and in skeletal muscle: studies using positron emission tomography. Diabetes **44:** 31–36.

50. FERRANNINI, E., A. NATALI, P. BELL, *et al.* 1997. Insulin resistance and hypersecretion in obesity. J. Clin. Invest. **100:** 1166–1173.
51. ZAMBONI, M., F. ARMELLINI & M.P. MILANI. 1992. Body fat distribution in pre- and post-menopausal women: metabolic and anthropometric variables and their inter-relationships. Int. J. Obes. Relat. Metab. Disord. **16:** 495–504.
52. BONORA, E., S. DEL PRATO, G. BONADONNA, *et al.* 1992. Total fat content and fat topography are associated differently with *in vivo* glucose metabolism in nonobese and obese nondiabetic women. Diabetes **41:** 1151–1159.
53. FERRANNINI, E. & B. BALKAU. 2002. Insulin: in search of a syndrome. Diabetic Med. **19:** 724–729.
54. WILLIAMS, C.M. 2004. Lipid metabolism in women. Proc. Nutr. Soc. **63:** 153–160.
55. CENTERS FOR DISEASE CONTROL AND PREVENTION. 2005. Available at: www.cdc.gov/nccdphp/burdenbook2004/index.htm.
56. MAJOR CARDIOVASCULAR DISEASE (CVD) DURING 1979–1999 AND MAJOR CVD HOSPITAL DISCHARGE RATES IN 1997 AMONG WOMEN WITH DIABETES –UNITED STATES. Available at www.cdc.gov/mmwr/preview/mmwrhtml/mm5043a2.htm.
57. AMERICAN HEART ASSOCIATION. Heart disease and stroke statistics-2005 update. Available at http//www.americanheart.org.
58. LERNER, D.J. & W.B. KANNEL. 1986. Patterns of coronary heart disease morbidity and mortality in the sexes: a 26-year follow up of the Framingham population. Am. Heart J. **111:** 383–390.
59. FRIEDMAN, D.S., J.D. OTVOS, F.J. JEYARAJAH, *et al.* 2004. Sex and age differences in lipoprotein subclasses measured by nuclear magnetic resonance spectroscopy: The Framingham Study. Clin. Chem. **50:** 1189–1200.
60. CUI, Y., R.S. BLUMENTHAL, J.A. FLAWS, *et al.* 2001. Non-high-density lipoprotein cholesterol level as a predictor of cardiovascular disease mortality. Arch. Intern. Med. **161:** 1413–1419.
61. HOKANSON, J.E. & M.A. AUSTIN. 1996. Plasma triglyceride level is a risk factor for cardiovascular disease independent of high-density lipoprotein level: a meta analysis of population-based prospective studies. J. Cardiovasc. Risk **3:** 213–219.
62. ISOMAA, B., P. ALMGREN, T. TUOMI, *et al.* 2001. Cardiovascular morbidity and mortality associated with the metabolic syndrome. Diabetes Care **24:** 683–689.
63. POPE, J.H., T.P. AUFDERHEIDE, R. RUTHAZER, *et al.* 2003. Missed diagnosis of acute cardiac ischemia in the emergency department. N. Engl. J. Med. **342:** 1163–1170.
64. BAIREY MERZ, C.N., S.F. KELSEY, C.J. PEPINE, *et al.* 1999. The Women's Ischemia Syndrome Evaluation (WISE) study: protocol design methodology and feasibility report. J. Am. Cardiol. **33:** 1453–1461.
65. PEPINE, C.J., R.S. BALABAN, R.O. BONOW, *et al.* 2004. Women's Ischemic Syndrome Evaluation: current status and future research directions. Report of the National Heart, Lung, and Blood Institute Workshop: October 2–4, 2002. Section 1: Diagnosis of stable ischemia and ischemic heart disease. Circulation **109:** 44e–46e.
66. SHAW, L., C.N. BAIREY METZ, C.J. PEPINE, *et al.* 2006. Insights from the NHLBI-Sponsored Women's Ischemia Syndrome Evaluation (WISE) Study Part = 1: gender differences in traditional and novel risk factors, symptom evaluation, and gender-optimized diagnostic strategies. J. Am. Coll. Cardiol. **47**(Suppl S): 4S–20S.

67. PANZA, M., A. JULIE, R. LAURIENZO, *et al.* 1997. Investigation of the mechanism of chest pain in patients with angiographically normal coronary arteries using transesophageal dobutamine stress echocardiography. J. Am. Coll. Cardiol. **29:** 293–301.

68. CHEN, Q., S.E. REIS, C.M. KAMMERER, *et al.* 2003. APOE polymorphism and angiographic coronary artery disease severity in the Women's Ischemia Syndrome Evaluation (WISE) study. Atherosclerosis **169:** 159–167.

69. WONG, N.D., M.G. SCIAMMARELLA, D. POLK, *et al.* 2003. The metabolic syndrome, diabetes and subclinical atherosclerosis assessed by coronary calcium. J. Am. Coll. Cardiol. **41:** 1547–1553.

70. KIP, K.E., O.C. MARROQUIN & D.E. KELLEY. 2004. Clinical importance of obesity versus the metabolic syndrome in cardiovascular risk in women : a report from the Women's Ischemia Syndrome Evaluation (WISE). Circulation **109:** 706–713.

71. MAROQUIN, O.C., K.E. KIP, D. KELLEY, *et al.* 2004. The metabolic syndrome modifies the cardiovascular risk associated with angiographic coronary heart disease in women: a report from WISE. Circulation **1009:** 714–721.

72. POELHAM, E.T. 2002. Menopause, energy expenditure and body composition. Acta Obstet. Gynecol. Scand. **3:** 603–611.

73. RUTTER, M.K., B. MEIGS, L. SULLIVAN, *et al.* 2005. Insulin resistance, the metabolic syndrome, and incident cardiovascular events in the Framingham Offspring Study. Diabetes **54:** 3252–3257.

74. KAHN, R., J. BUSE, E. FERRANNINI & M. STERN. 2005. The metabolic syndrome: time for a critical appraisal: joint statement from the American Diabetes Association and the European Association for the Study of Diabetes. Diabetes Care **28:** 2289–2304.

75. SMITH, S.R. & J.J. ZACHWIEJA. Visceral adipose tissue: a critical review of intervention strategies. Int. J. Obes. **23:** 329–335.

76. VISSER, M., L.M. BOUTER, G.M. MCQUILLAN, *et al.*1999. Elevated C-reactive protein levels in overweight and obese adults. JAMA **282:** 2131–2135.

77. ZICCARDI, P., F. NAPPO, G. GIUGLIANO, *et al.* 2002. Reduction of inflammatory cytokine concentrations and improvement of endothelial functions in obese women after weight loss over one year. Circulation **105:** 804–809.

78. AMERICAN HEART ASSOCIATION. Heart disease and stroke statistics—2005 update. Available at http//www.americanheart.org.

79. KIMM, S., W. GLYNN & A. KRISKA. 2002. Decline in physical activity in black girls and white girls during adolescence. N. Engl. J. Med. **347:** 709–715.

80. PATE, R.R., M. PRATT, S.N. BLAIR, *et al.* 1995. Physical activity and public health: a recommendation from the Centers for Disease Control and Prevention and the American College of Sports Medicine. JAMA **273:** 402–407.

81. HIGGINS, M., W. KANNEL, R. GARRISON, *et al.* 1988. Hazards of obesity—the Framingham experience. Acta Med. Scand. **723**(Suppl): 23–36.

82. MANSON, J., P. GREENLAND, A. LACROIX, *et al.* 2002. Walking compared to vigorous exercise for the prevention of cardiovascular events in women. N. Engl. J. Med. **347:** 716–725.

83. BALKAU, B., E. VIERRON, M. VERNAY, *et al.* 2006. D.E.S.I.R Study Group. The impact of 3-year changes in lifestyle habits on metabolic syndrome parameters: the D.E.S.I.R study. Eur. J. Cardiovasc. Prev. Rehabil. **13:** 334–340.

84. TUOMILEHTO, J., J. LINDSTROM, J. ERRIKSON, *et al.* 2001. Prevention of type 2 diabetes mellitus by changes in lifestyle among subjects with impaired glucose tolerance: the Diabetes Prevention Study (DPS) in Finland. N. Eng. J. Med. **344:** 1343–1350.
85. DPP RESEARCH GROUP. 2002. Reduction in the incidence of type 2 diabetes with lifestyle intervention or metformin. N. Engl. J. Med. **346:** 393–403.

From Menarche to Regular Menstruation

Endocrinological Background

IOANNIS E. MESSINIS

Department of Obstetrics and Gynecology, University of Thessalia,
Medical School, Larissa, Greece

ABSTRACT: Marked changes in hormone secretion occur from childhood to adulthood. Prior to puberty gonadotropin-releasing hormone (GnRH) secretion is markedly suppressed. At the onset of puberty, the hypothalamic gonadostat is derepressed and the amplitude of GnRH pulses increases. Follicle-stimulating hormone (FSH) and luteinizing hormone (LH) levels increase gradually during puberty stimulating follicle maturation and estrogen production in the ovaries. Only the negative feedback mechanism is powerful before puberty, while the positive feedback mechanism becomes active for the first time in late puberty. As a result, normal cyclicity is usually established at that time. During normal menstrual cycle, steroidal and nonsteroidal hormones mediate the effect of the ovaries on the hypothalamic-pituitary system. Estradiol and progesterone are important regulators of FSH and LH secretion, while inhibins play a role in the control of FSH secretion. Gonadotropin surge attenuating factor (GnSAF) is a nonsteroidal ovarian substance that controls the amplitude of the midcycle LH surge by antagonizing the sensitizing effect of estradiol on the pituitary.

KEYWORDS: menarche; puberty; pituitary; FSH; LH; estradiol; ovary

INTRODUCTION

The passage from childhood to puberty is characterized by changes in hormonal dynamics within the hypothalamic-pituitary system that lead to the onset of ovarian function. Menarche is one of the main manifestations of puberty occurring on average at the age of 12.8 years in Western countries. Prior to puberty, circulating levels of Follicle-stimulating hormone (FSH) and luteinizing hormone (LH) are very low due to minimal secretion of these hormones from the pituitary. This is attributed to the suppression of gonadotropin-releasing hormone (GnRH) secretion from the hypothalamus via two possible mechanisms, that is, a central inhibitory mechanism that has not been specified

Address for correspondence: Ioannis E. Messinis, Department of Obstetrics and Gynecology, University of Thessalia, Medical School, 22 Papakiriazi Street, 41222 Larissa, Greece. Voice: +30-2410-682795; fax: +30-2410-670096.
e-mail: messinis@med.uth.gr

Ann. N.Y. Acad. Sci. 1092: 49–56 (2006). © 2006 New York Academy of Sciences.
doi: 10.1196/annals.1365.004

yet and a peripheral mechanism that mediates the negative feedback effect of gonadal steroids. It has been hypothesized that during childhood the hypothalamus is extremely sensitive to the negative feedback effect of the very low circulating concentrations of estrogen.[1] Therefore, for puberty to start, reactivation of the hypothalamic-pituitary system is required, which increases the secretion of GnRH and gonadotropins. This is achieved via inhibition of the two inhibitory mechanisms and derepression of the gonadostat.[2]

The first indication that reactivation of the hypothalamic-pituitary system has started is the increased pulsatility of LH and FSH that occurs initially during the night and as puberty, progresses also during the day. Increased pulsatility of the two gonadotropins during the night as compared to the daytime is also evident prior to puberty, but with the onset of puberty the pulses are amplified with no alterations in frequency.[3] These changes in gonadotropin pulses reflect increased pulsatile secretrion of GnRH because administration of a GnRH antagonist to pubertal girls either eliminates or attenuates gonadotropin pulses.[3] Circulating levels of FSH and LH increase gradually during puberty and stimulate follicle maturation and estrogen synthesis in the ovaries.

Estradiol values that are very low during childhood increase gradually throughout puberty and stimulate proliferation of the endometrium that leads to the first menstruation. However, the levels of estradiol may be rather low even at Tanner stage 5 (about 60 pg/mL)[4] and therefore, inadequate to exert a positive feedback mechanism. Consequently, the first cycles that follow menarche may be anovulatory.

Apart from the described changes, the secretion of other hormones, such as inhibins, is also altered. These changes may not be directly related to the puberty itself but to the changes in the function of the hypothalamic-pituitary-ovarian axis. Following the rise of FSH, the levels of inhibin B increase gradually during the early stages of puberty, while those of inhibin A increase at a later stage.[5] At the beginning of puberty, there are positive correlations between the levels of gonadotropins and inhibins, while following the end of puberty a negative correlation between inhibin A and FSH is established, suggesting that this protein is gradually becoming part of the negative feedback mechanism.[5]

From the time the positive feedback mechanism becomes active, normal cyclicity is established, which is characterized by the occurrence of the mid-cycle LH surge.[6] The ovaries exert their effects on the hypothalamic-pituitary system via the secretion of various steroidal and nonsteroidal substances. However, the extent to which each of these substances contributes to the feedback mechanisms has not been clarified, although recent data have provided new information that will be discussed in the following sections (FIG. 1).

NEGATIVE FEEDBACK MECHANISM

When exogenous estrogens are given to normal women during the early follicular phase of the cycle, the levels of both FSH and LH are suppressed.[7]

GONADAL AXIS IN FEMALES

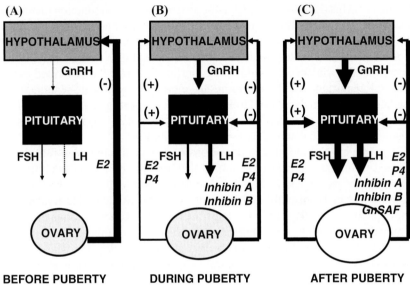

FIGURE 1. Changes in the secretion of GnRH and gonadotropins from childhood to puberty. Relationships between the ovarian hormones and the hypothalamic-pituitary system within the context of the feedback mechanisms.

The percentage decrease of FSH is similar to that of LH, suggesting at that stage of the cycle these two hormones are equally sensitive to the estradiol-suppressing effect.[7]

In normal premenopausal women, marked changes in the secretion of reproductive hormones occur following ovariectomy. For instance, during the first three days after the operation, performed either in the follicular or in the luteal phase of the cycle, serum estradiol, progesterone, and inhibin concentrations decline markedly, while those of FSH and LH increase gradually.[8] In a study in which exogenous estradiol was given to the women following ovariectomy in the luteal phase of the cycle, the expected increase in FSH and LH levels was postponed for 2–3 days supporting that this steroid is an important component of the negative feedback mechanism, but not the only factor that controls FSH and LH secretion during that period of the cycle.[9] When progesterone was added to the estradiol regimen, the increase in FSH and LH levels was postponed further indicating that during the luteal phase of the cycle these two steroids are important regulators of FSH and LH secretion.[9]

During the follicular phase, it appears that the two gonadotropins are controlled by different ovarian mechanisms. In a recent study in which a simulated follicular and a simulated luteal phase were created after the administration of exogenous estradiol and progesterone to postmenopausal women, basal gonadotropin levels, especially those of LH, decreased significantly.[10]

However, during a s ubsequent simulated follicular phase, the values of FSH remained stable, while those of LH increased despite the rising estradiol concentrations.[10] This demonstrates that in the absence of ovarian function increasing estradiol levels as in the normal follicular phase are inadequate to maintain low levels of LH, suggesting that the ovaries during the follicular phase of the normal menstrual cycle produce a factor that contributes to the control of LH secretion. This factor is possibly progesterone.[10] Under the described experimental conditions, FSH concentrations, although suppressed, remained at a higher level than in the normal follicular phase, suggesting that the functioning ovaries contribute to the control of FSH secretion not only via the steroids but also via nonsteroidal substances, possibly inhibin B.[10]

The role of inhibin in the normal menstrual cycle has not been fully investigated in humans. So far only animal data provide direct evidence that the two inhibins participate in the control of FSH secretion *in vivo*. The results of a study in which normally cycling premenopausal women were treated with clomiphene for 15 days have demonstrated that LH concentrations increased gradually and continuously during the administration of this compound, while FSH levels increased for the first 5 days and then declined.[11] These results support the notion that for the control of FSH secretion a role is also played by nonestrogenic mechanisms.

Inhibin may also play a role in the control of FSH secretion during the luteal-follicular transition. At that time, the intercycle rise of FSH takes place. The latter is also named "FSH window" and is responsible for the selection of the dominant follicle in the normal menstrual cycle. Marked changes in hormone secretion occur during that period of time. In particular, a significant decrease in inhibin A, estradiol, and progesterone concentrations takes place in late luteal phase, that is, before the onset of the FSH intercycle rise, suggesting that these hormones contribute to the negative feedback effect of the ovaries on FSH secretion in the luteal phase.[12] Following the increase in FSH, an increase in inhibin B starts, which in turn suppresses FSH levels.[12] It is possible therefore that the two inhibins are important for the intercycle rise of FSH with inhibin A participating in the mechanisms that "open" and inhibin B in the mechanisms that "close" the FSH window. From these and other data, it is clear that the two gonadotropins are differentially controlled by the ovaries both in the follicular and the luteal phase of the cycle.[13] In the follicular phase, the most important regulators of FSH secretion are estradiol and inhibin B and of LH secretion estradiol and progesterone. During the luteal phase, an important role is played by estradiol, progesterone, and inhibin A for FSH and by estradiol and progesterone for LH secretion.

POSITIVE FEEDBACK MECHANISM

Estradiol is the main component of the positive feedback mechanism that sensitizes the pituitary to GnRH and facilities the self-priming effect of GnRH on the gonadotrophs.[14] The role of progesterone is rather unclear, although it is possible that this hormone amplifies the estradiol positive effect and therefore the amplitude of the LH surge. The sensitizing effect of estradiol on the pituitary is evident from the time puberty starts. After the onset of puberty, a change in the pattern of pituitary response to GnRH takes place. In particular, during childhood FSH response to a single GnRH dose is greater than that of LH, while during puberty it is LH that is predominantly secreted under the stimulation by GnRH.[3]

It has been assumed that under the influence of GnRH the two gonadotropins are secreted from two separate pools of the pituitary gonadotrophs.[14] The first is the "releasable" pool that releases gonadotropins immediately after the stimulation by GnRH and the second is the "reserve" pool that requires a longer stimulation by GnRH to secrete gonadotropins. A functional differentiation between the two pools can be performed *in vivo* with the intravenous injection of two submaximal doses of GnRH, 10 μg each.[14] The response to the first GnRH dose is maximal at 30 min and represents gonadotropins secreted from the first pool. This also shows the "pituitary sensitivity" to GnRH, while the whole area under the curve represents the secretion from the second pool and shows the "pituitary reserve."

It has been demonstrated that the size of the two gonadotropin pools increases from the early to late follicular phase of the normal menstrual cycle.[14] However, investigation of the pituitary sensitivity to GnRH on a daily basis during the follicular phase of the cycle has demonstrated an unchanged pattern during the early and midfollicular phase despite the significant increase in estradiol concentrations.[15] This suggests that at that stage of the cycle the ovaries produce a substance that antagonizes the sensitizing effect of estradiol on the pituitary. A significant increase in the pituitary sensitivity to GnRH occurs only in late follicular phase.[15] These data are supported by a recent study demonstrating that in postmenopausal women the induction within 15 days of estradiol levels similar to those in the follicular phase of the normal cycle after the exogenous administration of estrogen resulted in a significant increase in the pituitary sensitivity to GnRH during the whole period of estradiol increase.[10] This pattern of changes in pituitary sensitivity differs from that described above during the follicular phase of the normal menstrual cycle and suggests that the premenopausal ovaries produce a factor that antagonizes the sensitizing effect of estradiol on the pituitary.

Progesterone is excluded from being such a factor because the administration of mefepristone to normal women during the follicular phase of the cycle has resulted in a reduction of both the pituitary sensitivity and the reserve.[16] It is probable, therefore, that progesterone sensitizes the pituitary to GnRH and that the missing factor in postmenopausal women is gonadotropin surge attenuating factor (GnSAF).[10] This factor is produced particularly during superovulation induction in women and attenuates the endogenous LH surge in such patients.[17] GnSAF acts via a significant reduction of the pituitary response to GnRH attenuating both the pituitary sensitivity and the reserve as well as the self-priming effect of GnRH on the pituitary.[18,19]

According to data in women, purification of GnSAF from human follicular fluid has demonstrated identity to the carboxyl-terminal fraction of human serum albumin.[20] This is supported by the data of a recent study in which recombinant products of human serum albumin corresponding to residues 490–585 (subdomain IIIB) were produced using the expression-secretion system of *pichia pastoris* GS 115.[21] When these fragments were tested in an vitro bioassay system using rat pituitary cells in culture, a significant suppression of GnRH-induced LH secretion was found, suggesting the expression of GnSAF bioactivity.[21] These data were supported by a more recent study in which the mRNA of human serum albumin was expressed in human granulosa cells.[22] However, although in the nucleus the whole molecule was expressed, in the cytoplasm only the amino- and the carboxyl-terminal fractions were detected, supporting the notion that the latter fragment is a potential GnSAF candidate.[22]

It is clear from these data that estradiol and GnSAF interact on the pituitary gonadotrophs in the context of the positive feedback mechanism. It is assumed that estradiol sensitizes the pituitary to GnRH, while GnSAF antagonizes the sensitizing effect of this steroid. Based on the existing knowledge, a hypothesis has been developed that the activity of GnSAF is higher during the early and midfollicular phases and lower in the late follicular phase and at midcycle.[13] Therefore, during the early and midfollicular phase the response of LH to GnRH is maintained at a low level and is markedly enhanced during the late follicular phase aiming at the full expression of the midcycle LH surge. The latter is required for luteinization and follicle rupture and for the maturation of the oocyte.

CONCLUSIONS

Marked changes in gonadal function occur in women from the onset to the end of puberty. In particular, before puberty despite the low concentrations of estrogen, it is the negative feedback mechanism that is extremely powerful suppressesing the hypothalamus and the pituitary. At the same period, the positive feedback mechanism is not active. During puberty, the negative feedback effect of estrogen is attenuated but more substances, such as inhibins, are incorporated into the system. Toward the end of puberty, the positive feedback mechanism becomes active and normal cyclicity starts. Finally, after puberty the two feedback mechanisms are the main determinants of the relationships between the ovaries and the hypothalamic-pituitary system.

REFERENCES

1. WINTER, J.S. & C. FAIMAN. 1973. The development of cyclic pituitary-gonadal function in adolescent females. J. Clin. Endocrinol. Metab. **37:** 714–718.

2. FOSTER, D.L. & K.D. RYAN. 1979. Endocrine mechanisms governing transition into adulthood: a marked decrease in inhibitory feedback action of estradiol on tonic secretion of luteinizing hormone in the lamb during puberty. Endocrinology **105:** 896–904.

3. APTER, D., T.L. BUTZOW, G.A. LAUGHLIN & S.S. YEN. 1993. Gonadotropin-releasing hormone pulse generator activity during pubertal transition in girls: pulsatile and diurnal patterns of circulating gonadotropins. J. Clin. Endocrinol. Metab. **76:** 940–949.

4. GRUMBACH, M.M. 1975. Onset of puberty. *In* Puberty. S.R. Berenberg, H.E. Stenfert & B.V. Kroese, Ed.:1–21, Leiden, Netherlands.

5. SEHESTED, A., A.A. JUUL, A.M. ANDERSSON, *et al*. 2000. Serum inhibin A and inhibin B in healthy prepubertal, pubertal, and adolescent girls and adult women: relation to age, stage of puberty, menstrual cycle, follicle-stimulating hormone, luteinizing hormone, and estradiol levels. J. Clin. Endocrinol. Metab. **85:** 1634–1640.

6. MESSINIS, I.E. & A.A. TEMPLETON. 1988. The endocrine consequences of multiple folliculogenesis. J. Reprod. Fertil. Suppl. **36:** 27–37.

7. MESSINIS, I.E. & A.A. TEMPLETON. 1990. Effects of supraphysiological concentrations of progesterone on the characteristics of the oestradiol-induced gonadotrophin surge in women. J. Reprod. Fertil. **88:** 513–519.

8. ALEXANDRIS, E., S. MILINGOS, G. KOLLIOS, *et al*. 1997. Changes in gonadotrophin response to gonadotrophin releasing hormone in normal women following bilateral ovariectomy. Clin. Endocrinol. (Oxf.) **47:** 721–726.

9. MESSINIS, I.E., S. MILINGOS, E. ALEXANDRIS, *et al*. 2002. Evidence of differential control of FSH and LH responses to GnRH by ovarian steroids in the luteal phase of the cycle. Hum. Reprod. **17:** 299–303.

10. DAFOPOULOS, K., C.G. KOTSOVASSILIS, S. MILINGOS, *et al*. 2004. Changes in pituitary sensitivity to GnRH in estrogen-treated post-menopausal women: evidence that gonadotrophin surge attenuating factor plays a physiological role. Hum. Reprod. **19:** 1985–1992.

11. MESSINIS, I.E. & A. TEMPLETON. 1988. Blockage of the positive feedback effect of oestradiol during prolonged administration of clomiphene citrate to normal women. Clin. Endocrinol. (Oxf). **29:** 509–516.

12. GROOME, N.P., P.J. ILLINGWORTH, M. O'BRIEN, *et al*. 1996. Measurement of dimeric inhibin B throughout the human menstrual cycle. J. Clin. Endocrinol. Metab. **81:** 1401–1405.

13. MESSINIS, I.E. 2006. Ovarian feedback, mechanism of action and possible clinical implications. Hum. Reprod. 12: 557–571.

14. HOFF, J.D., B.L. LASLEY, C.F. WANG & S.S.C. YEN. 1977. The two pools of pituitary gonadotropin: regulation during the menstrual cycle. J. Clin. Endocrinol. Metab. **44:** 302–312.

15. MESSINIS, I.E., D. LOLIS, K. ZIKOPOULOS, *et al*. 1994. Effect of an increase in FSH on the production of gonadotrophin-surge-attenuating factor in women. J. Reprod. Fertil. **101:** 689–695.

16. KAZEM, R., L.E. MESSINIS, P. FOWLER, *et al*. 1996. Effect of mifepristone (RU486) on the pituitary response to gonadotrophin releasing hormone in women. Hum. Reprod. **11:** 2585–2590.

17. MESSINIS, I.E., A. TEMPLETON & D.T. BAIRD. 1985. Endogenous luteinizing hormone surge during superovulation induction with sequential use of clomiphene citrate and pulsatile human menopausal gonadotropin. J. Clin. Endocrinol. Metab. **61:** 1076–1080.

18. MESSINIS, I.E. & A.A. TEMPLETON. 1989. Pituitary response to exogenous LHRH in superovulated women. J. Reprod. Fertil. **87:** 633–639.
19. MESSINIS, I.E. & A. TEMPLETON. 1991. Attenuation of gonadotrophin release and reserve in superovulated women by gonadotrophin surge attenuating factor (Gn-SAF). Clin. Endocrinol. (Oxf.). **34:** 259–263.
20. PAPPA, A., K. SEFERIADIS, T. FOTSIS, *et al.* 1999. Purification of a candidate gonadotrophin surge attenuating factor from human follicular fluid. Hum. Reprod. **14:** 1449–1456.
21. TAVOULARI, S., S. FRILLINGOS, P. KARATZA, *et al.* 2004. The recombinant subdomain IIIB of human serum albumin displays activity of gonadotrophin surge-attenuating factor. Hum. Reprod. **19:** 849–858.
22. KARLIGIOTOU, E., P. KOLLIA, A. KALLITSARIS & I.E. MESSINIS. 2006. Expression of human serum albumin (HSA) mRNA in human granulosa cells: potential correlation of the 95 amino acid long carboxyl terminal of HSA to gonadotrophin surge-attenuating factor. Hum. Reprod. **21:** 645–650.

Presence or Absence of Menstruation in Young Girls

MARGARET REES

Nuffield Department of Obstetrics and Gynaecology, Level 4, Women's Centre, John Radcliffe Hospital, Oxford, UK

ABSTRACT: Menstruation is a periodic discharge of sanguinous fluid and sloughing of the uterine lining in the female. It is an event characteristic of the reproductive cycle in humans and most subhuman primates and has no known biological function. However, it is an integral part of a woman's experience throughout her reproductive life. This article will examine menstrual patterns and concerns in young girls. The section on absent menstruation will concentrate on premature ovarian failure.

KEYWORDS: menstruation; adolescents; menarche; dysmenorrhea; menstrual blood loss; premature ovarian failure

INTRODUCTION

Menstruation is a periodic discharge of sanguinous fluid and sloughing of the uterine lining in the female. It is an event characteristic of the reproductive cycle in humans and most subhuman primates and has no known biological function.[1] However, it is an integral part of a woman's experience throughout her reproductive life.

The menarche occurs between the ages of 10 and 16 years in most girls in developed countries.[2] There has been a secular trend to earlier menarche over the past century with a decrease of about 3 to 4 months per decade in industrialized countries. Thus the average age of menarche in 1840 was 16.5 years and now averages 13 years. The age of menarche is determined by a combination of factors, which include genetic influences, socioeconomic conditions, general health and well-being, nutritional status, certain types of exercise, and family size.[2,3] This article will examine menstrual patterns and concerns in young girls. The section on absent menstruation will concentrate on premature ovarian failure.

Address for correspondence: M. Rees, Nuffield Department of Obstetrics and Gynaecology, Level 4, Women's Centre, John Radcliffe Hospital, Oxford, OX3 9DU UK. Voice: 00-44-1865-220024/221546; fax: 00-44-1865-769141.
e-mail: margaret.rees@obs-gyn.ox.ac.uk

Ann. N.Y. Acad. Sci. 1092: 57–65 (2006). © 2006 New York Academy of Sciences.
doi: 10.1196/annals.1365.005

Menstruating girls are concerned about the amount of blood loss, frequency, and duration of menstruation and menstrual pain.[4]

AMOUNT OF MENSTRUAL BLOOD LOSS

The amount of blood loss at each menstruation has been measured in several population studies such as that undertaken by Hallberg *et al* in the 1960s in Gothenberg in Sweden in women aged 15 years to 50 years.[5] They found that overall menstrual blood loss (MBL) shows a skewed distribution with the mean of about 43 mL. Furthermore, in teenagers menstrual blood loss is about 1–2 mL less than that found in women aged 20–45 years. MBL is considered excessive if it is greater than 80 mL: without treatment such a loss leads to iron deficiency, anemia, and constitutes objective menorrhagia. Ninety percent of blood is lost within the first 3 days of menstruation fitting in with patients' description of a tap being turned on and off. Menstrual blood loss may vary between ethnic groups and in Chinese women the mean is 56 mL.[6]

CYCLE LENGTH AND DURATION OF MENSTRUATION

Menstrual cycle length is the number of days from the start of one menstrual bleeding period to the start of the next. Duration of bleeding is the number of days from the start of menstrual bleeding until the start of the next bleed-free interval. There is a large degree of variability in cycle length that is compatible with good health. The so-called "ideal" 28-day cycle is not experienced by a majority of women. Cycle length varies across the reproductive life span with greatest variation immediately after the menarche and shortly before menopause. Both periods are characterized by an increased frequency of both very long and very short cycles as well as by an increased range of cycle lengths. For example, Treloar *et al*.[7] found that during the first year, menstruation cycle lengths range from 18 to 83 days with a median of 29 days. By the fifth year post menarche the median is 28 days and the range is 22–40 days. The average duration of menstruation is 4–6 days in a series of studies undertaken throughout the world with Hong Kong women bleeding the longest[8–10] (TABLE 1).

MENSTRUAL PAIN

Menstrual pain or dysmenorrhea is common and may limit school activities.[11,12] For example, a study 388 female students in Australia found that the reported prevalence of dysmenorrhea was 80%; 53% of those girls with dysmenorrhea reported that it limited their activities. In particular, 37% said that dysmenorrhea affected their school activities.[11] In the United States a study

TABLE 1. Regional variation in duration of menstruation

Study	Country	Mean duration (days)
WHO, 1981	Mexico	4.0
	India	4.4
	Egypt	4.4
	Yugoslavia	4.8
	UK	5.3
Belsey et al., 1988	Mexico	4.0
	Europe	5.9
WHO, 1986	Hong Kong	6.0

of 88 female high school adolescents found a prevalence of dysmenorrhea in 91%.[12]

ABSENCE OF MENSTRUATION

Premature menopause is not uncommon even in young girls. Overall, premature ovarian failure (POF) is responsible for 4–18% of cases of secondary amenorrhea and 10–28% of primary amenorrhea. It is estimated to affect 0.1% of women under 30 years of age.[13]

PRIMARY POF

Primary POF can present as primary or secondary amenorrhea. In the great majority of cases, no cause can be found. Although these women generally are considered to be infertile, spontaneous ovarian activity may occur with the resulting implications of fertility and pregnancy. Traditional texts have concentrated on describing ovarian failure as being associated with a deficient number of primordial follicles from the onset of menarche, accelerated follicle atresia, or follicles resistant to stimulation by gonadotrophins. In the absence of a noninvasive test to differentiate between follicular depletion or dysfunction, the only alternative is laparoscopic ovarian biopsy. The validity of single biopsies has been questioned, with pregnancies occurring despite histological lack of follicles in the biopsy material.[14] The causes of primary POF are listed in TABLE 2.

Chromosome Abnormalities

The requirement for two intact X chromosomes for normal follicular development was determined in the 1960s.[14] A critical region on the X chromosome (POF1), which ranges from Xq13 to Xq26, relates to normal ovarian function

TABLE 2. Causes of primary ovarian failure in young girls

Primary
   Chromosome abnormalities
   Follicle-stimulating hormone receptor gene polymorphism and inhibin B mutation
   Enzyme deficiencies
   Autoimmune disease
Secondary
   Chemotherapy and radiotherapy
   Bilateral oophorectomy
   Infection

that has been identified, as has a second gene of paternal origin (POF2), which is located at Xq13.3–q21.1. Idiopathic POF can be familial or sporadic, and the familial pattern of inheritance is compatible with X-linked with incomplete penetrance or an autosomal dominant mode of inheritance. In Turner syndrome, complete absence of one X chromosome (45XO) results in ovarian dysgenesis and primary ovarian failure. Familial POF has been linked with fragile X permutations.[15] Fragile X mutations occur at least 10 times more often in women with POF than the general population. Women with Down's syndrome (Trisomy 21) also have an early menopause.[16] The BEPS syndrome is a rare autosomal dominant condition that leads to congenital abnormalities of the eye, including blepharophimosis, ptosis, and epicanthus inversis.[17] In BEPS I, eyelid malformation cosegregates with POF and has been mapped to chromosome 3q.17.

Follicle-Stimulating Hormone Receptor Gene Polymorphism and Inhibin B Mutation

Resistance to the action of gonadotrophins can lead to the clinical features of POF, and this has been shown in a cohort of Finnish families.[18] This is a very rare cause. In addition, a mutation in the inhibin gene that has a frequency 10-fold higher than in control patients (7% vs. 0.7%) has been identified.[19]

Enzyme Deficiencies

A number of enzyme deficiencies have been found to be associated with an increased risk of POF.[13] The most common of these is the autosomal recessive condition of galactosemia in which there is a deficiency in the enzyme galactose-1-phosphate uridyltransferase. Accumulation of galactose results in damage to the liver, eyes, and kidneys. The risk of POF has been found to be as high as 81% in affected females and the cause seems to be a galactose-induced reduction in total germ–cell development during oogenesis. Other proposed mechanisms include accelerated follicular atresia and biologically inactive isoforms of follicle-stimulating hormone (FSH). Other enzyme abnormalities associated with POF include deficiencies of 17-α-hydroxylase, 17–20 desmolase, and cholesterol desmolase. Deficiency of 17-α-hydroxylase can prevent estradiol synthesis, which leads to primary amenorrhea and elevated levels of gonadotrophins, even though developing follicles are present. Patients with a deficiency of cholesterol desmolase are not able to produce biologically active steroids and rarely survive to adulthood.

Autoimmune Disease

POF frequently is associated with autoimmune disorders, particularly hypothyroidism (25%), Addison's disease (3%), and diabetes mellitus (2.5%).[20] Other coexisting conditions may include Crohn's disease, vitiligo, pernicious anemia, systemic lupus erythematosus, or rheumatoid arthritis. Addison's disease may be present as part of a polyglandular failure syndrome. The type I syndrome, which is associated with adrenal failure, hypoparathyroidism, and chronic mucocutaneous candidiasis, and mainly occurs in children, is also associated with POF. The type II syndrome may present much later with hypothyroidism and is less consistently associated with POF.

The prevalence of antibodies directed against the ovary has been the subject of significant research. Circulating antiovarian antibodies have been found in 10–69% of women with POF but also in a significant number of controls. Antigonadotrophin receptor antibodies have been isolated, but their significance remains unclear. Antibodies directed against steroid-producing cells have proved most promising in terms of predicting which patients may develop ovarian failure as part of the polyglandular syndrome; however, these women constitute a minority of those with POF.

SECONDARY POF

Secondary POF is becoming more important as survival after the treatment of childhood malignancy continues to improve. The development of techniques to conserve ovarian tissue or oocytes before therapy is instigated, however, should help with maintenance of fertility.[21]

The likelihood of ovarian failure after chemotherapy or radiotherapy depends on the agent used, dosage levels, interval between treatments and, particularly, the age of the patient, which probably reflects the age-related progressive natural decline in the oocyte pool.[13,22,23] The prepubertal ovary is relatively resistant to the effects of chemotherapeutic alkylating agents. Attempts to suppress the ovarian activity of women of reproductive age with oral contraceptives or gonadotrophin hormone-releasing analogues to mimic this protection have produced conflicting results.

Radiation-induced ovarian failure usually results in sterility when the total dose exceeds 6 Gy.[23] As with chemotherapy, however, prepubertal girls are more resistant to irradiation. Normal menstruation after treatment does not necessarily mean the ovaries are unaffected and premature menopause can occur, resulting in a shorter reproductive span. Surgical transposition of the ovaries outside of the direct field of treatment has been described.[21] A successful term pregnancy also depends on a normal uterine environment that is not only receptive to implantation but also able to accommodate normal growth of the fetus. The degree of damage to the uterus depends on the total dose of radiation and the site of irradiation.[23] The prepubertal uterus is more vulnerable to the effects of pelvic irradiation, with doses of radiation of 14–30 Gy likely to result in uterine dysfunction. High-dose pelvic radiotherapy in young women will have long-term effects on the uterine vasculature and development. Adverse pregnancy outcomes have been described for women treated with total body irradiation and include an increased risk of early pregnancy loss, preterm birth, and delivery of infants with low or very low birth weights. An excess risk of infants of low birth weight and preterm birth also exists among mothers who received abdominal irradiation for Wilms' tumor in childhood. Surgical oophorectomy is extremely rare in young girls.

Tuberculosis and mumps are infections that have been implicated most commonly in POF.[13] The increasing incidence of tuberculosis and the emergence of multidrug-resistant strains of bacilli is of concern. In most cases, normal ovarian function returns after infection with mumps. Malaria, varicella, and shigella infections have also been implicated in POF.

CONSEQUENCES OF POF

Young girls with untreated premature menopause are at increased risk of developing osteoporosis and cardiovascular disease but at lower risk of breast malignancy.[13,24] Mean life expectancy in women with menopause before the age of 40 years is 2.0 years shorter than that in women with menopause after the age of 55 years.[25] Premature menopause can lead to reduced peak bone mass.[26] The increased risk of coronary heart disease has been noted especially in smokers.[27,28]

MANAGEMENT

Girls and their parents must be provided with adequate information. Young girls may find it a difficult diagnosis to accept, especially if they wish to have children. They may also feel isolated from their peers and prematurely aged. National and international self-support groups for POF exist and these provide helpful psychological support. The possibility that ovulation may occur again, often intermittently, and cyclical menstrual bleeding or even pregnancy can result should be discussed.

Estrogen replacement therapy is the mainstay of treatment for young women with POF and is recommended until the average age of natural menopause. This view is endorsed by regulatory bodies and menopause societies.[29] No evidence shows that estrogen replacement increases the risk of breast cancer to a level greater than that found in normally menstruating women. Hormone replacement therapy (HRT) or the combined estrogen and progestogen contraceptive pill may be used. No clinical trial evidence attests the efficacy or safety of the use of non-estrogen-based treatments such as bisphosphonates, strontium ranelate, or raloxifene, in these women.[29]

A commonly adopted form of treatment in young girls is the combined oral contraceptive pill. The latter has the psychological benefit of being a treatment used by many of the patient's peer group. There is a paucity of controlled trial data on how to base treatment decisions.[13] The only direct comparison of ethinylestradiol and conjugated equine estrogen is a study of 17 women with Turner syndrome.[30] In this short study, no difference was seen between the two estrogens with respect to effect on the endometrium, hyperinsulinemia, or lipid profile. Ethinylestradiol had a more potent effect on markers of bone turnover and suppression of gonadotrophins.

CONCLUSION

Menstruation is an integral part of a woman's experience throughout her reproductive life. The average age of the menarche in industrialized countries is 13 years. In young girls there is a wide variation in menstrual cycle length. A major concern in girls with oligomenorrhea or amenorrhea is POF, especially if they have been treated for cancer.

REFERENCES

1. SCOMMEGNA, A. & W.P. DMOWSKI. 1973. Dysfunctional uterine bleeding. Clin. Obstet. Gynecol. **16:** 221–254.
2. GLUCKMAN, P.D. & M.A. HANSON. 2006. Evolution, development and timing of puberty. Trends Endocrinol. Metab. **17:** 7–12.
3. PARENT, A-S. *et al.* 2003. The timing of normal puberty and the age limits of sexual precocity: variations around the world, secular trends, and changes after migration. Endocr. Rev. 24: 668–693.
4. HARLOW, S. 1995. "What we do and do not know about the menstrual cycle; or, questions scientists could be asking," Robert H. Ebert Program on Critical Issues in Reproductive Health Publication Series. New York: Population Council. http://www.popcouncil.org/pdfs/ebert/MenstrualPaper.pdf accessed 26 April 2006.

5. HALLBERG, L. *et al.* 1966. Menstrual blood loss—a population study. Variation at different ages and attempts to define normality. Acta Obstet. Gynecol. Scand. **45:** 320–351.

6. JI, L.L.Y. *et al.* 1991. Menstrual blood loss in healthy Chinese women. Contraception **23:** 591–601.

7. TRELOAR, A.E. *et al.* 1967. Variation of the human menstrual cycle through reproductive life. Int. J. Fertil. **12:** 77–126.

8. WORLD HEALTH ORGANIZATION TASK FORCE ON PSYCHOSOCIAL RESEARCH IN FAMILY PLANNING, SPECIAL PROGRAMME OF RESEARCH, DEVELOPMENT AND RESEARCH TRAINING IN HUMAN REPRODUCTION. 1981. Women's bleeding patterns: ability to recall and predict menstrual events. Studies in Family Planning. **12:** 17–27.

9. WORLD HEALTH ORGANIZATION TASK FORCE ON ADOLESCENT REPRODUCTIVE HEALTH. 1986. World Health Organization Multicenter Study on menstrual and ovulatory patterns in adolescent girls. J. Adolesc. Health Care **7:** 236–244.

10. BELSEY, E.M. & S. PEREGOUDOV. 1988. Determinants of menstrual bleeding patterns among women using natural and hormonal methods of contraception. I. Regional variations. Contraception **38:** 227–242.

11. HILLEN, T.I. *et al.* 1999. Primary dysmenorrhea in young Western Australian women: prevalence, impact, and knowledge of treatment. J. Adolesc. Health **25:** 40–45.

12. WILSON, C.A. & W.R. KEYE, JR. 1989. A survey of adolescent dysmenorrhea and premenstrual symptom frequency. A model program for prevention, detection, and treatment. J. Adolesc. Health Care **10:** 317–322.

13. TUCKER, D. 2005. Premature ovarian failure. *In* The Abnormal Menstrual Cycle. M. Rees, S. Hope & V. Ravnikar, Eds.: 111–122. Taylor and Francis. Abingdon, UK.

14. NELSON, L.M., S.N. COVINGTON & R.W. REBAR. 2005. An update: spontaneous premature ovarian failure is not an early menopause. Fertil. Steril. **83:** 1327–1332.

15. CONWAY, G.S. *et al.* 1998. Fragile X permutation screening in women with premature ovarian failure. Hum. Reprod. **13:** 1184–1187.

16. SALAMANCA-GOMEZ, F., L. BUENTELLO & F. SALAMANCA-BUENTELLO. 2001. Reduced ovarian complement, premature ovarian failure, and Down syndrome. Am. J. Med. Genet. **99:** 168–169.

17. AMATI, P. *et al.* 1996. A gene for premature ovarian failure associated with eyelid malformation maps to chromosome 3q22-q23. Am. J. Hum. Gen. **58:** 1089–1092.

18. AITTOMAKI, K. *et al.* 1996. Mutation in the follicle-stimulating hormone receptor gene causes hereditary hypergonadotrophic ovarian failure. Cell **82:** 959–968.

19. SHELLING, A.N. *et al.* 2000. Inhibin: a candidate gene for premature ovarian failure. Hum. Reprod. **15:** 2644–2649.

20. HOEK, A., J. SCHOEMAKER & H.A. DREXHAGE. 1997. Premature ovarian failure and ovarian autoimmunity. Endocr. Rev. **18:** 107–134.

21. BEERENDONK, C.C. & D.D. BRAAT. 2005. Present and future options for the preservation of fertility in female adolescents with cancer. Endocr. Dev. **8:** 166–175.

22. HOWELL, S. & S. SHALET. 1998. Gonadal damage from chemotherapy and radiotherapy. Endocrinol. Metab. Clin. North Am. **27:** 927–943.

23. WALLACE, W.H. *et al.* 2005. Predicting age of ovarian failure after radiation to a field that includes the ovaries. Int. J. Radiat. Oncol. Biol. Phys. **62:** 738–744.

24. TITUS-ERNSTOFF, L. *et al.* 1998. Menstrual factors in relation to breast cancer risk. Cancer Epidemiol. Biomarkers Prev. **7:** 783–789.

25. OSSEWAARDE, M.E. *et al*. 2005. Age at menopause, cause-specific mortality and total life expectancy. Epidemiology **16:** 556–562.

26. REES, M. & D.W. PURDIE, Eds. 2006. Management of the Menopause. Royal Society of Medicine Press. London, UK.

27. HU, F.B. *et al*. 1999. Age at natural menopause and risk of cardiovascular disease. Arch Intern. Med. **159:** 1061–1066.

28. JACOBSEN, B.K., S.F. KNUTSEN & G.E. FRASER. 1999. Age at natural menopause and total mortality and mortality from ischemic heart disease: the Adventist Health Study. J. Clin. Epidemiol. **52:** 303–307.

29. PITKIN, J. *et al*. & BRITISH MENOPAUSE SOCIETY COUNCIL. 2005. Managing the menopause: British Menopause Society Council consensus statement on hormone replacement therapy. J. Br. Menopause Soc. **11:** 152–156.

30. GUTTMAN, H. *et al*. 2001. Choosing an oestrogen replacement therapy in young adult women with Turner syndrome. Clin. Endocrinol. **54:** 159–164.

A Behind-the-Scenes Look at the Safety Assessment of Feminine Hygiene Pads

MIRANDA A. FARAGE

The Procter and Gamble Company, Feminine & Family Care Clinical Sciences, Cincinnati, Ohio, USA

ABSTRACT: Forms of menstrual protection have evolved with time. Today's disposable feminine hygiene products, notably sanitary pads, include a wide range of designs and features to meet women's needs for reliable, discreet, and comfortable protection. Manufacturers support substantive research and testing programs to ensure the safety of these products. The premarket safety assessment of feminine hygiene pads is a systematic, stepwise process that includes toxicological evaluation of the raw materials, the conduct of prospective, controlled clinical trials to assess product safety-in-use, and, in some cases, independent scientific review. A broad clinical database, developed over the past 20 years, substantiates that modern, feminine hygiene pads are not associated with significant gynecological, dermatological, or microbiological effects. Postmarket surveillance provides reassurance that the products are acceptable to consumers worldwide.

KEYWORDS: sanitary pads; safety assurance; toxicological testing; skin patch tests; quantitative risk assessment; prospective clinical trials; postmarket surveillance

BRIEF HISTORY OF FEMININE HYGIENE PRODUCTS

Menstruation necessitates some form of sanitary protection; to meet this need, various approaches have been devised over time. Egyptian records dating back to the 15th century BCE reveal that the wealthy women employed internal plugs of wool or soft papyrus while poorer women used softened aquatic grasses. In various regions of the world, the indigenous cultures adapted mosses, flax, seaweed, and various native plant fibers to this purpose.[1-3] The advent of textiles made it possible to wash and reuse external protection made of cloth, an option that remains popular in the developing world for reasons of economy, culture, and tradition.

Address for correspondence: Dr. Miranda A. Farage, The Procter and Gamble Company, Winton Hill Technical Center, 6110 Center Hill Road Box 136, Cincinnati, OH 45224, USA. Voice: 513-634-5594; fax: 513-634-7364.

e-mail: farage.m@pg.com

Ann. N.Y. Acad. Sci. 1092: 66–77 (2006). © 2006 New York Academy of Sciences.
doi: 10.1196/annals.1365.006

1896	First commercial disposable sanitary pad, developed by Johnson & Johnson (USA) – Lister®
1921	First commercially successful, disposable sanitary pad in the USA, marketed by Kimberly-Clark Corporation – Kotex®
1926	First disposable sanitary pad introduced in Germany, by Vereinigten Papierwercke – Camelia®
1936	Disposable tampons with applicators commercialized in the USA, by the Tambrands Company[a] – Tampax®
1950	Disposable digitally-inserted tampons, commercialized in Germany by Johnson & Johnson – o.b.®
1970s	Sanitary pads with panty-fastening adhesive, introduced in the USA by Johnson & Johnson – Stayfree Maxipads®
1970s	Mini pads and panty liners commercialized in North America and Europe by several manufacturers, e.g., Kimberly-Clark – Carefree®
1983	Sanitary pads with perforated film topsheets, introduced in the USA by Procter & Gamble – Always with Dri-weave®
1986	Sanitary pads with side panty-shields, introduced in the USA and Europe by Procter & Gamble – Always with Wings®
1989	Ultra-thin superabsorbent menstrual pads, introduced in Japan by Procter & Gamble – Whisper Ultra®
early 1990s	Thick menstrual pads with a concave conformation induced by side-elastics, commercialized[b] in the USA by Kimberly-Clark Corporation – Kotex Natural Curves®
late 1990s	Small, disposable interlabial pad for light flow or tampon backup, commercialized in the USA by A-Fem Medical Corporation - InSync Miniform®
late 1990s	Disposable intravaginal menses collection cups, commercialized in North America by Ultra-Fem, Inc – INSTEAD Soft cups®
2001	Cloth-like perforated film topsheets introduced in Europe by Procter & Gamble – Always®

FIGURE 1. Milestones in the history of modern feminine hygiene products.
[a]Tambrands is now a part of the Procter and Gamble Co.
[b]Design no longer marketed

FIGURE 1 describes the development of modern disposable sanitary protection from the 1800s to the present day. Cultural acceptance of disposable pads and tampons took considerable time. Although invented in 1896, disposable pads were not successfully commercialized until 1921, and two more decades passed before such products supplanted the use of cloth in Western industrialized countries.[1] Tampons were controversial for almost three decades after commercial introduction due to concerns about a possible impact on virginity and sexuality and the perceived potential for sepsis. Tampons gained broader acceptance during World War II because they provided women more freedom to participate actively in the workplace.

The safety of modern sanitary pads and tampons is supported by substantive historical and ongoing research programs undertaken by major manufacturers.

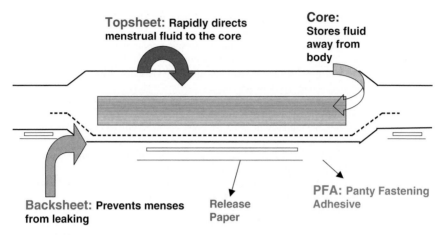

FIGURE 2. Cross-section and description of a sanitary pad.

The following discussion will focus on the design and safety assurance of external sanitary pads.

SANITARY PAD DESIGNS

FIGURE 2 illustrates the basic design of a sanitary pad

1. The surface layer (topsheet) acquires fluid and rapidly distributes it to the absorbent core.
2. The core stores fluid away from the body.
3. The moisture-impervious back layer (backsheet) prevents fluid leakage.
4. A panty-fastening adhesive (PFA) allows for attachment to the undergarment. The adhesive is covered by a removable release paper until use.

Sanitary pads have evolved from standard thick, belted products to a wide variety of designs tailored to different needs (FIG. 3). Innovative features introduced since the 1970s include: (a) PFA, which eliminated the need for belts and pins; (b) perforated film topsheets, which keep the pad surface clean and dry; (c) side panty-shields that minimize soiling; (d) pads with ultra-thin (3 mm) superabsorbent cores designed to be as effective but more comfortable and discreet than thick (20 mm) products; (e) variations in pad shape, width, and length to accommodate different body frames and flow levels (including day and nighttime use); (f) smaller panty liners for light protection with shapes and colors tailored to undergarment fashion; (g) odor-absorbing technologies; and (h) next-generation "breathable" materials to enhance comfort.

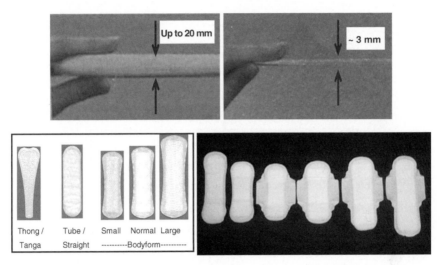

FIGURE 3. Sanitary pad designs and features. Adapted with permission from Farage et al.[20]

THE SAFETY ASSURANCE OF SANITARY PADS

Because sanitary pads are considered ordinary consumer products to be disposed of after use, the average person may not be aware that the major manufacturers implement rigorous research programs to ensure product safety. For perspective, The Procter & Gamble Company employs more than 24 personnel, including more than 15 PhD research scientists, responsible for product safety and regulatory compliance for the feminine hygiene category of products and spends around U.S. $0.5 million per year on safety-related pad research and testing. Our historical database includes more than 200 clinical trials on sanitary pads alone (published and unpublished data). This may seem like overkill for products that are typically considered inert; yet, we consider our approach essential to ensure that our products are safe for their intended use wherever in the world they are sold. Our toxicological and clinical research programs give us a high level of confidence that a practical assurance of safety has been built into every new product. The research also provides reliable scientific data to address health or safety questions that may arise.

FIGURE 4 illustrates a four-step, systematic approach to the safety assessment of sanitary pads. The four steps are

1. raw material safety assessment;
2. clinical evaluation of safety during use;
3. premarket independent review; and
4. postmarket surveillance.

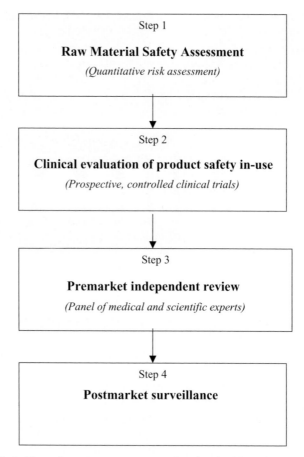

FIGURE 4. The safety assurance process. Reprinted with permission from Farage et al.[20]

The first three steps provide a thorough investigation of safety before commercial introduction; the final step monitors safety after the product has been commercialized.

Raw Material Safety Assessment

Step 1 involves an assessment of the potential toxicological effects of each raw material used in the product. Most sanitary pad components have well-established toxicological profiles and a long history of safe use. Nevertheless, any changes in the characteristics of the raw materials, the levels, or the formulation to be incorporated are scrutinized to ensure that there will not be an adverse impact on safety under anticipated conditions of use.

The most relevant toxicological and clinical endpoints for this product category are acute or cumulative skin irritation, the induction of delayed contact hypersensitivity, and the potential for acute or subchronic systemic effects. Sources of toxicological information include the medical and scientific literature, safety reviews conducted by government or trade organizations, and the results of historical testing of the individual ingredients or structurally related compounds. Once the available ingredient information has been analyzed, additional toxicological testing may be conducted if needed to address data gaps. Most materials used in sanitary products have a well-established toxicological profile and do not require substantial new testing.

The concentration of each material that can be used safely in the product is determined by conducting a quantitative risk assessment. This scientific paradigm, detailed elsewhere, is used to assess health risks of chemicals that display dose-dependent effects.[4,5] In brief, a quantitative estimate of exposure to the raw material components arising from product use is compared to a previously established, safe, benchmark dose. This benchmark dose, also known as the Reference Value,[6] is derived from historical toxicological or clinical data on relevant routes of exposure and incorporates a significant margin of safety (10- to 1,000-fold) to account for any limitations related to extrapolating from experimental results. The quantitative exposure estimate is based on chemical analysis of raw material components and an understanding of consumer habits and practices. A comparison of consumer exposure to the benchmark Reference Value allows systematic decisions to be made about the levels of raw materials that can safely be incorporated into the product. Consumer exposures to product ingredients are usually substantially lower than the safe Reference Value.

Additional testing may be performed beyond the quantitative risk assessment to further enhance the safety assessment. FIGURE 5 shows the result of a 21-day cumulative irritation patch test[7] in human subjects designed to evaluate skin irritation after prolonged exposure to a sanitary pad topsheet. The topsheet was compared to standard irritant (surfactant, Sodium Lauryl Sulfate at 0.05%) and nonirritant (physiologic saline) controls. It was found to be comparable to the nonirritant control under the test conditions, demonstrating the skin mildness of this component.

Because vulvar tissue may be more permeable than keratinized skin,[8,9] we use a more conservative, quantitative risk assessment process to assess the risk of induction of contact sensitization associated with topical vulvar exposures.[10] Moreover, with this in mind, we have developed a modified human repeat insult patch test protocol for evaluating contact sensitization potential of materials or products that contact the vulva.[11] For ethical reasons, this test is not used for hazard assessment but rather to substantiate the risk assessment conclusion that the potential for inducing sensitization is negligible.

Test protocols have also been developed to assess potential chemical irritation combined with mechanical irritation from physical contact (friction,

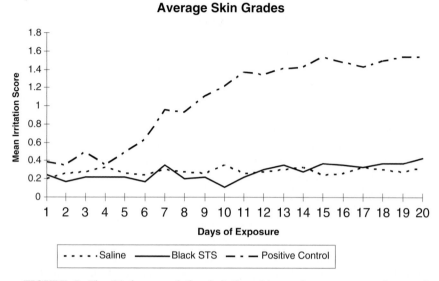

FIGURE 5. The 21-day cumulative irritation skin patch test on a sanitary pad topsheet.

chaffing, occlusion).[12,13] FIGURE 6 compares skin irritation resulting from application of two products to the popliteal fossae under a sports bandage for five consecutive days ("behind-the-knee" protocol). This test method, which employs occlusive contact in the context of physical motion, demonstrated that the potential for chemical and mechanical irritation associated with a novel product under the test conditions was comparable to the levels induced by a commercial product with a history of acceptable use in the marketplace.

Clinical Evaluation of Safety during Use

The safety of significant product innovations, such as the introduction of unique raw materials or the substantial modification of a product design, are assessed by conducting prospective, randomized trials under practical or exaggerated conditions of use. The clinical trials are conducted according to the International Committee on Harmonization/Good Clinical Practice (ICH/GCP) guidelines and approved by the Institutional Review Board or ethical committee of the pertinent institution. Participation in a prospective trial is voluntary with informed consent.

Several of our protocols were developed with the input of academic and medical experts in obstetrics and gynecology, dermatology, and microbiology. Regional consumer habits and practices influenced each protocol design to ensure that representative conditions of use are employed.

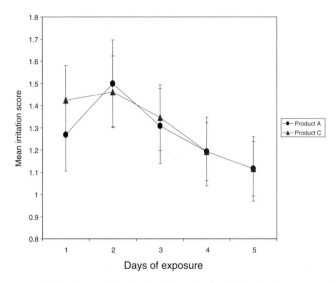

FIGURE 6. Evaluation of chemical and mechanical irritation by application to the popliteal fossa ("behind-the-knee" test).

The clinical trials are examiner-blind. Independent academic physicians in obstetrics and gynecology or dermatology serve as study investigators. Depending on the study objectives, gynecological, dermatological, and/or microbiological outcome measures may be included (FIG. 7).[14–17] For example, standardized objective, numerical scales are used to assess skin irritation and the condition of the external genitalia;[7,18] analysis of the isolation frequencies and cell densities of selected vulvo-vaginal microbes is used currently to determine microbiological effects;[17] moreover, our scientists are developing state-of-the-art, noncultivation-based techniques to refine our ability to detect such flora.[19] Group sizes are chosen to achieve at least 80% statistical power and less than a 5% risk of statistical differences occurring by chance alone. A review of 12 such trials performed in North America and Europe over the last 20 years has been published in the peer-reviewed literature.[20] When needed, our clinical studies are conducted at different clinical sites around the world to ensure we take into consideration different geographies' needs. This takes into consideration the regional consumer habits' and practices' differences to ensure that conditions of use are representative of target populations. Our most recent example study was performed in Greece, which addresses and demonstrates such a need.[21]

Premarket Independent Review

Before a major product innovation is introduced into the marketplace, a panel of independent experts may be invited to assist in study design and to critically review the results of the safety assurance program. Over the past two decades, we have relied extensively on the input of experts who are internationally renowned in their respective disciplines. Representatives from various geographic regions may participate. The premarket independent review provides an added level of confidence that the most up-to-date information and best scientific judgment are reflected in the study designs and interpretation. Moreover, the process is a source of objective feedback to confirm that all critical variables have been considered and satisfactorily addressed prior to marketing.

Postmarket Surveillance

Many manufacturers employ postmarket surveillance to monitor consumers' experience and satisfaction. At our company, a global team is solely responsible to continually monitor and analyze health-related questions and comments from around the globe. Consumers provide feedback by telephone (toll free), by letter, and increasingly, through manufacturer's web sites. This information is found on each package in each region of the world. The record of many years of postmarket surveillance serves as a reference for the types and levels of comments that can be expected for different product categories. Ongoing surveillance also serves as an alert system for unanticipated issues or unusual trends.

⤶ **Dermatological assessments**
- Skin irritation (erythema, edema, and vesicular or papular eruptions)
- Skin condition (normal, fissured, scaly, increased moisture, macerated)
- Diagnostic patch tests (induction of allergic contact hypersensitivity)

⤶ **Gynecological evaluation**
- Vaginal discharge (odor, appearance, consistency)
- Vaginal pH
- Clinical diagnosis of dermatitis, dermatoses, or infection (if present)
- Pap smear

⤶ **Vaginal and vulvar microbiology**
- Microbial isolation frequencies (representative endogenous flora and selected pathogens)
- Semi-quantitative or quantitative microbial cell densities (cfu/mL vaginal fluid or cfu/cm2 skin)[a]

⤶ **Objective measurements (investigative)**
- Skin barrier function/wetness (trans-epidermal water loss and other instruments)
- Pad loading (weight of absorbed fluid)

---

[a] More robust cultivation independent methods are under development[19]

FIGURE 7. Typical outcome measures in prospective clinical trials of sanitary pads. Reprinted with permission from Farage *et al.*[20]

Every health-related comment is either acted upon by the monitoring team or referred to scientists in our safety assurance organization for further follow-up. Alleged irritant or allergic effects are the most common type of health-related comment for external feminine hygiene products. With the help of the consumer, every effort is made to determine the cause of her problem and, if needed, to offer medical follow-up at manufacturer's expense. For a complaint of irritation or allergy, medical follow-up includes evaluation by an independent, board-certified dermatologist near her place of residence, with diagnostic patch-testing if contact sensitization is suspected. However, product-related adverse events are very rare: IKW German statistics for the category of absorbent hygiene products from 1997 to 1999 reveal not a single medically confirmed case of allergic contact dermatitis; the incidence of low-grade skin irritation was less than 1 case in 9 million products sold.[22] Incidents are most often found to be unrelated to product use, not reproducible, or secondary to another problem such as a preexisting dermatitis, dermatosis, or infection. Consumers usually find that they are able to use the product again without incident once the primary cause of their problem has been determined and addressed.

Our company's brands of feminine hygiene products are sold in most countries around the world: approximately 115 million women worldwide rely on them for feminine protection. While no sanitary product widely used in the marketplace can claim to be devoid of minor complaints of irritation or discomfort, the widespread use and consumer acceptance of these modern products is testimony to the rigor of the safety assurance process described herein.

CONCLUSION

Women who choose disposable sanitary pads for menstrual protection expect to be confident of their safety and effectiveness. We have described a systematic, stepwise approach for evaluating the safety of feminine hygiene pads that includes (i) raw material safety assessments based on quantitative risk assessment principles; (ii) the evaluation of safety-in-use by means of prospective, randomized clinical trials; (iii) independent review of significant innovations by independent experts; and (iv) postmarket surveillance. Our rigorous "behind-the-scenes" research programs offer a high level of confidence that a practical assurance of safety has been built into each product from the start. More than 20 years of toxicological and clinical research on two continents have produced a substantial, objective, reliable database to support the safety of modern feminine hygiene pads.

ACKNOWLEDGMENTS

The author is grateful to Deborah Hutchins, of Hutchins and Associates, LLC (Cincinnati, OH) for her technical input.

REFERENCES

1. FRIEDMAN, N. 1981. "Invented by a doctor": a medical and social history of tampons. *In* Everything You Must Know About Tampons. Berkley Publishing Group. New York, NY.
2. MCCALMAN, I. 1968. Menstrual practices of the Amandebele people in the Essexvale area. Cent. Afr. J. Med. **14:** 111.
3. THORNTON, M.J. 1943. Use of vaginal tampons for absorption of menstrual discharges. Am. J. Obstet. Gynecol. **46:** 259.
4. FELTER, S.P., C.A. RYAN, D.A. BASKETTER, *et al.* 2003. Application of the risk assessment paradigm to the induction of allergic contact dermatitis. Regul. Toxicol. Pharmacol. **37:** 1–10.
5. HOPPER, L.D. & F.W. OEHME. 1989. Chemical risk assessment: a review. Vet. Hum. Toxicol. **31:** 543–554.
6. U.S. Environmental Protection Agency. Integrated Risk Information System (IRIS). Glossary of IRIS terms. Revised September 2003, July 2005. Available at http://www.epa.gov/iris/gloss8.htm#r. Accessed August 31, 2005.
7. PHILLIPS, L., II, M. STEINBERG, H.I. MAIBACH, *et al.* 1972. A comparison of rabbit and human skin response to certain irritants. Toxicol. Appl. Pharmacol. **21:** 369–382.
8. LESCH, C.A., C.A. SQUIER, A. CRUCHLEY, *et al.* 1989. The permeability of human oral mucosa and skin to water. J. Dent. Res. **68:** 1345–1349.
9. van der Bijl, P., I.O. THOMPSON & C.A. SQUIER. 1997. Comparative permeability of human vaginal and buccal mucosa to water. Eur. J. Oral Sci. **105:** 571–575.
10. FARAGE, M.A., D.L. BJERKE, C. MAHONY, *et al.* 2003. Quantitative risk assessment for the induction of allergic contact dermatitis: uncertainty factors for mucosal exposures. Contact Dermatitis **49:** 140–147.
11. FARAGE, M.A., D.L. BJERKE, C. MAHONY, *et al.* 2003. A modified human repeat insult patch test for extended mucosal tissue exposure. Contact Dermatitis **49:** 214–215.
12. FARAGE, M.A., S. MEYER & D. WALTER. 2004. Development of a sensitive test method to evaluate mechanical irritation potential on mucosal skin. Skin Res. Technol. **10:** 85–95.
13. FARAGE, M.A., D.A. GILPIN, N.A. ENANE, *et al.* 2001. Development of a new test for mechanical irritation: behind the knee as a test site. Skin Res. Technol. **7:** 193–203.
14. HANKE-BAIER, P., J. JOHANNIGMANN, R.J. LEVIN, *et al.* 1994. Evaluation of vaginal and perineal area during the use of external sanitary protection throughout the menstrual cycle. Acta Obstet. Gynecol. Scand. **73:** 486–491.
15. VOSS, A., C. WALLRAUCH-SCHWARZ, D. MILATOVIC, *et al.* 1993. Quantitative study of vaginal flora during the menstrual cycle. Geburtshilfe Frauenheilkd **53:** 543–546.
16. FARAGE, M.A., N.A. ENANE, S. BALDWIN, *et al.* 1997. A clinical method for testing the safety of catamenial pads. Gynecol. Obstet. Invest. **44:** 260–264.
17. FARAGE, M.A. *et al.* 1997. Labial and vaginal microbiology: effects of extended panty liner use. Infect. Dis. Obst. Gynecol. **5:** 252–258.
18. PATRICK, E. & H.I. MAIBACH. 1989. Dermatotoxicology. *In* Principles and Methods of Toxicology. A.W. Hayes, Ed.: 383–406. Raven Press. New York, NY.
19. ZHOU, X., S.J. BENT, M.G. SCHNEIDER, *et al.* 2004. Characterization of vaginal microbial communities in adult healthy women using cultivation-independent methods. Microbiology **150:** 2565–2573.

20. FARAGE, M.A., A. STADLER, P. ELSNER, *et al.* 2004. Safety evaluation of modern feminine hygiene pads: two decades of use. Female Patient **29:** 23–30.
21. FARAGE, M.A., A. KATSAROU, E. TSAGRONI, *et al.* 2005. Cutaneous and sensory effects of two sanitary pads with distinct surface materials: a randomized prospective trial. J. Toxicol. Cutaneous. Ocular. Toxicol. **24:** 227–241.
22. IKW (INDUSTRIEVERBAND FÜR KÖRPERPFLEGE UND WASCHMITTEL E.V.) 2001 Hygieneprodukte — unentbehrlich im täglichen Leben, 1. Auflage, S. 46, Frankfurt/Main.

Contraception in Adolescence

EFTHIMIOS DELIGEOROGLOU, PANAGIOTIS CHRISTOPOULOS, AND GEORGE CREATSAS

Division of Pediatric-Adolescent Gynecology and Reconstructive Surgery, 2nd Department of Obstetrics and Gynecology, University of Athens, Medical School, "Aretaieion" Hospital, Athens, Greece

ABSTRACT: Adolescents, due to the lack of knowledge, experience, and counseling, may confront serious social and health-related problems, such as out-of-wedlock pregnancies and sexually transmitted diseases (STDs). The age of the first sexual intercourse has declined recently. Unintended pregnancies often force adolescents into unwanted marriage or limit their opportunities to further education or employment while predisposing them to long-term welfare dependence. To be most effective, sex education programs should be developed through a process of collaboration between families, health care professionals, educators, government officials, and youth themselves. The contraceptive choices during adolescence are the male condom, the use of spermicides, combined oral contraceptives (COCs), the depomedroxyprogesterone acetate (DMPA), the female condom, the vaginal sponge, implants and patches, male hormonal contraception, and others. Issues of emergency contraception (EC) are also discussed.

KEYWORDS: contraception; adolescence

INTRODUCTION

Adolescents, due to the lack of knowledge, experience, and counseling, may confront serious social and health-related problems, such as out-of-wedlock pregnancies and/or sexually transmitted diseases (STDs). The age of the first sexual intercourse has declined recently. On the contrary, the percentage of American adolescents who are sexually active has increased significantly in recent years.[1] It is reported that 56% and 73% of girls and boys, respectively, have had sexual intercourse before the age of 18 years.[2] A report from the National Survey of Family Growth in the United States in 2002 estimates that about 47% of teenagers (4.7 million) had sexual intercourse at least once.[3]

Address for correspondence: Panagiotis Christopoulos, M.D., 1 Hariton street, Kifissia, 11528 Athens, Greece. Voice/fax: 2108074687.
e-mail: dr_christopoulos@yahoo.gr

Ann. N.Y. Acad. Sci. 1092: 78–90 (2006). © 2006 New York Academy of Sciences.
doi: 10.1196/annals.1365.007

Annually, approximately 75 million unwanted pregnancies occur worldwide, mainly because of nonuse of contraception. An estimated 19 million unsafe abortions occur worldwide each year, resulting in the deaths of about 70,000 women of all reproductive ages.[4] Unintended pregnancies often force adolescents into unwanted marriage or limit their opportunities to further education or employment while predisposing them to long-term welfare dependence. In developed countries, 7.5–10% of adolescent women get pregnant (27% worldwide).[5] Approximately 51% of adolescent pregnancies result in a live birth, 35% of them end with an abortion with several complications, while 14% end in miscarriage or stillbirth.[2,6] A total of 52% of adolescents use noneffective contraception.[2] Most U.S. teenage pregnancies are unintended, partly because of inconsistent or no use of contraception.[7] Although a general reduction of births was noticed in the United States, the frequency of pregnancy increased for the ages between 14–17 years old. Approximately 31% of adolescents used no contraception at first intercourse, mostly those who had just met their sexual partner.[8] Hopefully, according to a more recent report from the National Survey of Family Growth in the United States in 2002, teenagers showed increased rates in the use of contraceptives.[3] About three out of four teenagers used a method of contraception at their first intercourse. About 91% of males and 83% of females used a method at their most recent sex.[3]

In Sweden, the abortion rate among teenagers increased by 25% over the last years. Teenage abortion rates have gone up, from 17/1,000 in 1995 to 22.5/1,000 in 2001. Genital chlamydial infections have increased from 14,000 cases in 1994 to 22,263 cases in 2001, 60% occurring among young people, basically among teenagers.[9]

Efforts are made to increase contraceptive use among sexually active adolescents, and especially the condom, which protects from both pregnancy and STDs. Recent studies have found that allowing access to sexual knowledge or birth control in school-based clinics did not affect rates of sexual activity or intercourse at a younger age but did increase use of condoms.[10] The majority of parents believe sex education should include information on birth control methods, should be provided by the family, and supplemented by schools before students reach the seventh grade, and that receiving a regular newsletter regarding teenage sexual issues could be of great help in communication with their children.[11] To be most effective, sex education programs should be developed through a process of collaboration between families, health care professionals, educators, government officials, and youth themselves.

The contraceptive choices during adolescence are the male condom, the use of spermicides, combined oral contraceptives (COCs), the Depo-Medroxyprogesterone Acetate (DMPA), the female condom, the vaginal sponge, implants and patches, male hormonal contraception, and others. Matters of emergency contraception (EC) are also discussed.

THE MALE CONDOM

COCs should be consistently used in combination with the condom as a method providing complete protection against unwanted pregnancy as well as STDs. Unfortunately, adolescents' dual use of condoms and hormonal contraceptives is very low.[12] Although the incidence rate of pelvic inflammatory disease (PID) shows over 50% decrease in pill users, the incidence of chlamydial and mycoplasmal cervical infections is slightly increased. Unfortunately, the pill offers no protection against viral infections, such as HIV. It is estimated that in the United States, approximately 3 million adolescents acquire an STD each year including both bacterial (e.g., gonorrhea, chlamydia) and viral infections (e.g., herpes, HIV). The rate of STDs among adolescents is increasing. It is reported that 21% of the American adolescents have had more than four partners.[13]

Most male condoms are made of latex. Beginning in the 1990s, nonlatex male condoms made of polyurethane film or synthetic elastomers also became available for use as alternative male barrier methods. Although the nonlatex condoms are associated with higher rates of failure than latex condoms, they still provide an acceptable alternative for users with allergies, sensitivities, or preferences that might prevent the consistent use of latex condoms.[14] Natural condoms (made of lamb intestine) may be permeable to microorganisms.

Consistent condom use is reported by less than half of all sexually active adolescents.[15] A study, among all 18-year-old girls and boys in four cities in northern Sweden, found several male and female factors associated with noncondom use, where the usage of oral contraception was the strongest indicator for noncondom use.[16] Breakage and slippage rates of the male condom have each been estimated to be less than 2%, although rates vary among the various studies and according to the user's experience.[17] Condom failure is about 10 times higher among teenagers as compared to adults.[18] It means that condoms cannot be 100% effective, with a theoretical annual failure rate around 2%. Actual failure rates range from 5% to 20%.[19] Goldman et al.[20] reported first year failure rates as low as 2–4% in adolescents. The literature findings show that condom use appears to decrease but does not fully eliminate the rate of transmission of most STDs.

SPERMICIDE

Spermicides contain an active ingredient (most commonly nonoxynol-9) and a formulation used to disperse the product, such as foam or vaginal suppository. A review examined all known randomized controlled trials of a spermicide used alone for contraception. In the largest trial, the gel containing the lowest dose of nonoxynol-9 (52.5 mg) was significantly less effective in preventing pregnancy than were gels with higher doses of the same agent (100 mg and 150 mg). Gel was liked more than the film or vaginal suppository in the largest trial.[21] Spermicides had been recommended as a mean of improving the efficacy of condom use.[19] In favor of contemporaneous use were findings of killing or inactivating not only sperm but also a great number of often isolated other pathogens, but no studies ever proved the effectiveness of spermicides on STD or HIV transmission. Furthermore, spermicides have been accused to cause vaginal irritation in some cases.[22]

COMBINED ORAL CONTRACEPTIVES

Hormonal contraceptives are among the most popular reversible contraceptives in current use worldwide.[23] More than 150,000,000 women-users are under 30 years old. In some European countries it is used by 50% of women and is considered an appropriate contraceptive method for adolescents. Apart from the protection against an unplanned pregnancy, other advantages of the use of the pill during adolescence are the decrease of menorrhagia[24] (which is very important when anemia coexists), reduction of benign breast disease, lowering the severity of endometriosis, suppression of ovarian functional cysts, decrease of ovarian and endometrial cancer,[25] and reduction of the incidence of ectopic pregnancy. Other important positive effects of hormonal contraception are the relief of dysmenorrhea,[26] the regulation of menstruation, and the inhibition of rheumatoid arthritis progression from mild to severe. The major benefits of modern low-dose oral contraceptives include relative safety and a high degree of efficacy; decreasing the need for abortion or surgical sterilization; lowering risks of bacterial (but not viral) PID; and when low-dose combination (not progestogen only) oral contraceptives are used, improvement of acne, hirsutism, and polycystic ovaries syndrome.[27] OCs are relatively safe and effective when used for years; they control fertility in women and facilitate spontaneous sexual activity. Furthermore, the pill may postpone menstruation over a certain period of time, such as school exams or during holidays, when bleeding or dysmenorrhea can create problems.

The COCs' undesired side effects depend on the dosage of estrogen or the quality of progestogen and they could be: headache, nausea, and breast pain, vaginal bleeding (found in pills with low estrogen dose), depression in young girls when other psychological problems coexist, galactorrhea or amenorrhea (in less than 1% of users), after the interruption of the COCs use.[28] Weight gain is often considered a side effect and can limit its use. However, three placebo-controlled, randomized trials did not find evidence supporting a causal association between combination oral contraceptives or a combination skin patch and weight gain.[29]

The risks associated with OC use are mostly cardiovascular, particularly in carriers of the coagulation factor V Leiden mutation. The risk of arterial thrombosis, such as myocardial infarction or stroke, may be directly related to estrogen dose (the risk decreases as the dosage of ethinyl estradiol decreases), particularly in women who have hypertension, smoke ≥25 cigarettes/day, or are over 35 years old.[27] Hormonal contraception should not be prescribed in the following cases: cardiovascular problems, venous thrombosis,[30] liver disease, focal migraine, depression, excessive obesity, and undiagnosed breast mass. Clinical tests concerning metabolism and lipid profiles are rarely necessary during adolescence. In some cases, blood coagulating factors and the hepatic functional tests are occasionally needed. A previous study evaluated the effects of two third-generation preparations of COCs, on seven natural inhibitors and hemostatic variables, such as prothrombin time, fibrinogen, antithrombin III activity, protein C activity, total protein S antigen, plasminogen activity, and lupus anticoagulant, but found no differences between the two studied groups.[30] Incorrect perception that hormonal contraceptive methods are dangerous may originate from breast and pelvic examination during the first consultation that might cause psychological problems. The only truly needed areas that need to be examined are the medical history and the measurement of blood pressure. For most women, no further evaluation is necessary.[31] Despite their high theoretical effectiveness, typical use results in much lower effectiveness. This disparity reflects difficulties in adherence to the contraceptive regimen and low rates for long-term continuation. Most studies to date have shown no benefit of strategies to improve adherence and continuation.[23] In comparison with older women, a higher rate of failure is noted during adolescence due to higher frequency of sexual relationships, ideal fertility conditions, but most of all, due to lower compliance to the method and its abandon or inappropriate use. An explanation to this may be the lack of experience and the young girls' immaturity.

DEPOMEDROXYPROGESTERONE ACETATE

Since its introduction, DMPA provides a highly effective, reversible method for pregnancy prevention, and it does not require daily administration or use at the time of coitus. It offers the longest contraceptive activity after a single injection every 13 weeks and can be reversed simply by discontinuing injections. DMPA is given in a standard dose of 150 mg intramuscularly every 3 months and yields a rate of 0–5.2 pregnancies per 1,000 women-years.[20] DMPA suppresses the preovulatory surge of luteinizing hormone and follicle-stimulating hormone and thereby inhibits ovulation. It is the most suitable method of pregnancy prevention for many women, such as adolescent and adult women who have experienced contraceptive failures or dissatisfaction with other methods. Despite its excellent safety and efficacy profiles, the method has failed to achieve its potential for widespread use as a result of negative publicity and litigation concerning its side effects. Bleeding irregularities was the main discontinuation reason. The dropout rate was high (approximately 70%)

during the first year.[32] Preinsertion counseling seems to play an important role in satisfaction and side effect tolerance.

Although combination injectable contraceptives are used in many countries, their acceptability could be limited by method characteristics, such as the need to obtain a monthly injection or bleeding pattern changes. Combination injectable contraceptives include 25 mg DMPA plus 5 mg estradiol cypionate (E_2C), as well as 50 mg norethisterone enanthate (NET-EN) plus 5 mg estradiol valerate (E_2V). These combination injectable contraceptives resulted in lower rates of early study discontinuation due to amenorrhea or other bleeding problems, but had higher rates of discontinuation due to other reasons than the progestin-only contraceptives.[33]

EMERGENCY CONTRACEPTION

A few years ago, in case of need of EC, such as rape or preservative rupture, a high dose of estrogens was in common use but was associated with a high frequency of nausea and vomiting. Yuzpe regimen is effective and much better tolerated. Danazol on the other hand, is not so highly effective. Mifepristone has an adverse-effect profile similar to that of the Yuzpe regimen. Furthermore, there is no experience on the use of Mifepristone (RU-486).[20] During the last years, the efficacy of the progestogen-only pill "levonorgestrel," used as an emergency contraceptive method, has been proposed. Levonorgestrel has better results with fewer side effects than previous methods. A 0.75 mg levonorgestrel pill taken as soon as possible after the insecure intercourse and a second one, 12 h later, is efficient. The efficacy depends on the time span between coitus and pill administration (95% for the first 24 h, 85% if taken 24–48 h later, 58% between 48 and 72 h later, and nearly no efficacy if more than 72 h have passed). Adolescents tolerate the medication well, experiencing transient side effects, including nausea, fatigue, and vomiting. A total of 90% of participants reported they would recommend EC to a friend or relative if needed.[34]

Awareness of EC is high among school-age students but knowledge of specific details, such as the recommended time window of effectiveness, is poor. Appropriate use of EC could prevent up to 75% of unplanned pregnancies.[35,36]

However, lack of knowledge on the method use is responsible for the failure of the method. Debate as to whether EC should be available to teenagers without a prescription is of great interest. Many teenagers appear to have problems using condoms correctly while others are taking chances by not using any method of contraception.[37] Data from 10,918 anonymously self-administered questionnaires among school-attending adolescents in Mexico has shown that experience with EC has no adverse effects on condom use, but is rather associated with an increased probability of condom use and an increased perceived capacity to negotiate condom use.[38] Data on young adolescents with increased, over-the-counter access to EC supported that teenagers aged younger than 16 years behaved no differently in response to increased access to EC from the other age groups. As with adults, EC use was greater among adolescents in advance provision, who used the method more frequently when needed, than in clinic access, while other behaviors and situations such as unprotected intercourse, condom use, sexually transmitted infection acquisition, pregnancy, or unwanted sexual activity, remained unchanged.[39]

Sexually active women, especially teenagers, seeking emergency hormonal contraception find that a special Unit of Family Planning for adolescents inside or independent to community hospitals, offers convenience and confidentiality.[40] On the other hand, EC should not be considered an alternative regular contraceptive method. The clinician should ensure that the woman uses an effective contraceptive thereafter.

FEMALE CONDOM

The female condom is made by polyurethane and can be used as an alternative in cases of latex allergy. The device is promoting healthy behaviors and increases sexual self-confidence and autonomy. Unfortunately, the method is not popular during adolescence.

VAGINAL SPONGE

The contraceptive vaginal sponge was developed as an alternative to other barrier methods. It is made of polyurethane and releases 125 mg of the spermicide "nonoxynol-9" over 24 h of use. It can be used for more than one intercourse within 24 h without changing or adding spermicide and does not require a prescription or fitting from a health care provider. Other advantages of this method are the control by the woman rather than her partner, the lack of side effects, antibacterial and antiviral properties, including protection from the HIV[19] as well as less medical contraindications. Unfortunately, the sponge is less effective in preventing pregnancy.[41] Similarly, high discontinuation and allergic-type reactions rates have been reported.[42]

IMPLANTS AND PATCHES

Implants carrying progestin are made of two types of polymers. Immediately after insertion, they begin to release the progestin in a consistent mode. Their effective life varies from 6 to 84 months but pharmaceutical industry experiments on extending this recommended maximum duration of use.[43]

The transdermal contraceptive patch delivers ethinylestradiol and norelgestromin over 7 days (one patch/week for 3 weeks, followed by 1 week of no treatment), that results in a similar cycle control efficacy and side effect profile to oral contraceptives. Excessive body weight is associated with lower efficacy. Attachment of the patch is not affected by warm humid climates, vigorous exercise, or exposure to saunas or water baths. A major advantage of this method compared to other methods, even to oral contraceptives, offers nearly 90% perfect compliance to the dosing schedule across all ages, which may be due to the once-a-week dosing and the simplicity of use of this system. The transdermal delivery approach minimizes the "peaks and troughs" of hormone concentrations associated with daily oral administration and avoids hepatic first-pass metabolism. Side effects are similar to those seen with OCs with the exception of application site reactions that are obviously unique to transdermal delivery.[44] All girls reported regular menstrual periods and about one-third reported a decrease. About one-third of those with a history of recurrent headaches and about one-third of those with acne at initiation reported a decrease while on patch. No significant BMI changes and no pregnancies were reported.[45]

Determination of the ovulation inhibition efficacy of a new, transparent, transdermal, combined hormonal contraceptive patch (area 10 cm^2) containing 0.9 mg ethinylestradiol and 1.9 mg gestodene resulted from an open-label study of 199 healthy, young female volunteers. This study showed that this new, combined contraceptive patch was highly effective in reversibly inhibiting ovulation, well tolerated, and regarded as "very convenient" by the majority of users.[46]

The purpose of another study was to examine implications of increased incidence of correct use on the cost-effectiveness of the contraceptive patch compared with low-estrogen-dose COCs. The base-case analysis showed that use of the patch resulted in a savings of U.S. $249 and 0.03 pregnancies per woman over 2 years compared with COCs.[47]

MALE HORMONAL CONTRACEPTION

New methods for male hormonal fertility control will come in practice probably within the next few years. Spermatogenesis is dependent on the pituitary gonadotropins. Administration of high-dosage of testosterone suppresses gonadotropins and spermatogenesis with an efficacy comparable to female oral contraceptives, resulting in reversible azoospermia in normal men. Combined administration of lower dosage of testosterone similar to physiological replacement doses plus a progestin or a gonadotropin-releasing hormone (GnRH) analogue has demonstrated a further suppression. Most of these male hormonal contraceptives have been associated with modest weight gain and suppression of serum high-density cholesterol levels.[48] The method has not been tested for adolescents. Male hormonal contraceptive methods (MHCM) are in Phase I clinical trials in the United States. Overall, participants had positive impressions about male MHCM (67% male; 67% female) and female partner trust of males' use was high (85%), as were males' intentions (60%).[49]

Nonhormonal drugs for contraception in men, such as gossypol and Tripterygium, which are derived from plants, may have advantages over hormonal methods, such as more rapid onset and less interference with androgen-dependent functions. Gossypol had problems with low efficacy and toxicity. Although sperm density was lower among those taking Tripterygium, later reports indicated some toxicity. Clinical trials studied injecting styrene maleic anhydride into the vas deferens, but no comparative data were provided. At this time, no safe and effective nonhormonal drug is available for contraception in men.[50]

OTHER CONTRACEPTIVE METHODS

Finally, intrauterine devices are not suggested during adolescence. Unless a pregnancy has occurred, other barrier methods such as caps and diaphragms are not in use during adolescence. Unfortunately, many adolescents have un-protected intercourse or use ineffective methods such as periodic abstinence (coitus interruptus or withdrawal prior to ejaculation). Fertility awareness-based methods of family planning estimate the fertile days of the menstrual cycle whether by observing fertility signs, such as cervical secretions and basal body temperature or by monitoring cycle days.[51] The Pearl index of these methods may be as high as 16. This is why abortion remains so frequent during adolescence.

CONCLUSIONS

The transition from childhood to reproductive age is signaled by a number of important events, such as menarche and acceleration of body development. Current rates of sexuality, gestation, and STDs among teenagers are still a public health concern. Abstaining or postponing sexual relationships is the best prevention against STDs and unwanted pregnancy. Adolescent contraception continues to be a complex and perplexing issue for families, health care professionals, educators, government officials, and youth themselves. Psychological and social problems are frequent every time an adolescent is facing an unplanned pregnancy. The theory that sex education and promotion of contraception use encourages sexual activities is incorrect. Adolescents recognize friends and TV as the main source of knowledge about contraception due to communication problems between parents and children. In Sweden, family and sex education are taught in schools and abortions are legal on demand, and free contraceptive counseling is easily available at well-organized Family Planning Units and Youth Health Centers. Condoms and COCs are available at low cost and EC is sold over the counter. The above have as a result a low teenage childbearing rate. The development of Family Planning Clinics is of great importance. Most U.S. adolescent females seeking family planning services report that their parents are aware of their use of services.[52] The organization of Family Planning Centers for Adolescents is undoubtedly necessary and must become a government priority.

A vast variety of safe and effective contraceptive methods are available for teenagers. Beside abstinence, condoms and vaginal spermicides are recommended for all sexually active adolescents to reduce the risk for acquiring STDs. Currently available intrauterine devices are not recommended for most adolescents. Abortion is not considered as a contraceptive method.[53] The most popular contraceptive method in the United States in 2002 was the oral contraceptive pill, used by 11.6 million women; followed by female sterilization, used by 10.3 million women. The condom was the third-leading method, used by about 9 million women and their partners. The condom is the most frequent contraceptive choice at first intercourse when the pill is the most popular method among women under 30. Hopefully, over the 20 years from 1982 to 2002, the percentage who had ever had a partner who used the male condom increased from 52 to 90%.[54]

A cost-utility analysis compared 13 methods of contraception to nonuse of contraception with respect to health care costs and quality-adjusted life years. Every method of contraception dominates nonuse. Methods that require action by the user less frequently than daily are both less costly and more effective than methods requiring action on a daily basis.[55]

Almost 1 million American adolescents become pregnant each year. Up-to-date knowledge on contraception will help physicians to counsel adolescents, preferably prior to the onset of sexual activity. Detailed explanations over various contraceptive alternatives and their side effects will help young people to decide which is the best method for them thus improving the likelihood of adherence.[56]

REFERENCES

1. HAFFNER, D.W., Ed. 1995. Facing facts: sexual health for america's adolescents. The Report of the National Commission on Adolescent Sexual Health. Sexuality Information and Education Council of the United States. New York, NY.
2. AMERICAN ACADEMY OF PEDIATRICS. COMMITTEE ON ADOLESCENCE. 1999. Adolescent pregnancy—current trends and issues. Pediatrics **103:** 516–520.
3. ABMA, J.C., G.M. MARTINEZ, *et al.* 2002. Teenagers in the United States: sexual activity, contraceptive use, and childbearing. Vital Health Stat. **23:** 1–48.
4. GRIMES, D.A. 2003. Unsafe abortion: the silent scourge. Br. Med. Bull. **67:** 99–113.
5. PAUKKU, M., J. QUAN, *et al.* 2003. Adolescents' contraceptive use and pregnancy history: is there a pattern? Obstet. Gynecol. **101:** 534–538.

6. VENTURA, S.J., W.D. MOSHER, *et al.* 2000. Trends in pregnancies and pregnancy rates by outcome: estimates for the United States, 1976–1996. Vital Health Stat. 21 **56:** 1–47.

7. MANLOVE, J., S. RYAN & K. FRANZETTA. 2004. Contraceptive use and consistency in U.S. teenagers' most recent sexual relationships. Perspect. Sex. Reprod. Health **36:** 265–275.

8. MANNING, W.D., M.A. LONGMORE & P.C. GIORDANO. 2000. The relationship context of contraceptive use at first intercourse. Fam. Plann. Perspect. **32:** 104–110.

9. EDGARDH, K. 2002. Adolescent sexual health in Sweden. Sex. Transm. Infect. **78:** 352–356.

10. SCHUSTER, M.A., R.M. BELL, *et al.* 1998. Impact of a high school condom availability program on sexual attitudes and behaviors. Fam. Plann. Perspect. **30:** 67–72.

11. JORDAN, T.R., J.H. PRICE & S. FITZGERALD. 2000. Rural parents' communication with their teen-agers about sexual issues. J. Sch. Health **70:** 338–344.

12. OTT, M.A., NE. ADLER, *et al.* 2002. The trade-off between hormonal contraceptives and condoms among adolescents. Perspect. Sex. Reprod. Health **34:** 6–14.

13. INSTITUTE OF MEDICINE, COMMITTEE ON PREVENTION AND CONTROL OF SEXUALLY TRANSMITTED DISEASES. 1997. The Hidden Epidemic. T.R. Eng, W.T. Butler, Eds. National Academy Press (Centers for Disease Control and Prevention [CDC], 2000).Washington, DC

14. GALLO, M., D. GRIMES, *et al.* 2006. Non-latex versus latex male condoms for contraception. Cochrane Database Syst. Rev. 25 Jan. **1:** CD003550.

15. SONENSTEIN, F.L., L.C. KU, *et al.* 1998. Changes in sexual behavior and condom use among teenage males: 1988 to 1995. Am. J. Public Health **88:** 956–959.

16. NOVAK, D.P. & R.B. KARLSSON. 2005. Gender differed factors affecting male condom use. A population-based study of 18-year-old Swedish adolescents. Int. J. Adolesc. Med. Health **17:** 379–390.

17. SPRUYT, A., M.J. STEINER, *et al.* 1998. Identifying condom users at risk for breakage and slippage: findings from three international sites. Am. J. Public Health **88:** 239–244.

18. CREATSAS, G. 2004. Contraception for Adolescents 2003. *In* Pediatric and Adolescent Gynecology: Evidence-Based Clinical Practice. C. Sultan, Ed.: 225–232. Karger. Basel, Switzerland.

19. HATCHER, R.A., J. TRUSSELL, *et al.* 1998. Contraceptive Technology. 17th edition. Ardent Media. New York, NY.

20. GOLDMAN, J.A., D. DICKER, *et al.* 1985. Barrier contraception in the teenager: a comparison of four methods in adolescent girls. Pediatr. Adolesc. Gynecol. **3:** 59–76.

21. GRIMES, D.A., L. LOPEZ, *et al.* 2005. Spermicide used alone for contraception: Cochrane Database Syst. Rev. 19 Oct. **4:** CD005218.

22. VAN DAMME, L. 2000. Advances in topical microbicides. Paper presented at the XIII International AIDS Conference. Durban, South Africa.

23. HALPERN, V., D. GRIMES, *et al.* 2006. Strategies to improve adherence and acceptability of hormonal methods for contraception. Cochrane Database Syst. Rev. 25 Jan. **1:** CD004317.

24. DELIGEOROGLOU, E. 1997. Dysfunctional uterine bleeding. Ann. N. Y. Acad. Sci. **816:** 158–164.

25. DELIGEOROGLOU, E., E. MICHAILIDIS & G. CREATSAS. 2003. Oral contraceptives and reproductive system cancer. Ann. N. Y. Acad. Sci. **997:** 199–208.

26. DELIGEOROGLOU, E. 2000. Dysmenorrhea. Ann. N. Y. Acad. Sci. **900:** 237–244.
27. SHERIF, K. 1999. Benefits and risks of oral contraceptives. Am. J. Obstet. Gynecol. **180:** S343–S348.
28. CONEY, P., K. WASHENIK, *et al.* 2001. Weight change and adverse event incidence with a low-dose oral contraceptive: two randomized, placebo-controlled trials. Contraception. **63:** 297–302.
29. GALLO, M., L. LOPEZ, *et al.* 2006. Combination contraceptives: effects on weight. Cochrane Database Syst. Rev. 25 Jan. **1:** CD003987.
30. CREATSAS, G., I. KONTOPOULOU–GRIVA, *et al.* 1997. Effect of the monophasic and triphasic (gestodene-ethinylestradiol) oral contraceptives on natural inhibitor and other haemostatic variables. Eur. J. Contracept. Reprod. Health Care **2:** 31–38.
31. STEWART, F.H., C.C. HARPER, *et al.* 2001. Clinical breast and pelvic examination requirements for hormonal contraception: current practice vs. evidence. J. Am. Med. Assoc.2. **285:** 2232–2239.
32. THOMAS, A.G., S. KLIHR-BEALL, *et al.* 2005. Concentration of depot medroxyprogesterone acetate and pain scores in adolescents: a randomized clinical trial. Contraception. **72:** 126–129.
33. GALLO, M.F., D.A. GRIMES, *et al.* 2005. Combination injectable contraceptives for contraception. Cochrane Database Syst. Rev. 20 Jul. **3:** CD004568.
34. HARPER, C.C., C.H. ROCCA, *et al.* 2004. Tolerability of levonorgestrel emergency contraception in adolescents. Am. J. Obstet. Gynecol. **191:** 1158–1163.
35. WANNER, M.S. & R.L. COUCHENOUR. 2002. Hormonal emergency contraception. Pharmacotherapy **22:** 43–53.
36. ELLERTSON, C., J. TRUSSELL, *et al.* 2001. Emergency contraception. Seminars in reproductive medicine. **19:** 323–330.
37. JONES, S. 2005. Emergency contraception use by Irish teenagers. Eur. J. Contracept. Reprod. Health Care **10:** 26–28.
38. WALKER, D.M., P. TORRES, *et al.* 2004. Emergency contraception use is correlated with increased condom use among adolescents: results from Mexico. J. Adolesc. Health. **35:** 329–334.
39. HARPER, C.C., M. CHEONG, *et al.* 2005. The effect of increased access to emergency contraception among young adolescents. Obstet. Gynecol. **106:** 483–491.
40. HEARD-DIMYAN, J. 1999. Issue of emergency hormonal contraception through a casualty department in a community hospital. Br. J. Fam. Plann. **25:** 105–109.
41. CREATSAS, G., E. GUERRERO, *et al.* 2001. A multinational evaluation of the efficacy, safety and acceptability of the Protectaid contraceptive sponge. Eur. J. Contracept. Reprod. Health Care **6:** 172–182.
42. KUYOH, M.A., C. TOROITICH-RUTO, *et al.* 2004. Sponge versus diaphragm for contraception (Cochrane Review). The Cochrane Library. Issue 1.
43. CROXATTO, H.B. 2002. Progestin implants for female contraception. Contraception **65:** 15–19.
44. BURKMAN, R.T. 2004. The transdermal contraceptive system. Am. J. Obstet. Gynecol. **190** Suppl. 4: S49–S53.
45. HAREL, Z., S. RIGGS, *et al.* 2005. Adolescents' experience with the combined estrogen and progestin transdermal contraceptive method Ortho Evra. J. Pediatr. Adolesc. Gynecol. **18:** 85–90.
46. HEGER-MAHN, D., C. WARLIMONT, *et al.* 2004. Combined ethinylestradiol/gestodene contraceptive patch: two-center, open-label study of ovulation inhibition, acceptability and safety over two cycles in female volunteers. Eur. J. Contracept. Reprod. Health Care. **9:** 173–181.

47. SONNENBERG, F.A., R.T. BURKMAN, *et al.* 2005. Cost-effectiveness and contraceptive effectiveness of the transdermal contraceptive patch. Am. J. Obstet. Gynecol. **192:** 1–9.
48. ANAWALT, B.D. & J.K. AMORY. 2001. Advances in male hormonal contraception. Ann. Med. **33:** 587–595.
49. MARCELL, A.V., K. PLOWDEN & S.M. BOWMAN. 2005. Exploring older adolescents' and young adults' attitudes regarding male hormonal contraception: applications for clinical practice. Hum. Reprod. **20:** 3078–3084. [Epub July 8, 2005].
50. LOPEZ, L.M., D.A. GRIMES & K.F. SCHULZ. 2005. Nonhormonal drugs for contraception in men: a systematic review. Obstet. Gynecol. Surv. **60:** 746–752.
51. GRIMES, D.A., M.F. GALLO, V. GRIGORIEVA, *et al.* 2005. Fertility awareness-based methods for contraception: systematic review of randomized controlled trials. Contraception. **72:** 85–90.
52. JONES, R.K., A. PURCELL, *et al.* 2005. Adolescents' reports of parental knowledge of adolescents' use of sexual health services and their reactions to mandated parental notification for prescription contraception. JAMA. **293:** 340–348.
53. GREYDANUS, D.E., D.R. PATEL & M.E. RIMSZA. 2001. Contraception in the adolescent: an update. Pediatrics **107:** 562–573.
54. MOSHER, W.D., G.M. MARTINEZ, *et al.* 2004. Use of contraception and use of family planning services in the United States: 1982–2002. Adv. Data. **350:** 1–36.
55. SONNENBERG, F.A., R.T. BURKMAN, *et al.* 2004. Costs and net health effects of contraceptive methods. Contraception **69:** 447–459.
56. BROOKS, T.L. & L.A. SHRIER. 1999. An update on contraception for adolescents. Adolesc. Med. **10:** 211–219.

Open Issues in Anorexia Nervosa

Prevention and Therapy of Bone Loss

VINCENZINA BRUNI, MARIA FRANCESCA FILICETTI, AND
VALENTINA PONTELLO

*Department of Gynecology, Perinatology, and Human Reproduction,
University of Florence, Firenze, Italy*

ABSTRACT: Anorexia nervosa and diet-induced amenorrhea have an important impact not only on gynecological health but also on bone mass, especially if the disease is not promptly recognized and treated. This is particularly important because these conditions usually arise in adolescence, when peak bone mass is normally achieved. In this article we discuss the therapeutic issues related to bone loss associated with eating disorders.

KEYWORDS: anorexia nervosa; BMD; bone loss; osteoporosis; therapy

INTRODUCTION

The prevalence of anorexia nervosa in young women is about 0.3–1%, with an estimate of 8 new cases per year for every 100,000 women.[1,2] It is well known that a wide range of atypical eating disorders exists: it is estimated that about 50% of cases remain undiagnosed because of the tendency to deny the problem and to hide restrictive or purging behaviors.[3,4]

Bone mass reduction is an early process, which occurs in the first 12 months after diagnosis,[5] with an average annual loss of 1%. More than 50% of adolescent girls with anorexia nervosa have osteopenia and 25% have osteoporosis at lumbar and femoral sites, while total body dual energy X-ray absorption (DEXA) is usually normal. This indicates that trabecular bone is more affected than cortical bone, which is reduced only in the most severe cases.[6] Moreover, volumetric measures show that in anorexia nervosa patients there is a reduction not only in the mineral content of the bone, but also in its size, measured as vertebral body, and femoral neck width.[7] Anorexia nervosa patients with more than 6 years of amenorrhea have a 7-fold increase of fractures

Address for correspondence: Prof. Vincenzina Bruni, Department of Gynecology, Perinatology, and Human Reproduction, University of Florence, Ospedale di Careggi, viale Morgagni 85, 50134 Firenze, Italy. Voice: +39-055-4277551; fax: +39-055-218844.
    e-mail: vbruni@unifi.it

Ann. N.Y. Acad. Sci. 1092: 91–102 (2006). © 2006 New York Academy of Sciences.
doi: 10.1196/annals.1365.008

TABLE 1. Negative prognostic factors

Late onset
Duration of the disease
Extremely low body weight
Strenuous physical activity
Persistent alteration in body image
Comorbidity with anxiety and depressive disorders
Personality disorders
Relational difficulties

rate,[8,9] and studies of long-term outcome indicate that at 11 years follow-up 44% of unrecovered patients is osteoporotic.[10] Moreover, in a longitudinal study the cumulative incidence of any fracture at 40 years after the diagnosis of anorexia nervosa was 57%, and fractures of the hip, spine, and forearm were late complications, occurring on average 38, 25, and 24 years, respectively, after diagnosis.[11]

Studies about long-term outcomes of anorexia nervosa have shown that 30–55% of cases fully recover, 25–30% of cases still show psychological stigmata of the disease despite satisfactory weight recovery, and 18–25% remain chronically ill[12] (risk factors for chronicity are outlined in TABLE 1[13,14]). In some cases, recovery of body weight is not associated with resumption of menses (especially when psychological features, such as alteration in body image and obsessive thoughts about food persist[15]), and it is debatable if resumption of menses may be associated with full recovery of bone mass. Indeed, studies from the literature show discordant results: some authors claim that the damage on bone mass can regress,[16–18] especially in shorter duration of illness[19] and with better prognosis in younger patients.[20,21] On the contrary, others report a permanent damage on bone mass,[22–24] principally in chronically ill subjects.[25,26] Moreover, the efficacy of medical and endocrinal treatments against osteopenia is currently under debate.

PATHOGENESIS OF BONE LOSS IN ANOREXIA NERVOSA

Restrictive eating behaviors have important consequences on neuroendocrine factors with repercussion on bone mass:

- Reduction of GnRH and gonadotropin secretion, with consequences on ovarian estrogen and androgen production;[27,28]
- Increase of cortisol plasmatic levels, as a result of increased adrenal production and clearance reduction, with preserved circardian rhythm;[29]
- Reduction of free-T_3 (as a consequence of decreased peripheral conversion from T_4) with normal free-T4 and TSH;[30,31]
- Decreased hepatic synthesis of IGF1, despite normal or increased GH levels;[32]

- Decreased leptin levels, related to the reduction in adipose tissue.[33] Recent studies have shown that leptin acts as a regulator of bone remodeling processes, through a direct effect on osteoblast differentiation and an indirect effect through the ventromedial nucleus of the hypothalamus via sympathetic system;[34,35]
- Increased cathecolamines (as a result of adaptation to metabolic stress caused by fasting), that appear related with markers for bone production in young adults.[36]

The combination of these neuroendocrine changes, nutritional deficits (especially calcium and vitamin D[37]), metabolic acidosis (as a consequence of prolonged fasting[38]), and in some cases depression comorbidity[39] can have a negative effect on bone mass, with failure to achieve an adequate peak bone mass in adolescent patients. In particular, factors predictive of bone loss are early onset of illness (e.g., primary amenorrhoea[8,40]), duration of amenorrhoea,[25,41–45] low body mass index (BMI),[46] (in particular duration of emaciation below a BMI of 16 kg/m^2[47]), and decreased lean mass.[48–50]

Differently from postmenopausal osteoporosis, in which bone formation and resorption are increased simultaneously, anorexia nervosa appears to be a low turnover state, with decreased neoformation and increased bone resorption.[51–54] This happens because estrogen deficiency is not the only cause, but an additional one is the reduction in regulatory mediators of osteoblast proliferation and differentiation, in particular IGF-1.[32] Indeed, during adolescence there is a physiological increase in bone mass,[55–57] and the gap between normal subjects and anorexia nervosa patients tends to widen with amenorrhoea duration. Furthermore, there are some data indicating that bone resorption may be accelerated even in some of the recently rehabilitated patients.[58–59] This indicates that bone mineral density (BMD) should be monitored well beyond recovery of body weight.

PREVENTION AND THERAPY OF BONE LOSS ASSOCIATED WITH ANOREXIA NERVOSA

Nutritional Rehabilitation

Body weight recovery appears to be crucial for the treatment of osteopenia, as highlighted by the improvement in DEXA measurements, the changes in bone turnover markers, and the increase in vertebral size, as a result of periosteal bone apposition.[18,19,23,60] However, there are some data showing that although bone mass increases when weight returns to normal, many subjects show persistent osteopenia.[61–62] Furthermore, some authors report that a weight increase of 10 kg in 1 year is not sufficient to increase significantly BMD both at lumbar and femoral sites in severely underweight adolescent girls (initial mean BMI 14.2 kg/m^2, after 1 year mean BMI 17.6 kg/m^2).[63] The reason for such discrepancies is not clear; we can assume that data from the literature are biased toward more severity, and, as we said before, the recovery is not complete in about two-thirds of the cases, with persistence of controlled eating behaviors and obsessive thought about food even in weight-recovered patients. We know that there is a range of eating disorders, with 50% of cases that remain undiagnosed and get to the attention of the doctor as diet-induced amenorrhoea or hypothalamic amenorrhoea. Therefore, it is particularly important to recognize and treat precociously these conditions, as they arise in adolescence, a period in which peak bone mass may be at risk of compromise, but with more chances of catch-up if the dietary habits are corrected. Nutritional rehabilitation programs should be tailored to the needs of each subject, and should be associated with psychological support. There are some data showing the protective effect of weight-bearing exercise on bone density, measured at the proximal femur.[40] However, moderate physical activity should be encouraged only when a satisfying body weight is reached, to avoid the risk of traumatic fractures in subjects with severe osteoporosis and to discourage the patient to use strenuous exercise as purging behavior. DEXA mineralometry can help us to follow the progress not only in bone mass recovery, but also in body composition (as improvements in both fat and lean mass).[64] Indeed, the percentage of total body fat appears to be a better indicator of the nutritional state than BMI.

Usually compliance to treatment is poor if weight gain is too fast, so at first we should be satisfied even if the intake of carbohydrates and proteins is low (about 2 g/Kg a day for carbohydrates),[65] but enough to preserve lean mass. On the contrary, fat content of the diet should be kept low, because of possible interference with vitamin D absorption. It can be useful to integrate calcium and vitamin D in the diet, given that during fasting or parenteral nutrition there can be hypophosphataemia, which for itself favors bone resorption.[66–67] Indeed, the result of a study on 16 adolescent women, treated for 3 months with a hypercaloric diet with high calcium dose (2 g/day) and vitamin D, was not only an increase in BMI and leptin, but also in IGF-1 and markers for bone formation (procollagen, carboxy-terminal-propeptide, and bone alkalyne phosphatase) with reduction of markers for bone resorption (C-telopeptide).[68]

ESTROGEN–PROGESTIN TREATMENT

Patients with anorexia nervosa are often more worried by amenorrhoea than by low body weight. Having regular menses is perceived as "being healthy," and sometimes patients ask for estro-progestin contraceptives to feel like their peers. However, even high dose oral contraceptives (OCs) are not protective on bone mass if they are not associated with nutritional rehabilitation.[69–70] This is confirmed also by data from bone biopsies in four patients.[71] Nevertheless, there are some data indicating that estrogen replacement therapy could be partially protective on lumbar BMD, but not on femoral neck BMD in subjects with anorexia nervosa, not yet rehabilitated.[7,40,72] In particular, it seems that severely underweight patients (less than 70% ideal body weight) are those who benefit the most from estro-progestin supplementation.[73] Indeed, also in cases in which all the criteria for anorexia nervosa are met, except for amenorrhoea, lumbar and more pronouncedly femoral BMD are reduced compared to healthy controls. This indicates that even endogenous estrogens only partially protect bone mass at lumbar level, but not at the femoral level.[74]

Maybe estrogen dose should be higher or used for longer periods to have an impact on bone mass. Some authors advocate the superiority of transdermal to oral administration, explaining the better results with the increase in serum estradiol concentrations,[75] but, to our knowledge, there are no other studies that compare these different routes. As we said before, it is more likely that estrogen deficiency is only one of the factors contributing to bone loss. On the other hand, there are some data showing that spontaneous resumption of menses is essential to normalize reduced BMD.[73,76] Therefore we must conclude that weight recovery is indispensable for the normalization of bone mass, but not sufficient *per se* if not associated with normal estrogen level.

IGF-1

Low protein intake has a profound impact on bone turnover (through the GH-IGF1 system). Grinspoon *et al.*[77] randomized 60 osteopenic women with anorexia nervosa into 4 groups: recombinant human IGF-1 (30 μg/kg s.c. twice daily) and oral contraceptive (ethinyl-estradiol 35 μg and 0.4 mg norethindrone), IGF-1 alone, oral contraceptive alone, or placebo for 9 months. All subjects received calcium 1,500 mg/day and a standard multivitamin containing 400 UI of vitamin D. The study highlighted that OC and recombinant IGF-1 have synergistic effect on bone mass in the group of patients treated with both drugs, while OC alone showed a nonsignificant effect on bone mass. Recombinant IGF-1 administration is a surrogate for protein intake and it is unlikely to become one of the therapeutic options because of its cost. However, a diet rich in essential aminoacids can be of help in increasing the release of this modulator.[78]

DEHYDROEPIANDROSTERONE

It is thought that DHEA stimulates osteoblast cell proliferation, most likely acting through aromatization to estrogens in peripheral tissues. Indeed, DHEA administered per os for 3 months at the dose of 50 mg/day can reverse the abnormalities in bone turnover markers.[79] But more recent data state that 1 year treatment with DHEA is no more effective than estro-progestin supplementation (EE 20 mcg/levonorgestrel 100 mcg). In particular, femoral bone density increase does not reach statistical significance when corrected for weight increase in recovering patients. However, an improvement in specific psychological parameters has been reported in the group taking DHEA.[80]

VITAMIN K2

Menatetrenone (vitamin K2) promotes bone formation through activating osteoblasts to enhance calcification or acting as a coenzyme in the gamma-carboxylation of glutamyl residues in several bone proteins, such as Gla-osteocalcin. Furthermore, it prevents bone resorption by inhibiting osteoclasts. Indeed, its deficiency has been associated with an increased risk of hip fractures in an epidemiological study on healthy women.[81]

In anorexia nervosa patients, vitamin K2 at a dose of 45 mg/day is shown to slow the decrease in vertebral BMD, with increase in markers for bone formation (osteocalcin) and decrease in markers for bone resorption (urine deoxypyridinoline).[82]

BIPHOSPHONATES

Experiences of use of biphosphonates in adolescent patients are related to the treatment of osteopenia associated with chronic diseases, such as rheumatic diseases,[83,84] osteogenesis imperfecta,[85] renal transplant,[86] and during chronic corticosteroid therapy[87] with good results, as assessed by DEXA or ultrasound.

In anorexia nervosa there are some data highlighting the usefulness of alendronate 10 mg/day, associated with calcium and vitamin D, in increasing lumbar and femoral BMD after 1 year of therapy. However, the authors conclude that restoration of body weight is the most crucial factor for the recovery in BMD, and in particular in the subjects who had also resumption of menses, there was no additional benefit at the lumbar site of treatment with alendronate.[62] There are experiences about risedronate use (5 mg/day), showing a 4% increase in lumbar bone density even in unrecovered patients at 9 months of follow-up, but with greater efficacy in the first 6 months of treatment.[88] Finally, some recent data show the efficacy of 3 months of therapy with 200 mg/day of etidronate, a first generation biphosphonate, in increasing tibial bone density, as assessed by ultrasound techniques (speed of sound). No statistically significant difference was seen in the same study between the use of etidronate and the supplementation with calcium and vitamin D, associated with weight rehabilitation.[89]

Nevertheless, we must remember that the U.S. Food and Drug Administration has approved the use of biphosphonates only in subjects taking corticosteroids for chronic diseases. Indeed, long-term effects of these drugs have not been definitively established in women of reproductive age and their use should be avoided in subjects at risk of pregnancy for their teratogenic effect, as documented in animal models.[90] In particular, some data show that alendronate has a high affinity for hydroxyapatite, with a terminal half-life in the bone up to 10 years and effects on bone turnover for at least 5 years.[91,92] On the contrary, risedronate has a terminal half-life of about 20 days,[93] with a "fast off effect:" 12 months after discontinuation, bone turnover markers return to basal levels.[94] We can speculate that, if further data will confirm its efficacy and safety, risedronate could become a drug of choice for the reversibility of its effects especially in young subjects.

OTHER THERAPEUTIC OPTIONS

In the literature there is a report of the use of alprazolam, as inhbitor of corticotropin-releasing factor (CRH) activity in the brain, in six women with anorexia nervosa, who recovered weight, but with persisting stress-related anovulation. Alprazolam has shown to improve GnRH pulse generator activity, with positive effect on ovulation.[95] It is debatable if the reduction in cortisol level and the improvement in gonadal function may be beneficial to preserve bone mass in those subjects, who recovered weight, but in whom amenorrhoea persists. At present, there are no data available on this issue.

CONCLUSION

In conclusion, therapeutic strategies for anorexia nervosa and other eating disorders should be managed by a multidisciplinary team, that deals with nutritional rehabilitation, psychological well-being, and treatment of medical conditions associated with the disease. The use of estro-progestin contraceptives should be reserved to those cases in which, despite a satisfactory body weight, amenorrhoea persists. Dietary supplementation with calcium, vitamin D, and vitamin K2 can be useful, especially during refeeding. At present, other therapeutic tools, such as biphosphonates and DHEA, are not routinely used.

REFERENCES

1. HOEK, H.W. & D. VAN HOEKEN. 2003. Review of the prevalence and incidence of eating disorders. Int. J. Eat. Disord. **34:** 383–396.
2. FAVARO, A., S. FERRARA & P. SANTONASTASO. 2003. The spectrum of eating disorders in young women: a prevalence study in a general population sample. Psychosom. Med. **65:** 701–708.
3. LUCAS, A.R., C.M. BEARD, W.M. O'FALLON, *et al.* 1991. 50-year trends in the incidence of anorexia nervosa in Rochester, MN: a population-based study. Am. J. Psychiatry **148:** 917–922.

4. SERDULA, M.K., M.E. COLLINS, D.F. WILLIAMSON, *et al.* 1993. Weight control practices of U.S. adolescents and adults. Ann. Intern. Med. **119:** 667–671.
5. SERAFINOWICZ, E., R. WASIKOWA, Z. IWANICKA, *et al.* 2003. Bone metabolism in adolescent girls with short course of anorexia nervosa. Endokrynol. Diabetol. Chor. Przemiany. Materni. Wieku. Rozw. **9:** 67–71.
6. PAFUMI, C., L. CIOTTA, M. FARINA, *et al.* 2002. Evaluation of bone mass in young amenorrhoic women with anorexia nervosa. Minerva Ginecol. **54:** 487–491.
7. KARLSSON, M.K., S.J. WEIGALL, Y. DUAN, *et al.* 2000. Bone size and volumetric density in women with anorexia nervosa receiving estrogen replacement therapy and in women recovered from anorexia nervosa. J. Clin. Endocrinol. Metab. **85:** 3177–3182.
8. BILLER, B.M., V. SAXE, D.B. HERZOG, *et al.* 1989. Mechanisms of osteoporosis in adult and adolescent women with anorexia nervosa. J. Clin. Endocrinol. Metab. **68:** 548–554.
9. VESTERGAARD, P., C. EMBORG, R.K. STOVING, *et al.* 2003. Patients with eating disorders. A high-risk group for fractures. Orthop. Nurs. **22:** 325–331.
10. HERZOG, W., H. MINNE, C. DETER, *et al.* 1993. Outcome of bone mineral density in anorexia nervosa patients 11.7 years after first admission. J. Bone Miner. Res. **8:** 597–605.
11. LUCAS, A.R., L.J. MELTON, C.S. CROWSON, *et al.* 1999. Long-term fracture risk among women with anorexia nervosa: a population-based cohort study. Mayo Clin. Proc. **74:** 972–977.
12. VIRICEL, J., C. BOSSU, B. GALUSCA, *et al.* 2005. Retrospective study of anorexia nervosa: reduce mortality and stable recovery rates. Presse. Med. **34:** 1505–1510.
13. KEEL, P.K., D.J. DORER, D.L. FRANKO, *et al.* 2005. Post-remission predictors of relapse in women with eating disorders. Am. J. Psychiatry **162:** 2263–2268.
14. BULIK, C.M., P.F. SULLIVAN, F. TOZZI, *et al.* 2006. Prevalence, heritability, and prospective risk factors for anorexia nervosa. Arch. Gen. Psychiatry **63:** 305–312.
15. BRAMBILLA, F., P. MONTELEONE, F. BORTOLOTTI, *et al.* 2003. Persistent amenorrhoea in weight recovered anorexics: psychological and biological aspects. Psychiatry Res. **118:** 249–257.
16. TREASURE, J.L., G.F. RUSSELL, I. FOGELMAN, *et al.* 1987. Reversible bone loss in anorexia nervosa. Br. Med. J. **295:** 474–475.
17. VALLA, A., I.L. GROENNING, U. SYVERSEN, *et al.* 2000. Anorexia nervosa: slow regain of bone mass. Osteoporos. Int. **11:** 141–145.
18. WENTZ, E., D. MELLSTROM, C. GILLBERG, *et al.* 2003. Bone density 11 years after anorexia nervosa onset in a controlled study of 39 cases. Int. J. Eat. Disord. **34:** 314–318.
19. CASTRO, J., L. LAZARO, F. PONS, *et al.* 2001. Adolescent anorexia nervosa: the catch-up effect in bone mineral density after recovery. J. Am. Acad. Child Adolesc. Psychiatry **40:** 1215–1221.
20. CARRUTH, B.R. & J.D. SKINNER. 2000. Bone mineral status in adolescent girls: effects of eating disorders and exercise. J. Adolesc. Health **26:** 322–329.
21. JAGIELSKA, G., T. WOLANCZYK, J. KOMENDER, *et al.* 2001. Bone mineral content and bone mineral density in adolescent girls with anorexia nervosa-a longitudinal study. Acta. Psychiatr. Scand. **104:** 131–147.
22. RIGOTTI, N.A., R.M. NEER, S.J. SKATES, *et al.* 1991. The clinical course of osteoporosis in anorexia nervosa. A longitudinal study of cortical bone mass. JAMA **265:** 1133–1138.

23. BACHRACH, L.K., D.K. KATZMAN, I.F. LITT, *et al.* 1991. Recovery from osteopenia in adolescent girls with anorexia nervosa. J. Clin. Endocrinol. Metab. **72:** 602–606.
24. HARTMAN, D., A. CRISP, B. ROONEY, *et al.* 2000. Bone density of women who have recovered from anorexia nervosa. Int. J. Eat. Disord. **28:** 107–112.
25. ZIPFEL, S., M.J. SEIBEL, B. LOWE, *et al.* 2001. Osteoporosis in eating disorders: a follow-up study of patients with anorexia and bulimia nervosa. J. Clin. Endocrinol. Metab. **86:** 5227–5233.
26. SCHNEIDER, M., M. FISHER, S. WEINERMAN, *et al.* 2002. Correlates of bone density in females with anorexia nervosa. Int. J. Adolesc. Med. Health **14:** 297–306.
27. BEUMONT, P.J., G.C. GEORGE, B.L. PIMSTONE, *et al.* 1976. Body weight and the pituitary response to hypothalamic releasing hormones in patients with anorexia nervosa. J. Clin. Endocrinol. Metab. **43:** 487–496.
28. VAN BINSBERG, C.J., H.J. COELINGH BENNINK, J. ODINK, *et al.* 1990. A comparative and longitudinal study on endocrine changes related to ovarian function in patients with anorexia nervosa. J. Clin. Endocrinol. Metab. **71:** 705–711.
29. MISRA, M., K.K. MILLER, C. ALMAZAN, *et al.* 2004. Alterations in cortisol secretory dynamics in adolescent girls with anorexia nervosa and effects on bone metabolism. J. Clin. Endocrinol. Metab. **89:** 4972–4980.
30. DE ROSA, G., S. DELLA CASA, S.M. CORSELLO, *et al.* 1983. Thyroid function in altered nutritional state. Exp. Clin. Endocrinol. **82:** 173–177.
31. KIYOHARA, K., H. TAMAI, Y. TAKAICHI, *et al.* 1989. Decreased thyroidal triiodothyronine secretion in patients with anorexia nervosa: influence of weight recovery. Am. J. Clin. Nutr. **50:** 767–772.
32. MISRA, M., K.K. MILLER, J. BJORNSON, *et al.* 2003. Alterations in growth hormone secretory dynamics in adolescent girls with anorexia nervosa and effects on bone metabolism. J. Clin. Endocrinol. Metab. **88:** 5615–5623.
33. GRINSPOON, S., T. GULICK, H. ASKARI, *et al.* 1996. Serum leptin levels in women with anorexia nervosa. J. Clin. Endocrinol. Metab. **81:** 3861–3864.
34. ISAIA, G.C., P. D'AMELIO, S. DI BELLA, *et al.* 2005. Is leptin the link between fat and bone mass? J. Endocrinol. Invest. **28**(Suppl. 10): 61–65.
35. COHEN, M.M. 2006. Role of leptin in regulating appetite, neuroendocrine function, and bone remodelling. Am. J. Med. Genet. **140:** 515–524.
36. GALUSCA, B., C. BOSSU, N. GERMAIN, *et al.* 2006. Age-related differences in hormonal and nutritional impact on lean anorexia nervosa bone turnover uncoupling. Osteporos. Int. **17:** 888–896.
37. FONSECA, V.A., V. D'SOUZA, S. HOULDER, *et al.* 1988. Vitamin D deficiency and low osteocalcin concentrations in anorexia nervosa. J. Clin. Pathol. **41:** 195–197.
38. GRINSPOON, S.K., H.B. BAUM, V. KIM, *et al.* 1995. Decreased bone formation and increased mineral dissolution during acute fasting in young women. J. Clin. Endocrinol. Metab. **80:** 3628–3633.
39. KONSTANTINOWICZ, J., H. KADZIELA–OLECH, M. KACZMARSKI, *et al.* 2005. Depression in anorexia nervosa: a risk factor for osteoporosis. J. Clin. Endocrinol. Metab. **90:** 5382–5385.
40. SEEMAN, E., G.I. SZMULKELER, C. FORMICA, *et al.* 1992. Osteoporosis in anorexia nervosa: the influence of peak bone density, bone loss, oral contraceptive use and exercise. J. Bone. Miner. Res. **7:** 1467–1474.
41. HAY, P.J., A. HALL, J.W. DELAHUNT, *et al.* 1989. Investigation of osteopaenia in anorexia nervosa. Aust. N. Z. J. Psychiatry **23:** 261–268.

42. BRUNI, V., L. BIGOZZI, M. DEI, *et al*. 1997. Bone mineral metabolism in diet-induced amenorrhoea. Ann. N. Y. Acad. Sci. **816:** 250–252.
43. WEINBRENNER, T., A. ZITTERMANN, I. GOUNI-BERTHOLD, *et al*. 2003. Body mass index and disease duration are predictors of disturbed bone turnover in anorexia nervosa. A case–control study. Eur. J. Clin. Nutr. **57:** 1262–1267.
44. GORDON, C.M., E. GOODMAN, S.J. EMANS, *et al*. 2002. Physiologic regulators of bone turnover in young women with anorexia nervosa. J. Pediatr. **141:** 64–70.
45. SCHNEIDER, M., M. FISHER, S. WEINERMAN, *et al*. 2002. Correlates of low bone density in females with anorexia nervosa. Int. J. Adolesc. Med. Health **14:** 297–306.
46. GOEBEL, G., U. SCHWEIGER, R. KRUGER, *et al*. 1999. Predictors of bone mineral density in patients with eating disorders. Int. J. Eat. Disord. **25:** 143–150.
47. HOTTA, M., T. SHIBASAKI, K. SATO, *et al*. 1998. The importance of body weight history in the occurrence and recovery of osteoporosis in patients with anorexia nervosa: evaluation by dual X-ray absorptiometry and bone metabolic markers. Eur. J. Endocrinol. **139:** 276–283.
48. KOOH, S.W., E. NORIEGA, K. LESLIE, *et al*. 1996. Bone mass and soft tissue composition in adolescents with anorexia nervosa. Bone **19:** 181–188.
49. JACOANGELI, F., A. ZOLI, A. TARANTO, *et al*. 2002. Osteoporosis and anorexia nervosa: relative role of endocrine alterations and malnutrition. EWD **7:** 190–195.
50. BRUNI, V., M. DEI, M.F. FILICETTI, *et al*. 2006. Predictors of bone loss in young women with restrictive eating disorders. Ped. End. Rev. **3** (Suppl. 1): 219–221.
51. STEFANIS, N., C. MACKINTOSH, H.D. ABRAHA, *et al*. 1998. Dissociation of bone turnover in anorexia nervosa. Ann. Clin. Biochem. **35:** 709–716.
52. SOYKA, L.A., S. GRINSPOON, L.L. LEVITSKY, *et al*. 1999. The effects of anorexia nervosa on bone metabolism in female adolescents. J. Clin. Endocr. Metab. **84:** 4489–4496.
53. LENNKH, C., M. DE ZWAAN, U. BAILER, *et al*. 1999. Osteopenia in anorexia nervosa: specific mechanisms of bone loss. J. Psych. Res. **33:** 349–356.
54. HEER, M., C. MIKA, I. GRZELLA, *et al*. 2004. Bone turnover during inpatient nutritional therapy and outpatient follow-up in patients with anorexia nervosa compared with that in healthy control subjects. Am. J. Clin. Nutr. **80:** 774–781.
55. BONJOUR, J.P., G. THEINTZ, B. BUCHS, *et al*. 1991. Critical years and stages of puberty for spinal and femoral bone mass accumulation during adolescence. J. Clin. Endocrinol. Metab. **73:** 555–563.
56. MATKOVIC, V., T. JELIC, G.M. WARDLAW, *et al*. 1994. Timing of peak bone mass in Caucasian females and its implication for the prevention of osteoporosis. J. Clin. Invest. **93:** 799–808.
57. SABATIER, J.P., G. GUAYDIER-SOUQUIERS, D. LAROCHE, *et al*. 1996. Bone mineral acquisition during adolescence and early adulthood: a study in 574 healthy females 10-24 years of age. Osteoporos. Int. **6:** 141–148.
58. AUDÌ, L., D.M. VARGAS, M. GUSSINYE, *et al*. 2002. Clinical and biochemical determinants of bone metabolism and bone mass in adolescent female patients with anorexia nervosa. Ped. Res. **51:** 497–504.
59. VALTUENA, S., V. DI MATTEI, L. ROSSI, *et al*. 2003. Bone resorption in anorexia nervosa and in rehabilitated patients. Eur. J. Clin. Nutr. **57:** 260–265.
60. BOLTON, J.G.F., S. PATEL, J.H. LACEY, *et al*. 2005. A prospective study of changes in bone turnover and bone density associated with regaining weight in women with anorexia nervosa. Osteoporos. Int. **16:** 1955–1962.

61. WARD, A., N. BROWN & J. TREASURE. 1997. Persistent osteopenia after recovery from anorexia nervosa. Int. J. Eat. Disord. **22:** 71–75.
62. GOLDEN, N.H., E. IGLESIAS, M.S. JACOBSON, *et al.* 2005. Alendronate for the treatment of osteopenia in anorexia nervosa: a randomized double-blind controlled study. J. Clin. Endocrinol. Metab. **90:** 3179–3185.
63. COMPSTON, J.E., C. MCCONACHIE, C. STOTT, *et al.* 2006. Changes in bone mineral density, body composition and biochemical markers of bone turnover during weight gain in adolescents with severe anorexia nervosa: a 1-year prospective study. Osteoporos. Int. **17:** 77–84.
64. LASKEY, M.A. & D. PHIL. 1996. Dual energy X-ray absorptiometry and body composition. Nutrition **12:** 45–51.
65. SNYDER, D.K., D.R. CLEMMONS & L.E. UNDERWOOD. 1989. Dietary carbohydrate content determines responsiveness to growth hormone in energy-restricted humans. J. Clin. Endocrinol. Metab. **69:** 745–752.
66. WEINSIER, R.L. & C.L. KRUMDIECK. 1981. Death resulting from overzealous total parenteral nutrition: the refeeding syndrome revisited. Am. J. Clin. Nutr. **34:** 393–399.
67. MIKA, C., I GRZELLA, B. HERPERTZ-DAHLMANN, *et al.* 2002. Dietary treatment enhances bone formation in malnourished patients. J. Gravit. Physiol. **9:** P331–P332.
68. HEER, M., C. MIKA, I. GRZELLA, *et al.* 2002. Changes in bone turnover in patients with anorexia nervosa during eleven weeks of inpatient dietary treatment. Clin. Chem. **48:** 754–760.
69. MUNOZ, M.T., G. MORANTE, J.A. GARCIA-CENTENERA, *et al.* 2002. The effects of estrogen administration on bone mineral density in adolescents with anorexia nervosa. Eur. J. Endocrinol. **146:** 45–50.
70. GOLDEN, N.H., L. LANZKOWSKY, J. SCHEBENDACH, *et al.* 2002. The effect of estrogen–progestin treatment on bone mineral density in anorexia nervosa. J. Pediatr. Adolesc. Gynecol. **15:** 135–143.
71. KREIPE, R.E., D.G. HICKS, R.N. ROSIER, *et al.* 1993. Preliminary findings on the effects of sex hormones on bone metabolism in anorexia nervosa. J. Adolesc. Health **14:** 319–324.
72. MAUGARS, Y.M., J.M. BERTHELOT, R. FORESTIER, *et al.* 1996. Follow-up of bone mineral density in 27 cases of anorexia nervosa. Eur. J. Endocrinol. **135:** 591–597.
73. KLIBANSKI, A., B.M. BILLER, D.A. SCHENFELD, *et al.* 1995. The effects of estrogen administration on trabecular bone loss in young women with anorexia nervosa. J. Clin. Endocrinol. Metab. **80:** 898–904.
74. MILLER, K.K., S. GRINSPOON, S. GLEYSTEEN, *et al.* 2004. Preservation of neuroendocrine control of reproductive function despite severe undernutrition. J. Clin. Endocrinol. Metab. **89:** 4434–4438.
75. HAREL, Z. & S. RIGGS. 1997. Transdermal versus oral administration of estrogen in the management of lumbar spine osteopenia in an adolescent with anorexia nervosa. J. Adolesc. Health **21:** 179–182.
76. IKETANI, T., N. KIRIIKE, S. NAKANISHI, *et al.* 1995. Effects of weight gain and resumption of menses on reduced bone density in patients with anorexia nervosa. Biol. Psychiatry **37:** 521–527.
77. GRINSPOON, S., L. THOMAS, K. MILLER, *et al.* 2002. Effects of recombinant human IGF-1 and oral contraceptive administration on bone density in anorexia nervosa. J. Clin. Endocrinol. Metab. **87:** 2883–2891.

78. CLEMMONS, D.R., M.M. SEEK, L.E. UNDERWOOD, *et al*. 1985. Supplemental essential aminoacids augment the somatomedin-C/Insulin-like growth factor-response to refeeding after fasting. Metabolism **34:** 391–395.
79. GORDON, C.M., E. GRACE, S.J. EMANS, *et al*. 1999. Changes in bone turnover markers and menstrual function after short-term oral DHEA in young women with anorexia nervosa. J. Bone Miner. Res. **14:** 136–145.
80. GORDON, C.M., E. GRACE, S.J. EMANS, *et al*. 2002. Effects of oral Dehydroepiandrosterone on bone density in young women with anorexia nervosa: a randomized trial. J. Clin. Endocrinol. Metab. **87:** 4935–4941.
81. FESKANICH, D., P. WEBER, W.C. WILLETT, *et al*. 1999. Vitamin K intake and hip fractures in women: a prospective study. Am. J. Clin. Nutr. **69:** 74–79.
82. IKETANI, T., N. KIRIIKE, MURRAY, *et al*. 2003. Effect of menatetrenone (vitamin K2) treatment on bone loss in patients with anorexia nervosa. Psychiatry Res. **117:** 259–269.
83. CIMAZ, R., M. GATTORNO, M.P. SORMANI, *et al*. 2002. Changes in markers of bone turnover and inflammatory variables durino alendronate therapy in pediatric patients with rheumatic diseases. J. Rheumatol. **29:** 1786–1792.
84. FALCINI, F., G. BINDI, G. SIMONINI, *et al*. 2003. Bone status evaluation with calcaneal ultrasound in children with chronic rheumatic diseases. A one year follow-up study. J. Rheumatol. **30:** 179–184.
85. DIMEGLIO, L.A., L. FORD, C. MCCLINTOCK, *et al*. 2005. A comparison of oral and intravenous biphosphonate therapy for children with osteogenesis imperfecta. J. Pediatr. Endocrinol. Metab. **18:** 43–53.
86. EL-HUSSEINI, A.A., A.E. EL-AGROUDY, M.F. EL-SAYED, *et al*. 2004. Treatment of osteopenia and osteoporosis in renal transplant children and adolescents. Pediatr. Transplant. **8:** 357–361.
87. SAAG, K.G., R. EMKEY, T.J. SCHNITZER, *et al*. 1998. Alendronate for the prevention and treatment of glucocorticoid-induced osteoporosis. Glucocorticoid-induced osteoporosis intervention study group. N. Eng. J. Med. **339:** 292–299.
88. MILLER, K.K., K.A. GRIECO, J. MULDER, *et al*. 2004. Effects of risedronate on bone density in anorexia nervosa. J. Clin. Endocrinol. Metab. **89:** 3903–3906.
89. NAKAHARA, T., N. NAGAI, M. TANAKA, *et al*. 2006. The effects of bone therapy on tibial bone loss in young women with anorexia nervosa. Int. J. Eat. Disord. **39:** 20–26.
90. PATLAS, N., G. GOLOMB, P. YAFFE, *et al*. 1999. Transplacental effects of biphosphonates on fetal skeletal ossification and mineralization in rats. Teratology **60:** 68–73.
91. LIN, J.H. 1996. Biphosphonates: a review of their pharmacokinetic properties. Bone **18:** 75–85.
92. NANCOLLAS, G.H., R. TANG, R.J. PHIPPS, *et al*. 2006. Novel insights into actions of biphosphonates on bone: differences in interactions with hydroxyapatite. Bone **38:** 617–627.
93. WHITE, N.J. & C.M. PERRY. 2003. Risedronate once a week. Treat. Endocrinol. **2:** 415–420.
94. WATTS, N.B., W.P. OLSZYNSKI, C.D. MCKEEVER, *et al*. 2004. Effects of risedronate treatment discontinuation on bone turnover and BMD. 31st European Symposium on Calcified Tissues. Nice, France. 136.
95. JUDD, S.J., J. WONG, S. SALONIKLIS, *et al*. 1995. The effect of alprazolam on serum cortisol and luteinizing hormone pulsatility in normal women and in women with stress-related anovulation. J. Clin. Endocrinol. Metab. **80:** 818–823.

Diagnostic and Therapeutic Approach to Hypothalamic Amenorrhea

ALESSANDRO D. GENAZZANI, FEDERICA RICCHIERI,
CHIARA LANZONI, CLAUDIA STRUCCHI, AND VALERIO M. JASONNI

*Department of Obstetrics and Gynecology, Gynecological Endocrinology Center,
University of Modena and Reggio Emilia, Modena, Italy*

ABSTRACT: Hypothalamic amenorrhea (HA) is a secondary amenorrhea
with no evidence of endocrine/systemic causal factors, mainly related to
various stressors affecting neuroendocrine control of the reproductive
axis. In clinical practice, HA is mainly associated with metabolic, physical, or psychological stress. Stress is the adaptive response of our body
through all its homeostatic systems, to external and/or internal stimuli
that activate specific and nonspecific physiological pathways. HA occurs generally after severe stressant conditions/situations such as dieting, heavy training, or intense emotional events, all situations that can
induce amenorrhea with or without body weight loss and HA is a secondary amenorrhea with a diagnosis of exclusion. In fact, the diagnosis
is essentially based on a good anamnestic investigation. It has to be investigated using the clinical history of the patient: occurrence of menarche,
menstrual cyclicity, time and modality of amenorrhea, and it has to be
exclude any endocrine disease or any metabolic (i.e., diabetes) and systemic disorders. It is necessary to identify any stressant situation induced
by loss, family or working problems, weight loss or eating disorders, or
physical training or agonist activity. Peculiar, though not specific, endocrine investigations might be proposed but no absolute parameter can
be proposed since HA is greatly dependent from individual response to
stressors and/or the adaptive response to stress. This article tries to give
insights into diagnosis and putative therapeutic strategies.

KEYWORDS: hypothalamic amenorrhea; stress; GnRH; weight loss;
β-endorphin; hypogonadotropic amenorrhea; hypoestrogenism

INTRODUCTION

Hypothalamic amenorrhea (HA) is a secondary amenorrhea with no evidence of endocrine/systemic causal factors, mainly related to various stressors

Address for correspondence: Alessandro Genazzani, M.D., Ph.D., Clinica Ostetrica Ginecologica,
University of Modena and Reggio Emilia, Via del Pozzo 71, 41100 Modena, Italy. Voice: 39-059-
4222278; fax: 39-059-42224394.
e-mail: algen@unimo.it

Ann. N.Y. Acad. Sci. 1092: 103–113 (2006). © 2006 New York Academy of Sciences.
doi: 10.1196/annals.1365.009

affecting neuroendocrine control of the reproductive axis. The disappearance of menstrual cyclicity is related to a dysfunction of hypothalamic signals to the pituitary gland, resulting in a failure of the ovarian function with no ovulation. The term "hypothalamic" refers to the hypothalamus, an area at the base of the brain that acts as a "hormone control center" for the many biological functions and activities and among them is the control of the reproductive functions and ovarian function.

Typically, women who are affected by this condition have no structural abnormalities of the hypothalamus or of the rest of the reproductive axis (i.e., pituitary gland and ovaries). Usually, HA is also indicated as "functional amenorrhea" and the diagnosis is that of exclusion since women with this disorder have no systemic causal factors, no endocrine disease (such as thyroid or prolactin [PRL] dysfunctions), and no central nervous system (CNS) disease or lesion such as tumor or trauma. HA occurs with a random frequency not different throughout the fertile life, as reported in a group of randomly sampled postmenarcheal women.[1] In fact, this disorder is not limited to a restricted period of a woman's reproductive life but may occur at any age.

NEUROENDOCRINE DISORDERS IN MENSTRUAL CYCLICITY

In clinical practice, HA is mainly associated with metabolic, physical, or psychological stress. Stress is the adaptive response of our body through all its homeostatic systems, to external and/or internal stimuli that activate specific and nonspecific physiological pathways. HA generally occurs after severe stressant conditions/situations such as dieting, heavy training, or intense emotional events—all situations that can induce amenorrhea with or without body weight loss.[2] A specific correlation exists between loss of weight and amenorrhea[2] when loss of weight is below a critical point and the ratio between fat and muscular mass is severely reduced, and loss of menstrual cyclicity is a typical occurrence. In fact, after dieting as well as during intense training of dancers or runners (excessive consumption of energies) amenorrhea is a frequent symptom.[3] Indeed, the low ratio may be due both to high energy consumption and reduced food intake, since the best performance in athletics is also linked to an equilibrium between lean mass (i.e., muscles) and body weight, where body weight is usually kept at the lower levels. Psychological stressors such as emotional, familial, or working problems may have a negative impact on food intake. Reduced food intake can induce amenorrhea through specific metabolic signals, which amplify the stress response to fasting.[4] Associated with psychological stressor(s) recorded as heavy negative event(s), many patients often show affective disorders (neuroticism, somatization, anxiety) and this mix of situations leads to the disruption of the hypothalamus–pituitary activity controlling the ovarian function.[5]

These cascades of situations negatively affect gonadotropin-releasing hormone (GnRH) release and the reproductive axis, activating or inhibiting hypothalamic and/or extra-hypothalamic areas in the brain as well as acting in the periphery. In particular, one of the key events of this modulatory action is played by neurotransmitters and neuropeptides produced in the central nervous system. These neuronal pathways are sensitive to external and internal environmental change (light–dark cycle, temperature), as well as to cognitive, social, cultural, and emotional events. Each of these signals may become stressor agents when acute changes occur, and through integration with the hormonal signals they can stimulate while adapting responses.

On the basis of what has been described above, the ovarian failure typically occurring in patients affected by HA represents the adaptive mechanism to stress, so that the reproductive axis activity is reduced/blocked. Such a blockade of the reproductive function is reversible but it occurs in such critical conditions that reproduction is not considered essential for the survival of those women. Poly- or oligomenorrhea are some intermediate steps that can anticipate the occurrence of the amenorrheic condition, which is the last and worst stage of this clinically adaptive response to stress.

PHYSIOPATHOLOGY OF STRESS-INDUCED HYPOTHALAMIC AMENORRHEA

HA[6–8] is a model of hypogonadism characterized by several neuroendocrine aberrations that occur after a relatively long period of exposure to a repetitive and/or chronic stressor(s) so as to affect the neuroendocrine hypothalamic activity[9,10] as well as the release of several hypophyseal hormones.[8,10–14] The reproductive axis is severely altered in these patients and both the opioid and dopaminergic systems have been proposed as potential mediators of stress-related amenorrhea in humans.[15,16]

As demonstrated in experimental studies in monkeys and rats, the common response to stressors is the increase of adrenocorticotropin hormone (ACTH) and cortisol plasma levels that activate lipolysis and glycogenolysis-like compensatory mechanisms. In animals it has been demonstrated that the intraventricular injection of corticotropin-releasing hormone (CRF) reduces GnRH and luteinizing hormone (LH) release.[17,18] Since the corticotropin-releasing hormone (CRF) is the specific hypothalamic stimulating factor for ACTH, elevation of ACTH in response to stress is anticipated by the elevation of CRF stimulation. Evidence of a central site of action for CRF in blocking GnRH-induced LH release is demonstrated by the fact that CRF antagonists reverse the stress-induced LH decrease in rats.[17] CRF elevation as an adaptive response to stress is also responsible for the increase of central β-endorphin (βEP) release. This last is probably the most important peptide of the endogenous opioid peptides (EOPs) family and is a potent inhibitor of GnRH-LH secretion. Because of this evidence a connection has been suggested between the activation of the hypothalamus–pituitary–adrenal (HPA) axis and the stress inhibition of the hypothalamus—pituitary–gonadal (HPG) axis.[11] Since naloxone, a specific opiod receptor antagonist, is able to counteract the CRF-induced LH secretory blockade,[19] opiod peptides have been considered the key factors in the stress-induced inhibition of the HPG axis. Moreover, the stress-induced hyperactivation of the CRF–ACTH–adrenal axis is able to determine an exaggerated secretion of cortisol from the adrenal glands. Such a situation induces higher cortisolemia in patients affected by HA and negatively modulates adrenal response to stress. In fact, it has been reported that these patients, though showing hypercortisolemia in basal condition, resulted in having a reduced response to exogenous ACTH stimulation.[20] Such data confirmed that though in baseline conditions the adrenal gland is overstimulated, the maximum response of cortisol to external stimuli remains the same. This means that the delta, which is the difference between the maximal cortisol response to the stimulation and the baseline level before the stimulation, is reduced. Clinically, this means that the adrenal gland produces a lower amount of cortisol when the stressant situation hits.

Peripheral hormonal signals, such as glucocorticoid hormones or PRL, are also activated by stress and are able to act as stress-induced hormonal signals. In fact, cortisol itself exerts a suppressive effect on GnRH-stimulated LH release[21] and such action mainly takes place at the pituitary level but it cannot be concluded that an additional negative effect may be present in extrapituitary areas, indirectly inhibiting LH secretion.[22] Also, PRL increases and responds to external stimuli such as emotional and physical events as well as internal rhythms such as sleep. This mechanism has been extensively studied in the rat[23] and is mediated by the activation of several stimulating factors like thyrotropin-releasing hormone, vasoactive intestinal peptide, oxytocin, or by the failure of the dopaminergic control that antagonizes prolactin. The final result of stress-related hormone responses is a negative effect both on gonadotropin secretion and gonadal steroid biosynthesis.

HORMONAL PROFILE IN HYPOTHALAMIC AMENORRHEA

HA is a secondary hypogonadism characterized by several aberrations in the hypophyseal and ovarian hormones' plasma levels, as well as in their release. The typical hypogonadal situations are sustained by reduced LH plasma levels, in part activated by stress-induced endogenous opioid hypertone. Typically, in these HA patients FSH plasma levels results are normal. Women affected by HA are usually characterized by two possible situations: (1) hypogonadotropinism, with LH equal or less than 3 mLU/mL or (2) normogonadotropinism, with LH more than 3 mLU/mL.

Usually, in HA patients, especially in hypogonadotropic patients, LH pulsatile secretion is characterized by a pulse amplitude significantly reduced while pulse frequency is higher than what can be observed in eumenorrheic women.[8] In some HA patients LH pulses can only be observed during the night as in prepuberal girls. In addition, LH response to exogenous GnRH may be lower than that in women with normal menstrual cycles.

These alterations in the secretion of hypophyseal hormones deeply influence ovarian activity, inducing the blockade of follicular maturation and the typical condition of hypoestrogenism. In these women most of the circulating estrogens derive from peripheral conversion of androgens, especially in the muscle tissue. The hypoestrogenic condition, especially if present for several months up to 1 year, might induce metabolic consequences, affecting, in particular, specific tissues such as bone tissue. In fact, bone mass peak might be affected and reduced so that showing osteopenia may expose the patient to the risk of reduced bone mass density during fertile life and perimenopausal period, which results in a major risk of pathological fractures. Hypoestrogenism also induces the increase of total cholesterol, VLDL, LDL, and triglyceride levels and the reduction of sex hormone binding globulin (SHBG) synthesis and release. This latter event can induce a higher rate of unbound androgen, which is biologically active. This condition of relative hyperandrogenism can easily induce the occurrence of mild/severe hirsutism and acne.

When stressant conditions are chronic, the HPA axis might be activated at higher levels for a long time interval. It can frequently be observed that in a discreet group of patients with HA there might be high and steady levels of cortisol, higher than 25 mg/L. Chronic activation of adrenal pathways determines a lower response of adrenal gland to endogenous as well as exogenous ACTH (i.e., ACTH stimulation test) in amenorrheic women than in eumenorrheic women, and this is due to the fact that in HA patients the adrenal gland is already highly activated and the adrenal response to ACTH cannot be higher than what has been observed as the maximal response.[24]

In HA PRL levels are normal or lower than in women with normal cyclicity, and this can be explained by the dopaminergic hypertone that inhibits PRL secretion. Moreover, in women with HA, and in particular in women with anorexia or with excessive restrictive feeding, hypothyroidism with low plasma levels of fT3 and fT4 and a relative increase of TSH plasma levels are frequent. These features characterize the so-called "low fT3 syndrome" where fT3 is reduced due to the fact that "reverse" T3, the biologically inactive analogue of fT3, is produced in a higher amount. The reverse T3 is not able to induce metabolic effects on the cells and this is a defensive system, especially for patients with feeding restriction or excessive energy consumption. In addition, the thyroid gland shows that lower basal metabolism is also reduced and limits the energy dispersion for heat production. In fact, these patients typically have cooler skin and wear heavy dresses in comparison to the other (eumenorrheic) subjects.

DIAGNOSTIC APPROACH

HA is a secondary amenorrhea with a diagnosis of exclusion. In fact, the diagnosis is essentially based on a good anamnestic investigation. The clinical history of the patient—occurrence of menarche, menstrual cyclicity, time and modality of amenorrhea—is investigated. Any endocrine disease or any metabolic (i.e., diabetes) and systemic disorders are excluded and it is important to identify any stressant situation induced by loss, family or working problems, weight loss, or eating disorders, resulting from physical training or agonist activity. All these are the main causal factors of stress-induced HA. Obviously, a clinical check is important for evaluating weight and body composition, computing body mass index (BMI = weight in kg/height in m^2), looking for physical signs of weight loss/anorexia like deterioration, hirsutism, hypoproteinemia, hypothermia, thin skin, and face and legs edema (these latter are induced by hypoproteinemia). It is important to exclude other kinds of amenorrhea such as hyperandrogenic amenorrhea (the signs are acne, hirsutism, seborrhea), hyperPRL (the signs are galactorrhea, cephalalgia), and visual disorders (that lead to the suspicion of pituitary micro/macro adenomas).

The third step is the evaluation of the hormonal profile in the baseline condition. It is important to evaluate LH, FSH, estradiol, androgens (testosterone, androstenedione, DHEA, DHEAS), cortisol, prolactin, thyroid hormones (TSH, fT3, fT4), and thyroid autoantibodies (anti-TPO, anti-TG, and anti-TSHr). The hepatic function, total proteins, albumin, sideremia, amylase, and lipid profile must also be evaluated. Though most of the diagnostic approach can be performed with a simple baseline determination, in some cases additional investigation might be more helpful to better study the physiopathological condition for that single patient. These kinds of exams can be done in specific centers where the dynamic endocrine stimulation tests can be organized. Among them the most useful are: the pulsatility study of LH and FSH (sampling every 10–15 min for 4–6 h) to assess the gonadotropin profile and to classify the type of LH pulses and the type of amenorrhea (normo- or hypogonadotropinemic); the GnRH test to evaluate LH and FSH pituitary responses; and the naloxone test to assess whether the opioidergic tone is responsible of the gonadotropin dysfunction. In women with stress-induced HA, LH response to naloxone infusion is considered positive when LH is increased more than two times the baseline levels. It is also necessary to mention that a negative response does not exclude the presence of the opioidergic hypertone since this might be so high that the amount of naloxone infused is not effective in counteracting it.

THERAPEUTIC STRATEGIES

The approach to HA must always be considered as stereoscopic, in the sense that more than one factor is always involved in the genesis of the functional blockage of the reproductive system. Therefore, more than one therapeutical approach might be needed.

If eating disorders are present, it is important to reduce the negative modulation/action induced by starvation, energy imbalance, and/or training as well as all the psychological disturbances. Obviously, it is very important to increase the quality of food with more proteins in the diet and probably psychological support might be suggested.

In case opioidergic hypertone is suspected as one of the pathogenetic mechanisms of HA, the therapeutic administration of an opioid receptor blocker, such as naltrexone cloridrate, might be proposed. Naltrexone is usually administered at a dose of 50 mg/die per os for several weeks (up to 3–6 months). Some clinical trials have reported the occurrence of menstrual cyclicity within 2–6 months.[35] It is important to note that a higher rate of success has been demonstrated in patients that are responsive to the naloxone test.[33]

Another possible therapeutic strategy is the use of acetyl-L-carnitine (ALC). In fact, ALC has been reported to act on the central cholinergic, serotoninergic, and dopaminergic systems[25–27] and to modulate some neuronal activities. For this reason ALC administration has also been used to improve the central nervous activities in patients affected by dementia.[28] The results of some studies[33] showed that ALC is active on the HPG axis function in hypogonadotropinemic patients. A 6 months ALC administration was able to induce the increase of both LH and PRL plasma levels and the LH pulse amplitude. The effect on PRL in hypogonadotropic amenorrhea supports the positive modulation of ALC either directly on pituitary function or through the increased estrogen milieu.[33] Indeed, ALC administration has been reported to increase GnRH-induced LH response in rats[29] as well as in women.[33] These observations support the fact that ALC is active in those hypothalamic areas involved in the activation/maturation of the hypothalamo-pituitary axis. It has been proposed that these effects might be due to the fact that carnitine derived from ALC increases the amount of the intra-mitochondrial carnitine, improving the transportation of free fatty acids in Krebb's cycle. This observation might explain the higher rate of success on patients with hypogonadotropic HA and weight loss and/or high energy consumption.

Among the mediator(s) of opiatergic and/or dopaminergic systems[30–35] in HA, a role has also been proposed for gamma-aminobutyric acid (GABA), an important modulator of the physiological response to stress or anxiety.[36] In fact, various acute and chronic stressors have been shown to produce a rapid decrease in the activity of GABAergic pathways in primates and in humans.[37,38] The fact that stress and anxiety stimulate both the secretion of corticotropin-releasing factor (CRF) and modulate GABAergic neurons, suggests a possible functional interaction between these two systems. Indeed, GABAergic or benzodiazepine receptor-mediated mechanisms inhibit CRF release,[39] and anxiolytic benzodiazepines can reverse or antagonize in experimental animals several CRF-mediated behavioral effects that are thought to be related to stress.[40,41]

Recently, a new neurotropic compound, pivagabine (PVG), a hydrophobic-4 aminobutyric acid derivative,[42] has been shown to exert specific effects on stress-induced activities in rats.[42,43] Experimental data also showed specific inhibitory actions of PVG on some behavioral parameters in rats exposed to various stressors,[47] probably acting indirectly on GABA receptor type A (GABA$_A$).[37,38] Since PVG prevents the reduction of hypothalamic contents of CRF and its discharge from hypothalamic neurons[44] in rats, it has been supposed that PVG might modulate the adaptative response to stress. When PVG was administered to a group of patients with HA specific modulation of GH, ACTH and cortisol secretions were observed.[53] These data sustained the role of anti-stress activity of this compound in patients with highly activated HPA axis[45] and quite often in the presence of a disturbed metabolic balance,[46] all of them being causal factors of the reproductive failure of these patients. In addition, PVG has been reported to reduce anxiety and depression in post-menopausal women.[48] Probably, PVG modulates the release of hypothalamic CRF and/or pituitary ACTH, and this last observation is in agreement with the fact that the increased GH release might also be related to the PVG-induced decrease of the CRF hypothalamic tone. In fact, CRF is involved in GH regulation and acute CRF administration inhibits GHRH-induced GH secretion probably through a higher somatostatin release.[52,53]

In conclusion, HA is quite a complex syndrome. Diagnostic criteria are not so easy to identify since any other systemic causal factors that might be the basis of the amenorrheic condition have to be excluded. It must be kept in mind that all kinds of stressors (physical, metabolic, and psychological) are always deeply and tightly involved in the genesis of the reproductive failure and it is almost impossible to exclude their combination. This means that HA needs a stereoscopic diagnosis, with a balanced analysis of all clinical and anamnestic data. Endocrinological as well as gynecological and psychological evaluation are important, thus confirming that the gynecologist of this modern era also needs to be well trained in fields close to gynecology or reproductive medicine such as internal medicine and psychology.

REFERENCES

1. BATRINOS, M.L., C. PANITSA-FAFLIA, N. COURCOUTSAKIS & V. CHATZIPAVLOU. 1990. Incidence, type, and etiology of menstrual disorders in the age group 12–19 years. Adolesc. Pediatr. Gynecol. **3:** 149–153.
2. FRISCH, R.E. & J.W. MCARTHUR. 1974. Menstrual cycles: fatness as a determinant of minumun weight for height necessary for their maintenance or onset. Science **185:** 949–951.
3. VELDHUIS, J.D., W.S. EVANS & L.M. DEMERS. 1985. Altered neuroendocrine regulation of gonadotropin secretion in women distance runners. J. Clin. Endocrinol. Metab. **61:** 557–562.

4. CAMERON, J.L., D.L. HELMREICH & D.A. SCHREIHOFER.1993. Modulation of reproductive hormone secretion by nutritional intake: stress signals versus metabolic signals. Hum. Reprod. **8:** 162–167.
5. FACCHINETTI, F., M. FAVA, L. FIORONI, *et al.* 1993. Stressful life events and affective disorders inhibit pulsatile LH secretion in hypothalamic amenorrhea. Psychoneuroendocrinology **18:** 397–404.
6. CANNAVO, S. & F. TRIMARCHI. 2001. Exercise-related female reproductive dysfunction. J Endocrinol Invest **24:** 823–832.
7. AMERICAN PSYCHIATRIC ASSOCIATION. 1995. Diagnostic and Statistical Manual of Mental Disorders, 4th ed. American Psychiatric Association. Washington, DC.
8. GENAZZANI, A.D., F. PETRAGLIA, G. FABBRI, *et al.* 1990. Evidence of luteinizing hormone secretion in hypothalamic amenorrhea associated with weight loss. Fertil. Steril. **54:** 222–226.
9. VIGERSKY, R.A., A.E. ANDERSEN, R.H. THOMPSON & D.L. LAURIAUX. 1977. Hypothalamic dysfunctuion in secondary amenorrhea associated with weight loss. N. Engl. J. Med. **297:** 1141–1146.
10. BERGA, S.L., S.F. MORTOLA, L. GIRTON, *et al.* 1989. Neuroendocrine aberrations in women with functional hypothalamic amenorrhea. J. Clin. Endocrinol. Metab. **68:** 301–308.
11. GENAZZANI, A.D., F. PETRAGLIA, M. GASTALDI, *et al.* 1993. FSH secretory pattern and degree of concordance with LH in amenorrheic, fertile and postmenopausal women. Am. J. Physiol. **264:** E776–E781.
12. GENAZZANI, A.D., F. PETRAGLIA, R. BENATTI, *et al.* 1991. Luteinizing hormone (LH) secretory burst duration is independent from LH, prolactin, or gonadal steroid plasma levels in amenorrheic women. J. Clin. Endocrinol. Metab. **72:** 1220–1225.
13. GENAZZANI, A.D., F. PETRAGLIA, M. GASTALDI, *et al.* 1994. Episodic release of prolactine in women with weight loss releated amenorrhea. Gynecol. Endocrinol. **8:** 95–100.
14. FIORONI, L., M. FAVA, A.D. GENAZZANI, *et al.* 1994. Life events impact in patients with secondary amenorrhea. J. Psychosom. Res. **6:** 617–622.
15. QUIGLEY, M.E., K.L. SHEEHAN, R.F. CASPER & S.S. YEN. 1980. Evidence for increased dopaminergic and opioid activity in patients with hypothalamic hypogonadotropic amenorrhea. J. Clin. Endocrinol. Metab. **50:** 949–954.
16. PETRAGLIA, F., A.E. PANERAI, C. RIVIER, *et al.* 1988. Opioid control of gonadotropin secretion. *In* Brain and Female Reproductive Function. A.R. Genazzani, U. Montemagno, C. Nappi, F. Petraglia, Eds.: 65–72. Parthenon. Carnforth, UK.
17. RIVIER, C., V. RIVIER & W. VALE. 1986. Stress-induced inhibition of reproductive functions: role of endogenous corticotropin-releasing factor. Science **231:** 607–609.
18. PETRAGLIA, F., S. SUTTON, W. VALE & P. PLOTSKY. 1987. Corticotropin-releasing factor decrease plasma luteinizing hormone levels in female rats by inhibiting gonadotropin-releasing hormone release into hypophyseal portal circulation. Endocrinology **120:** 1083–1088.
19. PETRAGLIA, F., W. VALE & C. RIVIER. 1986. Opioids act centrally to modulate stress-induced decrease in luteinizing hormone in the rat. Endocrinology **119:** 2445–2450.
20. NAPPI, R.E., F. PETRAGLIA, A.D. GENAZZANI, *et al.* 1993. Hypothalamic amenorrhea: evidence for a central derangement of hypothalamic-pituitary-adrenal cortex axis activity. Fertil. Steril. **59:** 571–576.

21. RINGSTROM, S.J., D. SUTER, J. D'AGOSTINO, *et al.* 1991. Effects of glucocorticoids on the hypothalamic-pituitary-gonadal axis. *In* Stress and Related Disorders from Adaptation to Dysfunction. A.R. Genazzani, G. Nappi, F. Petraglia and E. Martignoni, Eds.: 297–305. Parthenon. Carnforth, UK.

22. KAMEL, F. & C.L. KUBAJAK. 1987. Modulation of gonadotropic secretion by corticosterone interaction with gonadal steroids and mechanism of action. Endocrinology **121:** 561–568.

23. GALA, R.R. 1990. The physiology and mechanisms of stress-induced changes in prolactine secretion in rat. Life Sci. **46:** 1407–1410.

24. BLAZEJ, M., A. TONETTI, P. MONTELEONE, *et al.* 2000. Hypothalamic amenorrhea with normal body weight: ACTH, allopregnanolone and cortisol responses to corticotropinreleasing hormone test. Eur. J. Endocrin. **142:** 280–285.

25. ONOFRJ, M., I. BODIS-WOLLNER, P. POLA & M. CALVANI. 1983. Central cholinergic effects of levo-acetyl-carnitine. Drugs. Exp. Clin. Res. **9:** 161–167.

26. JANIRI, L. & E. TEMPESTA. 1983. A pharmacological profile of the effects of carnitine and acetyl-L-carnitine on the central nervous system. Int. J. Clin. Pharmacol. Res. **3:** 295–306.

27. TEMPESTA, E., L. JANIRI, C. PIRRONCELLI. 1985. Stereospecific effects of acetyl-L-carnitine on the spontaneous activity of brain stem neuronesa and their responses to acethylcoline and serotonin. Neuropharmacology **24:** 43–50.

28. TESTA, G. & C. ANGELINI. 1981. A preliminary trial with acetyl-L-carnitine (A-Cn) in dementia. Current Reports in Neurology **5:** 4–16.

29. KRSMANOVIC, L.Z., M.A. VIRMANI, S.S. STOJIKOVIC & K.J. CATT. 1992. Actions of acetyl-L-carnitine on gonadotrophin secretion. Gynecol. Endocrinol. **6** (Suppl 1): **11**.

30. QUIGLEY, M.E. & S.S.C. YEN. 1980. The role of endogenous opiates on LH secretion during the menstrual cycle. J. Clin. Endocrinol. Metab. **51:** 179–181.

31. PETRAGLIA, F., G. D'AMBROGIO, G. COMITINI, *et al.* 1985. Impairment of opiod control of luteinizing hormone secretion in menstrual disorders. Fertil. Steril. **43:** 535–540.

32. PETRAGLIA, F., C. PORRO, F. FACCHINETTI, *et al.* 1986. Opioid control of LH secretion in humans: menstrual cycle, menopause and aging reduce effect of naloxone but not of morphine. Life Sci. **38:** 2103–2110.

33. GENAZZANI, A.D., F. PETRAGLIA, I. ALGERI, *et al.* 1991. Acetyl-L-carnitine as possible drug in the treatment of hypothalamic amenorrhea. Act. Obstet. Gynecol. Scand. **70:** 487–492.

34. WILDT, L., G. LEYENDECKER, T. SIR-PETERMANN & S. WAIBEL-TREBER. 1993. Treatment with naltrexone in hypothalamic ovarian failure: induction of ovulation and pregnancy. Hum. Reprod. **8:** 350–358.

35. GENAZZANI, A.D., F. PETRAGLIA, M. GASTALDI, *et al.* 1995. Naltrexone treatment restores menstrual cycles in patients with weight loss related amenorrhea. Fertil. Steril. **64:** 951–956.

36. BIGGIO, G., E. SANNA, M. SERRA, E. COSTA. 1995. GABAa receptors and anxiety. In Advances in Biochemistry and Psychopharmacology, G. Biaggio, **vol 48**. Raven Press, New York, NY.

37. BIGGIO, G., A. CONCAS, M.G. CORDA, *et al.* 1990. GABAergic and dopaminergic trasmission in the rat cerebral cortex: effect of stress, anxiolytic and anxiogenic drugs. Pharmacol. Ther. **48:** 121–142.

38. CONCAS, A., M. SERRA, T. ATSOGGIU & G. BIGGIO. 1988. Foot shock and anxuiogenic beta-carbolines increase t-[35S]-butylbicyclophosphorotionate binding in

the rat cerebral cortex, an effect opposite to anxiolytic and gamma-aminobutyric acid mimetics. J. Neurochem. **51**: 1868–1876.

39. KALOGERAS, K.T., A.E. CALOGERO, T. KURIBAYIASHI, *et al.* 1990. *In vitro* and *in vivo* effects of triazolobenzodiazepine alprazolam and hypothalamic-pituitary-adrenal function: pharmacological and clinical implications. J. Clin. Endocrinol. Metab. **70**: 1462–1471.

40. IMAKI, T. & W. VALE. 1993. Chordiazepoxide attenuates stress-induced accumulation of corticotropin releasing factor mRNA in paraventricularnucleous. Brain Res. **623**: 223–228.

41. IMAKI, T., W. XIAO-QUAN, Y. SHIBASAKI, *et al.* 1995. Chlordiazepoxide attenuates stress-induced activation of neurons, corticotropin-releasing factor (CRF), gene transcription and CRF biosynthesis in the paraventricular nucleus (PVN). Mol Brain Res. **32**: 261–270.

42. GALZIGNA, L., L. GARBIN, M. BIANCHI & A. MARZOTTO. 1978. Properties of two derivatives of gamma-aminobutyric acid (GABA) capable of abolishing Cardiazol- and bicuculline-induced convulsions in the rat. Arch. Int. Pharmacodyn. Ther. **235**: 73–85.

43. ESPOSITO, G. & M.R. LUPARINI. 1997. Pivagabine: a novel psychoactive drug. Arzneim Forsch Drug Res. **47**: 1306–1309.

44. SERRA, M., A. CONCAS, M.C. MOSTALLINO, *et al.* 1999. Antagonism by pivagabine of stress-induced changes in GABAa receptor function and corticotropin-releasing factor concentrations in rat brain. Psychoneuroendocrinology **24**: 269–284.

45. M. FERIN. 1999. Stress and the reproductive cycle. J Clin Endocrinol Metab **84**: 1768–1774.

46. CAMERON, J.L. 1996. Regulation of reproductive hormone secretion in primates by short-term changes in nutrition. Rev. Reprod. **1**: 117–126.

47. SCAPAGNINI, U. & M. MATERA. 1997. Effects of pivagabine on psychophysical performance and behavioural response in experimental models of stress. Arznein Forsch Drug Res. **47**: 1310–1317.

48. GIGLIOLI, B., A. MULTINU & V.R. LAI. 1997. Role of pivagabine in the treatment of climacteric syndrome. Arzneim Forsch Drug Res. **47**: 1317–1321.

49. BRITTON, K.T., G. LEE & G.F. KOOB. 1988. Corticotropin releasing factor and amphetamine exaggerate partial agonist properties of benzodiazepine antagonist Ro 15-1788 in the conflict test. Psychopharmacolgy **94**: 306–311.

50. DE BOER, S.F., J.L. SLANGER & J. VAN DE GUTNER. 1995. Brain benzodiazepine receptor control of stress hormones. *In* Stress, Neuroendocrine and Molecular Approaches. R. Kvetnasky, R. Mc Carty, J. Axelrod, Eds.: 719–734. Gordon and Breach. New York, NY.

51. OWENS, M.J., G. BISSETTE & C.B. NEMEROFF. 1989. Acute effects of alprazolam and adinazolam on the concentrations of corticotropin-releasing factor in the rat brain. Synapse **4**: 196–202.

52. BARBARINO, A., S.M. CORSELLO, S. DELLA CASA, *et al.* 1990. Corticotropin-releasing hormone inhibition of growth hormone-releasing hormone-induced growth hormone release in man. J. Clin. Endocrinol. Metab. **71**: 1368–1374.

53. GENAZZANI, A.D., M. STOMATI, C. BERSI, *et al.* 2000. Pivagabine decreases stress-related hormone secretion in women with hypothalamic amenorrhea. J. Endocrinol. Invest. **23**: 526–532.

Use of Cognitive Behavior Therapy for Functional Hypothalamic Amenorrhea

SARAH L. BERGA AND TAMMY L. LOUCKS

*Department of Gynecology and Obstetrics, Emory University School of
Medicine, Atlanta, Georgia, USA*

ABSTRACT: Behaviors that chronically activate the hypothalamic-
pituitary-adrenal (HPA) axis and/or suppress the hypothalamic-
pituitary-thyroidal (HPT) axis disrupt the hypothalamic-pituitary-
gonadal axis in women and men. Individuals with functional
hypothalamic hypogonadism typically engage in a combination of behaviors that concomitantly heighten psychogenic stress and increase
energy demand. Although it is not widely recognized clinically, functional forms of hypothalamic hypogonadism are more than an isolated
disruption of gonadotropin-releasing hormone (GnRH) drive and reproductive compromise. Indeed, women with functional hypothalamic
amenorrhea display a constellation of neuroendocrine aberrations that
reflect allostatic adjustments to chronic stress. Given these considerations, we have suggested that complete neuroendocrine recovery would
involve more than reproductive recovery. Hormone replacement strategies have limited benefit because they do not ameliorate allostatic endocrine adjustments, particularly the activation of the adrenal and the
suppression of the thyroidal axes. Indeed, the rationale for the use of sex
steroid replacement is based on the erroneous assumption that functional
forms of hypothalamic hypogonadism represent *only or primarily* an alteration in the hypothalamic-pituitary-gonadal axis. Potential health consequences of functional hypothalamic amenorrhea, often termed stress-
induced anovulation, may include an increased risk of cardiovascular
disease, osteoporosis, depression, other psychiatric conditions, and dementia. Although fertility can be restored with exogenous administration
of gonadotropins or pulsatile GnRH, fertility management alone will not
permit recovery of the adrenal and thyroidal axes. Initiating pregnancy
with exogenous means without reversing the hormonal milieu induced
by chronic stress may increase the likelihood of poor obstetrical, fetal, or
neonatal outcomes. In contrast, behavioral and psychological interventions that address problematic behaviors and attitudes, such as cognitive
behavior therapy (CBT), have the potential to permit resumption of full
ovarian function along with recovery of the adrenal, thyroidal, and other
neuroendocrine aberrations. Full endocrine recovery potentially offers
better individual, maternal, and child health.

Address for correspondence: Dr. Sarah L. Berga, Department of Gynecology and Obstetrics,
Emory University School of Medicine, 1639 Pierce Drive, Room 4208-WMB, Atlanta, GA 30322.
Voice: 404-727-8600; fax: 404-727-8609.
 e-mail:sberga@emory.edu

Ann. N.Y. Acad. Sci. 1092: 114–129 (2006). © 2006 New York Academy of Sciences.
doi: 10.1196/annals.1365.010

KEYWORDS: stress; amenorrhea; anovulation; hypothyroidism; allostasis

CLINICAL AND PHYSIOLOGICAL BACKGROUND

The notion of a bidirectional interaction between behavior and reproductive function has been assumed by many (FIG. 1). Our expanding scientific knowledge permits us to refine our conceptualization of this interaction as well as to suggest holistic interventions intended to mitigate acute and chronic health burden. Because we can monitor the endocrine responses to thoughts, feelings, and behaviors, we now can specify how attitudes and behaviors gate hypothalamic-pituitary-gonadal and other neuroendocrine function.

Gonadal function depends directly upon secretion from the hypothalamus of gonadotropin-releasing hormone (GnRH). If a marked decline in endogenous pulsatile GnRH secretion occurs, pituitary secretion of luteinizing hormone (LH), and follicle-stimulating hormone (FSH) fall accordingly. In women, compromised folliculogenesis with luteal insufficiency or anovulation may result. Decreased GnRH pulsatility has been shown to be a common cause of anovulation and amenorrhea.[1] Decrements in central GnRH-LH/FSH drive exist on a continuum, however, and may vary from day to day.[2] Because of this potential variability in GnRH secretion, ovarian compromise exists as a spectrum and may manifest as amenorrhea, polymenorrhea, oligomenorrhea, or luteal phase deficiency with a preserved menstrual interval and luteal length. Clinically, decreased ovarian function can be occult or obvious. In men,

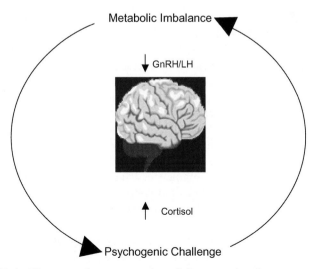

FIGURE 1. Diagrammatic representation of the synergism between metabolic and psychogenic stressors in the perpetuation of functional hypothalamic amenorrhea (FHA).

decreased central GnRH drive may cause oligoasthenozoospermia. Typically, gonadal compromise in men is clinically occult unless fertility is sought and the compromise is sufficiently significant to cause infertility. However, severe hypothalamic hypogonadism in men may present as decreased libido, diminished muscle mass, or altered hair growth.

The most common cause of reduced GnRH drive is functional; that is, it is not due to identifiable organic causes, such as hypothalamic tumors or pituitary adenomas. Functional hypothalamic hypogonadism can be defined as a common and theoretically reversible form of gonadal compromise in which psychophysiological and behavioral responses to life events activate central neuroregulator networks such that there is concomitant metabolic mobilization and reproductive suppression due to disruption of the GnRH pulse generator.[3] The GnRH pulse generator refers to a network of GnRH neurons diffusely distributed in the medial basal hypothalamus. Most, but not all, GnRH axons project to the median eminence, allowing pulses of GnRH to be released into the portal vasculature. GnRH neurons communicate with one another via synapses. Although GnRH neurons are endogenously pulsatile, their activity must be synchronized by GnRH-to-GnRH synapses for the GnRH bolus released into the portal vasculature to be of sufficient magnitude to trigger pituitary release of LH and FSH. The GnRH pulse generator is active during fetal and neonatal life [4] and then is inhibited or desynchronized by poorly defined central processes until the onset of puberty.[5–7] Puberty and ovulation are centrally driven processes that can be achieved by providing exogenous pulses of GnRH at a frequency of one pulse every 60 to 90 min [8–10] or by stimulating the dormant GnRH neuronal network with excitatory amino acids.[11]

The mechanisms that modulate the activity of the GnRH neuronal network or GnRH pulse generator are largely unknown. GnRH neurons have been demonstrated to receive synapses from neurons that contain GnRH, the endogenous opioid peptide β-endorphin,[12] NPY,[13] and catecholamines.[14–16] Other factors that modulate the frequency or activity of the GnRH pulse generator are thought to exert their effects indirectly by acting through the neuronal systems that have direct synaptic connections or by interacting with glial cells that interpose between synapses. For instance, progesterone slows the frequency of pulsatile GnRH release by increasing hypothalamic opioidergic tone. Peripheral substances may gain access to the GnRH neuronal network via specialized neurovascular cells that line the fenestrated blood–brain barrier at the level of the hypothalamus and median eminence.[17] It appears that the brain–gut axis communicates the metabolic state of an individual to the hypothalamic GnRH neurons, but the exact nature of these mechanisms remains to be better elucidated.[18]

Quantifying GnRH drive is tedious. In humans, GnRH pulsatile secretion can be inferred only from the pattern of LH secretion in the circulation. Blood samples must be obtained via an indwelling intravenous catheter at intervals of 10 to 15 min for durations of 12 to 24 h. Even so, inherent limitations

TABLE 1. Putative modulators of GnRH drive

• CRH	• Metabolic signals
• Opioids	• Sex steroids
• Adrenergic	• Gonadal peptides
• GABA	• Growth factors
• Dopamine	• Glial cells
• Serotonin	• GnRH
• Immune	• Other

exist in estimating GnRH secretion from peripheral LH patterns. Given these considerations, it is not surprising that documentation of the role of disturbed central GnRH drive as a cause of reduced ovarian function was accomplished only relatively recently.[19]

Technical limitations also plague recognition and quantification of stress and metabolic mobilization. The accuracy of psychometric inventories for assessing and quantifying stress, mood, and cognitive patterns is inherently constrained by reporting biases, while biochemical and biophysical indices of stress and metabolic mobilization are technically cumbersome and expensive to collect. Two primary systems that mediate the stress response are the hypothalamic corticotrophin-releasing hormone (CRH) and the locus coruleus–noradrenergic (LC-NE) neuronal networks and their respective effector systems, the pituitary–adrenal axis and the autonomic pathways.[20] While innumerable animal studies have demonstrated that activation of the hypothalmic-pituitary-adrenal (HPA) axis by a variety of stressful paradigms induces reproductive compromise, only a few studies have elucidated the mechanisms mediating the disruption of GnRH drive. Direct evidence exists for CRH, β-endorphin, dopamine, and vasopressin.[12,14,22–28] Recently, neuropeptide Y has been implicated as serving a neuromodulatory link between metabolic deficits induced by diet and exercise and reduced GnRH drive.[29] A key inhibitory neurotransmitter system in the brain uses γ-aminobutyric acid (GABA). GABA opens the same potassium channels in neurons of the mediobasal hypothalamus as μ-opioid receptor agonists, such as β-endorphin. GABA inhibited GnRH gene expression in rats [30] and suppressed pubertal GnRH increase in juvenile female rhesus monkeys,[31] but the role of GABA in human hypothalamic hypogonadism remains unclear. There are many metabolic signals that also might communicate the metabolic status of an individual to the hypothalamus. The exact role of these signals in functional hypothalamic hypogonadism also remains to be elucidated. A partial list of putative neuromodulators of GnRH activity or synchronicity is shown in TABLE 1.

PATHOGENESIS OF FHA

The best biochemical evidence supporting the concept that stress impairs ovarian function in women is the consistent demonstration that women with hypogonadotropic hypogonadism not due to defined organic conditions have higher cortisol levels than eumenorrheic, ovulatory women.[3,32,33] There is direct evidence that this relationship holds in women with athletic amenorrhea as well.[34,35] Loucks *et al.* observed an inverse relationship between the degree of ovarian compromise and the increase in circulating 24-h cortisol levels.[34] When compared with eumenorrheic but sedentary women, eumenorrheic athletes had less luteal progesterone secretion as evidenced by lower urinary levels of pregnanediol–glucuronide, fewer LH pulses in a day, and higher cortisol levels. Furthermore, amenorrheic athletes that were anovulatory had the fewest LH pulses in a day and the highest cortisol levels.

An inverse relationship holds between HPA axis activation, independent of the life events or behaviors that initiate or sustain this activation, and suppression of the hypothalamic GnRH drive to the ovary, as evidenced by marked reduction in the 24-h LH pulse frequency in women with functional forms of hypothalamic amenorrhea.[3,32,33,36] Other hypothalamic outputs also are altered in women with functional hypothalamic amenorrhea (FHA). Given the neuroanatomical integration of the hypothalamus, this is predictable. The purpose of the hypothalamus is to generate an "endocrine action plan" to preserve the organism in the face of challenge. Part of the action plan involves metabolic mobilization. However, metabolic mobilization involves more than an increase in cortisol secretion. In FHA, the HPT axis differs from that of eumenorrheic women in that TSH is not increased in response to decrements in thyronine and thyroxine. This pattern indicates an altered hypothalamic set point akin to what is seen in hospitalized patients who develop what is referred to as "sick euthyroid syndrome."[3] In athletic women, a similar alteration in the HPT was seen only in those who had compromised ovarian function.[37] The secretory patterns of growth hormone, prolactin, and melatonin also differed in FHA from those in eumenorrheic women.[3,38] The constellation of neuroendocrine aberrations that accompany FHA strongly suggests that central neurotransmission has been altered so as to allow homeostatic hypothalamic responses and, when chronic, a new allostatic state. The aim of these compensatory adjustments is to equip the individual to cope with actual and perceived challenge. In this context, then, the hypothalamus links the external environment, the internal milieu, and gonadal function.

The process of recovering from the allostatic state of FHA is less well documented. FHA is theoretically reversible. We first showed that women in the process of spontaneously recovering from FHA displayed cortisol levels comparable to those of eumenorrheic women before there was complete recovery of GnRH drive.[36] Further, a marked increase in TSH occurred before increases in thyroxine and thyronine. We then used cognitive behavior therapy (CBT) to catalyze reproductive recovery and showed that reproductive recovery did not require weight gain. This leaves open the question as to whether reproductive recovery is accompanied by full metabolic recovery. To date, there is limited data suggesting that hypothalamic recovery involves a sequence of interlinked adjustments starting with HPA restoration, return of GnRH pulsatility and reproductive recovery, and lastly remission of hypothalamic hypothyroidism.

The characteristic hypothalamic alterations associated with FHA only become problematic when ongoing challenges elicit a chronic (allostatic) rather than acute (homeostatic) response. The long-term consequences of persistent HPA activation have been studied in animal models and hippocampal neuron loss has been documented.[39] Further, persistent stress has been linked to acute and chronic health burden in humans.[40] For instance, recent data obtained in women with weight-restored anorexia nervosa who remained amenorrheic indicated that exogenous sex steroid replacement was unable to stimulate appropriate bone accretion.[41,42] Hormone exposure alone fails to compensate for the catabolic state induced by ongoing metabolic derangements, such as increased cortisol exposure, altered growth hormone action, or hypothalamic hypothyroidism. Because of the concomitant endocrine and metabolic disturbances, hypothalamic hypogonadism must be regarded as a condition deserving clinical attention even when fertility is not an immediate goal.

The central neuromodulators responsible for the initiation and maintenance of the disruption of GnRH are difficult to identify in humans. First, the factors that initiate the disruption may differ from neuroregulators that maintain the disruption. To study the initiating factors, one would need to intensely monitor populations at risk for the development of hypothalamic hypogonadism or try to induce hypothalamic hypogonadism in a nonhuman primate model. Once a chronic hypogonadal state had been reached, it theoretically would be possible to identify the agents that maintain this disruption by administering antagonists that cross the brain–blood barrier, by performing lumbar punctures and obtaining cerebrospinal fluid, or by performing neuroimaging studies with an appropriate ligand. To date, efforts to identify these neuromodulators in humans have yielded inconsistent results. Thus, naloxone, an opioidergic blocker, increased LH pulse frequency or levels in some, but not all, women with FHA.[43,44] Also, infusion of metoclopramide, a dopamine receptor blocker, to women with FHA accelerated LH pulse frequency in our laboratory, while that of eumenorrheic women remained constant.[45] To explore the hypothesis that the reduction in GnRH drive was maintained by CRH, vasopressin, β-endorphin, or a combination of these factors, we performed lumbar punctures to obtain rostral cerebrospinal fluid in women with FHA and those with eumenorrhea. This approach has revealed increased CRH in subjects with depression and anorexia nervosa, but we found that CRH levels were identical in women with FHA and eumenorrhea.[46] Vasopressin levels were similar, and surprisingly, β-endorphin levels were lower in women with FHA. These data argue against the suspected role for CRH or opioids in the maintenance of FHA and suggest that other factors may play a role once FHA has been established. One group reported that a single 2 mg dose of alprazolam, a GABA receptor agonist, decreased cortisol levels and increased LH pulse frequency from 0.8 to 2.0 pulses/8 h in women with stress-related anovulation, while its administration decreased LH pulse frequency in eumenorrheic women in the follicular phase.[47] We recently showed, using a monkey model, that stress-sensitive monkeys with reproductive compromise displayed altered prolactin and cortisol responses to the serotonergic agonist, fenfluramine, indicating an underlying reduction in serotonergic tone.[48] Further, stress-sensitive monkeys demonstrated increased cortisol secretion when behaviorally challenged, underscoring the notion that "stressfulness" is more of a characteristic of the individual than the stimulus. Other data suggest a possible indirect role for GABA neurons in the stress-induced neuromodulation of GnRH pulsatility. More recently, we have been interested in how metabolic challenge and energy deficits may alter the brain and induce vulnerability, including reproductive compromise, to subsequent psychogenic stressors. It appears that undernutrition heightens reactivity to subsequent psychosocial challenge, but the neural mechanisms mediating this relationship are not clear. Not surprisingly, the neurochemistry of stress and/or FHA is far from simple, and firm conclusions are not possible at present.

BEHAVIORAL CAUSES OF STRESS-INDUCED ANOVULATION

The variables that activate the adrenal axis and suppress the thyroidal axis while leading to reproductive quiescence are not always readily identifiable. It has been suggested that different stressors and behaviors elicit somewhat different central mechanisms, such that the signals that alter hypothalamic function are specific to the type of stressor. Indeed, this variability may well explain in part why the neurochemistry of stress is so complex. Psychosocial dilemmas are seen as activating those central pathways subserving perception, whereas exercise and weight loss are generally viewed as disturbing metabolic regulation. Although it seems logical that there is specificity in the neural or peripheral cascades that mediate the response to specific stressors, we have no method for clearly differentiating psychogenic from metabolic stress. Psychogenic stress has a metabolic cost and metabolic stressors, such as food restriction and excessive exercise, are often initiated to cope with psychogenic stress. However, until proven otherwise, the safest assumption is that stress comes in flavors and that some individuals are more sensitive than others to the same stressor or set of stressors.

The notion that stress comes in neurochemical flavors is supported by animal studies suggesting that there are subtle but distinct differences in the neuroendocrine responses to different stress paradigms.[49] Further, neuroendocrine and metabolic responses to acute exercise were greater in men whose HPA axis did not suppress when they were given dexamethasone before the exercise challenge.[50] These data indicate that the degree of HPA activation potentiates the neuroendocrine and metabolic responses to subsequent challenge. Conversely, Altemus et al. showed that lactating women are hyporesponsive to exercise challenge.[51] Taken together, these data buttress the notion that responses to a given stressor are gated not only by the stressor type, but also by the organism's preexisting hormonal and metabolic state. Thus, some individuals are more, and some less, reactive to similar stressors. Even the same individual may vary in terms of stress sensitivity, depending on prevalent nutrition and psychosocial status. Obviously, emotional valence and expectation also determine the extent to which psychosocial variables serve as psychogenic stressors. Our preliminary investigations in women who developed FHA unrelated to weight loss, excessive exercise, and definable psychiatric disorders indicated that a primary factor that distinguished women with FHA from those with definable causes of anovulation and those who were ovulatory was the presence of unrealistic expectations.[52] Fioroni [53] also found the women with FHA, as compared to eumenorrheic women or those with other causes of anovulation, held more negative attributions about recent life events. Kirschbaum[54] found that men who did not habituate when exposed to repeated psychogenic challenge viewed themselves as less attractive, had lower self-esteem, and reported being in a depressed mood more often. Apparently, unachievable ambitions or other cognitive distortions create vulnerability to life's inevitable challenges and likely heighten responsivity to metabolic stressors, such as exercise or food restriction. Potentially, the converse is true. Metabolic mobilization may augment reactivity to psychogenic stressors.

There can be no doubt that weight loss and exercise serve as metabolic stressors. In monkeys trained to run, it was shown that caloric supplementation reversed the anovulation induced by training.[55] Interestingly, the monkeys did not spontaneously develop a compensatory increase in appetite and had to be "bribed" with colorful candy to consume more calories. On the other hand, modest dietary restriction accompanied by small amounts of exercise greatly increased the proportion of monkeys who become anovulatory when presented with social stress. A prospective study of unselected women demonstrated that exercise and weight loss caused anovulation.[56] Likely, sufficient exercise and weight loss, independent of psychogenic stress, can alter metabolism to the point that GnRH pulsatility is disrupted. Loucks and Thurma [57] recently quantified the amount of energy restriction needed to impact GnRH drive by studying eumenorrheic women in the follicular phase. Energy balance was achieved by providing 45 kcal/kg of lean body mass (LBM) per day. Graded daily energy deficits of 10, 25, and 35 kcal/kg were then experimentally induced for 5 days. An energy deficit of 33% had no impact on LH pulse frequency whereas an energy deficit of about 75% induced a decline in LH pulse frequency of about 40%. The induction of an energy deficit resulted in a graded increase in the 24-h cortisol level. At an energy availability of 10 kcal/kg of LBM (75% deficit), the mean 24-h cortisol was increased by about 30%, which is the amount of increase typically seen in women with FHA. Much like the stress-sensitive monkeys, women whose luteal phase progesterone levels were lowest at the initiation of the energy restriction showed the greatest response to the imposed metabolic challenge. In most real-life situations, except for extreme circumstances, such as war or famine, metabolic deficits are not imposed, but rather, initiated by individuals in response to self-imposed expectations. Most women with FHA, when carefully evaluated, display more than one trait, state, or behavior capable of activating stress response cascades or inducing a mild metabolic deficit, but most do not have a profound metabolic deficit that alone would explain the reduction in central GnRH drive. Many of the behaviors, such as exercise, that independently suppress central reproductive drive but only at more extreme levels, may be initiated as coping responses to psychosocial dilemmas. Because of the synergism between metabolic and psychogenic stressors, a combination of multiple, small magnitude, mixed stressors may be potentially more disruptive of reproductive function than a single large stressor limited to one category.

To better understand how a combination of seemingly minor psychogenic and metabolic stressors might synergistically disrupt GnRH drive as demonstrated in our monkey model,[58] we compared endocrine responses to submaximal exercise in women with FHA to those in eumenorrhea.[59] Women with FHA displayed a larger increase in cortisol than ovulatory eumenorrheic women in response to exercise. Further, glucose responses between the two groups were divergent in that women with FHA showed a 10% decrease in glucose and EW only a 3% increase. Interestingly, these two groups did not differ at baseline with regard to cortisol or glucose levels. The decrement in glucose seen in FHA but not EW suggests latent metabolic imbalance and indicates that FHA are unable to meet the energetic demands of ongoing activities. Further, it is likely that the drop in glucose activates the HPA axis and is at least partly responsible for the sustained hypercortisolemia characteristically seen in FHA. Since metabolic signals modulate GnRH pulsatility, exercise-induced metabolic imbalance also likely contributes to ongoing reproductive suppression. These results also reveal why the endocrine effects of a stressor, such as exercise, depend on the preexisting allostatic state of the individual.

TREATMENT CONSIDERATIONS

In women, functional hypothalamic hypogonadism may not be recognized unless the menstrual interval is markedly short, long, irregularly irregular, or absent. Similarly, luteal phase insufficiency due to decreased hypothalamic drive may not be noted unless infertility results. Even then, it is notoriously difficult to document unless it is recurrent. Based on the foregoing concepts, the more clinically evident the ovarian compromise, the greater is the hypothalamic challenge and the more profound are the associated adrenal and thyroid derangements and sex steroid deprivation.

If a woman with functional hypothalamic hypogonadism is seeking to become pregnant, ovulation induction can be accomplished technically with exogenous administration of pulsatile GnRH therapy[9,10] or gonadotropins.

The obvious advantage of exogenous GnRH therapy is that it diminishes the risk of ovarian hyperstimulation and multiple gestation associated with gonadotropins. Clominphene citrate can be tried, but it may not work because it has a hypothalamic site of action and the hypothalamus is already not responding to decreased sex steroid secretion. There also is some concern that ovulation induction may place women with FHA at risk for premature labor and intrauterine growth retardation.[60] The parenting skills of women with FHA may be impaired because they are already overwhelmed and stressed prior to pregnancy and delivery and thus their children may be at risk for poor psychosocial development.[61] Further, a recent study showed that children born to mothers with clinically occult hypothyroidism due to autoimmune thyroiditis had a mean full-scale intelligence quotient that was seven points lower than the control population.[62] The women with clinically silent hypothyroidism had a 30% reduction in thyroxine, which is roughly what is observed in women with FHA. It is important to remember that maternal thyroxine is the only source of fetal thyroxine in the first trimester and the predominant fetal source in the second and third trimesters. Because the fetal brain requires an appropriate amount of thyroxine for neurogenesis, even small deficits in thyroxine may induce neurodevelopmental deficits. Increased maternal cortisol may also have independent effects upon fetal neurodevelopment and organogenesis. Recent evidence showed that severe stress, such as that associated with the unexpected death of a child increased the risk of congenital anomalies of the cranial neural crest eightfold.[63] Further, stress and its endocrine concomitants have been implicated as a cause of preterm delivery. It is not known if the endocrine concomitants associated with FHA pose a similar risk, but this is clearly a potential hazard if ovulation induction is undertaken before amelioration of the allostatic changes in the adrenal and thyroidal axes.

A popular approach to a woman with FHA who is not seeking immediately to become pregnant is to offer her hormone replacement. This approach is based on the presumption that sex steroid deprivation is the primary therapeutic issue. There are inherent limitations with this approach, however. First, data indicate that exogenous sex steroid exposure does not fully promote bone accretion or cardioprotection in the presence of ongoing metabolic derangements.[41,42] Second, the ongoing insults to the brain from chronic amplification of stress cascades go unchecked. Further, estrogen therapy does not correct hypothalamic hypothyroidism.[64] In short, hormone therapy may mask potentially deleterious processes that are unlikely to be ameliorated by hormone exposure alone. It is critical to remember that FHA is more than a disorder of reduced GnRH secretion.

Hormone therapy per se is unlikely to be harmful, but more than hormone administration is needed. The stress process needs to be interrupted. Although psychopharmacologic approaches have not been well studied, they probably could be used on an interim basis in special circumstances. The study of Judd *et al.* suggested that a short course of alprazolam might be effective in reducing

HPA activation and permitting hypothalamic-pituitary-ovarian recovery.[47] However, this approach would not be the best recommendation in a woman hoping to conceive because of the risk of fetal exposure to benzodiazepines. The optimal intervention is to reverse the stress process so that the hypothalamus recovers and gonadal function resumes. An integral goal of the treatment plan for women with functional hypothalamic hypogonadism is to help them identify and ameliorate sources of psychogenic and metabolic stress and to provide emotional support while coping mechanisms other than dieting or exercising are learned. Nonpharmacologic interventions, such as stress management, relaxation training, or psychoeducation empower individuals by fostering self-care and competency. In this regard, nonpharmacologic therapies have the potential to produce long-term benefits upon psychological, and thereby, physical health. Behavioral therapies acknowledge the wisdom of the body and recognize that functional hypothalamic amenorrhea represents an endocrine adaptation that can be reversed with appropriate psychogenic and behavioral modifications.

Given these considerations, we recently studied whether CBT aimed at ameliorating problematic attitudes and behaviors would permit reproductive recovery in normal weight women with FHA.[65] Women with FHA were randomized to observation versus CBT. CBT consisted of 16 visits with a physician, therapist, or nutritionist over 20 weeks. The two groups were followed for return of menses for up to 8 weeks following the intervention. Regardless of menstrual pattern, estradiol and progesterone levels were monitored at weekly intervals for 4 weeks before and after observation versus CBT. About 88% of those who underwent CBT had evidence of ovulation whereas only 25% of those who were observed. FIGURE 2 illustrates the recovery of sex steroid secretion in a woman treated with CBT who showed ovarian recovery and in a woman randomized to observation who did not have recovery of ovarian function. Interestingly, when it occurred, ovarian recovery was not associated with significant weight gain. This does not mean that subjects did not alter food intake or energy expenditure, however.

SUMMARY

Functional hypothalamic hypogonadism is a clinical example of how attitudes, moods, and behaviors can have endocrine consequences and cause clinically evident reproductive compromise. Although a link between brain states and gonadal function has long been hypothesized, only recently have we been able to specify some of the mechanisms mediating this relationship. This understanding not only has concrete clinical implications, it also expands our appreciation of what it means to be healthy. Health truly depends upon developing healthy attitudes and healthy behaviors. Misattributions, negative images of self and others, unrealistic expectations, and emotional disharmony can cause neuroendocrine havoc. We must seek to develop healthy mindsets

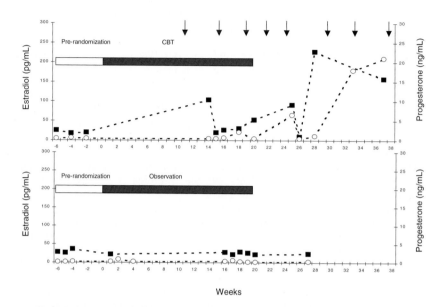

FIGURE 2. Estradiol (■) and progesterone (○) levels in a woman with functional hypothalamic amenorrhea (FHA) who had return of ovulatory menstrual cycles while undergoing CBT (*top panel*) and estradiol and progesterone levels in a woman with FHA who remained anovulatory and amenorrheic during observation for 20 weeks (*bottom panel*). Vaginal bleeding is indicated by ↓. (Reprinted from Berga *et al.*[65] with permission from the American Society for Reproductive Medicine.)

that permit us to meet life's innumerable challenges without overwhelming our coping mechanisms and without activating a chronic stress response. If we expect adversity and learn to cope well with it, then we likely will have more than just good reproductive functioning.

ACKNOWLEDGMENTS

Portions of the data presented were funded by grants from the National Institutes of Health (RO1-MH50748 to SLB and RR-00046 to the General Clinical Research Center at the University of Pittsburgh School of Medicine).

REFERENCES

1. BERGA, S.L. & T.L. DANIELS. 1991. Use of the laboratory in disorders of reproductive neuroendocrinology. J. Clin. Immunoassay **14:** 23–28.
2. REAME, N.E., S.E. SAUDER, G.D. CASE, *et al.* 1985. Pulsatile gonadotropin secretion in women with hypothalamic amenorrhea: evidence that reduced frequency of gonadotropin-releasing hormone secretion is the mechanism of persistent anovulation. J. Clin. Endocrinol. Metab. **61:** 851–858.

3. BERGA, S.L., J.F. MORTOLA, L. GIRTON, *et al.* 1989. Neuroendocrine aberrations in women with functional hypothalamic amenorrhea. J. Clin. Endocrinol. Metab. **68:** 301–308.
4. RASMUSSEN, D.D., J.H. LIU, P.H. WOLF & S.S.C. YEN. 1986. Gonadotropin-releasing hormone neurosecretion in the human hypothalamus: *in vitro* regulation by dopamine. J. Clin. Endocrinol. Metab. **62:** 470–483.
5. MEDHAMURTHY, R., V.L. GAY & T.M. PLANT. 1990. The prepubertal hiatus in gonadotropin secretion in the male rhesus monkey (Macaca mulatta) does not appear to involve endogenous opioid peptide restraint of hypothalamic gonadotropin-releasing hormone release. Endocrinology **126:** 1036–1042.
6. CONTE, F.A., M.M. GRUMBACK & S.L. KAPLAN. 1975. A diphasic pattern of gonadotropin secretion in patients with the syndrome of gonadal dysgenesis. J. Clin. Endocrinol. Metab. **40:** 670–674.
7. TERASAWA, E., W.E. BRIDSON, T.E. NASS, *et al.* 1984. Developmental changes in the luteinizing hormone secretory pattern in peripubertal female rhesus monkeys: comparison between gonadally intact and ovariectomized animals. Endocrinology **115:** 2233–2240.
8. WILDT, L., G. MARSHALL & E. KNOBIL. 1980. Experimental induction of puberty in the infantile female rhesus monkey. Science **207:** 1373–1375.
9. HURLEY, D.M., R. BRIAN, K. OUTCH, *et al.* 1984. Induction of ovulation and fertility in amenorrheic women by pulsatile low-dose gonadotropin-releasing hormone. N. Engl. J. Med. **301:** 1069–1074.
10. MILLER, D.S., R.R. REID, N.S. CETEL, *et al.* 1983. Pulsatile administration of low-dose gonadotropin-releasing hormone: ovulation and pregnancy in women with hypothalamic amenorrhea. JAMA **250:** 2937–2941.
11. PLANT, T.M., V.L. GAY, G.R. MARSHALL & M. ARSLAN. 1989. Puberty in monkeys is triggered by chemical stimulation of the hypothalamus. Proc. Natl. Acad. Sci. USA **86:** 2506–2510.
12. THIND, K.K. & P.C. GOLDSMITH. 1988. Infundibular gonadotropin-releasing hormone neurons are inhibited by direct opioid and autoregulatory synapses in juvenile monkeys. Neuroendocrinology **47:** 203–216.
13. DUDAS, B. & I. MERCHENTHALER. 2006. Three-dimensional representation of the neurotransmitter systems of the human hypothalamus: inputs of the gonadotropin hormone-releasing hormone neuronal systems. J. Neuroendocrinol. **18:** 79–95.
14. KULJIS, R.O. & J.P. ADVIS. 1989. Immunocytochemical and physiological evidence of a synapse between dopamine and luteinizing hormone releasing hormone-containing neurons in the ewe median eminence. Endocrinology **124:** 1579–1581.
15. LERANTH, C., N.J. MACLUSKY, M. SHANABROUGH & F. NAFTOLIN. 1988. Catecholaminergic innervation of luteinizing hormone-releasing hormone and glutamic acid decarboxylase immunopositive neurons in the rat medial preoptic area. Neuroendocrinology **48:** 581–602.
16. GOODMAN, R.L. 1989. Functional organization of the catecholaminergic neural system inhibiting luteinizing hormone secretion in anestrous ewes. Neuroendocrinology **47:** 203–250.
17. PREVOT, V., D. CROIX, S. BOURET, *et al.* 1999. Definitive evidence for the existence of morphological plasticity in the external zone of the median eminence during the rat estrous cycle: implication of neuro-glio-endothelial interactions in gonadotropin-releasing hormone release. Neuroscience **94:** 809–819.

18. BERGA, S.L. & S.S.C. YEN. 2004. Reproductive failure due to central nervous system-hypothalamic-pituitary dysfunction. In: Yen and Jaffe's Reproductive Endocrinology: Physiology, Pathophysiology, and Clinical Managements Strauss, & Barbieri (eds). Fifth edition. Elsevier Saunders, Philadelphia, PA. Chapter 18, pp. 564–569.

19. CROWLEY, W.F. JR., M. FILICORI, D.I. SPRATT & N. SANTORO. 1985. The physiology of gonadotropin-releasing hormone (GnRH) secretion in men and women. Recent Prog. Horm. Res. **41:** 473–526.

20. CHROUSOS, G.P. & P.W. GOLD. 1992. The concepts of stress and stress system disorders. JAMA **267:** 1244–1252.

21. MACLUSKY, N.J., F. NAFTOLIN & C. LERANTH. 1988. Immunocytochemical evidence for direct synaptic connections between corticotropin-releasing factor (CRF) and gonadotropin-releasing hormone (GnRH)-containing neurons in the preoptic area of the rat. Brain Res. **439:** 381–395.

22. WILLIAMS, C.L., M. NISHIHARA, J.C. THALABARD, et al. 1990. Corticotrophin-releasing factor and gonadotropin-releasing hormone pulse generator activity in the rhesus monkey. Neuroendocrinology **52:** 133–137.

23. PETRAGLIA, F., W. VALE & C. RIVIER. 1986. Opioids act centrally to modulate stress-induced decrease in luteinizing hormone in the rat. Endocrinology **119:** 2445–2450.

24. SAPOLSKY, R.M. & L.C. KREY. 1988. Stress-induced suppression of luteinizing hormone concentrations in wild baboons: role of opiates. J. Clin. Endocrinol. Metab. **66:** 772–776.

25. THIND, K.K. & P.C. GOLDSMITH. 1989. Corticotropin-releasing factor neurons innervate dopamine neurons in the periventricular hypothalamus of juvenile macaques. Neuroendocrinology **50:** 351–358.

26. HEISLER, L.E., A.J. TUMBER, R.L. REID & D.A. VAN VUGT. 1994. Vasopressin mediates hypoglycemia-induced inhibition of luteinizing hormone secretion in the ovariectomized Rhesus monkey. Neuroendocrinology **60:** 297–304.

27. THIND, K.K., J.E. BOGGAN & P.C. GOLDSMITH. 1991. Interactions between vasopressin and gonadotropin-releasing-hormone-containing neuroendocrine neurons in the monkey supraoptic nucleus. Neuroendocrinology **53:** 287–297.

28. WHITNALL, M.H. 1989. Stress selectively activates the vasopressin-containing subset of corticotropin-releasing hormone neurons. Neuroendocrinology **50:** 702–707.

29. TERASAWA, E. 1995. Control of luteinizing-hormone releasing hormone pulse generation in nonhuman primates. Cell. Mol. Neurobiol. **15:** 141–164.

30. LI,. S. & G. PELLETIER. 1996. Further studies on the mechanism of action of the endogenous benzodiazepine receptor ligand octadecaneuropeptide on gonadotropin-releasing hormone gene expression in the rat brain. Neuroendocrinology **64:** 79–84.

31. KASUYA, E., C.L. NYBERG, K. MOGI & E. TERASAWA. 1999. A role of γ-aminobutyric acid (GABA) and glutamate in control of puberty in female rhesus monkeys: effect of an antisense oligodeoxynucleotide for GAD67 messenger ribonucleic acid and MK801 on luteinizing hormone-releasing hormone release. Endocrinology **140:** 705–712.

32. SUH, B.Y., J.H. LIU, S.L. BERGA, et al. 1988. Hypercortisolism in patients with functional hypothalamic amenorrhea. J. Clin. Endocrinol. Metab. **66:** 733–739.

33. BILLER, B.M.K., J.H. FEDEROFF, J.I. KOENIG & A. KLIBANSKI. 1990. Abnormal cortisol secretion and responses to corticotropin-releasing hormone in women with hypothalamic amenorrhea. J. Clin. Endocrinol. Metab. **70:** 311–317.

34. LOUCKS, A.B., J.F. MORTOLA, L. GIRTON & S.S.C. YEN. 1989. Alternations in the hypothalamic-pituitary-ovarian and hypothalamic-pituitary-adrenal axes in athletic women. J. Clin. Endocrinol. Metab **68:** 402–411.
35. DE SOUZA, M.J., B.E. MILLER, A.B. LOUCKS, *et al.* 1998. High frequency of luteal phase deficiency and anovulation in recreational women runners: blunted elevation in follicle-stimulating hormone observed during luteal-follicular transition. J. Clin. Endocrinol. Metab. **83:** 4220–4232.
36. BERGA, S.L., T.L. DANIELS & D.E. GILES. 1997. Women with functional hypothalamic amenorrhea but not other forms of anovulation display amplified cortisol concentrations. Fertil. Steril. **67:** 1024–1030.
37. LOUCKS, A.B., G.A. LAUGHLIN, J.F. MORTOLA, *et al.* 1992. Hypothalamic-pituitary-thyroidal function in eumenorrheic and amenorrheic athletes. J. Clin. Endocrinol. Metab. **75:** 514–518.
38. BERGA, S.L., J.F. MORTOLA & S.S. YEN. 1988. Amplification of nocturnal melatonin secretion in women with functional hypothalamic amenorrhea. J. Clin. Endocrinol. Metab. **66:** 242–244.
39. STEIN-BEHRENS, B., M.P. MATTSON, I. CHANG, *et al.* 1994. Stress exacerbates neuron loss and cytoskeletal pathology in the hippocampus. J. Neurosci. **14:** 5373–5380.
40. MCEWEN, B.S.. 1998. Protective and damaging effects of stress mediators. N. Engl. J. Med. **338:** 171–179.
41. KLIBANSKI, A.N., B.M.K. BILLER, D.A. SCHOENFELD, *et al.* 1994. The effects of estrogen administration on trabecular bone loss in young women with anorexia nervosa. J. Clin. Endocrinol. Metab. **80:** 898–904.
42. GOLDEN, N.H., L. LANZKOWSKY, J. SCHEBENDACH, *et al.* 2002. The effect of estrogen-progestin treatment on bone mineral density in anorexia nervosa. J. Pediatr. Adolesc. Gynecol. **15:** 135–143.
43. KHOURY, S.A., N.E. REAME, R.P. KELCH & J.C. MARSHALL. 1987. Diurnal patterns of pulsatile luteinizing hormone secretion in hypothalamic amenorrhea: reproducibility and responses to opiate blockade and a α_2-adrenergic agonist. J. Clin. Endocrinol. Metab. **64:** 755–762.
44. QUIGLEY, M.E., K.L. SHEEHAN, R.F. CASPER & S.S.C. YEN. 1980. Evidence for increased dopaminergic and opioid activity in patients with hypothalamic hypogonadotropic amenorrhea. J. Clin. Endocrinol. Metab. **50:** 949–954.
45. BERGA, S.L., A.B. LOUCKS, W.G. ROSSMANITH, *et al.* 1991. Acceleration of LH pulse frequency in functional hypothalamic amenorrhea by dopaminergic blockade. J. Clin. Endocrinol. Metab. **72:** 151–156.
46. BERGA, S.L., T.L. LOUCKS-DANIELS, L.J. ADLER, *et al.* 2000. Cerebrospinal fluid levels of corticotropin-releasing hormone in women with functional hypothalamic amenorrhea. Am. J. Obstet. Gynecol. **182:** 776–784.
47. JUDD, S.J., J. WONG, S. SALONIKLIS, *et al.* 1995. The effect of alprozalam on serum cortisol and LH pulsatility in normal women and in women with stress-related anovulation. J. Clin. Endocrinol. Metab. **80:** 818–823.
48. BETHEA, C.L., F.K. PAU, S. FOX, *et al.* 2005. Sensitivity to stress-induced reproductive dysfunction linked to activity of the serotonin system. Fertil. Steril. **83:** 148–155.
49. ROMERO, L.M., P.M. PLOTSKY & R.M. SAPOLSKY. 1993. Patterns of adrenocorticotropin secretory release with hypoglycemia, novelty, and restraint after colchicine blockade of axonal transport. Endocrinology **132:** 199–204.

50. PETRIDES, J.S., G.P. MUELLER, K.T. KALOGERAS, et al. 1994. Exercise-induced activation of the hypothalamic-pituitary-adrenal axis: marked differences in the sensitivity to glucocorticoid suppression. J. Clin. Endocrinol. Metab **79:** 377–383.
51. ALTEMUS, M., P.A. DEUSTER, E. GALLIVEN, et al. 1995. Suppression of hypothalamic-pituitary-adrenal axis responses to stress in lactating women. J. Clin. Endocrinol. Metab. **80:** 2954–2959.
52. GILES, D.E. & S.L. BERGA. 1993. Cognitive and psychiatric correlates of functional hypothalamic amenorrhea: a controlled comparison. Fertil. Steril. **60:** 486–492.
53. FIORONI, L., M. FAVA, A.D. GENAZZANI, et al. 1994. Life events impact in patients with secondary amenorrhea. J. Psychosom. Res. **38:** 617–622.
54. KIRSCHBAUM, C., J.C. PRUSSNER, A.A. STONE, et al. 1995. Persistent high cortisol responses to repeated psychological stress in a subpopulation of healthy men. Psychosom. Med. **57:** 468–474.
55. CAMERON, J.L., C. NOSBISCH, D. HELMREICH & D.B. PARFITT. 1990. Reversal of exercise-induced amenorrhea in female cynomolgus monkeys (Macasa Fascicularis) by increasing food intake. Abstract 1042. Proc. 72nd Annual Meeting of the Endocrine Society. Atlanta, GA. 1285.
56. BULLEN, B.A., G.S. SKRINAR, I.Z. BETINS, et al. 1985. Induction of menstrual disorders by strenuous exercise in untrained women. N. Engl. J. Med. **312:** 1349–1353.
57. LOUCKS, A.B. & J.R. THURMA. 2003. Luteinizing hormone pulsatility is disrupted at a threshold of energy availability in regularly menstruating women. J. Clin. Endocrinol. Metab. **88:** 297–311.
58. WILLIAMS, N.L., S.L. BERGA & J.L. CAMERON. 1997. Mild metabolic stress potentiates the suppressive effects of psychological stress on reproductive function in female cynomolgus monkeys. Abstract P1-367, 79th Annual Meeting of The Endocrine Society, Minneapolis, MN, June 11–14.
59. LOUCKS, T.L., J. DUBE, K. LAYCHAK, et al. 2004. Metabolic and endocrine responses to submaximal exercise challenge in women with functional hypothalamic amenorrhea. Abstract 605. 51st Annual Meeting of the Society of Gynecologic Investigation, Houston, TX. March 24–27.
60. VAN DER SPUY, Z.M., P.J. STEER, M. MCCUSKER, et al. 1988. Outcome of pregnancy in underweight women after spontaneous and induced ovulation. Br. Med. J. **296:** 962–965.
61. PIKE, K.M. & J. RODIN. 1991. Mothers, daughters, and disordered eating. J. Abnorm. Psychol. **100:** 198–204.
62. HADDOW, J.E., G.E. PALOMAKI, W.C. ALLAN, et al. 1999. Maternal thyroid deficiency during pregnancy and subsequent neuropsychological development of the child. N. Engl. J. Med. **341:** 549–555.
63. HANSEN, D., H.C. LOU & J. OLSEN. 2000. Serious life events and congenital malformations: a national study with complete follow-up. Lancet **356:** 875–880.
64. GENAZZANI, A.D., O. GAMBA & F. PETRAGLIA. 1998. Estrogen replacement therapy modulates spontaneous GH secretion but does not affect GHRH-induced GH response and low T3 syndrome in women with hypothalamic amenorrhea associated to weight loss. J. Endocrinol. Invest. **21:** 353–357.
65. BERGA, S.L., M.D. MARCUS, T.L. LOUCKS, et al. 2003. Recovery of ovarian activity in women with functional hypothalamic amenorrhea who were treated with cognitive behavior therapy. Fertil. Steril. **80:** 976–981.

Ovarian and Adrenal Hyperandrogenism

ENRICO CARMINA

Department of Clinical Medicine, University of Palermo, Palermo, Italy

ABSTRACT: Because in normal women androgens are secreted in almost equal quantities by both adrenals and ovaries, for many years many studies have tried to distinguish the source of androgen excess. However, in the last 10–15 years, the diagnoses of ovarian or adrenal hyperandrogenism have almost disappeared. This is due to the lack of specificity of dynamic tests as well as to the emphasis given on clinical information and ovarian sonography for the diagnosis of hyperandrogenic syndromes. However, determination of the source of increased androgens may still be useful for improving the classification and the understanding of androgen excess disorders. The aim of this review is to examine the source of androgen excess in the three more common androgen excess disorders: polycystic ovary syndrome (PCOS), idiopathic hyperandrogenism; and nonclassic 21-hydroxylase deficiency (NCAH). The ovary is the main androgen source in PCOS and idiopathic hyperandrogenism while adrenal androgen secretion is prevalent in NCAH. However, androgen secretion from more than one source is common in all main forms of hyperandrogenism as is the case in 70–80% of patients with NCAH, in 35% of women with PCOS, and in 50% of patients with idiopathic hyperandrogenism. Secondary PCOS is the main cause of ovarian androgen excess in nonclassic 21-hydroxylase deficiency while adrenal hyperandrogenism in PCOS and idiopathic hyperandrogenism is probably the consequence of multiple factors including hyperinsulinemia, altered cortisol metabolism, and increased ovarian steroid production. The clinical image is not generally affected by the source of androgen excess. However, hyperandrogenic patients with increased dehydroepiandrosterone sulfate (DHEAS) tend to have lower body weight and insulin levels and a better metabolic profile.

KEYWORDS: polycystic ovary syndrome; PCOS; nonclassic 21-hydroxylase deficiency; NCAH; idiopathic hyperandrogenism; androgen excess

INTRODUCTION

Androgen excess is the most common endocrine disorder of adult women.[1] Several studies have shown that 6–8% of young adult women are affected

Address for correspondence: Enrico Carmina, M.D., Endocrine Unit, Department of Clinical Medicine, University of Palermo, Via delle Croci 47, 90139 Palermo, Italy. Voice: +39091328997; fax: +390916555995.

e-mail: enricocarmina@libero.it

Ann. N.Y. Acad. Sci. 1092: 130–137 (2006). © 2006 New York Academy of Sciences.
doi: 10.1196/annals.1365.011

by polycystic ovary syndrome (PCOS)[2,3] and that another 2–3% are affected by some other androgen disorder.[4] Because in normal women both adrenals and ovaries participate in almost equal quantities to androgen secretion, it is clear that both glands may be the source of increased androgen production.

In the past, many studies have been dedicated to the understanding of the source of androgen excess in hyperandrogenic syndromes.[5] However, during the last 15 years, there has been a lack of interest in this kind of research. This is probably due to loss of confidence in dynamic tests as well as to the emphasis given on clinical data and ovarian sonography for the diagnosis of androgen excess disorders. In most recent large studies, evaluation of androgen source has been limited to the diagnosis of nonclassic adrenal enzymatic deficiencies (i.e., by measurement of serum 17OHProgesterone) or of androgen-secreting tumors.[4,6,7] However, the knowledge of the source of increased androgens in different disorders may still be useful for improving the classification and the understanding of androgen excess syndromes. In this review, we will present the most recent evidence on the source of the androgens in the three most common androgen excess disorders: PCOS, idiopathic hyperandrogenism, and nonclassic 21-hydroxylase deficiency (NCAH).

ANDROGEN SOURCE IN PCOS

In the most common androgen excess disorder, PCOS, the ovary is the main androgen source.[8] Although no genetic ovarian enzymatic deficiency has been detected,[9] ovarian hyperandrogenism represents the main pathogenetic mechanism of the syndrome[10] and the increased androstenedione and testosterone production by the ovary results not only by increased luteinizing hormone (LH) (and insulin) drive but by increased primary androgen secretion by theca cells.[11,12] In fact, *in vitro* studies have demonstrated that theca cells from polycystic ovaries produce more androstenedione both in basal conditions and after gonadotropin stimulation.[11,12]

However, in many women with PCOS, there is more than one source of androgen hypersecretion. In fact, adrenal androgen secretion is also increased.[13] In the past, we have shown that about 50% of women with PCOS have elevated circulating levels of dehydroepiandrosterone sulfate (DHEAS) and 11β-hydroxy-androstenedione, two androgens that are almost exclusively secreted by zona reticularis of the adrenal glands.[14,15] Other authors studying different ethnic populations have reported that serum DHEAS is increased in about 20–30% of adult women with classic anovulatory PCOS.[16] More recently, we have reviewed the prevalence of increased DHEAS in women with PCOS and found that increased circulating levels of this steroid are present in 39.4% of women with classic anovulatory PCOS.[17] The prevalence is slightly lower in ovulatory PCOS and therefore, using European Society Human Reproduction/American Society Reproductive Medicine (ESHRE/ASRM) criteria for diagnosis of PCOS,[18,19] prevalence of adrenal hyperandrogenism in PCOS is about 37% in the southern Italian population.[17] It is possible that ethnic components influence the prevalence of adrenal hyperandrogenism in PCOS. The mechanisms for adrenal hyperandrogenism in PCOS are not well understood.

Brothers of women with PCOS have significantly higher DHEAS levels compared to controls suggesting an inherited abnormality in adrenal androgen secretion.[20] However, in PCOS, no genetic alterations of adrenal enzymatic activity have been found[21] and the most consistent abnormality is an increased adrenal androgen response to adrenocorticotropin hormone (ACTH).[22–24] Because circulating ACTH is normal,[22] it is probable that factors external to the adrenal gland are responsible for the increased adrenal androgen responsivity.[25]

It has been suggested that increased insulin may be the main determinant of increased adrenal androgen secretion in women with PCOS.[26] However, serum DHEAS tends to be lower in obese women with PCOS[27] and in hyperandrogenic women serum DHEAS presents a negative correlation with serum insulin.[17] Therefore, it is unlikely that hyperinsulinemia has a main role in determining increased DHEAS levels. It does not exclude a role of insulin in adrenal androgen excess in women with PCOS. In fact, we have demonstrated a significant correlation of serum insulin with the Δ_4 pathway and with adrenal androstenedione formation in particular.[28]

The increased DHEAS levels of women with PCOS are probably explained by the cumulative effect of different factors including elevated circulating unbound estradiol circulating levels[28,29] and altered cortisol metabolism. In fact, in PCOS, increased peripheral metabolism of cortisol due to enhanced inactivation of this steroid by 5-α-reductase or impaired reactivation of cortisol from cortisone by 11β-hydroxysteroid dehydrogenase type 1[30,31] has been observed. It would potentially result in decreased negative feedback on ACTH so that pituitary adrenal androgen axis activity would increase to maintain normal cortisol levels at the expense of AA excess.

Finally, in some women with PCOS, increased peripheral sulfatase activity has been found and it may have a role in the increase of serum DHEAS.[25]

As previously reported, in most patients adrenal hyperandrogenism is associated with excessive ovarian androgen production. Only few patients with PCOS present an isolated adrenal hyperandrogenism. In our experience, an isolated DHEAS increase is present only in 4.5% of women with PCOS.[17] In these instances, a pattern of enzymatic deficiency of 3β-hydroxysteroid-dehydrogenase may be found.[32] However, in patients who develop this form of hyperandrogenism during adult life, no specific genetic defects have been detected and it has been suggested that these patients may have a functional enzymatic deficiency.[33] In practice, these patients are considered affected by PCOS because they have the same phenotype of classic PCOS.[32,34]

ANDROGEN SOURCE IN IDIOPATHIC HYPERANDROGENISM

Idiopathic hyperandrogenism is the second most common androgen disorder.[7] It is a diagnosis of exclusion in hyperandrogenic patients who do not fulfill the criteria for diagnosis of PCOS, nonclassic adrenal enzymatic deficiencies, or other uncommon hyperandrogenic disorders (androgen-secreting tumors, Cushing's syndrome, HAIR-AN syndrome).[4,7]

Data regarding androgen source in these patients are few. In fact, while in the past many patients with similar phenotype have been studied,[5,35] many of those patients should now have a diagnosis of ovulatory PCOS.[4] We have recently reviewed the hormonal data of a group of patients with idiopathic hyperandrogenism[7,17] and will use these data in this review.

Adrenal hyperandrogenism is common in patients with idiopathic hyperandrogenism. In fact, almost 50% (48.3%) of the patients with idiopathic hyperandrogenism present elevated circulating DHEAS levels suggesting that adrenal hyperandrogenism may be more common in mild androgen disorder than in PCOS.[17]

As in PCOS, the androgen source in idiopathic hyperandrogenism is generally mixed (ovarian and adrenal): an isolated increase of serum DHEAS was present only in 7% of the patients with idiopathic hyperandrogenism.[17] Conversely, isolated increase of serum testosterone (probably indicating an exclusive androgen ovarian source) was present in 45% of these patients.[17] It suggests that an ovarian source of the androgens is present in about 90% of the patients with idiopathic hyperandrogenism and that in about a half the ovarian source is associated with an exaggerated adrenal production.

ANDROGEN SOURCE IN NCAH

NCAH constitutes the third most common androgen excess disorder.[6,7] While prevalence of NCAH largely varies between populations,[36] in our population (Sicily, Italy) 4% of women were referred because of clinical hyperandrogenism presenting this genetic disorder.[7]

As expected, in patients with NCAH the main androgen source is the adrenal gland.[37] Because of the partial enzymatic blockade, adrenal steroid biosynthesis is deviated to increased androgen production in an effort to maintain normal cortisol production. It regards particularly the Δ_4 androgens with an elevation of serum androstenedione and consequently (by peripheral transformation) of serum testosterone. In the past, we had demonstrated that 11β-hydroxyandrostenedione (a marker of adrenal androstenedione production) is increased in all patients with NCAH while only a minority of patients present also an increase of serum DHEAS.[38] Although the peripheral pattern of serum androgens is similar to that found in PCOS,[39–41] the mean serum levels of androstenedione and testosterone are generally higher in NCAH than in PCOS.[7]

Although the androgen source is mainly adrenal, in many patients with NCAH an ovarian androgen source is also present. In our recent study, 77% of adult women with NCAH present polycystic ovaries[7] and we have previously shown that prolonged GnRH administration (inhibiting ovarian secretion) reduces serum androstenedione and testosterone[42] suggesting that, in most adult NCAH, the androgen source is mixed probably because the prolonged hormonal perturbation may determine a secondary PCOS.[43]

INFLUENCE OF ANDROGEN SOURCE ON PHENOTYPE OF ANDROGEN EXCESS DISORDERS

In general, it is believed that the androgen source does not influence the phenotype of androgen excess disorders. While many differences in phenotype are present between the different androgen disorders and mainly between severe (PCOS) and mild syndromes,[4] these differences seem to be determined mostly by other characteristics of the syndrome (mainly insulin resistance). However, we have recently observed that hyperandrogenic patients with increased DHEAS, independently of the form of androgen excess disorder (PCOS or idiopathic hyperandrogenism), tend to be leaner and to have lower insulin levels and a better metabolic profile.[17] These data need to be confirmed but raise the possibility that increased DHEAS may have a protective effect on metabolism or on the contrary that increased insulin levels tend to suppress DHEAS secretion.

REFERENCES

1. CARMINA, E. & R.A. LOBO. 1999. Polycystic ovary syndrome (PCOS): arguably the most common endocrinopathy is associated with significant morbidity in women. J. Clin. Endocrinol. Metab. **84:** 1897–1899.
2. KNOCHENHAUER, E.S., T.J. KEY, W. KAHSAR-MILLER, et al. 1998. Prevalence of the polycystic ovary syndrome in unselected black and white women of the southeastern USA: a prospective study. J. Clin. Endocrinol. Metab. **83:** 3078–3082.
3. DIAMANTI-KANDARAKIS, E., C.R. KOULI, A.T. BERGIELE, et al. 1999. A survey of polycystic ovary syndrome in the Greek island of Lesbos: hormonal and metabolic profile. J. Clin. Endocrinol. Metab. **84:** 4006–4011.
4. CARMINA, E. 2006. Mild androgen disorders. Best Pract. Res. Clin. Endocrinol. Metab. **20:** 207–220.
5. MAROULIS, G.B. 1981. Evaluation of hirsutism and hyperandrogenemia. Fertil. Steril. **36:** 273–305.
6. AZZIZ, R., L.A. SANCHEZ, E.S. KNOCHENHAUER, et al. 2004. Androgen excess in women: experience with over 1000 consecutive patients. J. Clin. Endocrinol. Metab. **89:** 453–462.
7. CARMINA, E., F. ROSATO, A. JANNÌ, et al. 2005. Relative prevalence of different androgen excess disorders in 950 women referred because of clinical hyperandrogenism. J. Clin. Endocrinol. Metab. **91:** 2–6.

8. BARNES, R.B., R.L. ROSENFIELD, S. BURNSTEIN & D.A. EHRMANN. 1989. Pituitary-ovarian responses to nafarelin testing in the polycystic ovary syndrome. N. Engl. J. Med. **320:** 559–565.

9. ESCOBAR-MORREALE, H.F., M. LUQUE-RAMIREZ & J.L. SAN MILLAN. 2005. The molecular-genetic basis of functional hyperandrogenism and the polycystic ovary syndrome. Endocr. Rev. **26:** 251–282.

10. ABBOTT, D.H., D.K. BARNETT, C.M. BRUNS & D.A. DUMESIC. 2005. Androgen excess fetal programming of female reproduction: a developmental etiology for polycystic ovary syndrome? Hum. Reprod. Update **11:** 357–374.

11. GILLING-SMITH, C., D.S. WILLIS, R.W. BEARD & S. FRANKS. 1994. Hypersecretion of androstenedione by isolated theca cells from polycystic ovaries. J. Clin. Endocrinol. Metab. **79:** 1158–1165.

12. GILLING-SMITH, C., H. STORY, V. ROGERS & S. FRANKS. 1997. Evidence for a primary abnormality of theca cell steroidogenesis in the polycystic ovary syndrome. Clin. Endocrinol. (Oxf) **47:** 93–99.

13. CARMINA, E. 1997. Prevalence of adrenal androgen excess in PCOS. *In* Androgen Excess Disorders in Women. R.A. Azziz, J.B. Nestler & D. Dewailly, Eds.: 385–393. Lippincott-Raven. Philadelphia, PA.

14. CARMINA, E., F. ROSATO & A. JANNÌ. 1986. Increased DHEAS levels in PCO syndrome: evidence for the existence of two subgroups of patients. J. Endocrinol. Invest. **9:** 5–10.

15. STANCZYK, F.Z., L. CHANG, E. CARMINA, *et al.* 1991. Is 11β-hydroxyandrostenedione a better marker of adrenal androgen excess than dehydroepiandrosterone sulfate? Am. J. Obstet. Gynecol. **165:** 1837–1842.

16. KUMAR, A., K.S. WOODS, A.A. BARTOLUCCI & R. AZZIZ. 2005. Prevalence of adrenal androgen excess in patients with the polycystic ovary syndrome (PCOS). Clin. Endocrinol. (Oxf) **62:** 644–649.

17. CARMINA, E. & R.A. LOBO. Prevalence and characteristics of adrenal androgen secretion in patients with different forms of androgen excess disorders. Hum. Reprod. In press.

18. ROTTERDAM ESHRE/ASRM SPONSORED PCOS CONSENSUS WORKSHOP GROUP. 2004. Revised 2003 consensus on diagnostic criteria and long-term health risks related to polycystic ovary syndrome. Fertil. Steril. **81:** 19–25.

19. ROTTERDAM ESHRE/ASRM SPONSORED PCOS CONSENSUS WORKSHOP GROUP. 2004. Revised 2003 consensus on diagnostic criteria and long-term health risks related to polycystic ovary syndrome. Hum. Reprod. **19:** 41–47.

20. LEGRO, R.S., A.R. KUNSELMAN, L. DEMERS, *et al.* 2002. Elevated dehydroepiandrosterone sulfate levels as the reproductive phenotype in the brothers of women with polycystic ovary syndrome. J. Clin. Endocrinol. Metab. **87:** 2134–2138.

21. AZZIZ, R.A. 1997. Abnormalities of adrenocortical steroidogenesis in PCOS. *In* Androgen Excess Disorders in Women. R.A. Azziz, J.B. Nestler & D. Dewailly, Eds.: 403–414. Lippincott-Raven. Philadelphia, PA.

22. CARMINA, E. & R.A. LOBO. 1990. Pituitary-adrenal responses to ovine corticotropin-releasing hormone in polycystic ovary syndrome and in other hyperandrogenic patients. Gynecol. Endocrinol. **4:** 225–232.

23. AZZIZ, R., V. BLACK, G.A. HINES, *et al.* 1998. Adrenal androgen excess in the polycystic ovary syndrome: sensitivity and responsivity of the hypothalamic-pituitary-adrenal axis. J. Clin. Endocrinol. Metab. **83:** 2317–2323.

24. MORAN, C., R. REYNA, L.S. BOOTS & R.A. AZZIZ. 2004. Adrenocortical hyperresponsiveness to corticotropin in polycystic ovary syndrome patients with adrenal androgen excess. Fertil. Steril. **81:** 126–131.
25. CARMINA, E. 1997. The role of extra-adrenal factors in adrenal androgen excess: *in vivo* studies. *In* Androgen Excess Disorders in Women. R.A. Azziz, J.B. Nestler & D. Dewailly, Eds.: 425–434. Lippincott-Raven. Philadelphia, PA.
26. MOGHETTI, P., R. CASTELLO, C. NEGRI, *et al.* 1996. Insulin infusion amplifies 17a-hydroxyxorticosteroid intermediate response to adrenocorticotropin in hyperandrogenic women. Apparent relative impairment of 17,20 lyase activity. J. Clin. Endocrinol. Metab. **81:** 881–886.
27. MORAN, C., E. KNOCHENHAUER, L.R. BOOTS & R.A. AZZIZ. 1999. Adrenal androgen excess in hyperandrogenism: relation to age and body mass. Fertil. Steril. **71:** 671–674.
28. CARMINA, E., F. GONZALEZ, A. VIDALI, *et al.* 1999. The contribution of oestrogen and growth factors to increased adrenal androgen secretion in polycystic ovary syndrome. Hum. Reprod. **14:** 307–311.
29. DITKOFF, E.C., F. FRUZZETTI, L. CHANG, *et al.* 1995. The impact of estrogen on adrenal androgen sensitivity and secretion in polycystic ovary syndrome. J. Clin. Endocrinol. Metab. **80:** 603–607.
30. WALKER, B.R., A. RODIN, N.F. TAYLOR & R.N. CLAYTON. 2000. Endogenous inhibitors of 11beta-hydroxysteroid dehydrogenase type I do not explain abnormal cortisol metabolism in polycystic ovary syndrome. Clin. Endocrinol. (Oxf) **52:** 77–80.
31. TSILCHOROZIDOU, T., J.W. HONOUR & G.S. CONWAY. 2003. Altered cortisol metabolism in polycystic ovary syndrome: insulin enhances 5alpha-reduction but not the elevated adrenal steroid production rates. J. Clin. Endocrinol. Metab. **88:** 5907–5913.
32. LOBO, R.A. & U. GOEBELSMANN. 1981. Evidence for reduced 3β-ol-hydroxysteroid dehydrogenase activity in some hirsute women thought to have polycystic ovary syndrome. J. Clin. Endocrinol. Metab. **53:** 394–400.
33. ZERAH, M., E. RHEAUME, P. MANI, *et al.* 1994. No evidence of mutations in the genes for type I and type II 3β-hydroxysteroid dehydrogenase (3β-HSD) in nonclassical 3β-HSD deficiency. J. Clin. Endocrinol. Metab. **79:** 1811–1817.
34. CARBUNARU, G., P. PRASAD, B. SCOCCIA, *et al.* 2004. The hormonal phenotype of nonclassic 3 beta-hydroxysteroid dehydrogenase (HSD3B) deficiency in hyperandrogenic females is associated with insulin-resistant polycystic ovary syndrome and is not a variant of inherited HSD3B2 deficiency. J. Clin. Endocrinol. Metab. **89:** 783–794.
35. STEINBERGER, E., K.D. SMITH & L.J. RODRIGUEZ-RIGAU. 1984. Testosterone, dehydroepiandrosterone, and dehydroepiandrosterone sulfate in hyperandrogenic women. J. Clin. Endocrinol. Metab. **59:** 471–477.
36. NEW, M.I. & P.W. SPEISER. 1986. Genetics of adrenal steroid 21-hydroxylase deficiency. Endocr. Rev. **7:** 331–349.
37. AZZIZ, R., D. DEWAILLY & D. OWERBACH. 1994. Nonclassic adrenal hyperplasia: current concepts. J. Clin. Endocrinol. Metab. **78:** 810–815.
38. CARMINA, E., F.Z. STANCZYK, L. CHANG, *et al.* 1992. The ratio of androstenedione: 11b-hydroxyandrostenedione is an important marker of adrenal androgen excess in women. Fertil. Steril. **58:** 148–152.

39. LOBO, R.A. & U. GOEBELSMANN. 1980. Adult manifestations of congenital adrenal hyperplasia due to incomplete 21-hydroxylase deficiency mimicking polycystic ovarian disease. Am. J. Obstet. Gynecol. **138:** 720–726.

40. CARMINA, E., A.M. GAGLIANO, F. ROSATO, *et al.* 1984. The endocrine pattern of late onset adrenal hyperplasia (21-hydroxylase deficiency). J. Endocrinol. Invest. **7:** 89–92.

41. DEWAILLY, D., M.C. VANTYGHEM-HAUDIQUET, C. SAINSARD, *et al.* 1986. Clinical and biological phenotypes in late-onset 21-hydroxylase deficiency. J. Clin. Endocrinol. Metab. **63:** 418–423.

42. CARMINA, E. & R.A. LOBO. 1994. Ovarian suppression reduces clinical and endocrine expression of late-onset congenital adrenal hyperplasia due to 21-hydroxylase deficiency. Fertil. Steril. **62:** 738–743.

43. LEVIN, J.H., E. CARMINA & R.A. LOBO. 1991. Is the inappropriate gonadotropin secretion of patients with polycystic ovary syndrome similar to that of patients with adult-onset congenital adrenal hyperplasia? Fertil. Steril. **56:** 635–640.

Causes of Intrauterine Growth Restriction and the Postnatal Development of the Metabolic Syndrome

GEORGE VALSAMAKIS,[a] CHRISTINA KANAKA-GANTENBEIN,[b] ARIADNE MALAMITSI-PUCHNER,[a] AND GEORGE MASTORAKOS[a]

[a]Endocrine Unit and Neonatal Division, Second Department of Obstetrics and Gynaecology, Aretaieion Hospital, Medical School, University of Athens, Athens, Greece

[b]Unit of Endocrinology, Diabetes and Metabolism, First Department of Paediatrics, Aghia Sofia Children's Hospital, Medical School, University of Athens, Athens, Greece

ABSTRACT: The term intrauterine growth restriction (IUGR) is assigned to newborns with a birth weight and/or birth length below the 10th percentile for their gestational age and whose abdominal circumference is below the 2.5th percentile with pathologic restriction of fetal growth. IUGR is usually due to maternal, fetal, or placental factors. However, many IUGR cases have unknown underlying cause. Recent studies focus on new factors that can influence fetal development and birth outcome like the timing and the type of fetal nutrition, maternal psychosocial stress and personality variables, 11β-hydroxysteroid dehydrogenase type 2 placental activity, the activity of the neuroendocrine system that mediates the effects of psychosocial stress, and the role of proinflammatory cytokines and of oxidative stress. Data have shown that IUGR is associated with a late life increased prevalence of metabolic syndrome, a condition associating obesity with hypertension, type 2 diabetes mellitus (DM2), and cardiovascular disease. Recent data demonstrated that the diabetes-associated mortality appears to be disproportionately concentrated among individuals of abnormal birth weight.

KEYWORDS: IUGR; SGA; fetal origin; metabolic syndrome; cardiovascular disease

INTRODUCTION

During the last years, evidence has emerged showing that low birth weight is associated with raised prevalence of cardiovascular disease in adult life including

Address for correspondence: Dr. George Valsamakis, Leoforos Pendelis 37A, 15235 Vrilissia, Athens, Greece. Voice/fax: +30-210-6137330.
e-mail: geodimval@hotmail.com

Ann. N.Y. Acad. Sci. 1092: 138–147 (2006). © 2006 New York Academy of Sciences.
doi: 10.1196/annals.1365.012

raised blood pressure, glucose intolerance, and dyslipidemia. The clustering of these metabolic abnormalities constitutes the metabolic syndrome.[1-3] A low birth weight baby is defined as an infant with ≤2 standard deviations (SD) of weight for the gestational age, although this definition is not adequate for all groups, especially in developing countries.[4] Intrauterine life prepares the fetus to arrive mature in postnatal life and be able to face postnatal insults. During intrauterine life the organism passes through critical periods of rapid tissue growth with increased cell division. Affection of the organism in these critical periods might lead to permanent changes in individual organs. Increased maternal insulin resistance in the second half of pregnancy facilitates transfer of nutrients to the baby by reducing their utilization by the mother. Programming according to Lucas[5] is said to occur "when an early stimulus or insult, operating at a critical or sensitive period, results in permanent or long-term changes in the structure or function of the organism."

Normal fetal growth takes place in phases. The first phase consists of proliferation, organization, and differentiation of the embryo (embryonal life) while the second one consists of continuing growth and functional maturation of the different tissues and organs of the fetus (fetal life).[6] Fetal growth depends on genetic, placental, and maternal factors. The fetus is thought to have an inherent growth potential that, under normal circumstances, yields a healthy newborn of appropriate size. The maternal-placental-fetal unit acts in harmony to provide the needs of the fetus, while supporting the physiologic changes of the mother. Fetal growth restriction is the second leading cause of perinatal morbidity and mortality preceded only by prematurity.[7] The term intrauterine growth restriction (IUGR) is assigned to newborns with a birth weight and/or length below the 10th percentile for their gestational age and whose abdominal circumference is below the 2.5th percentile with pathologic restriction of fetal growth.[4] The incidence of IUGR is estimated to be approximately 5% in the general obstetric population.[8] Small for gestational age (SGA) babies are defined based on birth weight and/or length of ≤2 SD the mean for gestational age, although data on intrauterine growth are not always available and therefore it is rather a descriptive definition. However, taking into account only size at birth, SGA also includes "short-normal" babies with no pathological fetal growth restriction. This subgroup of "short-normal" SGA babies is not at increased risk for later development of metabolic abnormalities, as is the case for the IUGR babies.[9,10] The development of different somatometric parameters of fetal growth such as length and weight takes place during different stages of the intrauterine life. Growth in length occurs early in prenatal life while accumulation of weight occurs later during prenatal life.[6] According to the time of adverse intrauterine nutrition, an IUGR fetus may be classified as symmetric or asymmetric. Symmetric growth restriction indicates a fetus whose entire body is proportionally small (small weight, length, and head circumference). In this case the adverse environment is usually present early during gestation and the growth impairment is multifactorial, being the result of either genetic factors or congenital infections, congenital syndromes, or toxic effects in early gestation.[4] In symmetric IUGR fetuses, cell division and cell growth are diminished and postnatal catch-up growth is rarely seen. On the contrary, asymmetric growth restriction indicates an undernourished fetus (usually later during intrauterine life). In this case most of the energy is directed to growth maintenance of vital organs such as the heart and the brain at the expense of the liver, muscle, and fat (normal length but small weight).[11] This type of growth restriction is usually the result of placental insufficiency. Asymmetric IUGR presents with normal head circumference but small abdominal circumference, scrawny limbs, and thinned skin due to decreased liver size, muscle mass, and subcutaneous fat, respectively.

CAUSES OF IUGR

In IUGR fetuses, one-third of birth weight variations are determined by genetic factors, while two-thirds by environmental ones.[12] However, in many cases the underlying cause is unknown. During recent years significant progress has been made in the understanding of IUGR-associated pathophysiology. The effect of the genetic determinant is believed to be the consequence of early programming altered by intrauterine undernutrition and to work in concert with prenatal effects.[13] During intrauterine life brain growth seems to have a priority over the growth of other organs. This is apparent in IUGR fetuses. In this case brain growth is promoted by increased blood flow at the expense of the circuit that supplies the viscera including heart, liver, kidneys, pancreas, and bulk of the muscle in the lower limbs.[11,14] It is apparent, from epidemiological studies, that the timing of maternal nutrient restriction has a major influence on outcome in terms of predisposing the offspring to adult obesity. If nutrient restriction happens during the second and third trimester the future development of type 2 diabetes mellitus (DM2) is facilitated.[15] To investigate the role of fetal undernutrition Fernandez-Twinn et al. employed a rat model of maternal protein restriction throughout gestation and lactation, which imposed changes in maternal levels of glucose, insulin, prolactin, progesterone, estradiol, and leptin. Offspring in that study were born smaller than controls and developed diabetes, hyperinsulinemia, and tissue insulin resistance in adulthood. The authors concluded that these changes could influence the programming of eventual adult disease in the developing fetus.[16] A similar study suggested that early maternal protein restriction leads to skeletal muscle insulin resistance in rats due to reduced expression of protein kinase C zeta isoform.[17] The fetuses of alcoholic mothers represent another IUGR model. Alcohol-induced endocrine imbalances during pregnancy may contribute to the reprogramming of the hypothalamus-pituitary-adrenal (HPA) axis and the concept of fetal programming. Alcohol crosses the placenta and can directly affect developing fetal cells and tissues.[18]

Poor placental function has been associated with fetal undernutrition and IUGR.[12,19] Measurements of maternal placental and umbilical blood flows show that blood flows are reduced on both sides of the placenta in growth-restricted fetuses. Decreased placental exchange of important nutrients such as amino acids has been demonstrated in IUGR both *in vitro* and *in vivo*. It has been hypothesized that placenta may function as a nutrient sensor matching fetal growth rate to available nutrient resources by altering transport function, thus explaining fetal growth restriction and possibly growth enhancement in pregnancies with gestational diabetes (GD).[20] Placental dysfunction in IUGR is associated with decreased secretion of placental growth hormone (PGH) and IGF-1, both important determinants of fetal growth.[21] Under normal circumstances access to maternal endogenous glucocorticoids by the fetus is low because of the synthesis of 11β-hydroxysteroid dehydrogenase (11β-HSD) type 2 in the placenta. This enzyme interconverts active cortisol and corticosterone to inactive cortisone and 11-dehydrocorticosterone. There are two isoforms of 11βHSD, type 1, which acts bidirectionally and type 2, which acts unidirectionally (cortisol to cortisone). Studies showed an attenuated 11βHSD type 2 placental activity in IUGR suggesting that glucocorticoids may contribute to impaired fetal growth as it is generally accepted that placental 11βHSD type 2 is of primary importance in excluding maternal glucocorticoids from the fetus.[22,23]

Recent studies in humans suggest that alterations in the activity of the neuroendocrine system mediate the effects of psychosocial stress on fetal development and birth outcome. Chronic maternal distress compromises normal regulation of hormonal activity during pregnancy and elevated free circulating corticotropin-releasing hormone (CRH), probably of placental origin, occurs before its normal increase at term. Excess of CRH and other hormones such as cortisol that pass through the placenta can reduce birth weight and slow growth rate in prenatally stressed infants.[24]

In a study it has been shown that prenatal psychosocial stress and personality variables are associated with neuroendocrine parameters during human pregnancy implying a possible mechanism linking features of the maternal psychosocial environment to the fetal brain development.[25] Stress will lead to many cardiovascular and endocrine changes in the mother including increases in the secretion of ACTH, β-endorphin, glucocorticoids, and catecholamines. Catecholamines constrict placental blood vessels and cause fetal hypoxia, which in its turn will activate fetal HPA axis.[26] The impact of maternal stress on placental 11βHSD type 2 synthesis is not known. However, placental 11βHSD type 2 activity is reduced in IUGR pregnancies.[23]

Endocrine-related causes can lead to IUGR. The most important endocrine determinant of fetal growth is the insulin-like growth factor (IGF) system.[27,28] The IGFs are detectable in many different fetal tissues from the first trimester and their concentrations in the fetal circulation increase during pregnancy. The most important regulator of fetal IGF-1 concentrations is the availability of adequate glucose across the placenta. There are observations that umbilical cord blood IGF-1 levels correlate with birth weight.[29] Woods *et al.* reported a patient with a homozygous partial deletion of the gene encoding IGF-1 resulting in IGF-1 deficiency who had severe IUGR and postnatal growth failure.[30] There is an inverse correlation between fetal IGF binding protein (BP) 1 concentrations and birth weight from as early as 16 weeks gestation. IGFBP-1 is inversely related to insulin concentration and its secretion is regulated by insulin suggesting that hypoinsulinemia could be responsible for the increased IGFBP-1 concentrations in IUGR.[31] Finally, IUGR is associated with a state of growth hormone (GH) resistance.[29] A case-control study of 76 full-term gestations of which 31 were diagnosed as IUGR showed lower TSH, IGF-1, insulin, cholesterol, and albumin levels but higher GH levels compared to controls.[32] Furthermore, a recent study provided further evidence of dysregulation of the HPA axis in people who were born SGA by having significantly lower pituitary-adrenal responses in the dynamic dexamethasone-suppressed CRH test.[33]

The role of the oxidative stress and of proinflammatory cytokines in the outcome of IUGR is still under investigation. Recent data show that GD is associated with increased 8-isoprostane release—a marker of oxidative stress[34] compared to normal pregnancies. Oxidative stress can cause vascular dysfunction in the placenta, leading to fetal compromise.[35] Elevations in 8-isoprostane secretion from the placenta in women with GD may induce pathophysiological effects that contribute to adverse pregnancy outcomes. Other data show elevated levels of inflammatory cytokines in maternal serum and peritoneal washing during arrested labor.[36] Kotani *et al.* have shown that cord blood concentrations of adiponectin were positively correlated with both birth weight and fetal fat mass.[37]

IUGR AND THE METABOLIC SYNDROME

Data have shown that IUGR is associated with a late life increased prevalence of metabolic syndrome, a condition associating obesity with hypertension and DM2. Barker first associated birth size and later development of metabolic syndrome in adult life.[38] Carrying out a study on more than 20,000 newborns delivered between 1911 and 1930 in Hertfordshire County, he was able to demonstrate that the smaller the birth weight or the weight at 1 year of age the greater was the prevalence of metabolic syndrome in adult life. This relationship was continuous across the birth weight categories with those men who were smallest at birth (<2.5 kg), being nearly seven times more likely to have impaired glucose tolerance or DM2 than were those who were heaviest at birth (>4.3 kg).[19] One of the striking relationships observed in the Hertfordshire cohort was between birth weight and current presence of the metabolic syndrome. The prevalence of the metabolic syndrome increased with decreasing birth weight so that those men who were smallest at birth were 18 times more likely to have the metabolic syndrome at the time of the study than were those who were heaviest at birth.[39] Lipid abnormalities corresponding to the atherogenic profile and clotting factors' anomalies observed in adulthood were as well, directly correlated with low birth weight.

Woods *et al.* described a relation between postnatal lack of catch-up growth and development of insulin resistance.[30] Connection of low birth weight and insulin resistance or diabetes in adulthood may be a result of fetal malnutrition (the thrifty phenotype hypothesis) due to poor nutritional reserves of the mother, not adequate flow of the blood in uterus, or destruction of nutrients in the placenta.[40] Malnutrition then acts on insulin-sensitive tissues like liver, skeletal muscles, or pancreas. As an answer to malnutrition fetal insulin secretion decreases and adrenaline and cortisol levels increase to adjust fetal and placental metabolism for maximal utilization of nutrients, allocation of blood supply, and alteration of growth speed. Indeed, hormones have programmed functions and target effects in specific periods of development and their impairment may cause defect in physiological functions later in life.[40] Hofman *et al.* showed that short prepubertal IUGR children have a specific impairment in insulin sensitivity compared to their normal birth weight peers.[41] Furthermore, Yaznik *et al.* later described that for a given BMI Indians have a higher percentage of body fat and visceral fat than members of other populations.[42] Babies who are thin at birth lack muscle, a deficiency that will persist because the crucial period for muscle growth is ~30 weeks *in utero*, and there is little cell replication after birth. If they gain weight rapidly in childhood, they are liable to put on fat rather than muscle, leading to a disproportionately high fat mass in later life. This might be associated with the development of insulin resistance.[39] Ozanne *et al.* found decreased expression of specific insulin-signaling proteins in low birth weight subjects compared to controls.[43] Children born small for gestational age have been found to have reduced adiponectin levels, an adipocytokine with insulin-sensitizing and antiatherogenic properties, inversely related to postnatal catch-up growth.[44] Studies in Europe, North America, and India have shown association between coronary heart disease and small size at birth.[45] A very recent study demonstrated that birth weight was associated with total coronary artery diameter in 9-year-old children, independent of current weight and height, suggesting that growth during fetal life may have lasting effect on coronary artery size. Those who have been born SGA had smaller diameter of coronary arteries than those born appropriate for gestational age (AGA), bearing therefore a further risk factor for cardiovascular events besides their higher risk for the occurrence of the metabolic syndrome.[46] In the Helsinki cohort in men and women born between 1934 and 1944 the cumulative incidence of hypertension requiring medication fell from 20.2% in those weighing <3 kg at birth to 12.3% in those weighing >4 kg.[47]

Further to the possible links between low birth weight and the development of the metabolic syndrome later in life, and given the known associations between small alterations in adrenocortical activity and features of the metabolic syndrome such as raised blood pressure and glucose intolerance studies show that children with low birth weight have increased salivary cortisol responses to stress compared to controls.[48] Recently, a large epidemiological study among all 2,508 residents in Rochester, Minnesota, who met research criteria for adult onset DM2 found that the excess mortality observed for diabetes appeared disproportionately concentrated among abnormal birth weight individuals identifying a subset of at-risk diabetic individuals and reinforcing the importance of normal birth weight deliveries.[49]

CONCLUSIONS

In conclusion, an adverse intrauterine milieu can cause IUGR and this seems to be associated with the development of the metabolic syndrome later in life. As the metabolic syndrome is a major risk factor for the development of the epidemic of DM2 and cardiovascular disease, special attention should be paid to the metabolic endometrial environment, avoiding any adverse effects that could affect fetal growth with long-standing postnatal metabolic consequences.

REFERENCES

1. BARKER, D.J.P. 1998. Mothers, babies, and health in later life. Second edition. Barker, D.J.P., Ed.: Churchill Livingstone, New York.
2. PHILIPS, D.I.W. 2002. Endocrine programming and fetal origins of adult disease. Trends Endocrinol. Metab. **13:** 363.
3. KANAKA-GANTENBEIN C, G. MASTORAKOS & G.P. CHROUSSOS. 2003. Endocrine related causes and consequences of intrauterine growth retardation. Ann. N. Y. Acad. Sci. **997:** 150–157.
4. WOLLMANN, H.A. 1998. Intrauterine growth restriction: definition and etiology. Horm. Res. **49.** (Suppl 2): 1–6.
5. LUCAS, A. 1991. Programming by early nutrition in man. The childhood environment and adult disease. *In* CIBA Foundation Symposium 156. John Wiley, Chinchester 38–55.
6. RAPPAPORT, R. 1993. Fetal growth in pediatric endocrinology: physiology, pathophysiology and clinical aspects. Second edition. J. Bertrand, R. Rappaport & P.C. Sizonenko, Eds.: Williams and Wilkins, Baltimore, MD.
7. BERNSTEIN, I. & S.G GABBE. 1996. Intrauterine growth restriction. *In* S.G. Gabbe, J.R. Niebyl, J.L. Simpson, G.L. Annas, *et al.*, Eds.: 863–886. Obstetrics: normal and problem pregnancies. Third edition. Churchill Livingstone, New York.
8. NEERHOF, M.G. 1995. Causes of intrauterine growth restriction. Clin. Perinatol. **22:** 375–385.
9. LEE, P.A., S.D. CHERNAUSEK, A.C. HOKKEN KOELEGA & P. CHERNICHOW. 2003. International Small for Gestational Age Advisory Board consensus development conference statement: management of small children born small for gestational age April 24-October 1, 2001. Paediatrics. **112:** 180–182.

10. GARDOSI, J. 2006. New definition of small for gestational age based on fetal growth potential. Horm. Res. **65**(Suppl 3): 15–18.
11. DESAI, M., N.J. CROWTHER, A. LUCAS & C.N. HALES. 1996. Organ-selective growth in the offspring of mothers protein-restricted. Br. J. Nutr. **76**: 591–603.
12. BRYAN S.M. & P. HINDMARSH. 2006. Normal and abnormal fetal growth. Horm. Res. **65** (Suppl 3): 19–27.
13. SZITANYI, P., J. JANDA & R. POLDENE. 2003. Intrauterine undernutrition and programming as a new risk of cardiovascular disease in later life. Physiol. Res. **52**: 389–395.
14. GARROW, J.S., K. FLETCHER & D. HALLIDAY.1965. Body composition in severe infantile malnutrition. J. Clin. Invest. **44**: 417–425.
15. SYMONDS, M.E., S. PEARCE, J BISPHAM, *et al.* 2004. Timing of nutrient restriction and programming of fetal adipose tissue. Proceedings of the Nutrition Society. **63**: 397–403.
16. FERNANDEZ-TWINN D.S., S.E. OZANNE & S. EKIZOGLOU. 2003. The maternal endocrine environment in the low protein model of intrauterine growth restriction. Br. J. Nutr. **90**: 815–822.
17. OZANNE, S.E., G.S. OLSEN & L.L. HANSEN. 2003. Early growth restriction leads to down regulation of protein kinase zeta and insulin resistance in skeletal muscle. J. Endocrinol. **177**: 235–241.
18. ZHANG, X., J.H. SLIWOWSKA & J. WEINBERG. 2005. Prenatal alcohol exposure and fetal programming: effects on neuroendocrine and immune function. Exp. Biol. Med. **230**: 376–388.
19. OZANNE, S.E. & N. HALES. 2002. Early programming of glucose insulin metabolism. Trends Endocrinol. Metab. **13**: 368–373.
20. GLAZIER, J.D., I. CETIN, G. PERUGINO, *et al.* 1997. Association between the activity of the system A amino acid transporter in the microvillous plasma membrane of the human placenta and severity of fetal compromise in intrauterine growth restriction. Paediatr. Res. **42**: 514–519.
21. MC INTYRE H.D., R. SEREK, D.I. CRANE, *et al.* 2000. Placental growth hormone, GH-binding, and insulin like growth factor axis in normal, growth retarded and diabetic pregnancies: correlations with fetal growth. J. Clin. Endocrinol. Metab. **85**: 1143–1150.
22. SHAMS, M., M.D. KILBY & D.A SOMERSET. 1998. 11beta-hydroxysteroid dehydrogenase type 2 activity in human pregnancy and reduced expression in intrauterine growth restriction. Hum. Reprod. **13**: 799–804.
23. MCTERNAN, C.L., N. DRAPER, H. NICHOLSON, *et al.* 2001. Reduced placental 11β-hydroxysteroid dehydrogenase type 2 mRNA levels in human pregnancies complicated by intrauterine growth restriction: an analysis of possible mechanisms. J. Clin. Endocrinol. Metab. **86**: 4979–4983.
24. WEINSTOCK, M. 2005. The potential influence of maternal stress hormones on development and mental health of the offspring. Brain Behav. Immun. **19**: 296–308.
25. WADHWA, P.D., C DUNKEL-SCHETTER, A. CHIEZ-DE MET, *et al.* 1996. Prenatal psychosocial factors and the neuroendocrine axis in human pregnancy. Psychosom. Med. **58**: 432–446.
26. CHALLIS, J.R.C. 2000. Endocrine and paracrine regulation of birth at term and preterm. Endocr. Rev. **21**: 514–550.
27. GLUCKMAN, P.D. & J.E HARDING. 1997. The physiology and pathophysiology of intrauterine growth retardation. Horm. Res. **48**: 11–16.

28. GICQUEL, C. & Y. LE BOUC. 2006. Hormonal regulation of fetal growth. Horm. Res. **65**(Suppl 3): 28–33.
29. GLUCKMAN, P.D. 1997. Endocrine and nutritional regulation of prenatal growth. Acta Paediatr. **423**: 153–157.
30. WOODS, K.A., C. CAMACHO-HUBNER, M.O. SAVAGE & A. CLARK. 1996. Intrauterine growth retardation and postnatal growth failure associated with deletion of the insulin-like growth factor-1 gene. N. Engl. J. Med. **335**: 1363–1367.
31. CUTFIELD, W.S., P.L. HOFMAN, M. VICKERS, et al. 2002. IGFs and binding proteins in short children with intrauterine growth retardation. J. Clin. Endocrinol. Metab. **87**: 235–239.
32. NIETO-DIAZ A, J. VILLAR, R MATORRAS-WEINIG & P VALENZUELA-RUIZ. 1996. Intrauterine growth retardation at term: association between antropometric and endocrine parameters. Acta Obstet. Gynecol. Scand. **75**: 127–131.
33. WARD, A.M., H.E. SYDDALL, P.J. WOOD, et al. 2004. Fetal programming of the hypothalamic-pituitary-adrenal axis: low birth weight and cer HPA regulation. J. Clin. Endocrinol. Metab. **89**: 1227–1233.
34. LAPPAS, M., M. PERMEZEL & G.E. RICE. 2004. Release of proinflammatory cytokines and 8-isoprostane from placenta, adipose tissue and skeletal muscle from normal pregnant women and women with gestational diabetes mellitus. J. Clin. Endocrinol. Metab. **89**: 5627–5633.
35. MYATT, L., W. KOSSENJANS, R SAHAY, et al. 2000. Oxidative stress causes vascular dysfunction in the placenta. J. Maternal Fetal Neonatal Med. **9**: 79–82.
36. ABRAMOV, Y., Y. EZRA, U. ELCHALAL, et al. 2004. Markedly elevated levels of inflammatory cytokines in maternal serum and peritoneal washing during arrested labor. Acta Obstet. Scand. **83**: 358–363.
37. KOTANI, Y., I. YOKOTA, S. KITAMURA, et al. 2004. Plasma adiponectin levels in newborns are higher than those in adults and positively correlated with birth weight. Clin. Endocrinol. **61**: 418–423.
38. BARKER D.J.P., P.D. GLUCKMAN, K.M. GODFREY, et al. 1993. Fetal nutrition and cardiovascular disease. Lancet **341**: 938–941.
39. BARKER D.J.P., C.N. HALES, C.H. FALL, et al. 1993. Type 2 (non-insulin-dependent) diabetes mellitus, hypertension and hyperlipidaemia (syndrome X): relation to reduced fetal growth. Diabetologia **36**: 62–67.
40. JAQUET, D., J. LEGER, P. CSERNICHOW & C LEVY-MARCHAL. 2002. The effect of in utero undernutrition on the insulin resistance syndrome. Curr. Diab. Rep. **2**: 77–82.
41. HOFMAN, P.L., W.S. CUTFIELD, E.M. ROBINSON, et al. 1997. Insulin resistance in short children with intrauterine growth retardation. J. Clin. Endocrinol. Metab. **82**: 402–406.
42. YAZNIK, C.S. 2004. Early life origins of insulin resistance and type 2 diabetes in India and other Asian countries. J. Nutr. **134**: 205–210.
43. OZANNE, S.E., C.B. JENSSEN, K.J. TINGEY, et al. 2005. Low birthweight is associated with specific changes in muscle insulin-signalling protein expression. Diabetologia **48**: 547–552.
44. CIANFARANNI, S., C. MARTINEZ, A. MAIORANA, et al. 2004. Adiponectin levels are reduced in children born small for gestational age and are inversely related to postnatal growth catch-up. J. Clin. Endocrinol. Metab. **89**: 1346–1351.
45. FRANKEL, S., P. ELWOOD, P. SWEETNAM, et al. 1996. Birthweight, body mass index in middle age and incident coronary heart disease. Lancet **348**: 1478–1480.

46. JIANG, B., K.M. GODFREY, C.N. MARTYN & C.R. GALE. 2006. Birth weight and cardiac structure in children. Paediatrics **117:** 257–261.
47. BARKER D.J.P., T. FORSEN, J.E. ERIKSSON & C. OSMOND. 2002. Growth and living conditions in childhood and hypertension in adult life: longitudinal study. J. Hypertension **20:** 1951–1956.
48. JONES, A., K.M. GODFREY, P. WOOD, *et al*. 2006. Fetal growth and the adrenocortical response to psychological stress. J. Clin. Endocrinol. Metab. **91(5):** 1868–1871.
49. LEIBSON, C.L., J.P. BURKE, B.S. RANSOM, *et al*. 2005. Relative risk of mortality associated with diabetes as a function of birth weight. Diab. Care **28:** 2839–2845.

Premature Adrenarche Leads to Polycystic Ovary Syndrome?

Long-Term Consequences

ELENI KOUSTA

Consultant in Endocrinology and Diabetes, Corfu, Greece

ABSTRACT: Premature adrenarche is characterized by an early increase in adrenal androgen production that results in the development of pubic hair before the age of 8 years in girls and 9 years in boys, with or without axillary hair, and with no other signs of sexual development. Premature adrenarche has no adverse effects on the onset and progression of gonadarche and final height. However, it can no longer be considered a benign condition as it has been associated with hyperinsulinemia, dyslipidemia, and obesity already in the prepubertal period and polycystic ovary syndrome (PCOS) at adolescence. Furthermore, a possible association between premature adrenarche and metabolic and endocrine abnormalities with low birth weight has been postulated. PCOS, as recently redefined, is the most common endocrine disorder to affect women of reproductive age and has been associated with increased risk for type 2 diabetes and increased prevalence of cardiovascular risk factors at an earlier age than expected. Premature adrenarche and PCOS share similar metabolic disturbances. It may be that metabolic abnormalities start very early in life during the prenatal or prepubertal period and premature adrenarche may be a forerunner of PCOS and the metabolic syndrome in some girls. Large long-term epidemiological studies are needed to allow clear association of the two conditions and assessment of the risk of disease in later life.

KEYWORDS: premature adrenarche; polycystic ovaries; long-term consequences

INTRODUCTION

Adrenarche is the puberty of the adrenal gland and is characterized by the activation of adrenal androgen production and by increases in dehydroepiandrosterone (DHEA) and dehydroepiandrosterone sulfate (DHEAS), both products

Address for correspondence: Dr. Eleni Kousta, M.D., Ph.D., 6, S. Arvanitaki, Corfu 49100, Greece. Voice: +30-26610-80561; fax: +30-26610-80562.
  e-mail: lkousta@otenet.gr

Ann. N.Y. Acad. Sci. 1092: 148–157 (2006). © 2006 New York Academy of Sciences.
doi: 10.1196/annals.1365.013

of the zona reticularis of the adrenal gland.[1] The descriptive clinical term *pubarche* indicates the appearance of pubic hair, which may be accompanied by axillary hair. This process is considered premature if it occurs before the age of 8 years in girls and 9 years in boys.[1] Premature adrenarche can no longer be considered a benign condition in girls. It has metabolic consequences such as polycystic ovary syndrome (PCOS), insulin resistance, and dyslipidemia in later life; some of these metabolic abnormalities are already recognized in childhood or adolescence.[1] Premature adrenarche in boys was not associated with endocrine-metabolic abnormalities by some authors,[2] but was associated with decreased insulin sensitivity, independent of obesity, by others.[3]

PCOS is the most common endocrine disorder to affect women of reproductive age.[4] The clinical and biochemical features of the syndrome are heterogeneous and the combination and degree of expression of these features vary between individuals. In the last few years, it became clear that PCOS is not simply a combination of hyperandogenemia and anovulation, but has been associated with increased risk for type 2 diabetes and increased prevalence of cardiovascular risk factors.[5]

Premature adrenarche and PCOS share similar metabolic disturbances and it has been postulated that premature adrenarche precedes the development of ovarian hyperandrogenemia.[1] In this review, metabolic consequences and the association between the two conditions are discussed.

PREMATURE ADRENARCHE

Premature adrenarche refers to an early increase in adrenal androgen production that results in the development of pubic hair before the age of 8 years in girls and 9 years in boys, with or without axillary hair and pubertal odor, and with no other signs of sexual development.[1] Premature adrenarche is a diagnosis of exclusion. Children with premature adrenarche need to be evaluated to exclude late-onset congenital adrenal hyperplasia, precocious puberty, Cushing's disease, a virilizing adrenal or gonadal tumor, and iatrogenic androgen administration.[1] As in precocious puberty, girls are much more frequently affected than boys, with a ratio of almost 10:1.[6]

The exact prevalence of premature adrenarche is not known. There are significant racial differences in the prevalence of premature adrenarche. In a cross-sectional study involving 17,077 girls, where though no endocrine evaluations were carried out, 9.5% and 34.3% of black girls at 6 and 8 years of age, respectively, had at least Tanner stage 2 pubic hair, whereas 1.4% and 7.7% of white girls, at the same ages, respectively, had pubic hair.[7] In another study of Lithuanian schoolgirls the prevalence of premature adrenarche was found to be much lower (0.8%).[8]

Nutritional status has been postulated to be a regulator of adrenarche[9] and obesity has been associated with a higher incidence of premature adrenarche.[10]

Pathophysiology

In premature adrenarche there is an early isolated maturation of the adrenal gland, the cause of which remains unclear.[11] Baseline serum levels of adrenal androgens, particularly DHEA, DHEAS, androstenedione, and testosterone are moderately increased for chronological age, but are in the range of those found in early puberty.[11,12] However, DHEAS levels may exceed those of pubertal controls.[12] In some patients, the early development of pubic hair is associated with normal androgen levels for chronological age suggesting increased peripheral sensitivity.[13] Gonadotropins do not play a role in the development of premature adrenarche just as in normal adrenarche.[14]

Onset of Puberty and Final Height

Premature adrenarche causes a transient acceleration in growth and bone maturation.[15,16] Growth velocity may be increased and bone maturation may be moderately advanced ($<\pm2$ standard deviation [SD], but correlating with the height age).[15,17] However, premature adrenarche is not associated with a significant alteration in the timing of the child's subsequent pubertal development; the initiation of gonadarche (Tanner breast stage 2) is comparable to maternal and population data.[15] Final height in girls with premature adrenarche correlates well with height prognosis at the time of diagnosis and at onset of puberty and is generally above midparental heights, following the secular trend.[15] Therefore, although premature adrenarche appears to cause an acceleration in bone maturation, it has no adverse effects on the onset and progression of gonadarche and final height.

Premature Adrenarche and PCOS

Although premature adrenarche does not influence the timing of puberty, it has been associated with ovulatory dysfunction and functional ovarian hyperandrogenism. An increased incidence of hirsutism and PCOS was initially observed in peripubertal and postpubertal girls with premature adrenarche during childhood.[18] In a subsequent study, the prevalence of polycystic appearance of the ovaries on ultrasound in girls with premature adrenarche throughout childhood and puberty has been shown to be greater than would be expected for their age.[19] In another study, 16 out of 35 adolescents with a history of premature adrenarche showed hirsutism, oligomenorrhea, and elevated baseline testosterone and/or androstenedione levels.[20] The assessment of ovulatory function by frequent measurements of salivary progesterone and urinary luteinizing hormone (LH) in girls with a history of premature adrenarche, studied 3 years after menarche, has shown decreased ovulation rates compared with the normal population.[21] These observations suggest increased incidence of PCOS among the girls with (a history of) premature adrenarche.

Premature Adrenarche and Metabolic Risk Factors

Hyperinsulinemia after an oral glucose load was documented among lean girls with premature adrenarche before and also during pubertal development compared with bone age- and Tanner stage-matched control white girls.[22] In the same study increased free androgen indexes and lower serum sex hormone binding globulin (SHBG) and insulin growth factor binding protein (IGFBP)-1 levels were also found at most pubertal stages in girls with premature adrenarche.[22] It has been postulated that hyperinsulinemia in premature adrenarche may be directly related to the degree of androgen excess.[23] Similarly to Caucasian subjects, nearly 50% of prepubertal Black African and Caribbean girls with premature adrenarche had significant decrease in insulin sensitivity during the frequently sampled intravenous (i.v.) glucose tolerance test.[24] Thus, hyperinsulinemia is a common feature among girls with premature adrenarche and may be related to the degree of hyperandrogenemia.

Premature adrenarche has been associated with several other atherosclerosis risk factors. Body mass index (BMI) is higher among girls with premature adrenarche than control girls.[25] Both systolic and diastolic blood pressure (BP), total cholesterol, LDL-C, VLDL-C, and TC/HDL-C were higher among girls with premature adrenarche compared to control girls.[25] HDL-Cholesterol was found to be decreased in African American and Caribbean Hispanic girls with premature adrenarche compared to control girls.[26] Increased serum triglyceride levels throughout all stages of pubertal development, independent of obesity, were observed in girls with premature adrenarche.[27]

Increased prevalence of type 2 diabetes and impaired glucose tolerance in first-degree relatives of Caucasian, African American, and Caribbean Hispanic girls with premature adrenarche were observed compared to a control population.[24,28]

Premature Adrenarche and Reduced Fetal Growth

Barker et al. reported increased rates of cardiovascular disease and type 2 diabetes mellitus in adults born with intrauterine growth retardation.[29] According to Barker's hypothesis, the growth-retarded fetus adapts to undernutrition and survives by altering endocrine and metabolic set points that appear to remain altered postnatally (see the chapter by Valsamakis et al. in the same volume).

Girls with premature adrenarche have significantly lower birth scores compared to control girls of similar gestational ages.[30,31] Furthermore, the degree

of prenatal growth restriction is more pronounced among those girls with premature adrenarche who display hyperandrogenemia and hyperinsulinemia.[30]
It could be that premature adrenarche and the metabolic syndrome in some
girls may have an early origin with low birth weight serving as a marker.[1]

PCOS

Although the first description of PCOS occurred almost 70 years ago,[32]
there has been no universal agreement about its definition. Recently, the European Society for Human Reproduction and Embryology and the American
Society for Reproductive Medicine (ESHRE/ASRM) achieved a new consensus regarding the definition of PCOS.[5] This is now defined as the presence
of any two of the following three criteria: (a) polycystic ovaries on ultrasound
scan; (b) oligo- and/or anovulation; and (c) clinical or biochemical evidence of
hyperandrogenism, provided other etiologies (congenital adrenal hyperplasia,
androgen-secreting tumors, Cushing's syndrome) have been excluded. Furthermore, the ultrasound diagnostic criteria for PCO morphology have been
redefined as the presence of 12 or more follicles in each ovary measuring
2–9 mm in diameter, and/or increased ovarian volume (>10 mL).[5] The prevalence of PCOS varies according to the definition used and the reference population.[4,33]

Disagreement about diagnostic criteria has, up to now, made it difficult to
compare epidemiological studies of long-term health risks, however, it is now
well accepted that PCOS has been associated with metabolic disorders and
increased risk factors for cardiovascular disease.[5]

IMPAIRED INSULIN ACTION AND SECRETION, INCREASED RISK OF OBESITY, AND TYPE 2 DIABETES IN PCOS

Women with PCOS, even when lean, have a greater frequency and degree
of both hyperinsulinemia and insulin resistance than matched controls.[34] Hyperinsulinemia itself may contribute to the mechanism of anovulation and the
expression of PCOS.[35] Defects in insulin secretion in addition to insulin resistance were documented among women with PCOS.[36] It has been postulated
that metabolic abnormalities in PCOS start very early in life, during the prenatal
or prepubertal period, and an early exposure to androgens during development
may affect body fat distribution and insulin action.[35]

A significant proportion of women with PCOS are affected by obesity.[37] The
cause of obesity among women with PCOS is unknown, but the presence of
obesity in PCOS women has not only important metabolic but also reproductive
consequences including anovulation, infertility, and miscarriage.[38]

The overall risk of developing type 2 diabetes was found to be increased
3–7 times among PCOS women[39,40,41] and mortality from the complications

of diabetes among women with PCOS is increased.[42] The onset of glucose intolerance in PCOS women seems to occur at an early age, typically in the third to fourth decade of life.[39,40] Abnormalities in both insulin action and secretion and glucose intolerance have been observed even in adolescents with PCOS.[43,44]

Other Markers of Cardiovascular Risk in PCOS: Hyperlipidemia, Hypertension, Endothelial Dysfunction, and Premature Atherosclerosis

Dyslipidemia is common among women with PCOS, even after controlling for obesity.[41,45] Data on BP in women with PCOS are controversial. BP has been reported to be raised among PCOS women compared with control women, even after adjusting for BMI[41] by some but not all investigators.[46]

Decreased endothelial function and raised endothelin-1 were shown among women with PCOS, even when young, normotensive, nonobese, and nondyslipidemic women were studied, suggestive of an early vascular impairment among them.[47] CRP concentrations were significantly increased in women with PCOS compared to BMI-matched control women, suggestive of low-grade inflammation and endothelial dysfunction.[48] Greater carotid intima-media thickness, a marker of an increased risk for atherosclerosis was shown among young PCOS women compared to age and BMI-matched control subjects.[47] These observations are indicative of the early stages of atherosclerosis at an earlier age than expected in women with PCOS. It is not known whether the cause of these abnormalities can be attributed to PCOS *per se* or to the metabolic disturbances of the syndrome.

Cardiovascular Events in PCOS

Although cardiovascular risk factors are increased among women with PCOS, increased prevalence of cardiovascular events has not been confirmed. In a large retrospective study of 786 women with PCOS in the UK mortality or morbidity rates from cardiovascular disease are not higher than expected.[42] There was an increased number of deaths where type 2 diabetes was a complicating factor.[42] A more detailed subsequent study by the same research group showed increased history of cerebrovascular disease among women with PCOS and higher levels of several cardiovascular and metabolic risk factors such as diabetes, hypertension, hypercholesterolemia, hypertriglyceridemia, and increased waist/hip.[41] However, the subjects studied were middle-aged at the time of observation and it cannot be excluded that as the cohort ages, there will be a divergence between PCOS and control groups in the incidence of coronary heart disease. Further, long-term epidemiological studies are needed before definite conclusions can be drawn.

SUMMARY

In premature adrenarche there is an early isolated maturation of the adrenal gland, the clinical manifestation of which is the development of pubic hair, with or without axillary hair, before the age of 8 years in girls and 9 years in boys. Premature adrenarche is a diagnosis of exclusion and children with premature adrenarche need to be evaluated to exclude other causes of excess androgen production. There is now evidence to suggest that premature adrenarche can no longer be considered a benign condition in girls. Although premature adrenarche has no adverse effects on the onset and progression of gonadarche and final height, it has been associated with hyperinsulinemia, dyslipidemia, and obesity already in the prepubertal period and PCOS at adolescence, indicating long-term follow-up of these in girls into adulthood. Premature adrenarche may precede the development of PCOS and may have an early origin with low birth weight serving as a marker.

Women with PCOS have increased levels of cardiovascular risk factors, but the level of risk of cardiovascular disease is uncertain. This adverse cardiovascular risk profile may start at an early age and may lead to premature atherosclerosis. The overall risk of developing type 2 diabetes among women with PCOS was found to be increased 3–7 times and mortality from the complications of diabetes is also increased.

These observations taken together suggest that it may be that metabolic abnormalities start very early in life during the prenatal or prepubertal period; premature adrenarche may be a forerunner of PCOS and the metabolic syndrome in some girls. Importantly, there are, as yet, no large long-term studies of girls with premature adrenarche and of well-characterized women with PCOS that will allow clear association of the two conditions and assessment of the risk of disease in later life. Such epidemiological studies are needed to assess the risk of long-term health consequences, to identify the subgroups of girls and women, which need to be targeted, and determine the timing and nature of measures for intervention and prevention.

REFERENCES

1. IBANEZ, L., et al. 2000. Premature adrenarche—normal variant or forerunner of adult disease? Endocr. Rev. **21:** 671–696.
2. POTAU, N., et al. 1999. Pronounced adrenarche and precocious pubarche in boys. Horm. Res. **51:** 238–241.
3. DENBURG, M.R., et al. 2002. Insulin sensitivity and the insulin-like growth factor system in prepubertal boys with premature adrenarche. J. Clin. Endocrinol. Metab. **87:** 5604–5609.
4. FRANKS, S. 1995. Polycystic ovary syndrome. N. Engl. J. Med. **333:** 853–861.
5. THE ROTTERDAM ESHRE/ASRM-SPONSORED PCOS CONSENSUS WORKSHOP GROUP. 2004. Revised 2003 consensus on diagnostic criteria and long-term health risks related to polycystic ovary syndrome (PCOS). Hum. Reprod. **19:** 41–47.

6. SIGURJONSDOTTIR, T.J. & A.S. HAYLES. 1968. Premature pubarche. Clin. Pediatr. (Phila.) **7:** 29–33.
7. HERMAN-GIDDENS, M.E., *et al.* 1997. Secondary sexual characteristics and menses in young girls seen in office practice: a study from the Pediatric Research in Office Settings Network. Pediatrics **99:** 505–512.
8. ZUKAUSKAITE, S., *et al.* 2005. Onset of breast and pubic hair development in 1231 preadolescent Lithuanian schoolgirls. Arch. Dis. Child. **90:** 932–936.
9. REMER, T. & F. MARZ. 1999. Role of nutritional status in the regulation of adrenarche.. J. Clin. Endocrinol. Metab. **84:** 3936–3944.
10. JABBAR, M., *et al.* 1991. Excess weight and precocious pubarche in children: alterations of the adrenocortical hormones. J. Am. Coll. Nutr. **10:** 289–296.
11. VOUTILAINEN, R., J. PERHEENTUPA & D. APTER. 1983. Benign premature adrenarche: clinical features and serum steroid levels. Acta Paediatr. Scand. **72:** 707–711.
12. IBANEZ, L., N. POTAU & A. CARRASCOSA. 1997. Androgens in adrenarche and pubarche. *In* Androgen Excess Disorders. R.A. Women, J.E. Nestler & D. Dewailly, Eds.: 73–84. Lippincott-Raven. Philadelphia.
13. ROSENFIELD, R.L. 1994. Normal and almost normal precocious variations in pubertal development: premature pubarche and premature thelarche revisited. Horm. Res. **41:** 7–13.
14. LEE, P.A. & F.J. GAREIS. 1976. Gonadotropin and sex steroid response to luteinizing-hormone-releasing hormone in patients with premature adrenarche. J. Clin. Endocrinol. Metab. **43:** 195–197.
15. IBANEZ, L., *et al.* 1992. Natural history of premature pubarche: an auxological study. J. Clin. Endocrinol. Metab. **74:** 254–257.
16. PERE, A., *et al.* 1995. Follow-up of growth and steroids in premature adrenarche. Eur. J. Pediatr. **154:** 346–352.
17. SAENGER, P. & E.O. REITER. 1992. Premature adrenarche: a normal variant of puberty? J. Clin. Endocrinol. Metab. **74:** 236–238.
18. YEN, S.S.C. 1986. Chronic anovulation caused by peripheral endocrine disorders. *In* Reproductive Endocrinology. S.C.C. Yen & R.B. Jaffe, Eds.: 441–499. Saunders. Philadelphia.
19. BRIDGES, N.A., *et al.* 1995. Ovaries in sexual precocity. Clin. Endocrinol. (Oxf.) **42:** 135–140.
20. IBANEZ, L., F. DE ZEGHER & N. POTAU. 1993. Postpubertal outcome in girls diagnosed of premature pubarche during childhood: increased frequency of functional ovarian hyperandrogenism. J. Clin. Endocrinol. Metab. **76:** 1599–1603.
21. IBANEZ, L., *et al.* 1999. Anovulation after precocious pubarche: early markers and time course in adolescence. J. Clin. Endocrinol. Metab. **84:** 2691–2695.
22. IBANEZ, L., *et al.* 1997. Hyperinsulinemia and decreased insulin-like growth factor binding protein-1 are common features in prepubertal and postpubertal girls with a history of premature pubarche. J. Clin. Endocrinol. Metab. **82:** 2283–2288.
23. IBANEZ, L., *et al.* 1996. Hyperinsulinemia in postpubertal girls with a history of premature pubarche and functional ovarian hyperandrogenism. J. Clin. Endocrinol. Metab. **81:** 1237–1243.
24. VUGUIN, P., *et al.* 1999. The role of insulin sensitivity, insulin-like growth factor-I and insulin-like growth factor binding proteins 1 and 3 in the hyperandrogenism of African American and Caribbean Hispanic girls with premature adrenarche. J. Clin. Endocrinol. Metab. **84:** 2037–2042.
25. GUVEN, A., P. CINAZ & A. BIDECI. 2005. Is premature adrenarche a risk factor for atherogenesis? Pediatr. Int. **47:** 20–25.

26. DiMartino-Nardi, J. 1999. Premature adrenarch: findings in prepubertal African-American and Caribbean-Hispanic girls. Acta Paediatr. Suppl. **433:** 1–6.
27. Ibanez, L., *et al.* 1998. Hyper-insulinemia, dyslipidemia and cardiovascular risk in girls with a history of premature pubarche. Diabetologia **41:** 1057–1063.
28. Ibanez, L., *et al.* 1999. Increased prevalence of unknown type 2 diabetes mellitus and impaired glucose tolerance in first-degree relatives of girls with a history of precocious pubarche. Clin. Endocrinol. (Oxf.) **51:** 395–401.
29. Barker, D.J.P., *et al.* 1993. Type 2 diabetes mellitus, hypertension and hyperlipi-daemia (syndrome X): relation to reduced fetal growth. Diabetologia **36:** 62–67.
30. Ibanez, L., *et al.* 1998. Precocious pubarche, hyperinsulinism and ovarian hyper-androgenism in girls: relation to reduced fetal growth. J. Clin. Endocrinol. Metab. **83:** 3558–3662.
31. Neville, K.A. & J.L. Walker. 2005. Precocious pubarche is associated with SGA, prematurity, weight gain, and obesity. Arch. Dis. Child. **90:** 258–261.
32. Stein, I.F. & M.L. Leventhal. 1935. Amenorrhea associated with bilateral poly-cystic ovaries. Am. J. Obstet. Gynecol. **29:** 181–191.
33. Knochenhauer, E.S., *et al.* 1998. Prevalence of the polycystic ovary syndrome in unselected black and white women of the southeastern United States: a prospec-tive study. J. Clin. Endocrinol. Metab. **83:** 3078–3082.
34. Dunaif, A. 1997. Insulin resistance and the polycystic ovary syndrome: mechanism of action and implications for pathogenesis. Endocr. Rev. **18:** 774–800.
35. Abbott, D.H., D.A. Dumesic & S. Franks. 2002. Developmental origin of poly-cystic ovary syndrome—a hypothesis. J. Endocrinol. **174:** 1–5.
36. Dunaif, A. & D.T. Finegood. 1996. Beta-cell dysfunction independent of obesity and glucose intolerance in the polycystic ovary syndrome. J. Clin. Endocrinol. Metab. **81:** 942–947.
37. Asuncion, M., *et al.* 2000. A prospective study of the prevalence of the polycystic ovary syndrome in unselected Caucasian women from Spain. J. Clin. Endocrinol. Metab. **85:** 2434–2438.
38. Hamilton-Fairley, D., *et al.* 1992. Association of moderate obesity with a poor pregnancy outcome in women with polycystic ovary syndrome treated with low dose gonadotrophin. Br. J. Obstet. Gynaecol. **99:** 128–131.
39. Ehrmann, D.A., *et al.* 1999. Prevalence of impaired glucose tolerance and diabetes in women with polycystic ovary syndrome. Diabetes Care **22:** 141–146.
40. Legro, R.S., *et al.* 1999. Prevalence and predictors of risk for type 2 diabetes mel-litus and impaired glucose tolerance in polycystic ovary syndrome: a prospective, controlled study in 254 affected women. J. Clin. Endocrinol. Metab. **84:** 165–169.
41. Wild, S., *et al.* 2000. Cardiovascular disease in women with polycystic ovary syndrome at long-term follow-up: a retrospective cohort study. Clin. Endocrinol. (Oxf.). **52:** 595–600.
42. Pierpoint, T., *et al.* 1998. Mortality of women with polycystic ovary syndrome at long-term follow-up. J. Clin. Epidemiol. **51:** 581–586.
43. Lewy, V.D., *et al.* 2001. Early metabolic abnormalities in adolescent girls with polycystic ovarian syndrome. J. Pediatr. **138:** 38–44.
44. Palmert, M.R., *et al.* 2002. Screening for abnormal glucose tolerance in adoles-cents with polycystic ovary syndrome. J. Clin. Endocrinol. Metab. **87:** 1017–1023.
45. Talbott, E., *et al.* 1998. Adverse lipid and coronary heart disease risk profiles in young women with polycystic ovary syndrome: results of a case-control study. J. Clin. Epidemiol. **51:** 415–422.

46. MATHER, K.J., F. KWAN & B. CORENBLUM. 2000. Hyperinsulinemia in polycystic ovary syndrome correlates with increased cardiovascular risk independent of obesity. Fertil. Steril. **73:** 150–156.
47. ORIO, F.J., *et al*. 2004. Early impairment of endothelial structure and function in young normal-weight women with polycystic ovary syndrome. J. Clin. Endocrinol. Metab. **89:** 4588–4593.
48. KELLY, C.C., *et al*. 2001. Low grade chronic inflammation in women with polycystic ovarian syndrome. J. Clin. Endocrinol. Metab. **86:** 2453–2455.

Polycystic Ovary Syndrome

A Multifaceted Disease from Adolescence to Adult Age

RENATO PASQUALI AND ALESSANDRA GAMBINERI

Endocrinology Unit, Department of Internal Medicine, S. Orsola-Malpighi Hospital, University of Bologna, Bologna, Italy

ABSTRACT: Polycystic ovary syndrome (PCOS), one of the most common causes of ovulatory infertility, affects 4–7% of women. Although it was considered that PCOS may have some genetic component and that clinical features of this disorder may change throughout a life span, starting from adolescence to postmenopausal age, no effort has been made to define differences in the phenotype and clinical presentation according to age. Indeed, it has been widely recognized in the last decade that several features of metabolic syndrome (MS), particularly insulin resistance and hyperinsulinemia, are inconsistently present in the majority of women with PCOS. This represents an important factor in the evaluation of PCOS throughout life, which implies that PCOS by itself may not be a hyperandrogenic disorder exclusively related to young and fertile-aged women, but may also have some health implications later in life. In young women with PCOS, hyperandrogenism, menses irregularities, and insulin resistance may occur together, emphasizing the pathophysiological role of excess androgen and insulin on PCOS. Hyperandrogenism and infertility represent the major complaints of PCOS in adult fertile age. In addition, obesity and MS may affect more than half these women. Later in life, it becomes clear that the association of obesity (particularly the abdominal phenotype) and PCOS renders affected women more susceptible to develop type 2 diabetes mellitus (T2DM), with some difference in the prevalence rates among countries, suggesting that environmental factors are important in determining individual susceptibility. Little is known about ovarian morphology and androgen production in women with PCOS after menopause. Some studies found that morphological ultrasonographic features consistent with polycystic ovaries are very common in postmenopausal women, and that these features are associated with higher than normal testosterone levels and metabolic alterations. There is an obvious need for further research in this area. Identification of major complaints and features of PCOS during the different ages

Address for correspondence: Renato Pasquali. U.O. di Endocrinologia, Dipt. Medicina Interna, Osp. S.Orsola-Malpighi, via Massarenti 9, 40138 Bologna, Italy. Voice: 0039-0-51-6364147; fax: 0039-0-51-6363080.
e-mail: renato.pasquali@unibo.it

Ann. N.Y. Acad. Sci. 1092: 158–174 (2006). © 2006 New York Academy of Sciences.
doi: 10.1196/annals.1365.014

of an affected woman may help, in fact, to plan individual therapeutic strategies, and, possibly, prevent long-term chronic metabolic diseases.

KEYWORDS: polycystic ovary syndrome (PCOS); hyperandrogenism; hyperinsulinemia; infertility; obesity

DEFINITION OF THE POLYCYSTIC OVARY SYNDROME

PCOS, one of the most common causes of ovulatory infertility, affects 4–7% of women.[1] Over the years, after the first description by Stein and Leventhal in 1935,[2] this syndrome has been defined in different ways. In 1990 the National Institutes of Health (NIH) established the new diagnostic criteria for this disorder, which were based on the presence of hyperandrogenism and chronic oligoanovulation, with the exclusion of other causes of hyperandrogenism such as adult onset congenital adrenal hyperplasia, hyperprolactinemia, and androgen-secreting neoplasms.[3] More recently, a consensus conference held in Rotterdam, 2003, reexamined the 1990 criteria and admitted the opportunity of including ultrasound morphology of the ovaries as a potential criterion to define PCOS.[4] On the other hand, it was also established that at least two of the following criteria—oligo and/or anovulation, clinical and/or biochemical signs of hyperandrogenism, and polycystic ovaries at ultrasound—are sufficient for the diagnosis. Although it was considered that PCOS may have some genetic component and that clinical features of this disorder may change throughout a life span, starting from adolescence to postmenopausal age, no effort has been made to define differences in the phenotype and clinical presentation according to age (FIG. 1). This can be considered an important problem both in research and clinical practice. Indeed, it has been widely recognized in the last decade that several features of "metabolic syndrome (MS)," particularly insulin resistance and hyperinsulinemia, are inconsistently present in the majority of women with PCOS. This represents an important factor in the evaluation of PCOS throughout life and implies that PCOS is not only a hyperandrogenic disorder related to young and fertile-aged women, but may also have some health implications later in life.[5] In addition, obesity is a very common clinical feature in women affected by PCOS, more than 50–60% of PCOS women being obese. This suggests a pathogenetic role of obesity in the subsequent development of the syndrome.[6] Finally, very few studies have examined the functional role of the polycystic ovaries in postmenopausal women, as no data are yet available on the role of androgens in the pathophysiology of chronic metabolic and cardiovascular diseases (CVDs) in older PCOS women.

This short review aims to define the clinical, hormonal, and metabolic features of women with PCOS at the different ages. This may be of great importance because therapeutic approaches should be targeted on primary complaints according to women's expectations and modify the natural history of this disorder.

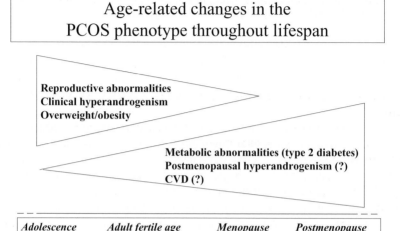

FIGURE 1. Age-related changes in the PCOS phenotype throughout a life span. The question marks identify still debatable topics.

PCOS PHENOTYPE IN ADOLESCENCE AND YOUNG WOMEN

At the age of approximately 10 years, a 20-fold increase in luteinizing hormone (LH) concentrations occurs over 1 year's time in girls,[7] followed by a 5- to 10-fold increase in serum androgen and estradiol levels over the following few years. Furthermore, the pubertal increase of growth hormone leads to a 30% decrease in insulin sensitivity, an increase in insulin levels, and a significant decrease in circulating sex hormone-binding globulin (SHBG).[8] Anovulation is undetectable in childhood, whereas in the perimenarcheal phase, adolescent women exhibit a transient state of anovulation, characterized by accentuated 24-h LH levels.[9] However, making a correct clinical diagnosis of ovarian dysfunction at this age represents a difficult task and another 2 or 3 years may be needed. In fact, the menstrual cycle is rather long and variable during the first few years after menarche[9] and the establishment of regular ovulatory cycles is a slow process in physiological conditions. Using sequential progesterone measurements, it has been shown that more than 80% of cycles are anovulatory during the first year after menarche, 60% during the third, and 25% after the sixth year were still anovulatory.[9] On the other hand, there are data supporting the finding that anovulatory pubertal or postpubertal girls may have higher testosterone, androstenedione, and LH levels than their ovulatory counterparts.[9,10] These young girls therefore appear to be characterized by endocrine features resembling PCOS, although it cannot be excluded that even "physiological" anovulation during and after puberty may be associated with transient hyperactivity of the hypothalamic-pituitary-gonadal axis leading, in turn, to increased androgen production. Moreover, in early puberty, ovarian hyperandrogenism is rarely detected, but it becomes more common after the age of 14–15 years.[15] On the other hand, the persistence of the high LH level profile in hyperandrogenic adolescent girls may be responsible for anovulation and therefore for irregular menses.[11] This should be appropriately considered in clinical practice. In fact, the typical clinical manifestations of PCOS occurring at puberty and adolescent age include irregular menses, particularly oligomenorrhea, increased LH levels, and signs of androgen excess. The most distinctive clinical expression of androgen excess is hirsutism.[12,13] The face and chin are the sites most commonly involved, and the rate of hair growth is gradual over time. Hirsutism might start during pubertal development or right after it; however, it can be expressed earlier, even during midchildhood, where it is often described as a premature adrenarche characterized by the appearance and progressive development of pubic and/or axillary hair.[13] Other manifestations of hyperandrogenemia include acne oily skin, and sometimes male-pattern balding or alopecia. Before gonadarche, acne and the appearance of pubic hair are due mostly to premature or exaggerated adrenarche.[14]

The difficulty of diagnosing PCOS during the adolescent period is not only due to physiological anovulation, but also to the fact that puberty is characterized by a physiological increase in insulin resistance and rising LH levels, both features associated with the development of PCOS.[17] It is in fact estimated that approximately two-thirds of adult women with PCOS have insulin resistance, which is independent of body weight.[1,17,18] The direct clinical manifestation of insulin resistance may be the appearance of *acanthosis nigricans*, which is quite common, particularly in overweight or obese PCOS women. Therefore, it appears that hyperandrogenism, menses irregularities, and insulin resistance may occur together in well-characterized young PCOS women. This emphasizes that androgens and insulin play a pivotal role in the pathophysiology of PCOS at the beginning of the natural history of the disorder.[17,18]

Overweight and obesity represent a rapidly growing threat to the health of populations and an increasing number of countries worldwide present this problem.[19] As expected, there is an increasing prevalence of overweight and obesity not only in the general population, but also in adolescent and young women with PCOS.[13] Whether the high prevalence of obesity in PCOS women may depend, at least in part, on the increasing epidemic of obesity by itself in the world is unknown, although it represents an attractive hypothesis. This obviously implies the absolute need for national and/or international epidemiological prospective studies to investigate this potential association. The association between obesity and alterations of the reproductive functions in women had been recognized a long time ago. In Stein and Leventhal's original description, obesity, together with hirsutism and infertility, represented one of the characteristics of the eponymous syndrome.[2] Much later, Rogers and Mitchell[20] demonstrated that 43% of women affected by various menstrual disorders, infertility, and recurrent miscarriages were overweight or obese. Furthermore, Hartz and colleagues[21] showed that the presence of anovulatory cycles, oligoamenorrhea, and hirsutism, separately or in association, were significantly higher in obese than in normal-weight women. In addition, the same authors found that the incidence of obesity during puberty and early adolescence was greater in adult married women without children than in those having had one or multiple pregnancies, thus confirming the existence of a correlation between obesity and infertility. Similar findings have subsequently been reported by others.[22] The relationship between excess body fat and reproductive disturbances appears to be stronger for early onset obesity, although this still represents a controversial issue, largely due to the heterogeneity of the overweight or obese preadolescent or adolescent populations investigated.[23] There are several epidemiological studies that suggest changes in body weight and/or body composition are critical factors regulating pubertal development in young women.[22] The discovery of leptin provided a unique explanation in this complex circuit, leptin being a main product of body fat[24] and, at the same time, regulating the gonadotropin surge which initiates the development of pubertal stages.[25] Indirect confirmation of this concept derives from evidence that the reproductive system remains prepubertal in leptin deficient *ob/ob* mouse.[26] Several studies have repeatedly reported that the age of menarche,[27,28] as well as the onset of ovarian failure and increased production of follicle-stimulating hormone (FSH) at menopause,[29,30] generally occur at a younger age in obese than in normal-weight women. Moreover, in adolescent and young women the age of onset of obesity and that of menstrual irregularities are significantly correlated (FIG. 2).[31] There are also data indicating that the association with menstrual disorders may be more frequent in girls with onset of excess body weight during puberty than in those who were obese during infancy. These findings were substantially confirmed in a large study performed in approximately 6,000 women by Lake *et al.*,[32] who found that obesity in childhood and the early twenties increased the risk of menstrual problems. It is therefore likely that overweight and obesity do contribute to a significant proportion of menstrual disorders in young women.

Finally, Cresswell *et al.* suggested an intrauterine origin of a particular phenotype of PCOS, based on mother and their childbirth weight.[33] The history of weight gain frequently precedes the onset of the menstrual disorder and hyperandrogenism, suggesting a pathogenetic role of obesity in the subsequent development of PCOS.[31] Moreover, obesity has been associated with premature adrenarche and subsequent development of PCOS.[34] This supports the concept that a different hormonal environment might distinguish obese PCOS adolescents from their normal-weight counterparts. The mechanisms by which obesity may promote or maintain PCOS are complex and still under debate, and have been reviewed recently.[6,35]

CLINICAL MANIFESTATIONS OF PCOS DURING THE FERTILE AGE

Hyperandrogenism and infertility represent the major complaints of PCOS in the adult fertile age. These features are however frequently influenced by

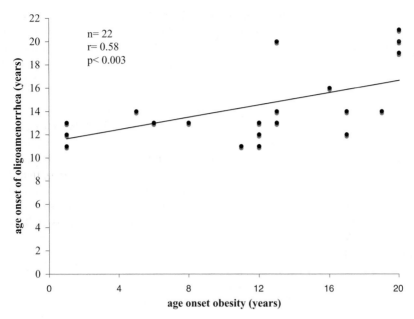

FIGURE 2. Relationship between onset of obesity and onset of oligo- or amenorrhea in a group of young women with PCOS.[31]

several factors that may emphasize or reduce their clinical relevance. Many patients, in fact, undergo pharmacological treatments with oral contraceptives with or without antiandrogens for many years after adolescence. This may obviously change the natural history of hyperandrogenic symptoms, particularly acne and hirsutism. In addition, at the present time, many women with PCOS, while complaining of aesthetic symptoms, undergo many cosmetic procedures, in search of definitive advantages otherwise unachievable without adequate behavioral and/or pharmacological interventions. Another important confounding factor is represented by the growing prevalence of overweight and obesity, very common in adult PCOS women, being present in more than half patients. It is noteworthy that most of these women develop an abdominal phenotype of fat distribution, as a consequence of both hyperandrogenic state and insulin resistance.[35] The impact of obesity on the hyperandrogenic state in adult women with PCOS has been investigated by several studies. They uniformly demonstrate that obese PCOS women are characterized by significantly lower SHBG plasma levels and worsened hyperandrogenism[35] in comparison with their normal-weight counterparts. Moreover, it has been repeatedly described that a higher proportion of obese PCOS women complained of hirsutism and menstrual disturbances than normal-weight women.[23,35] Therefore, there is consistent evidence that the increase of body weight may favor worsening of hyperandrogenic state in women with PCOS.

With increasing obesity and accompanied insulin resistance, *acanthosis nigricans* also becomes more frequent. This dermatological sign should therefore be looked for in all PCOS women, regardless of their hyperandrogenic state, because its presence can unmask subtle metabolic alterations. PCOS women are in fact characterized by a high prevalence of several metabolic abnormalities that are strongly influenced by the presence of obesity. Adequate confirmation on the genuine role of obesity in determining hyperinsulinemia and insulin resistance in women with PCOS derives from studies comparing groups of normal-weight and obese PCOS women. Both fasting- and glucose-stimulated insulin concentrations are in fact significantly higher in obese than in nonobese PCOS subgroups.[18,35] Accordingly, studies examining insulin sensitivity by using different methods, such as the euglycemic hyperinsulinemic clamp technique, the frequent sample intravenous glucose test, and the insulin test, further demonstrated that obese PCOS women had significantly lower insulin sensitivity than their nonobese PCOS counterparts and, therefore, a more severe insulin resistant state.[18,35] The percentage of women affected by PCOS and obesity presenting glucose intolerance is also rather high, ranging from 20 to 49%,[18] therefore substantially above the prevalence rates reported in premenopausal women in population-based studies. On the contrary, glucose intolerance in normal-weight PCOS women is uncommon.[18] Altogether, this may indicate that obesity *per se* plays an important role in altering the insulin-glucose system in PCOS. In a 10-year follow-up study we found that both fasting- and glucose-stimulated insulin and C-peptide spontaneously increased in PCOS women, suggesting that insulin resistance tended to worsen with time.[36] Although PCOS *per se* may be associated with alterations of both lipid and lipoprotein metabolism, the coexistence of obesity usually leads to a more atherogenic lipoprotein pattern. A greater reduction of high-density lipoproteins together with a higher increase of both triglycerides and total cholesterol levels were in fact observed in obese with respect to normal-weight PCOS women (see Ref. 36 for revision).

Although signs and symptoms of hyperandrogenism continue to be a cardinal clinical feature of PCOS in adult PCOS women, nonetheless the major complaints of these women are represented by menstrual alterations and infertility. PCOS is in fact one of the most common causes of anovulation and endocrine infertility in women, worsened by the coexistence of obesity.[23,36] Several studies have in fact clearly demonstrated that abnormal menses are more frequent in obese than normal-weight PCOS women.[21,37] There is evidence that a reduced incidence of pregnancy and blunted responsiveness to pharmacological treatments to induce ovulation may be more common in obese PCOS.[38] Both insulin resistance and hyperinsulinemia may be responsible for the alteration of both spontaneous and induced ovulation observed in normal-weight and more in obese PCOS women. This concept is indirectly supported by the demonstration that insulin sensitizing agents, such as metformin and thiazolinidediones, are efficient in ameliorating menstrual cycles and both spontaneous and clomiphene-induced ovulation in PCOS women.[39] There-fore, infertility in PCOS is particularly associated with obesity, as a worse pattern of insulin resistance and hyperinsulinemia is present.

THE TRANSITION PHASE OF PCOS TOWARD METABOLIC AND CARDIOVASCULAR DISORDERS IN THE ADULT AGE AND AFTER MENOPAUSE

The presence of insulin resistance in all obese women with PCOS and in at least half of normal-weight women indicates that most affected women may have MS. This complex dysmetabolic condition represents the major causative factor of the changing picture of PCOS throughout a life span.

The National Cholesterol Education Program Adult Treatment Panel (ATPIII)[40] guidelines define MS as having three or more of the following abnormalities: waist circumference in females >88 cm, fasting serum glucose ≥110 mg/dL, fasting serum triglycerides ≥150 mg/dL, serum HDL cholesterol <50 mg/dL, and systolic and diastolic blood pressure ≥130 and 85 mm/Hg, respectively. There is consistent evidence that the MS is associated with a high risk for developing type 2 diabetes mellitus (T2DM)[41] and CVDs,[42] as well as with cardiovascular mortality.[43] The ATPIII criteria were used to ascertain the prevalence of MS in a representative adult sample of the United States using data from the Third National Health and Nutrition Examination Survey (NHANES III).[44] In this sample, the prevalence of MS among women in age groups of 20–29 and 30–39 years was 6% and 15%, respectively.[45] Some recent studies used the ATPIII criteria to assess the prevalence of MS also in PCOS women. Korhonen et al.[46] conducted a cross-sectional population-based study and reported that serum concentrations of some sex hormones differed between premenopausal women with or without ATPIII-defined MS. Glueck et al.[47] studied 138 PCOS patients and found a prevalence rate of 46%, whereas, more recently, Apridonidze et al.[48] found a prevalence of 43% by retrospectively reviewing the medical charts of 106 PCOS attending the Endocrine Clinic of Richmond, VA. Both these studies therefore described a prevalence of MS in PCOS nearly twofold higher than that reported in the general population inves-tigated in the cited NHANES III report,[9] matched for age and BMI. Moreover, Apridonidze et al.[48] described higher free testosterone and lower SHBG levels in those women with MS with respect to those without it, other than a higher prevalence of *acanthosis nigricans* and a tendency toward a greater family history of PCOS. We recently analyzed a large cohort of 200 selected PCOS women of the Mediterranean area where we found that 18% were characterized by the absence of any criteria of MS, 51% had at least two criteria, and 31% met the three criteria according to the ATPIII recommendations.[49] Therefore, collectively, 82% of PCOS women had at least one feature of MS, a finding consistent with a large presence of single or grouped metabolic abnormalities

TABLE 1. Prevalence of the metabolic syndrome (MS) according to the ATPIII criteria in PCOS women in Richmond, VA,[40] and in Bologna, Italy (unpublished data)

Features of metabolic syndrome	Richmond (%)	Bologna (%)
No criteria	–	18
Less than 2 criteria	57	51
Three or more criteria	43	31

in this disorder. Compared to those without any criteria, the other two groups were progressively more obese and had a higher prevalence of the abdominal pattern of fat distribution. In addition, those presenting with MS were characterized by higher systolic and diastolic blood pressure, higher pulse rate, greater frequency of liver enzyme abnormalities, worsened insulin resistance, higher glycosylated haemoglobin, and a more severe hyperandrogenemia (higher free androgen index and lower SHBG concentrations). Taken together, these findings demonstrate that the prevalence of MS in women with PCOS is higher than that of the general population, regardless of ethnicity and geographical area (TABLE 1). They also indicate a strong association between MS and the hyperandrogenic state.

Compared to the general population, studies in American,[50,51] Asian,[52] and Italian[53] subjects have also shown that women with PCOS have an increased risk for the selective development of impaired glucose tolerance (IGT) and T2DM, with a tendency to an early development of glucose intolerance states during life.[18] The close connection between PCOS and glucose intolerance is further emphasized by the finding of a high prevalence of polycystic ovarian morphology on ultrasound scans both in premenopausal women with T2DM[54] and in those with previous gestational diabetes.[55] Similar to what occurs in the general population,[56] there is evidence that insulin resistance may play a major pathophysiological role in the development of glucose intolerance also in PCOS women. The decrease of insulin sensitivity in PCOS appears in fact to be quite similar to that found in patients with T2DM and to be relatively independent of obesity, fat distribution, and lean body mass.[17,18] On the other hand, there is strong evidence that obesity, particularly the abdominal phenotype, *per se*, represents an important independent risk factor for glucose intolerance in PCOS women.[18,35] Moreover, an impaired early phase insulin secretion should play a role in the development of glucose intolerance in obese PCOS, at least in Hispanic American subgroups,[18,57] particularly when they have a positive family history for diabetes.[57,58] The prevalence of IGT and T2DM described by our group in the PCOS women living in different cities of Italy[53] was significantly higher than that described in the general population with a similar age,[59] but somewhat lower with respect to that reported in previous studies cited above performed in the United States or in Asia (TABLE 2).[50–52] This suggests that environmental factors may play a dominant role in determining individual susceptibility to metabolic

TABLE 2. Prevalence of IGT or type 2 diabetes mellitus (T2DM) in premenopausal women with PCOS living in different geographical areas in the world

Reference	Ethnicity	IGT (%)	T2DM (%)	Age range (years)
Legro et al.[50]	Hispanic Americans	31.1	7.5	14–44
Ehrmann et al.[51]	Hispanic Americans	35	10	13.5–40
Weerakiet et al.[52]	Asian Thai	22.8	17.7	15–40
Gambineri et al.[53]	Italians	15.7	2.5	14–37

disorders, which is probably more important than genetic background, as suggested by recent long-term epidemiological studies demonstrating that the appearance of T2DM can be prevented by adequate lifestyle intervention, focusing on dietary habits and increased physical activity.[60,61] Moreover, in our study performed in Italian women, we found that although all PCOS women with glucose intolerance were obese, nearly 80% of obese PCOS women had, conversely, normal glucose tolerance,[53] which clearly supports the concept that although obesity increases the susceptibility of PCOS women to develop T2DM, it does not represent, *per se*, a specific condition responsible for this disorder.

Women with PCOS are often assumed, *a priori*, to be at increased risk for CVD, given the high prevalence of MS among them. There is, however, no single definition of PCOS in the studies that have analyzed its association with CVD, and for that reason a comparison of these studies is impossible. Long-term studies of well-characterized women with PCOS are also lacking, and the link of this syndrome to primary cardiovascular events, such as stroke or myocardial infarction, remains more speculative than substantive. Epidemiological studies that have focused on isolated signs and stigmata of PCOS, such as polycystic ovaries, hyperandrogenism, or chronic anovulation, have found mixed results.[62,63] There are studies that suggest a slight increase in cardiovascular events in women with polycystic ovaries, with perhaps stronger evidence of an increased risk of cardiovascular events in women with menstrual irregularities. However, there is little evidence for an association between hyperandrogenism *per se* and cardiovascular events. Furthermore, there are less data to substantiate an increased risk of events in women with PCOS identified on the basis of a combination of signs and symptoms, such as hyperandrogenic chronic anovulation.[63] The existing data suggest that PCOS may adversely affect or accelerate the development of an adverse cardiovascular risk profile, and even of subclinical signs of atherosclerosis, but it does not appear to decrease the time of clinical presentation to a premenopausal age.[63]

Recent studies investigating well-defined PCOS women have extensively documented, however, that many markers of the risk for CVD frequently aggregate in women with PCOS. As reported above, they include not only classical features of MS, but also other markers of vessel damage, endothelial dysfunction, proinflammatory state, and hemocoagulative factors. In the previous paragraph it was reported that more than one-third of women with PCOS develop IGT or overt T2DM, a finding that is consistently seen across several geographic areas and ethnic groups. In addition, a mild increase in diastolic blood pressure could represent an additional factor involved in the change in cardiac morphology. PCOS women have also been shown to present with some alterations of diastolic dysfunctions.[64,65] Interestingly, these alterations can occur at a young age, in both obese and normal-weight PCOS women.[66] There are many other observations regarding other potential risk factors, widely discussed in a review by Legro.[63] Whether the high prevalence of risk factors in PCOS may have some pathophysiological role in the development of CVD in PCOS women should still be considered a hypothesis, because there are no data demonstrating that these patients have higher adverse outcomes (such as myocardial infarction, stroke, etc.) later in life. There is therefore a need for long-term, well-designed, prospective trials to prove this hypothesis. At present, it is our opinion that susceptibility to develop CVD in women with PCOS may depend on the high prevalence of metabolic abnormalities and T2DM, rather than PCOS status *per se*.

PCOS AFTER MENOPAUSE: A STILL UNDEFINED ENDOCRINOLOGICAL ENTITY

In normal women, the transition to postmenopause involves not only decreases in ovarian estrogen formation but also a reduction of androgen (androstenedione, not testosterone) production rates, and therefore of androstenedione circulating levels.[67,68] It should be pointed out that there are very few studies, however, in which longitudinal changes in the hormonal status of women reaching postmenopausal age have been evaluated. Little is known about what happens to ovarian morphology and androgen production in women with PCOS after menopause.[69,70] In one study analyzing a group of postmenopausal women, it was found that 42–44% had morphological ultrasonographic features consistent with polycystic ovaries.[70] Moreover, the comparison between the group with and that without polycystic ovaries showed that postmenopausal women with polycystic ovaries had higher serum concentrations of testosterone and triglycerides than postmenopausal women with normal ovaries. These findings strongly resemble PCOS features and indicate that this disorder is probably higher than expected in postmenopausal women. On the other hand, it should be also considered that hyperandrogenism appears to partly resolve before menopause in women with PCOS. In fact, one study found that total and non-SHBG-bound testosterone levels were reduced by approximately 50% among women of 42–47 years with respect to 20–42 years of age and remained stable in women older than 47 years of age.[70] When PCOS women were compared to controls, testosterone levels were similar between the two groups in the age range of 42–47 years, whereas they were significantly

TABLE 3. Major characteristics of the PCOS phenotype according to age

Age	Features	Comments
Childhood	- None	- Search for the presence of PCOS (or related features) in the family; gestational diabetes in the mother; low birthweight; early adiposity
Early adolescence	- Early menarche	- Irregular menses, increased testosterone and LH may represent a "physiological" phase during the first years after menarche
	- Irregular menses (oligoamenorrhea)	- Clinical hyperandrogenism should alert to the presence of PCOS
	- Hirsutism or acne	- US examination of the ovaries is not pathognomonic in the absence of other criteria
	- Overweight or obesity	- A long follow-up is needed
	- Increased testosterone and LH	
	- Mild metabolic abnormalities	
Late adolescence	- Irregular menses (oligoamenorrhea)	- Persistent oligoanovulation (or oligoamenorrhea) in the presence of hyperandrogenism (clinical or biochemical), strongly suggest PCOS
	- Hirsutism, acne	- PCO morphology at US supports the diagnosis
	- Persistent hyperandrogenemia	- Consider potential role of excess body weight
	- Overweight or obesity	
	- Metabolic alterations	
Adult fertile age	- Hyperandrogenism (hirsutism, acne, alopecia)	- Infertility, hyperandrogenism, and obesity are the major complaints of adult women having PCOS
	- Hyperandrogenemia	- Search for the presence of MS or T2DM in all PCOS women with obesity.
	- Irregular menses (particularly oligo- or amenorrhea)	
	- Infertility	
	- Overweight or obesity	
	- Features of MS and T2DM	
	- PCO at US	
Postmenopause	- PCO at US	- Include androgen measurement in all women with a previous diagnosis of PCOS
	- Mild hyperandrogenemia	- Provide adequate reference values for androgens in postmenopause
	- Metabolic alterations and T2DM (?)	- US examination of the ovaries needed? (no data available)
		- Great relevance to metabolic and cardiovascular disease (CVD) risk factors in the presence of hyperandrogenism.

NOTE: US: ultrasound. The question marks identify still debatable topics.

higher in PCOS than controls under or above this range. The assumption that hyperandrogenism tends to improve during late fertile age in PCOS women may explain the tendency of women with PCOS to cycle regularly as they grow older.

CONCLUSION

It is quite clear that there is a need for further research in this field for several reasons. First, the investigation of the phenotypes(s) of PCOS after menopause could make it possible to define the natural history of this disorder, therefore improving both pathophysiological knowledge and clinical management (TABLE 3). Second, as reported in the previous paragraph, an increasing number of studies support the concept that PCOS may represent a risk factor for CVD later in life, although no definitive demonstration of this assumption exists as yet. Therefore, the long-term evaluation of PCOS up to postmenopausal age should provide important information regarding the prevalence of CVD in PCOS women. Third, the identification of high-risk subgroups of PCOS women for long-term chronic metabolic diseases could permit new therapeutic strategies in the prevention of glucose intolerance states. This represents an exciting scientific challenge for the next few years.

REFERENCES

1. EHRMANN, D.A. 2005. Polycystic ovary syndrome. N. Engl. J. Med. **352:** 1223–1236.
2. STEIN, I.F. & M.L. LEVENTHAL. 1935. Amenorrhea associated with bilateral polycystic ovaries. Am. J. Obstet. Gynecol. **29:** 181.
3. GOUDAS, V.T. & D.A. DUMESIC. 1997. Polycystic ovary syndrome. Endocrinol. Metab. Clin. North Am. **26:** 893–912.
4. THE ROTTERDAM ESHRE/ASRM-SPONSORED PCOS CONSENSUS WORKSHOP GROUP. 2004. Revised 2003 consensus on diagnostic criteria and long-term health risks related to polycystic ovary syndrome (PCOS). Hum. Reprod. **19:** 41–47.
5. DAHLGREN, E., S. JOHANSSON, G. LINDSTEDT, et al. 1992. Women with polycystic ovary syndrome wedge resected in 1956 to 1965: a long term follow-up focusing on natural history and circulating hormones. Fertil. Steril.**57:** 505–513.
6. PASQUALI, R. & F. CASIMIRRI. 1993. The impact of obesity on hyperandrogenism and polycystic ovary syndrome in premenopausal women. Clin. Endocrinol. (Oxf.) **39:** 1–16.
7. APTER, D. 1997. Pubertal development in PCOS. *In*: Androgen Excess Disorders in Women. R. Azziz, J.E. Nestler & D. Dewailly, Eds.: 327–338. Lippincot-Raven Publishers. Philadelphia, PA.
8. APTER, D. & I. SIBILA. 1993. Development of children and adolescence: physiological, pathophysiological, and therapeutic aspects. Curr. Opin. Obstet. Gynecol. **5:** 764–773.

9. IBANEZ, L., F. DE ZEGHER & N. POTAU. 1999. Anovulation after precocious pubarche: early markers and time course in adolescence. J. Clin. Endocrinol. Metab. **84:** 2691–2695.
10. APTER, D. & R. VIHKO. 1985. Hormonal patterns of first menstrual cycles. In Adolescence in Females. S. Venturoli, C. Flamigni & J.R. Givens, Eds.: 215–238.Year Book Medical Publishers. Chicago, IL.
11. VENTUROLI, S., E. PORCU, R. FABBRI, et al. 1992. Longitudinal evaluation of the different gonadotropin pulsatile patterns in anovulatory cycles of young girls. J. Clin. Endocrinol. Metab.**74:** 836–841.
12. YOUNG, R.L. & J.W. GOLDZIEHER. 1988. Clinical manifestations of polycystic ovarian disease. Endocrinol. Metab. Clin. North Am. **17:** 621–635.
13. PELUSI, C. & R. PASQUALI. 2003. Polycystic ovary syndrome in adolescence. Pathophysiology and treatment. Treat. Endocrinol. **2:** 215–230.
14. CARA, J.F. & R.L. ROSENFIELD. 1994. Androgens and the adolescent girl. In Pediatric Adolescent Gynecology. J.S. Sanfilippo, D. Muram, P.A. Lee & J. Dewhurst, Eds.: 250–277. WB Saunders. Philadelphia, PA.
15. DRAMUSIC, V., H.H. GOH, M. YANG, et al. 1991. Menstrual dysfunction in adolescence. Singapore J. Obstet. Gynecol. **22:** 69–75.
16. YEN, S.S. 1980. The polycystic ovary syndrome. Clin. Endocrinol. (Oxf.) **12:** 177–207.
17. PORETSKY, L., N.A. CATALDO, Z. ROSENWAKS, et al. 1999. The insulin-related ovarian regulatory system in health and disease. Endocr. Rev.. **20:** 535–582.
18. DUNAIF, A. 1997. Insulin resistance and the polycystic ovary syndrome: mechanism and implications for pathogenesis. Endocr. Rev. **18:** 774–800.
19. WHO. 1997. Preventing and managing the global epidemic. Report of a WHO consultation on obesity. Geneva. WHO/NUT/NCD/98.1.
20. ROGERS, J. & G.W. MITCHELL. 1952. The relation of obesity to menstrual disturbances. N. Engl. J. Med. **247:** 53–56.
21. HARTZ, A.J., P.N. BARBORIAK, A. WONG, et al. 1979. The association of obesity with infertility and related menstrual abnormalities in women. Int. J. Obes. **3:** 57–77.
22. AZZIZ, R., E. EHRMANN, R.S. LEGRO, et al. 2001. Troglitazone improves ovulation and hirsutism in the polycystic ovary syndrome: a multicenter, double-blind, placebo-controlled trial. J. Clin. Endocrinol. Metab. **86:** 1626–1632.
23. PASQUALI, R., C. PELUSI, S. GENGHINI, et al. 2003. Obesity and reproductive disorders in women. Hum. Reprod. Up. **9:** 359–372.
24. CONSIDINE, R.V., M.K. SINHA, M.L. HEIMAN, et al. 1996. Serum immunoreactive leptin concentrations in normal-weight and obese humans. N. Engl. J. Med. **334:** 292–295.
25. FAROOQI, I.S., S.A. JEBB, G. LANGMACK, et al. 1999. Effects of recombinant leptin therapy in a child with congenital leptin deficiency. N. Engl. J. Med. **341:** 879–884.
26. O'RAILLY, S. 1998. Life without leptin. Nature **392:** 330–331.
27. MONTEMAGNO, U., F. CONTALDO, P. MARTINELLI, et al. 1979. Gynecological complications of obesity. In: Medical Complications of Obesity. M. Mancini, B. Lewis & F. Contaldo, Eds.: 227–283. Academic Press. London.
28. BRUNI, V., S. BUCCIANTINI, S. CARUSO, et al. 1985. Obesity in adolescence. In Adolescence in Females C. Flamigni, S. Venturoli & J.R. Givens, Eds.: 309–320. Year Book Medical Publisher. Chicago, IL.
29. BRAY, G.A. 1997. Obesity and reproduction. Hum. Reprod. **12:** 26–32.

30. NORMAN, R.J. & A.M. CLARK. 1998. Obesity and reproductive disorders: a review. Reprod. Fertil. Dev. **10:** 55–63.
31. PASQUALI, R., F. CASIMIRRI, D. ANTENUCCI, *et al.* 1985. Relationship between onset of obesity and onset of oligomenorrhea in females with obesity and polycystic ovaries. *In:* Adolescence in Females. C. Flamigni, S. Venturoli, J.R. Givens, Eds.: 363–365.Year Book Medical Publisher. Chicago, IL.
32. LAKE, J.K., C. POWER & T.J. COLE. 1997. Women's reproductive health—the role of body mass index in early and adult life. Int. J. Obes. Relat. Metab. Disord. **21:** 432–438.
33. CRESSWELL, I.I., D.J.P. BARKER & C. OSMOND. 1997. Fetal growth, length of gestation, and polycystic ovaries in adult life. Lancet **350:** 1131–1135.
34. JABBAR, M., M. PUGLIESE, P. FORT, *et al.* 1991. Excess weight and precocious pubarche in children: alterations of the adrenocortical hormones. J. Am. Coll. Nutr. **10:** 289–296.
35. GAMBINERI, A., C. PELUSI, V. VICENNATI, *et al.* 2002. Obesity and the polycystic ovary syndrome. Int. J. Obes. Relat. Metab. Disord. **26:** 883–896.
36. PASQUALI, R., A. GAMBINERI, B. ANCONETANI, *et al.* 1999. The natural history of the metabolic syndrome in young women with the polycystic ovary syndrome and the effect of long-term oestrogen-progestagen treatment. Clin. Endocrinol. (Oxf.) **50:** 517–527.
37. KIDDY, D.S., P.S. SHARP, D.M. WHITE, *et al.* 1990. Differences in clinical and endocrine features between obese and non-obese subjects with polycystic ovary syndrome: an analysis of 263 consecutive cases. Clin. Endocrinol. (Oxf.) **32:** 213–220.
38. GALTIER-DEREURE, F., P. PUJOL, D. DEWAILLY, *et al.* 1997. Choice of stimulation in polycystic ovarian syndrome: the influence of obesity. Hum. Reprod. **12:** 88–96.
39. DE LEO, V., A. LA MARCA & F. PETRAGLIA. 2003. Insulin-lowering agents in the management of polycystic ovary syndrome. Endocr. Rev. **24:** 633–667.
40. THIRD REPORT OF THE NATIONAL CHOLESTEROL EDUCATION PROGRAM (NCEP) Expert Panel on Detection, evaluation, and Treatment of High Blood Cholesterol in Adults. (Adult Treatment Panel III). Final Report. 2002. Circulation **106:** 3143–3421.
41. HAFFNER, S.M., R.A. VALDEZ, H.P. HAZUDA, *et al.* 1992. Prospective analysis of the insulin-resistance syndrome (syndrome X) Diabetes **41:** 715–722.
42. ISOMAA, B., P. ALMGREN, T. TUOMI, *et al.* 2001. Cardiovascular morbidity and mortality associated with the metabolic syndrome. Diabetes Care **24:** 683–689.
43. TREVISAN, M., J. LIU, F.B. BAHSAS, *et al.* 1998. Syndrome X and mortality: a population-based study. Risk Factor and Life Expectancy Research Group. Am. J. Epidemiol. **148:** 958–966.
44. U.S. DEPARTMENT OF HEALTH AND HUMAN SERVICES (DHHS). National Center for Health Statistics. 1996. Third National Health and Nutrition Examination Survey, NHANES III, 1988-1994. Hyattsville, MD: Center for Disease Control and Prevention.
45. FORD, E.S., W.H. GILES & W.H. DIETZ. 2002. Prevalence of the metabolic syndrome among US adults: findings from the third National Heath and Nutrition Examination Survey. JAMA **287:** 356–359.
46. KORHONEN, S., M. HIPPELAINEN, M. VANHALA, *et al.* 2003. The androgenic sex hormone profile is an essential feature of metabolic syndrome in premenopausal women: a controlled community-based study. Fertil. Steril.**79:** 1327–1334.

47. GLUECK, C.J., R. PAPANNA, P. WANG, et al. 2003. Incidence and treatment of metabolic syndrome in newly referred women with confirmed polycystic ovarian syndrome. Metabolism 52: 908–915.
48. APRIDONIDZE, T., P. ESSAH, M.J. IOURNO, et al. 2005. Pevalence and characteristics of the metabolic syndrome in women with PCOS. J. Clin. Endocrinol. Metab. 90: 1929–1935.
49. PASQUALI, R., L. PATTON, U. PAGOTTO, et al. 2005. Metabolic alterations and cardiovascular risk factors in the polycystic ovary sindrome. Min. Ginecol. 57: 79–85.
50. LEGRO, R.S., A.R. KUNSELMAN, W.C. DODSON, et al. 1999. Prevalence and predictions of the risk of type 2 diabetes mellitus and impaired glucose tolerance in polycystic ovary syndrome: a prospective, controlled study in 254 affected women. J. Clin. Endocrinol. Metab. 84: 165–169.
51. EHRMANN, D.A., R.B. BARNES, R.L. ROSENFIELD, et al. 1999. Prevalence of impaired glucose tolerance and diabetes in women with polycystic ovary syndrome. Diabetes Care 22: 141–146.
52. WEERAKIET, S., C. SRISOMBUT, P. BUNNAG, et al. 2001. Prevalence of type 2 diabetes mellitus and impaired glucose tolerance in Asian women with polycystic ovary syndrome. Int. J. Gynaecol. Obstet. 75: 177–184.
53. GAMBINERI, A., C. PELUSI, E. MANICARDI, et al. 2004. Glucose intolerance in a large cohort of Mediterranean women with polycystic ovary syndrome. Phenotype and associated factors. Diabetes 53: 2353–2358.
54. CONN, J.J., H.S. JACOBS & G.S. CONWAY. 2000. The prevalence of polycystic ovaries in women with type 2 diabetes mellitus. Clin. Endocrinol. (Oxf.) 52: 81–86.
55. HOLTE, J., G. GENNARELLI, L. WIDE, et al. 1998. High prevalence of polycystic ovaries and associated clinical, endocrine, and metabolic features in women with previous gestational diabetes mellitus. J. Clin. Endocrinol. Metab. 83: 1143–1150.
56. DE FRONZO, R.A. & E. FERRANNINI. 1991. Insulin resistance: a multifaceted syndrome responsible for NIDDM, obesity, hypertension, dyslipidemia, and atherosclerotic cardiovascular disease. Diabetes Care 14: 173–194.
57. EHRMANN, D.A., J. STURIS, M.M. BYRNE, et al. 1995. Insulin secretory defects in polycystic ovary syndrome. Relationship to insulin sensitivity and family history of non-insulin-dependent diabetes mellitus. J. Clin. Invest. 96: 520–527.
58. COLILLA, S., N.J. COX & D.A. EHRMANN. 2001. Heritability of insulin secretion and insulin action in women with polycystic ovary syndrome and their first degree relatives. J. Clin. Endocrinol. Metab. 86: 2027–2031.
59. HARRIS, M.I., W.C. HADDEN, W.C. KNOWLER, et al. 1987. Prevalence of diabetes and impaired glucose tolerance and plasma glucose levels in U.S. population aged 20-74 yr. Diabetes 36: 523–534.
60. NORRIS, S.L., X. ZHANG, A. AVENELL, et al. 2004. Long-term effectiveness of lifestyle and behavioral weight loss interventions in adults with type 2 diabetes: a meta-analysis. Am. J. Med. 117: 762–774.
61. KANAYA, A.M. & K.M. NARAYAN. 2003. Prevention of type 2 diabetes: data from recent trials. Prim. Care. 30: 511–526.
62. TALBOTT, E.O., D.S. GUZICK, A. CLERICI, et al. 1995. Coronary heart disease risk factors in women with polycystic ovary syndrome. Arterioscler. Thromb. Vasc. Biol. 15: 821–826.

63. LEGRO, R.S. 2003. Polycystic ovary syndrome and cardiovascular disease: a premature association? Endocr. Rev. **24:** 302–312.
64. YARALI, H., A. YILDIRIR, F. AYBAR, *et al*. 2001. Diastolic dysfunction and increased serum homocysteine concentrations may contribute to increased cardiovascular risk in patients with polycystic ovary syndrome. Fertil. Steril. **76:** 511–516.
65. TIRAS, M.B., R. YALCIN, V. NOYAN, *et al*. 1999. Alterations in cardiac flow parameters in patients with polycystic ovarian syndrome. Hum. Reprod. **14:** 1949–1952.
66. ORIO, F. JR, S. PALOMBA, L. SPINELLI, *et al*. 2004. The cardiovascular risk of young women with polycystic ovary syndrome: an observational, analytical, prospective case-control study. J. Clin. Endocrinol. Metab. **89:** 3696–3701.
67. PARKER, C.R. 1997. Possibile physiologic impact of altered androgen:estrogen relationship in menopause. *In* Androgen Excess Disorders in Women.R. Azziz, J.E. Nestler & D. Dewailly, Eds.: 93–99. Lippincot-Raven Publishers. Philadelphia, PA.
68. PAULI, S. & R.A. LOBO. 2004. Polycystic ovary syndrome after menopause: a case report. J. Reprod. Med. **49:** 491–494.
69. BIRDSHALL, M.A. & C.M. FARQUHAR. 1996. Polycystic ovary syndrome in pre- and post-menopausal women. Clin. Endocrinol. (Oxf.) **44:** 269–276.
70. Winters S.J., E. TALBOTT, D.S. GUZICK, *et al*. 2000. Serum testosterone levels decrease in middle age in women with the polycystic ovary syndrome. Fertil. Steril. **73:** 724–729.

Indices of Low-Grade Inflammation in Polycystic Ovary Syndrome

EVANTHIA DIAMANTI-KANDARAKIS, THOMAS PATERAKIS, AND HELEN A. KANDARAKIS

First Department of Medicine, Endocrine Section, University of Athens, Athens, Greece

ABSTRACT: Polycystic ovary syndrome (PCOS) is probably the most common endocrinopathy of reproductive age. PCOS represents a disorder that not only enhances the risk for type 2 diabetes (T2D) but is also associated with an increased number of cardiovascular risk factors known to facilitate atherogenesis. On the other hand, inflammation is thought to play an important role in the progression and development of complications of atherosclerosis. Evidence of low-grade chronic inflammation in PCOS is indicated by the presence of elevated C-reactive protein (CRP) levels, inflammatory cytokines (i.e., IL-6 and IL-18), and increased leucocyte count. CRP, a nonspecific marker of inflammation, has been proven to be one of the strongest predictors of the risk of cardiovascular events in patients with or without cardiovascular disease. The levels of the adhesion molecules (AM), sIVAM-1, sVCAM-1, and sE-selectin in serum reflect low-grade chronic inflammation of the endothelium and independently predict coronary heart disease (CHD) and T2D. In a recent study in a large number of PCOS women we demonstrated elevated levels of sIVAM-1 and sE-selectin and we further substantiated the existence of a low-grade chronic inflammatory process in PCOS. However, it remains to be assessed with long-term studies whether the early presence of markers of chronic inflammation in young women with this syndrome has clinical significance.

KEYWORDS: PCOS; inflammation indices; adhesion molecules; cytokinines; TNF-α; sVCAM; sICAM; Selectin E

INTRODUCTION

The polycystic ovarian syndrome (PCOS) is considered to be the most frequently encountered endocrinopathy of women in reproductive age. The prevalence of the syndrome, according to three major epidemiological studies

Address for correspondence: E. Diamanti-Kandarakis, M.D., Ph.D., First Department of Medicine, Endocrine Section, University of Athens, GR-115 27, Athens, Greece. Voice : 0030-210-8133318; fax: 0030-310-8130031.

e-mail: akandara@otenet.gr

Ann. N.Y. Acad. Sci. 1092: 175–186 (2006). © 2006 New York Academy of Sciences.
doi: 10.1196/annals.1365.015

employing NIH diagnostic criteria—chronic anovulation and clinical/or biochemical hyperandrogenemia—ranges from 6.5 to 5.7% in women of reproductive age.[1] Recently at a joint meeting, the European Society for Human Reproduction (ESHRE) and the American Society of Reproductive Medicine (ASRM) set new guidelines for the diagnosis of PCOS that included polycystic ovary morphology by intravaginal ultrasound. According to these guidelines the syndrome can be defined if two out of the three following criteria are present: (i) oligo- or anovulation, (ii) clinical and/or biochemical signs of hyperandrogenism, (iii) polycystic ovaries and exclusion of other etiologies (congenital adrenal hyperplasia, androgen-secreting tumors, Cushing's syndrome).[2]

PCOS is not considered a pure reproductive disorder because it is considered to be a metabolic one too. PCOS is associated with several major and minor metabolic aberrations such as obesity, insulin resistance, dyslipidemia,[3–7] increased serum levels of plasminogen-activator inhibitor 1 (PAI-1),[8] increased Endothelin-1 levels,[9] elevated plasma advanced glycation end-products levels (AGEs),[10] endothelial dysfunction, and echocardiographic abnormalities.[11,12] All these factors contribute to atherogenesis. Inflammation is now thought to play a key role in the pathophysiological mechanism of atherosclerosis and CVD.[13–16]

LOW-GRADE CHRONIC INFLAMMATION AND PCOS

Insulin resistance and hyperinsulinemia are present in up to 70% of women with PCOS. It is present in obese and nonobese PCOS patients and it seems to have a central role in the pathogenesis of hyperandrogenemia and anovulation.[4] Pathogenesis of insulin resistance in PCOS is still a matter of debate. A defect in intracellular signal transduction of insulin has been reported in PCOS patients.[17,18]

Dunaif et al. found that increased insulin receptor serine phosphorylation decreased its protein kinase activity. This intrinsic defect in insulin receptor signaling in PCOS independently of obesity leads to hyperinsulinemia.[19,20] The latter stimulates androgen production in the polycystic ovary from PCOS patients either directly by stimulating the theca cells (human ovaries have specific receptors for insulin),[21–24] or indirectly through stimulation of luteinizing hormone (LH) secretion and inhibition of IGF binding protein (IGFBP) and sex hormone-binding globulin (SHBG) synthesis and secretion. Insulin also stimulates adrenal androgen secretion.[25–31]

Additionally, insulin resistance has been increasingly recognized as having an important role in inflammatory pathways[32–35] and has been shown to have a negative impact on endothelial function. A supportive finding along these lines is that the therapeutic intervention with insulin-sensitizer has been proven beneficial.[36–38]

TABLE 1. Markers of low-grade inflammation in PCOS

Marker	Author	Journal
CRP	Kelly *et al.* 2001	J. Clin. Endocrinol. Metab. **86:** 2453–2455
CRP	Fenkci *et al.* 2003	Fertil. Steril. **80:** 123–127
CRP	Boulman *et al.* 2004	J. Clin. Endocrinol. Metab. **89:** 2160–2165
CRP	Tarkun *et al.* 2004	J. Clin. Endocrinol. Metab. **89:** 5592–5596
CRP	Talbott *et al.* 2004	J. Clin. Endocrinol. Metab. **89:** 6061–6067
CRP	Orio *et al.* 2005	J. Clin. Endocrinol. Metab. **90:** 2–5
CRP	Diamanti-Kandarakis *et al.* 2006	Hum. Reprod. **21:** 1426–1431
Leucocytes	Orio *et al.* 2005	J. Clin. Endocrinol. Metab. **90:** 2–5
IL-18	Escobar-Morreale *et al.* 2004	J. Clin. Endocrinol. Metab. **89:** 806–811
IL-6	Mohlig *et al.* 2004	Eur. J. Endocrinol. **150:** 525–532
TNF-α	Gonzalez *et al.* 1999	Metabolism **48:** 437–441
AM	Diamanti-Kandarakis *et al.* 2006	Hum. Reprod. **21:** 1426–1431

In the last decade, markers of systemic inflammation and certain components of the haemostatic system have been found to predict atherosclerotic risk in insulin resistance states in which PCOS is now included.[39,40]

PCOS associated with hyperandrogenemia, anovulation, and metabolic aberrations could be considered as a female subtype of metabolic syndrome carrying a potential preatherogenic load.[38] For example, 40% of obese PCOS women share diagnostic criteria for impaired glucose tolerance or type 2 diabetes (T2D) by the age of 26 years,[42] threefold increased prevalence of hypertension,[43] high low-density lipoprotein (LDL), and low high-density lipoprotein (HDL) cholesterol (LDL-C and HDL-C) levels compared with regularly menstruating women.[44] Thereafter, the need to identify the early presence of markers of chronic inflammation in young women with this syndrome is justified. A number of studies have demonstrated abnormal levels of several inflammatory indices (TABLE 1).

CRP as a Marker of Low-Grade Inflammation in PCOS

C-reactive protein (CRP) is a marker of inflammation shown in multiple prospective epidemiological studies to predict incidence of myocardial infarction, stroke, peripheral arterial disease, and sudden death.[45] CRP seems to be more potent as a predictor of cardiovascular events than LDL-C, and it adds prognostic information at all levels of calculated Framingham risk and at all levels of the metabolic syndrome.[39] Therefore, in light of its suggested potential to predict cardiovascular disease (CVD) in apparently healthy women with normal or high LDL-C, prone to cardiovascular morbidity and mortality, CRP may be an ideal marker for screening apparently healthy, young PCOS patients.[46–48]

The first study that examined low-grade chronic inflammation in women with PCOS by measuring CRP was conducted in 2001 by Kelly *et al.*[49] They showed that CRP concentrations, by highly sensitive assay, were significantly increased in women with PCOS ($n = 17$) relative to those in healthy women ($n = 15$) (geometric means, 2.12 and 0.67 mg/L, respectively; $P = 0.016$). They also noted that CRP concentrations in both PCOS and controls correlated with the degree of obesity and inversely with insulin sensitivity, although not with total testosterone concentrations. They proposed low-grade chronic inflammation as a novel mechanism contributing to the increased risk of coronary heart disease (CHD) and T2D in these women.

Two years later Fenkci et al. tried to determine whether oxidative stress is associated with increased risk of CVD in women with PCOS.[50] A total of 30 women with PCOS and 31 healthy women were enrolled in the study and CRP was measured in both populations. They found that CRP concentrations were higher in PCOS women compared to controls (means, 6.30 and 2.35 mg/L, respectively; $P = 0.004$).

Boulman et al. in 2004[48] in a retrospective, case–control, cross-sectional study compared the levels of CRP in a large group of PCOS patients ($n = 116$) and BMI-matched controls ($n = 94$). In this study they did not measure androgen levels in all patients or controls and PCOS was defined as menstrual irregularity due to oligomenorrhea (fewer than nine menstrual periods per year) or amenorrhea (no menstrual periods for 3 or more months) and clinical evidence of hyperandrogenism (hirsutism, acne, or male pattern balding). The mean age of the PCOS group was 27.5 ± 8 years, and the mean age of the controls was 30.4 ± 8 years. There were no other differences in patients' characteristics between the two groups. CRP measurements were determined by two different methods: highly sensitive CRP (hsCRP) and regular CRP (R-CRP). The hsCRP was used for the low-range levels (<5 mg/L). The mean ($\pm$SD) CRP concentration was 5.46 ± 7.0 mg/L in the PCOS group versus 2.04 ± 1.9 mg/L in the controls ($P < 0.001$). Whereas 36.8% of the PCOS patients had CRP levels above 5 mg/L, only 9.6% of the controls exhibited such CRP levels ($P < 0.001$). A total of 46.5% of the PCOS patients had CRP levels above 3 mg/L and only 27.7% of the BMI-matched controls exhibited such CRP levels ($P = 0.005$). Whereas most controls (72.4%) had CRP levels less than 3 mg/L, almost half (46.5%) of the PCOS patients had CRP greater than 3 mg/L, and more than one-third had levels above 5 mg/L. The mean CRP concentrations were significantly higher in the PCOS subgroups at normal BMI (<25) and in the obese group (BMI > 30) compared with the control subgroups of similar BMI ($P < 0.001$). For the subgroup of overweight PCOS and controls (BMI 25–29), the CRP was higher in the PCOS subgroup (3.55 vs. 2.08, respectively), but the difference did not reach statistical significance ($P = 0.07$), probably due to the smaller number of patients in this subgroup.

Tarkun et al.[51] in 2004 examined hsCRP levels in young women with PCOS with normal BMI. The geometric means for women with PCOS ($n = 37$) and the control group ($n = 25$) were 0.25 and 0.09 mg/dL, respectively ($P = 0.007$). The study showed that CRP concentrations measured using a highly sensitive assay were significantly increased in women with PCOS as compared to age- and BMI-matched healthy women. CRP was correlated only with BMI, insulin-sensitivity indices (HOMA and QUICKI), and flow-mediated dilatation (FMD). Interestingly, CRP concentrations were correlated with BMI although patients' mean BMI was within normal limits. Moreover, CRP concentrations were correlated with abdominal obesity. In conclusion, this study provided the first evidence that nonobese women with PCOS had higher hsCRP concentrations than age- and weight-matched healthy women.

Talbott *et al.*[52] in 2004 determined the circulating concentration of CRP among women with PCOS ($n = 47$) aged 45 years and older in comparison with controls ($n = 59$) of similar age (49.2 vs. 49.5 years, respectively). Significant differences were noted between PCOS cases and controls in BMI (32.4 vs. 26.0 kg/m^2; $P < 0.001$), waist circumference (94.2 vs. 81.6 cm; $P < 0.001$), waist/hip ratio (0.83 vs. 0.78; $P < 0.001$), and visceral fat (16,876 vs. 9,010 mm^2; $P < 0.001$). CRP levels were significantly elevated among PCOS patients compared with controls (3.4 vs. 2.1 mg/dL; $P = 0.002$). When stratified by BMI, CRP levels remained significantly increased in PCOS patients compared with controls in the BMI 25 or greater subgroups only (4.1 vs. 2.6 mg/dL, $P = 0.008$).

A year later in 2005, Orio *et al.*,[53] studying a large group of women ($n = 300$), 150 with PCOS and 150 controls, confirmed that a significantly higher concentration of CRP was demonstrated in PCOS women compared to controls (2 vs. 0.7 mg/L; $P < 0.0001$). PCOS and control groups were matched for age and BMI.

More recently Diamanti-Kandarakis *et al.*[54] studying hsCRP levels in 107 Greek Caucasian women (62 PCOS patients and 45 women with regular menstrual cycles, normal androgen levels, of similar age and BMI values) showed that PCOS women had significantly higher hsCRP levels compared to controls (1.31 ± 0.22 vs. 0.92 ± 0.27, $P = 0.014$).

In conclusion, the current data are all in agreement that PCOS women when matched for age, BMI, and fat distribution with the control groups, have elevated CRP levels, an independent marker for cardiovascular risk.

The Increase of Leukocytes as Marker of Low-Grade Chronic Inflammation in PCOS

Four years after the initial study of Kelly *et al.* who proposed low-grade chronic inflammation as a novel mechanism contributing to increased risk of CHD and T2D in PCOS women, because of the significant higher levels of CRP in these women, Orio *et al.*[53] proposed a new marker of low-grade inflammation in PCOS: the white blood cell count. They thought that because an elevated WBC count is a risk factor for atherosclerotic vascular disease,[55] the association of leukocyte count with cardiovascular risk factors may represent a manifestation of subclinical disease, or alternatively leukocyte count could be part of a chain of atherogenic factors, leading to atherosclerosis.[56] The leukocyte count was significantly higher in PCOS women compared with the control group, even though no case of leukocytosis was found in either group. Analyzing the leukocyte formula, a significant increase of lymphocytes and monocytes in PCOS women versus controls ($P < 0.0001$) was observed. In both groups, there was a significant association between leukocyte count and HOMA index (PCOS, $r = 0.94$ with $P < 0.0001$; controls, $r = 0.91$ with $P < 0.0001$).

Inflammatory Cytokines

For more than a decade a broad spectrum of proinflammatory cytokines in a deleterious cascade has been shown to paricipate in the atherogenetic process. IL-18, a proinflammatory cytokine, induces the production of tumor necrosis factor (TNF-α),[57] which in turn promotes the synthesis of IL-6.[58] The latter regulates the synthesis of CRP in the liver.[59] Like IL-6 and CRP, IL-18 is considered a strong risk marker for cardiovascular events.[60] Serum IL-18 concentrations strongly correlate with BMI in women[61] and moreover correlate with waist to hip ratio (WHR) and fasting insulin levels, indexes of insulin resistance, suggesting that the increase in serum IL-18 levels is related not only to obesity but also to insulin resistance.[61]

Escobar-Morreale et al.[62] measured serum levels of IL-18 in 60 PCOS women and compared them to 34 controls matched for BMI. Serum IL-18 concentrations were increased in lean and obese PCOS patients compared with their nonhyperandrogenic counterparts ($P = 0.031$). Obese women presented with increased IL-18 levels ($P = 0.018$) irrespective of the presence or absence of PCOS. It was suggested that both PCOS and obesity are independently associated with an increase in serum IL-18 levels. Because both lean and obese women with PCOS presented with increased WHR and decreased insulin sensitivity compared with their nonhyperandrogenic counterparts, the increase in IL-18 levels found in PCOS was attributed to visceral adiposity and insulin resistance, frequently found in PCOS patients.

However, there are studies which have not confirmed the elevated levels of cytokines but do agree that these molecules are positively correlated with BMI.[63] Another well-known inflammatory cytokine whose expression has been associated with insulin resistance was also detected in women with PCOS. TNF-α levels and its relationship with insulin levels and body weight was studied in women with PCOS.[64] Women with PCOS exhibited a significantly ($P < 0.02$) higher mean serum TNF-α concentration compared with controls. The serum TNF-α level and BMI were directly correlated in women with PCOS ($r = 0.48$, $P < 0.005$) and highly correlated in controls ($r = 0.78$, $P < 0.001$). The conclusions drawn from this study were that serum TNF-α is increased in normal-weight women with PCOS and is even higher in obese individuals regardless of the presence of PCOS. The authors suggested that factors other than obesity are the cause of elevated serum TNF-α in normal-weight women with PCOS.

The discovery of leptin confirmed that adipose tissue is no longer regarded as a mere reserve of fuel in the form of triglycerides but it functions as an endocrine organ that supervises energy metabolism. This seems to be partially accomplished by "adipocytokines," secreted substances that probably contribute to peripheral insulin sensitivity. Furthermore, it has been established that resistin, another cytokine, is almost exclusively produced in adipose tissue.[65–67] Considering the association of PCOS with impaired glucose tolerance, diabetes mellitus, and obesity, as well as inconsistent evidence pointing at resistin as a possible link between obesity and insulin resistance, Panidis *et al.* 2004[68] measured serum resistin levels in women with PCOS with normal body mass index (BMI < 25 kg/m^2) and with BMI > 25 kg/m^2, and assessed possible correlations between resistin and the hormonal and metabolic parameters of the syndrome. Resistin levels were significantly higher in women with PCOS and BMI >25 kg/m^2 compared with women with normal BMI, with or without PCOS. They did not find any difference in resistin levels between women with normal BMI. A significant positive correlation between resistin concentration in the serum and BMI was also observed. Women with PCOS and normal BMI did not have significantly higher serum resistin levels than ovulating women with normal BMI and without hyperandrogenism. Furthermore, no correlation of resistin levels to gonadotropin or androgen levels was found.

Adhesion Molecules

The levels of the adhesion molecules (AM), sIVAM-1, sVCAM-1, and sE-selectin in serum reflect low-grade chronic inflammation of the endothelium and independently predict the risk for CHD and T2D.[69–75]

Recently, Diamanti-Kandarakis *et al.*[54] measured sIVAM-1, sVCAM-1, and sE-selectin, in both groups in the serum of 107 Greek Caucasian women (62 PCOS patients and 45 women with regular menstrual cycles, normal androgen levels, of similar age and BMI values).

Plasma levels of sICAM-1 (ng/mL) and sE-selectin (ng/mL) were higher in PCOS compared with controls (301.21 ± 24.80 vs. 209.86 ± 17.05, $P = 0.025$; 57.37 ± 4.08 vs. 45.67 ± 4.62, $P = 0.045$, respectively). However, sVCAM-1 did not differ statistically between the two groups ($P = 0.896$). The relationship between hyperandrogenemia and inflammation is under investigation. Nevertheless, a positive correlation between hsCRP concentrations and hyperndrogenemia was found while a predictive value for PCOS presence was revealed by regression analysis on sICAM and sE-selectin levels. This finding is in conjunction with the genetic abnormalities, such as polymorphisms in inflammatory markers that have been identified in hyperandrogenic states and may be proved to be of clinical relevance.[76–79]

The elevated levels of AM demonstrated in the serum of women with PCOS could be of particular interest because they provide strong evidence that in the endothelium of these women there is an ongoing inflammatory process, which theoretically could lead to atheromatosis and CVD.

REFERENCES

1. DIAMANTI-KANDARAKIS, E., C.R. KOULI, A.T. BERGIELE, et al. 1999. A survey of the polycystic ovary syndrome in the Greek island of Lesbos: hormonal and metabolic profile. J. Clin. Endocrinol. Metab. **84:** 4006–4011.
2. The Rotterdam ESHRE/ASRM-Sponsored PCOS consensus workshop group revised 2003 consensus on diagnostic criteria and long-term health risks related to polycystic ovary syndrome. 2004. Fertil. Steril. **81:** 19–25.
3. ORIO, F. JR., S. PALOMBA, L. SPINELLI, et al. 2004. The cardiovascular risk of young women with polycystic ovary syndrome: an observational, analytical, prospective case–control study. J. Clin. Endocrinol. Metab. **89:** 3696–3701.
4. DUNAIF, A. 1997. Insulin resistance and the polycystic ovary syndrome: Mechanisms and implications for pathogenesis. Endocr. Rev. **18:** 774–800.
5. OVALLE, F. & R. AZZIZ. 2002. Insulin resistance, polycystic ovary syndrome, and type 2 diabetes mellitus. Fertil. Steril. **77:** 1095–1105.
6. CHRISTIAN, R.C., D.A. DUMESIC, T. BEHRENBECK, et al. 2003. Prevalence and predictors of coronary artery calcification in women with polycystic ovary syndrome. J. Clin. Endocrinol. Metab. **88:** 2562–2568.
7. TALBOTT, E., D. GUZICK, A. CLERICI, et al. 1995. Coronary heart disease risk factors in women with polycystic ovary syndrome. Artherioscler. Thromb. Vasc. Biol. **15:** 821–826.
8. DIAMANTI-KANDARAKIS, E., G. PALIONIKO, K. ALEXANDRAKI, et al. 2004. The prevalence of 4G5G polymorphism of plasminogen activator inhibitor-1 (PAI-1) gene in polycystic ovarian syndrome and its association with plasma PAI-1 levels. Eur. J. Endocrinol. **150:** 793–798.
9. DIAMANTI-KANDARAKIS, E., G. SPINA, C. KOULI, et al. 2001. Increased endothelin-1 levels in women with polycystic ovary syndrome and the beneficial effect of metformin therapy. J. Clin. Endocrinol. Metab. **86:** 4666–4673.
10. DIAMANTI-KANDARAKIS, E., C. PIPERI, A. KALOFOUTIS, et al. 2005. Increased levels of serum advanced glycation end-products in women with polycystic ovary syndrome. Clin. Endocrinol. (Oxf.) **62:** 37–43.
11. PARADISI, G., H.O. STEINBERG, A. HEMPFLING, et al. 2001. Polycystic ovary syndrome is associated with endothelial dysfunction. Circulation **103:** 1410–1415.
12. TIRAS, M.B., R. YALCIN, V. NOYAN, et al. 1999. Alterations in cardiac flow parameters in patients with polycystic ovarian syndrome. Hum. Reprod. **14:** 1949–1952.
13. ALEXANDER, R.W. 1994. Inflammation and coronary artery disease. N. Engl. J. Med. **331:** 468–469.
14. WILSON, P.W., W.B. KANNEL, H. SILBERSHATZ, et al. 1999. Clustering of metabolic factors and coronary heart disease. Arch. Intern. Med. **159:** 1104–1109.

15. LEE, C.D., A.R. FOLSOM, F.J. NIETO, *et al.* 2001. White blood cell count and incidence of coronary heart disease and ischemic stroke and mortality from cardiovascular disease in African-American and white men and women. Am. J. Epidemiol. **154:** 758–764.

16. PAI, J.K., T. PISCHON, J. MA, *et al.* 2004. Inflammatory markers and the risk of coronary heart disease in men and women. N. Engl. J. Med. **351:** 2599–2610.

17. FLIER, J.S., R.C. EASTMAN, K.L. MINAKER, *et al.* 1985. Acanthosis nigricans in obese women with hyperandrogenism. Characterization of an insulin-resistant state distinct from the type A and B syndromes. Diabetes **34:** 101–107.

18. JIALAL, I., P. NAIKER, K. REDDI, *et al.* 1987. Evidence for insulin resistance in nonobese patients with polycystic ovarian disease. J. Clin. Endocrinol. Metab. **64:** 1066–1069.

19. DUNAIF, A. 1995. Hyperandrogenic anovulation (PCOS): a unique disorder of insulin action associated with an increased risk of non-insulin-dependent diabetes mellitus. Am. J. Med. **98:** 33S–39S.

20. DUNAIF, A., X. WU, A. LEE, *et al.* 2001. Defects in insulin receptor signalling *in vivo* in the polycystic ovary syndrome (PCOS) Am. J. Physiol. Endocrinol. Metab. **281:** E392–E399.

21. PORETSKY, L., N.A. CATALDO, Z. ROSENWAKS, *et al.* 1999. The insulin-related ovarian regulatory system in health and disease. Endocr. Rev. **20:** 535–582.

22. PORETSKY, L., F. GRIGORESCU, M. SEIBEL, *et al.* 1985. Distribution and characterization of insulin and insulin-like growth factor I receptors in normal human ovary. J. Clin. Endocrinol. Metab. **61:** 728–734.

23. PORETSKY, L., D. SMITH, M. SEIBEL, *et al.* 1984. Specific insulin binding sites in human ovary. J. Clin. Endocrinol. Metab. **59:** 809–811.

24. WILLIS, D., H. MASON, C. GILLING-SMITH, *et al.* 1996. Modulation by insulin of follicle-stimulating hormone and luteinizing hormone actions in human granulosa cells of normal and polycystic ovaries. J. Clin. Endocrinol. Metab. **81:** 302–309.

25. BERGH, C., B. CARLSSON, J.H. OLSSON, *et al.* 1993. Regulation of androgen production in cultured human thecal cells by insulin-like growth factor I and insulin. Fertil. Steril. **59:** 323–331.

26. DULEBA, A.J., R.Z. SPACZYNSKI & D.L. OLIVE. 1998. Insulin and insulin-like growth factor I stimulate the proliferation of human ovarian thecainterstitial cells. Fertil. Steril. **69:** 335–340.

27. CARA, J.F. & R.L. ROSENFIELD. 1988. Insulin-like growth factor I and insulin potentiate luteinizing hormone-induced androgen synthesis by rat ovarian thecal-interstitial cells. Endocrinology **123:** 733–739.

28. HERNANDEZ, E.R., C.E. RESNICK, M.E. SVOBODA, *et al.* 1988. Somatomedin-C/insulin-like growth factor I as an enhancer of androgen biosynthesis by cultured rat ovarian cells. Endocrinology **122:** 1603–1612.

29. WRATHALL, J.H. & P.G. KNIGHT. 1995. Effects of inhibin-related peptides and oestradiol on androstenedione and progesterone secretion by bovine theca cells *in vitro.* J. Endocrinol. **145:** 491–500.

30. KRISTIANSEN, S.B., A. ENDOH, P.R. CASSON, *et al.* 1997. Induction of steroidogenic enzyme genes by insulin and IGF-I in cultured adult human adrenocortical cells. Steroids **62:** 258–265.

31. ADASHI, E.Y., C.E. RESNICK, A.J. D'ERCOLE, *et al.* 1985. Insulin-like growth factors as intraovarian regulators of granulosa cell growth and function. Endocr. Rev. **6:** 400–420.

32. DANESH, J., P. WHINCUP, M. WALKER, *et al.* 2000. Low-grade inflammation and coronary heart disease: a prospective study and updated metaanalyses. Br. Med. J. **321:** 199–204.
33. PICKUP, J.C., M.B. MATTOCK, G.D. CHUSNEY, *et al.* 1997. NIDDM as a disease of the innate immune system: association of the acute-phase reactants and interleukin 6 with metabolic syndrome X. Diabetologia **40:** 1286–1292.
34. PICKUP, J.C. & M.A. CROOK. 1998. Is type II diabetes a disease of the innate immune system? Diabetologia **41:** 1241–1248.
35. FERNANDEZ-REAL, J.M. & W. RICART. 2003. Insulin resistance and chronic cardiovascular inflammatory syndrome. Endocr. Rev. **24:** 278–301.
36. PARADISI, G., H. STEINBERG, M. SHEPARD, *et al.* 2003. Troglitazone therapy improves endothelial function to near normal levels in women with polycystic ovary syndrome. J. Clin. Endocrinol. Metab. **88:** 576–580.
37. WHEATCROFT, S.B., I.L. WILLIAMS, A.M. SHAH, *et al.* 2003. Pathophysiological implications of insulin resistance on vascular endothelial function. Diabet. Med. **20:** 255–268.
38. DIAMANTI-KANDARAKIS, E., K. ALEXANDRAKI, A. PROTOGEROU, *et al.* 2005. Metformin administration improves endothelial function in women with polycystic ovary syndrome. Eur. J. Endocrinol. **152:** 749–756.
39. RIDKER, P.M., C.H. HENNEKENS, J.E. BURING, *et al.* 2000. C-reactive protein and other markers of inflammation in the prediction of cardiovascular disease in women. N. Engl. J. Med. **342:** 836–843.
40. DANESH, J., J.G. WHEELER, G.M. HIRSCHFIELD, *et al.* 2004. C-reactive protein and other circulating markers of inflammation in the prediction of coronary heart disease. N. Engl. J. Med. **350:** 1387–1397.
41. SAM, S. & A. DUNAIF. 2003. Polycystic ovary syndrome: syndrome XX? Trends Endocrinol. Metab. **14:** 365–370.
42. TALBOTT, E.O., J.V. ZBOROWSKI, K. SUTTON-TYRRELL, *et al.* 2001. Cardiovascular risk in women with polycystic ovary syndrome. Obstet. Gynecol. Clin. North Am. **28:** 111–133.
43. TALBOTT, E., D. GUZICK, A. CLERICI, *et al.* 1995. Coronary heart disease risk factor in women with polycystic ovary syndrome. Arterioscler. Thromb. Vasc. Biol. **15:** 821–826.
44. WILD, R.A., P.C. PAINTER, P.B. COULSON, *et al.* 1985. Lipoprotein lipid concentration and cardiovascular risk in women with polycystic ovary syndrome. J. Clin. Endocrinol. Metab. **61:** 946–951.
45. RIDKER, P.M. 2003. Clinical application of C-reactive protein for cardiovascular disease: detection and prevention. Circulation **107:** 363–369.
46. PEARSON, T.A., G.A. MENSAH, R.W. ALEXANDER, *et al.* 2003. Markers of inflammation and cardiovascular disease: application to clinical and public health practice: a statement for healthcare professionals from the Center for Disease Control and Prevention and the American Heart Association. Circulation **107:** 499–511.
47. RIDKER, P.M., J.E. BURING, N.R. COOK, *et al.* 2003. C-reactive protein, the metabolic syndrome, and risk of incident cardiovascular events: an 8-year follow-up of 14719 initially healthy American women. Circulation **107:** 391–397.
48. BOULMAN, N., Y. LEVY, R. LEIBA, *et al.* 2004. Increased C-reactive protein levels in the polycystic ovary syndrome: a marker of cardiovascular disease. J. Clin. Endocrinol. Metab. **89:** 2160–2165.
49. KELLY, C.C., H. LYALL, J.R. PETRIE, *et al.* 2001. Low-grade chronic inflammation in women with polycystic ovarian syndrome. J. Clin. Endocrinol. Metab. **86:** 2453–2455.

50. FENKCI, V., S. FENKCI, M. YILMAZER, *et al.* 2003. Decreased total antioxidant status and increased oxidative stress in women with polycystic ovary syndrome may contribute to the risk of cardiovascular disease. Fertil. Steril. **80:** 123–127.

51. TARKUN, I., B.C. ARSLAN, Z. CANTURK, *et al.* 2004. Endothelial dysfunction in young women with polycystic ovary syndrome: relationship with insulin resistance and low-grade chronic inflammation. J. Clin. Endocrinol. Metab. **89:** 5592–5596.

52. TALBOTT, E.O., J.V. ZBOROWSKI, M.Y. BOUDREAUX, *et al.* 2004. The relationship between C-reactive protein and carotid intima-media wall thickness in middle-aged women with polycystic ovary syndrome. J. Clin. Endocrinol. Metab. **89:** 6061–6067.

53. ORIO, F. JR, S. PALOMBA, T. CASCELLA, *et al.* 2005. The increase of leukocytes as a new putative marker of low-grade chronic inflammation and early cardiovascular risk in polycystic ovary syndrome. J. Clin. Endocrinol. Metab. **90:** 2–5.

54. DIAMANTI-KANDARAKIS, E., T. PATERAKIS, K. ALEXANDRAKI, *et al.* 2006. Indices of low-grade chronic inflammation in polycystic ovary syndrome and the beneficial effect of metformin. Hum. Reprod. **21:** 1426–1431.

55. HASEGAWA, T., T. NEGISHI & M. DEGUCHI. 2002. WBC count, atherosclerosis and coronary risk factors. J. Atheroscler. Thromb. **9:** 219–223.

56. NIETO, F.J., M. SZKLO, A.R. FOLSOM, *et al.* 1992. Leukocyte count correlates in middle-aged adults: the Atherosclerosis risk in communities (ARIC) study. Am. J. Epidemiol. **136:** 525–537.

57. OKAMURA, H., H. TSUTSUI, S. KASHIWAMURA, *et al.* 1998. Interleukin-18: a novel cytokine that augments both innate and acquired immunity. Adv. Immunol. **70:** 281–312.

58. STEPHENS, J.M., M.D. BUTTS & P.H. PEKALA. 1992. Regulation of transcription factor mRNA accumulation during 3T3–L1 preadipocyte differentiation by tumour necrosis factor-a. J. Mol. Endocrinol. **9:** 61–72.

59. HEINRICH, P.C., J.V. CASTELL & T. ANDUS. 1990. Interleukin-6 and the acute phase response. Biochem. J. **265:** 621–636.

60. BLANKENBERG, S., L. TIRET, C. BICKEL, *et al.* 2002. Interleukin-18 is a strong predictor of cardiovascular death in stable and unstable angina. Circulation **106:** 24–30.

61. ESPOSITO, K., A. PONTILLO, M. CIOTOLA, *et al.* 2002. Weight loss reduces interleukin-18 levels in obese women. J. Clin. Endocrinol. Metab. **87:** 3864–3866.

62. ESCOBAR-MORREALE, H.F., J.I. BOTELLA-CARRETERO, G. VILLUENDAS, *et al.* 2004. Serum interleukin-18 concentrations are increased in the polycystic ovary syndrome: relationship to insulin resistance and to obesity. J. Clin. Endocrinol. Metab. **89:** 806–811.

63. MOHLIG, M., J. SPRANGER, M. OSTERHOFF, *et al.* 2004. The polycystic ovary syndrome per se is not associated with increased chronic inflammation. Eur. J. Endocrinol. **150:** 525–532.

64. GONZALEZ, F., K. THUSU, E. ABDEL-RAHMAN, *et al.* 1999. Elevated serum levels of tumor necrosis factor alpha in normal-weight women with polycystic ovary syndrome. Metabolism **48:** 437–441.

65. FRIEDMAN, J.M. & J.L. HALAAS. 1998. Leptin and the regulation of body weight in mammals. Nature **395:** 763–770.

66. UKKOLA, O. 2002. Resistin: a mediator of obesity-associated insulin resistance or an innocent bystander? Eur. J. Endocrinol. **147:** 571–574.

67. STEPPAN, C.M. & M.A. LAZAR. 2002. Resistin and obesity-associated insulin resistance. Trends Endocrinol. Metabol. **13:** 18–22.
68. PANIDIS, D., G. KOLIAKOS, A. KOURTIS, *et al.* 2004. Serum resistin levels in women with polycystic ovary syndrome. Fertil. Steril. **81:** 361–366.
69. LEY, K. & Y. HUO. 2001. VCAM-1 is critical in atherosclerosis. J. Clin. Invest. **107:** 1209–1210.
70. PAI, J.K., T. PISCHON, J. MA, *et al.* 2004. Inflammatory markers and the risk of coronary heart disease in men and women. N. Engl. J. Med. **351:** 2599–2610.
71. MEIGS, J.B., F.B. HU, N. RIFAI, *et al.* 2004. Biomarkers of endothelial dysfunction and risk of type 2 diabetes mellitus. JAMA **291:** 1978–1986.
72. ROLDAN, V., F. MARIN, G.Y. LIP, *et al.* 2003. Soluble E-selectin in cardiovascular disease and its risk factor. A review of the literature. Thromb. Haemost. **90:** 1007–1020.
73. CORTI, R., R. HUTTER, J.J. BADIMON, *et al.* 2004. Evolving concepts in the triad of atherosclerosis, inflammation and thrombosis. J. Thromb. Thrombolysis **17:** 35–44.
74. KOWALSKA, I., M. STRACZKOWSKI, M. SZELACHOWSKA, *et al.* 2002. Circulating E-selectin, vascular cell adhesion molecule-1, and intercellular adhesion molecule-1 in men with coronary artery disease assessed by angiography and disturbances of carbohydrate metabolism. Metabolism **51:** 733–736.
75. KADO, S. & N. NAGATA. 1999. Circulating intercellular adhesion molecule-1, vascular cell adhesion molecule-1, and E-selectin in patients with type 2 diabetes mellitus. Diabetes Res. Clin. Pract. **46:** 143–148.
76. PERAL, B., J.L. SAN MILLAN, R. CASTELLO, *et al.* 2002. Comment: the methionine 196 arginine polymorphism in exon 6 of the TNF receptor 2 gene (TNFRSF1B) is associated with the polycystic ovary syndrome and hyperandrogenism. J. Clin. Endocrinol. Metab. **87:** 3977–3983.
77. VILLUENDAS, G., J.L. SAN MILLAN, J. SANCHO, *et al.* 2002. The -597 G→A and -174 G→C polymorphisms in the promoter of the IL-6 gene are associated with hyperandrogenism. J. Clin. Endocrinol. Metab. **87:** 1134–1141.
78. ESCOBAR-MORREALE, H.F., R.M. CALVO, J. SANCHO, *et al.* 2001. TNF-alpha and hyperandrogenism: a clinical, biochemical, and molecular genetic study. J. Clin. Endocrinol. Metab. **86:** 3761–3767.
79. ESCOBAR-MORREALE, H.F., R.M. CALVO, G. VILLUENDAS, *et al.* 2003. Association of polymorphisms in the interleukin 6 receptor complex with obesity and hyperandrogenism. Obes. Res. **11:** 987–996.

The Retroperitoneal Approach
in Minimally Invasive Pelvic Surgery

JEAN-BERNARD DUBUISSON, YANNICK DE DYCKER,
AND MICHAL YARON

*Department of Obstetrics and Gynecology, Hôpitaux Universitaires de Genève,
Switzerland*

ABSTRACT: The retroperitoneal approach is a minimally invasive surgery
than can be performed through direct access or through indirect access,
with abdominal penetration. The choice of indirect transabdominal approach is appropriate when additional abdominal surgery is indicated
(radical hysterectomy, pelviabdominal exploration). The advantages of
the direct retroperitoneal access are the absence of risk of creating intra-
abdominal adhesions associated with those of intraperitoneal operative
laparoscopy.

KEYWORDS: Retroperitoneal; surgical procedures; minimally invasive;
pelvis

INTRODUCTION

Most abdominal gynecological operations are done with intraperitoneal approach. The retroperitoneal approach is a minimally invasive surgery that can
be performed through direct access (without penetration of the abdominal
cavity) or through indirect access (with abdominal penetration). The choice of
indirect transabdominal approach is appropriate when additional abdominal
surgery is indicated (radical hysterectomy, myomectomy, or pelvic-abdominal
exploration). The direct access is taken in specific indications, such as: pelvic
lymphadenectomy, treatment of urinary stress incontinence (as in Burch procedure), preventive occlusion of the uterine artery during myomectomies and
hysterectomies, treatment of uterine fibroids with laparoscopic bipolar coagulation of the uterine vessels, and retroperitoneal ovarian cystectomies where
severe adhesions are present. The advantages of the retroperitoneal approach
are numerous and are similar to the advantages offered by intraperitoneal operative laparoscopy approach.[1] The laparoscopic technique and parameters are
the same except for CO_2 pressure, which must be about 12 mm Hg lower. This

Address for correspondence: Jean-Bernard Dubuisson, M.D., Department of Obstetrics and Gynecology, Hôpitaux Universitaires de Genève, Switzerland. Voice: +41-0-22-382-68-16; fax +41-0-22-
382-44-24. e-mail: jean-bernard.dubuisson@hcuge.ch

Ann. N.Y. Acad. Sci. 1092: 187–198 (2006). © 2006 New York Academy of Sciences.
doi: 10.1196/annals.1365.016

defers complications related to hypercapnia and to CO_2 passage into tissues susceptible to emphysema.

PELVIC LYMPHADENECTOMY

Pelvic lymphadenectomy, performed laparoscopically, is done in a similar fashion to laparotomy.[2] Laparoscopic pelvic lymphadenectomy can be performed through direct retroperitoneal approach or by abdominal laparoscopy followed by peritoneal incision between the round ligament and the umbilical artery to access the iliac vessels. In the treatment of cancer, the latter approach is performed more frequently along with radical hysterectomy and salpingo-oophorectomy. In the retroperitoneal approach, a monopolar needle is used to make a vertical peritoneal incision, between the round ligament and the umbilical artery, consequently reaching the external iliac vessels. The lymphatic dissection begins along the medial part of the external iliac vein (FIG. 1). The dissection then proceeds to reach the pelvic wall, the obturator muscle, and the obturator pedicle. Posteriorly, the dissection of the external iliac lymph nodes advances to the iliac bifurcation after visualization of the ureter (FIG. 2). During the dissection, bipolar coagulation of the small vessels is mandatory to allow clear visualization. Precise dissection and perfect visualization ensure preservation of all the adjacent anatomical structures. Removal of the lymph nodes is then carried away through the 10–12 mm suprapubic trocar.

The indications for pelvic lymphadenectomy are gynecological malignancies such as, endometrial, cervical, and ovarian cancer.[3] Lymphadenectomy is indicated in endometrial cancer when myometrial invasion or endocervical extension is present. It is also indicated in stages IA2 and IB cervical cancer.

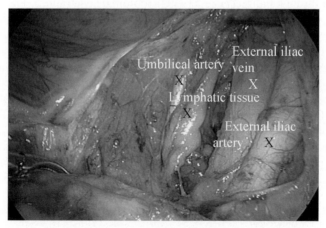

FIGURE 1. Right pelvic lymphadenectomy: dissection of the lymphatic tissue from the external iliac vein and pelvic wall.

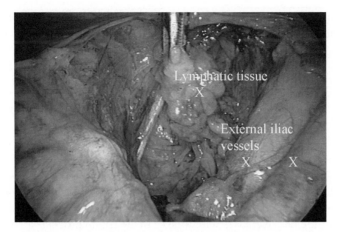

FIGURE 2. Right pelvic lymphadenectomy: dissection from the umbilical artery.

The mean number of excised lymph nodes varies among authors: 3–22 nodes (mean 8.7 nodes per patient) in Querleu's study,[4] 3–30 nodes (mean 14 nodes per patient) in Golfier's study,[5] 12–24 nodes (mean 14 nodes) in Primicero's study[6] and 23.9 ± 10.3 nodes in Lee's study.[7] Most publications limit the dissections to pelvic lymph nodes, except when macroscopically or palpable abnormal para-aortic lymph nodes are present.[8,9]

The complications of laparoscopic iliac lymphadenectomy are rare. Golfier reports 2 lymphoceles and 1 obturator nerve injury, out of 47 patients, which have resolved spontaneously.[5] Querleu *et al.* report 1 bleeding secondary to the umbilical artery injury and 1 hypercapnia out of 39 patients.[4] No complications were reported in Primicero's study out of 17 patients.[6] In a study by Lee, an aberrant obturator and iliac vein injuries were observed out of 70 patients.[7]

Para-aortic lymphadenectomy may be performed using a retroperitoneal approach through a left McBurney incision. Following a cutaneous incision, expansion of the retroperitoneal space is done digitally, which in turn is insufflated with CO_2 up to 12 mm Hg. Two additional left trocars are placed along the axillary line. The lymph node dissection begins below the left renal vein. The lymphadenectomy is performed from the aorta down to the left common iliac artery and includes the origin of the inferior mesenteric artery. The dissection comprises the left, the anterior, and posterior parts of the aorta and the left common iliac artery. The 4th and 5th lumbar arteries are occluded with a clip to allow access to the retroaortic space, the interaorticocave space, and to the anterior and posterior facets of the vena cava. Dargent *et al.* [10] consider the left retroperitoneal approach to be superior to the classical abdominal and laparoscopic approaches with less postoperative adhesions, better bowel mobility, and less complications post radiotherapy. In their study, 15 ± 3 aortic lymph nodes (range: 10–19 nodes) were removed.[10]

In cervical cancer, Dargent *et al.* recommend para-aortic lymphadenectomy only in cases in which the iliac lymph nodes appear macroscopically normal.[10] This allows for precise staging and better selection of the patients requiring brachytherapy. According to Hoskins *et al.*, para-aortic lymph node metastases are present in 6% of stage IB, 12% of stage IIB, 33% stage IIIA, 29% IIIB, and 30% of stage IV patients.[11]

BURCH PROCEDURE

The Burch retropubic colposuspension is a well-established procedure in the treatment of women with genuine stress incontinence (GSI) and it is considered to be an effective surgery.[12] However, it is well documented that the subjective cure rate decreases with time.[13] In the Burch procedure, the vaginal endopelvic fascia is fixed close to the bladder neck and the proximal portion of the urethra is fixed to Cooper's ligament. The procedure is classically done through a transversal suprapubic incision. Nowadays, most surgeons perform it laparoscopically. It has been demonstrated that the anatomic and clinical results after laparoscopic and open Burch colposuspension for primary SUI are the same.[14] Two different laparoscopic procedures give access to Retzius space. In the direct (retroperitoneal) approach, a trocar is introduced directly and medially through to Retzius space and CO_2 insufflation reaches up to of 12 mm Hg. In the second approach, the laparoscope is introduced through the umbilicus. The peritoneum is then opened above the bladder to give access to Retzius space (FIG. 3). The reported success rate of laparoscopic Burch colposuspension is 89% at 2-year follow-up.[15] Complications such as, hemorrhage, bladder injury, and hypercapnia may occur and result from the laparoscopic dissection of Retzius space. Postoperative infection of the Retzius space has also been reported. In a randomized trial, comparing laparoscopic Burch colposuspension versus tension-free vaginal tape (TVT), the complication rates were similar.[16]

We perform laparoscopic Burch procedure following a minimally invasive technique. After umbilical introduction of the laparoscope, a lateral vertical incision of the peritoneum, about 3 cm between the umbilical artery and the round ligament, is done on both sides. This incision gives access to Cooper's ligament. Then, Retzius space is minimally dissected, as well as, the vaginal endopelvic fascia close to the proximal urethra. Two nonabsorbable sutures are then placed between the vagina and Cooper's ligament and suspension of the periurethal tissue takes place without excessive tension. To avoid postoperative infections, the vaginal suture is extramucosal. The peritoneum is then closed using absorbable sutures. This is done to prevent postoperative bowel obstruction caused by bowel adhesions to the Retzius space.

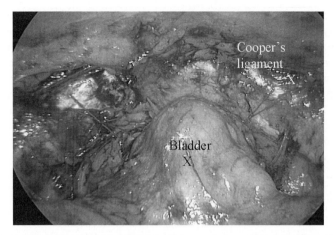

FIGURE 3. Burch procedure: bilateral colposuspension: placement of the first nonabsorbable suture.

LAPAROSCOPIC PREVENTIVE OCCLUSION OF THE UTERINE ARTERY COMBINED WITH MYOMECTOMY AND HYSTERECTOMY

Preventive occlusion of the uterine artery combined with laparoscopic myomectomy is an acceptable procedure to decrease uterine bleeding. Myomectomy may be performed by laparoscopy in selected cases, particularly when subserous and intramural fibroids are present.[17–19] The indications for laparoscopic myomectomy depend on the number, size, type, and localization of the fibroids. Most reports on laparoscopic myomectomy speak in favor of this technique when relatively few (1–3 per patient) and medium-sized fibroids (about 5–8 cm) are present.[20]

Myomectomy is a hemorrhagic operation. Enucleation of the fibroid and immediate suturing of the uterus usually reduces the amount of bleeding. The laparoscopic technique presents two advantages over laparotomy in terms of limiting the hemorrhagic risk during myomectomy. The pneumoperitoneal pressure of 15 mm Hg prevents extravasation of blood from intramyometrial capillaries and veins. In addition, the magnification, provided by the laparoscope lens, helps to identify more precisely the anatomical structures and enables selective coagulation of the small vessels feeding the fibroid. However, in highly vascularized fibroid these advantages are not sufficient in limiting blood loss.[21] In our series of 426 laparoscopic myomectomies, conversion rate to open procedures (either laparotomy or mini-laparotomy) was 11.3%. In the majority of cases, this was due to excessive bleeding during the laparoscopic procedure.[22]

In our center, we have modified laparoscopic myomectomy procedures by adding preventive occlusion of the uterine arteries using clips. Before January 2001, when encountering excessive bleeding during laparoscopic myomectomy, we occluded the uterine arteries to stop the hemorrhage. The decrease in bleeding was impressive and allowed us to resume laparoscopic myomectomy without any further complications. The postoperative course was uneventful in all cases. This observation prompted us to run a comparative study and enabled us to demonstrate the advantages of this procedure. We report a nonrandomized study comparing two equivalent groups of patients treated with laparoscopic myomectomy.[23] In one group (21 patients) laparoscopic myomectomy was combined with preventive occlusion of the uterine arteries; in the other group (21 patients) laparoscopic myomectomy was performed without any vascular occlusion.

The preventive occlusion of the uterine arteries is done as follows: a 3-cm longitudinal peritoneal incision is made with scissors on the upper part of the broad ligament, behind the round ligament. The umbilical artery is then dissected and followed reaching the origin of the uterine artery, which in turn is dissected away from the uterine vein. Close to the artery the ureter is visualized, adherent to the peritoneum. One nonabsorbable clip (Titanium ligaclip, Storz Company Tuttlingen, Germany) is placed at the origin of the uterine artery (FIG. 4). Hemostasis of small vessels is carried out if necessary. At the end of the procedure, the peritoneum of the broad ligament is closed using a 00 vicryl running suture.

In this study, the decrease in mean hemoglobin (preoperative and postoperative) was 1.8 ± 1.2 in the occlusion group (first group) compared with 2.1 ± 2.2 in the nonocclusion group (second group) ($P = 0.2374$). The postoperative hemoglobin level was 11.4 ± 1.5 g/dL for the first group and 10.6 ± 1.6 g/dL

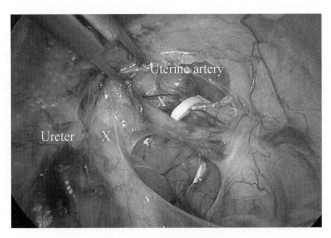

FIGURE 4. Preventive uterine artery occlusion. A clip is placed on the right artery.

for the second group ($P = 0.0169$). Hemoglobin decrease of more than 3 g/dL was observed in 2 of 48 patients in the first group and in 10 of 47 patients in the second group ($P = 0.0121$).

The uterine artery is clipped at its origin after exposing a few centimeters of its length. We report no complications using this technique. We do not use bipolar coagulation to dissect the artery to avoid thermal damage to the ureter located close by. Notably, this technique does not prolong the duration of the operation significantly.

In most cases (60%), the occlusion is performed on both sides. Unilateral occlusion is indicated when the fibroid is lateral with a selective vascularization coming from the ipsilateral uterine artery, documented by ultrasound prior to the operation. In such cases, the occlusion of one uterine artery is sufficient to decrease bleeding during hysterotomy.

Another advantage of this technique is that it makes myomectomy easy. The hysterotomy is carried out with moderate bleeding. The cleavage plane is clearly defined. After enucleating the fibroid, hemostasis of the hysterotomy edges usually takes place spontaneously and the use of bipolar coagulation is limited to few vessels. Moreover, the decrease in bleeding allows for more precise and faster suturing.

We also noted low rate of intramural hematoma formation. Only 3 of 43 patients (7%) had a hematoma documented by ultrasound 2–3 months postoperatively.

In cases of extensive vascularization of the fibroid, the myomectomy poses significant risk for perioperative hemorrhage. In our study, the number of cases with a hemoglobin drop of more than 3 g/dL was significantly lower in the group of patients treated with laparoscopic myomectomy combined with preventive occlusion of the uterine arteries compared with the group without vascular occlusion.

In the occlusion group we observed good scarring of the myometrium. This was evaluated by ultrasound, at approximately 2–3 months postoperatively. In 41.9% of the cases, the myomectomy incision was not visible, which suggests good healing. Quick revascularization of the uterus was confirmed postoperatively by color Doppler sonography.

We also measured blood flow impedance. The blood flow to the uterus was the same before and 2–3 months after preventive occlusion. During laparoscopy, the first few minutes following arterial occlusion, first the fibroid that turns pale, then the uterus. This selective blanching of the fibroid is suggestive of selective fibroid vascular changes. At the end of the myomectomy, the uterus reddens again. Such fast revascularization is explained by reestablishment of uterine vascularity.

Laparoscopic myomectomy combined with preventive occlusion of the uterine arteries has not yet been studied in women who wish to conceive. Theoretically, the permanent occlusion of both uterine arteries during laparoscopic myomectomy should alter the perfusion of a pregnant uterus and the placental

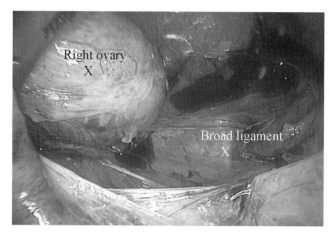

FIGURE 6. Retroperitoneal access of a right ovarian cyst: the cyst is dissected.

hysterectomies, laparoscopic bipolar coagulation of the uterine vessels in treatment of symptomatic fibroids, and retroperitoneal ovarian cystectomies where severe adhesions are present.

The laparoscopic retroperitoneal approach is reliable, feasible, and allows for excellent operative results. All gynecological surgeons should practice it regularly.

REFERENCES

1. SERACHIOLI, R., J.A. HOURCABIE, F. VIANELLO, *et al.* 2004. Laparoscopic treatment of pelvic floor defects in women of reproductive age. J. Am. Assoc. Gynecol. Laparosc. **11:** 332–335.
2. WATTIEZ, A., F. RAYMOND, M. CANIS, *et al.* 1993. External iliac lymphadenectomy by celioscopy surgical technique. Ann. Chir. **47:** 523–528.
3. NARDUCCI, F., B. OCCELLI, E. LEBLANC, *et al.* 2003. La lymphadénectomie interiliaque par coelioscopie. J. de Chirurgie **140:** 104–109.
4. QUERLEU, D., E. LEBLANC & B. CASTELAIN. 1991. Laparoscopic pelvic lymphadenectomy in the staging of early carcinoma of the cervix. Am. J. Obstet. Gynecol. **164:** 579–581.
5. GOLFIER, F., D. RAUDRANT, F. CHAMPION, *et al.* 1997. Laparoscopic external iliac lymphadenectomy in the treatment of cancer of the cervix uteri. J. Gynecol. Obstet. Biol. Reprod. (Paris) **26:** 590–596.
6. PRIMICERO, M., M. MONTANINO-OLIVA, A. CASA, *et al.* 1996. Laparoscopic lymphadenectomy and vaginal radical hysterectomy for the treatment of cervical cancer. J. Am. Assoc. Gynecol. Laparosc. **3**(Suppl.): S40–S41.
7. LEE, Y.S. 1999. Early experience with laparoscopic pelvic lymphadenectomy in women with gynecologic malignancy. J. Am. Assoc. Gynecol. Laparosc. **6:** 59–63.

8. SCRIBNER, D.R., J.L. WALKER, G.A. JOHNSON, *et al.* 2001. Laparoscopic pelvic and paraaortic lymph node dissection : analysis of the first 100 cases. Gynecol. Oncol. **82:** 498–503.

9. POSSOVER, M., N. KRAUSE, K. PLAUL, *et al.* 1998. Laparoscopic paraaortic and pelvic lymphadenectomy: experience with 150 patients and review of the literature. Gynecol. Oncol. **71:** 19–28.

10. DARGENT, D., Y. ANSQUER & P. MATHEVET. 2000. Technical development and results of left extraperitoneal laparoscopic paraaortic lymphadenectomy for cervical cancer. Gynecol. Oncol. **77:** 87–92.

11. HOSKINS, W.J., C. PEREZ & R. YOUNG. 1989. Gynecologic tumors. *In* Cancer Principles and Practice of Oncology. V.T. De Vita, S. Helman & S.A. Rosenberd, Eds: 1099–1161. 3rd ed. Lippincott: Philadelphia, PA.

12. BLACK, N.A. & S.H. DOWNS. 1996. The effectiveness of surgery for stress incontinence in women : a systematic review. Br. J. Urol. **78:** 497–510.

13. KJOLHEDE, P. 2005. Long-term efficacy of Burch colposuspension: a 14-year follow-up study. Acta Obstet. Gynecol. Scand. **84:** 767–772.

14. HUANG, W.C. & J.M. YANG. 2004. Anatomic comparison between laparoscopic and open Burch colposuspension for primary stress urinary incontinence. Urology **63:** 676–681.

15. ROSS, J.W. 1998. Multichannel urodynamic evaluation of laparoscopic Burch colposuspension for genuine stress incontinence. Obstet. Gynecol. **91:** 55–59.

16. PARAISO, M.F., M.D. WALTERS & M.M. KARRAM. 2005. Laparoscopic Burch colposuspension versus tension-free vaginal tape: a randomized trial. Obstet. Gynecol. Surv. **60:** 166–167.

17. DANIELL, J.G. & L.D. GURLEY. 1991. Laparoscopic treatment of clinically significant symptomatic uterine fibroids. J. Gynecol. Surg. **7:** 37–39.

18. DUBUISSON, J.B., F. LECURU, H. FOULOT, *et al.* 1991. Myomectomy by laparoscopy: a preliminary report of 43 cases. Fertil. Steril. **56:** 827–830.

19. HASSON, H.M., C. ROTMAN, N. RANA, *et al.* 1992. Laparoscopic myomectomy. Obstet. Gynecol. **80:** 884–888.

20. DUBUISSON, J.B., A. FAUCONNIER, K. BABAKI-FARD, *et al.* 2000. Laparoscopic myomectomy: a current view. Hum. Reprod. Update **6:** 558–594.

21. DUBUISSON, J.B., A. FAUCONNIER & C. CHAPRON. 2001. *In* An Atlas of Operative Laparoscopy and Hysteroscopy. J. Donnez & M. Nisolle, Eds.: 215–224. 2nd ed. The Parthenon Group Limited: New York, NY.

22. DUBUISSON, J.B., A. FAUCONNIER, V. FOURCHOTTE, *et al.* 2001. Laparoscopic myomectomy: predicting the risk of conversion to an open procedure. Hum. Reprod. **16:** 1726–1731.

23. DUBUISSON, J.B., C. MALARTIC, S. JACOB, *et al.* 2004. Preventive uterine artery occlusion combined with laparoscopic myomectomy: a valid procedure to prevent bleeding. J. Gynecol. Surg. **20:** 105–112.

24. MENGERT, W.F., R.C. BURCHELL, R.W. BLUMSTEIN, *et al.* 1969. Pregnancy after bilateral ligation of the internal iliac and ovarian arteries. Obstet. Gynecol. **34:** 664–666.

25. MORIKAWA, S. & H. TAKAMIZAWA. 1986. 1 case-report of small-for-gestational-age infant after bilateral ligation of the internal iliac arteries. Asia Oceania J. Obstet. Gynecol. **12:** 213–215.

26. DUBUISSON, J.B., X. CHAVET, C. CHAPRON, *et al.* 1995. Uterine rupture during pregnancy after laparoscopic myomectomy. Hum. Reprod. **10:** 1475–1477.

27. PELOSI, M. & M.A. PELOSI. 1997. Spontaneous uterine rupture at thirty-three weeks subsequent to previous superficial laparoscopic myomectomy. Am. J. Obstet. Gynecol. **11:** 1547–1549.
28. LIU, W.M., H.T. NG., Y.C. WU, *et al*. 2001. Laparoscopic bipolar coagulation of uterine vessels: a new method for treating symptomatic fibroids. Fertil. Steril. **75:** 417–422.
29. CHEN, Y.J., P.H. WANG, C.C. YUAN, *et al*. 2003. Pregnancy following treatment of symptomatic myomas with laparoscopic bipolar coagulation of uterine vessels. Hum. Reprod. **18:** 1077–1081.

Laparoscopic Management of Hydrosalpinx

JOHN N. BONTIS AND THEODOROS D. THEODORIDIS

First Department of Obstetrics and Gynecology, Aristotle University of Thessaloniki, Papageorgiou General Hospital, Nea Efkarpia, Thessaloniki, Greece

ABSTRACT: Hydrosalpinx is a common cause of female infertility. Lower implantation and pregnancy rates have been reported in women with hydrosalpinges. How hydrosalpinx exerts its negative effect on the implantation process is not clearly understood. Mechanical factors, toxicity of the hydrosalpingeal fluid, and receptivity dysfunction may explain the impaired IVF outcome in the presence of hydrosalpinx. Laparoscopic surgery has a place in the diagnosis and management of hydrosalpinx. Analysis of the results of laparoscopic management of hydrosalpinx underscores the positive role of laparoscopy in fertility outcomes in women with this pathological tubal disease. Laparoscopic salpingectomy should be offered in those women who have bilateral disease or in cases where hydrosalpinges are large enough to be visible on ultrasound. Further randomized trials are required to assess other surgical treatment options for hydrosalpinx, such as laparoscopic salpingostomy, laparoscopic or hysteroscopic tubal occlusion, and drainage of hydrosalpinx before or during oocyte retrieval.

KEYWORDS: hydrosalpinx; *in vitro* fertilization; laparoscopy; salpingectomy

INTRODUCTION

Tubal factor infertility resulting from various forms of tuboperitoneal damage remains an extremely common cause of female infertility, accounting for more than 35% of all cases of female infertility. Probably the most severe form of tubal pathology is hydrosalpinx. Hydrosalpinx is a Greek word that means a Fallopian tube filled with water or fluid. Patients with hydrosalpinges have been identified as a subgroup with significantly lower implantation and pregnancy rates than patients with other tubal pathologies. An increased risk for early pregnancy loss and increased risk for ectopic pregnancies was reported,

Address for correspondence: Theodoros D. Theodoridis, M.D., 8, Agias Theodoras St., 546 23, Thessaloniki, Greece. Voice/fax: +30-2310-240333.
e-mail: theodtheo@yahoo.gr

Ann. N.Y. Acad. Sci. 1092: 199–210 (2006). © 2006 New York Academy of Sciences.
doi: 10.1196/annals.1365.017

and many studies confirmed that the presence of hydrosalpinx significantly impairs *in vitro* fertilization (IVF) outcome as well.[1–4] Surgical management of hydrosalpinx improves pregnancy rates but patient selection is an important factor for successful surgery. Prognostic factors include the extent of adhesions, the nature of adhesions, the diameter of the hydrosalpinx, the macroscopic condition of the endosalpinx, and tubal wall thickness.[5] The success of pregnancy depends on the pathoanatomic condition of the tube, particularly on the degree of epithelial destruction, the flattened folds, the absence of cilia on the ciliated cells, and the deficiency of secretory cells particularly in the ampulla. These findings were confirmed obtaining microbiopsies before salpingostomy, which were studied by scanning and transmission electron microscopy.[6] According to the previous criteria most authors suggest four stages for the classification of hydrosalpinx: stages I, II, III, and IV. The success of pregnancy is higher in stages I and II but disappointing in stages III and IV. On the contrary, ectopic pregnancies are more often reported in patients with stages III and IV.[7] Microsurgical and laparoscopic salpingostomy results in the same conception rates but minimal access surgery has advantage over laparotomic microsurgery as shorter hospital stay, less postoperative pain, and less adhesion formation are reported after laparoscopy.[8–11]

ETIOLOGY AND DIAGNOSIS OF HYDROSALPINX

The main causes of hydrosalpinx are pelvic inflammatory disease, previous ectopic pregnancy, endometriosis, previous abdominal operations, and history of peritonitis and tuberculosis. In a series of 219 women with hydrosalpinx, 60 reported at least one termination of pregnancy, 55 had pelvic inflammatory disease, 43 had endometriosis, 32 had previous abdominal or pelvic operations, 5 had secondary location of tubal tuberculosis, and 24 had unknown etiology.[6]

Hydrosalpinx may be diagnosed with hysterosalpingography (HSG), transvaginal ultrasound, hydrosonography, laparoscopy, salpingoscopy, hydrolaparoscopy, chlamydia serology, and MRI HSG. HSG is the most widespread method of detecting hydrosalpinges, it does not need anesthesia, and is easily performed in outpatient setting. HSG findings can be used to stage tubal disease and the appearance of the intraluminal mucosal architecture is a good prognostic factor for a subsequent pregnancy.[12,13] Although hydrosalpinx has a characteristic appearance on HSG, transvaginal ultrasound better evaluates the volume of the dilated tubes while hydrosonography and air-contrast sonohysterography appear to be superior to HSG and comparable to laparoscopic diagnosis.[14,15] Laparoscopy with or without chromopertubation is the gold standard method of diagnosing hydrosalpinx and provides both the certain diagnosis and the treatment at the same time.[16,17] A meta-analysis of all the studies comparing HSG to laparoscopy showed the HSG to have a sensitivity of 65% and specificity of 83% in the diagnosis of tubal obstruction.[18,19]

Salpingoscopy is also an essential part of diagnostic and prognostic evaluation of the tubal mucosa. Although the degree of tubal mucosal damage does not always correlate with that of periadnexal adhesions, it does directly correlate with poor pregnancy outcome.[20-22] The appearance of mucosal folds at HSG, the appearance of tubal wall at laparoscopy, and the degree of distal tubal occlusion are the proposed factors that influence prognosis. When tubes are assessed with this scoring system, intrauterine pregnancies were significantly better for patients with mild-to-moderate damaged tubes as compared to those with severely damaged tubes.[23-25] It was also demonstrated that assessment of tubal mucosa may be the only factor that sufficiently estimates the prognosis.[25] In a prospective study relating tubal lesions to pregnancy outcome in hydrosalpinges, it was reported that thick-walled hydrosalpinges with wall fibrosis exclude intrauterine pregnancies and that among the different lesions of thin-wall hydrosalpinges, mucosal adhesions are the most important factor in determining fertility outcome.[26] New methods, such as transvaginal salpingoscopy and fertiloscopy, may be useful techniques of evaluating fallopian tubes.[27]

POOR IVF OUTCOME IN WOMEN WITH HYDROSALPINX

IVF was first developed as fertility treatment to overcome mechanical obstruction for women without functional fallopian tubes. In patients with hydrosalpinges poor IVF results have been reported compared to women with other tubal factor-related infertility. Hydrosalpinges adversely affect implantation and pregnancy rates and increase the preclinical miscarriages, spontaneous abortions, and ectopic pregnancies.

Strandell et al.[1] reported that women with unilateral or bilateral hydrosalpinges had a significantly lower pregnancy rate than women with tubal disease but without obstruction of tubal distal end. The IVF pregnancy rate was 13% in women with hydrosalpinges and 26% for women without hydrosalpinges. In another study, the pregnancy rate for the hydrosalpinx group was reported to be 6% but it reached 23% when hydrosalpinx was not present.[28] The success rate of IVF was significantly affected in women with hydrosalpinx of inflammatory etiology.[29] One of the biggest retrospective studies that was conducted by Katz et al.[30] included 1,766 cycles. Implantation and pregnancy rates were lower in the patients with hydrosalpinx than in patients with other tubal pathologies. Andersen et al.[2] reported a marked reduction in implantation rate when hydrosalpinges were visible on ultrasound, and they noted IVF pregnancy rates of 22% in cases of hydrosalpinx and 36% in cases with tubal disease of other origin, respectively. The miscarriage rate was 70% in the hydrosalpinx group, compared with 36% in the other group. Vandromme et al.[3] confirmed the findings of the previous authors with pregnancy rate of 10% in women with hydrosalpinx and 23% in women without hydrosalpinx. Freeman et al.[31] reported lower pregnancy rates in the presence of hydrosalpinx compared with diseases of other origin. These authors suggest that hydrosalpinx affects not only the implantation rate but the quality of the ovum as well. Even in nonstimulated cycles the implantation rate of the fertilized ovum was affected.[32] Hydrosalpinges visible on ultrasound may correlate with the decreased pregnancy rate.[33] In another retrospective study Ng et al.[34] reported similar implantation, pregnancy and clinical miscarriage rates in 43 women with hydrosalpinges compared with 101 women without hydrosalpinges. In the same study ectopic pregnancies were reported only in the hydrosalpinx group.

The first meta-analysis on the effect of hydrosalpinges on IVF demonstrated that hydrosalpinges decreased the chance for pregnancy by half when compared to other tubal factor infertility.[35] The implantation rate and the ongoing pregnancy rates were 50% lower in women with hydrosalpinges than in women without hydrosalpinges. On the contrary, the miscarriage rate was doubled. A second meta-analysis confirmed the above results.[36]

FACTORS AFFECTING IMPLANTATION IN THE PRESENCE OF HYDROSALPINX

The exact mechanism through which hydrosalpinx exerts its negative effects is still not clearly understood. Mechanical factors or embryotoxic properties of the hydrosalpinx fluid may play a negative role in implantation, but the most important factor seems to be the disturbance of endometrial receptivity.

Simple mechanical washout of the embryos[37,38] and interference of the fluid interface with apposition of the implanting embryo were suggested mechanisms affecting implantation in the presence of hydrosalpinx.[39,40] The presence of hydrometra proved to be a poor prognostic factor among women with hydrosalpinx undergoing IVF. Endometrial cavity fluid is associated with poor ovarian response and increased cancellation rates in IVF cycles.[41] Hill et al.[42] reported that hydrosalpinx may enlarge during ovarian stimulation protocols for IVF, thereby increasing tubal secretion. Aboulghar et al.[43] observed decreased ovarian response in ovarian stimulation with gonadotrophins, whereas drainage of the hydrosalpinx before IVF ensured a better ovarian response to stimulation. Another hypothesis that could explain the reduced implantation rate in cases with hydrosalpinx is a reflux phenomenon generated by a pressure gradient from tubal fluid accumulation that opposes the cervix-to-fundus intrauterine peristalsis.[44,45]

Mukherjee et al.[46] studied the influence of hydrosalpinx fluid on embryo development using a murine model and showed a concentration-dependent negative correlation between hydrosalpinx fluid and blastocyst development. Five out of eight published studies on mouse embryo culture in hydrosalpinx fluid described embryotoxicity at low concentrations and three studies demonstrated impaired development only in undiluted hydrosalpinx fluid.[47] There are two studies that evaluated the toxic properties of hydrosalpingeal fluid in human embryos and both do not demonstrate any toxic effect on embryo development.[48,49] In Strandell's study,[48] human embryos cultured in 50% expressed the same rate of blastocyst development as in control medium but undiluted hydrosalpinx fluid resulted in 50% reduction in blastocyst development rate as compared with control medium. Granot et al.[49] reported an unchanged blastocyst development rate regardless of hydrosalpinx concentration. It seems that there is no potent embryo toxic factor present, but rather a deficiency or dilution of nutritive substances.[48,50]

The negative effect of hydrosalpinx fluid in endometrial receptivity was reported in various studies. Integrin $a_v\beta_3$ acts both as a receptor for the embryo at the endometrial surface epithelium and a stimulator of trophoblastic penetration and invasion and therefore is a marker of endometrial receptivity during the implantation window in the luteal phase.[51,52] Meyer et al.[53] stated that the expression of integrin $a_v\beta_3$ was downregulated during the implantation period in women with hydrosalpinges. This was described as a possible explanation for IVF failure. Interestingly, after surgical correction of hydrosalpinges, integrin $a_v\beta_3$ expression was increased to normal levels.[53]

Irreversible endometrial damage simultaneously with the acute-phase tubal damage and the release of intrauterine cytokines, prostaglandins, leukotrienes, lymphocytes, and other inflammatory compounds directly to the endometrium or via the lymphatic system are proposed mechanisms by which hydrosalpinx decreases the success rates of implantation.[1,54] Chlamydia antibodies have been linked to the formation of antibodies against heat shock protein (HSP)60 in patients with hydrosalpinges. In these patients decreased pregnancy rates were reported.[55–57]

All the above-mentioned mechanisms may explain the impairment of embryo development in the presence of hydrosalpinx fluid, but it is most likely that the low implantation rate is caused by a mixture of these factors.[58,59]

THE PLACE OF LAPAROSCOPIC SURGICAL MANAGEMENT OF HYDROSALPINX PRIOR TO IVF

One of the first studies to prove that surgical management of the tubes improves pregnancy rates in IVF was performed by Vandromme et al.[3] The authors compared three groups of women with hydrosalpinx, salpingectomy, and normal tubes. The pregnancy rates were 10%, 22%, and 31%, respectively. Kassabji et al.[60] compared 118 patients with hydrosalpinges and 157 patients who underwent salpingectomy and found that the pregnancy rate after IVF was 18% and 31%, respectively. Murray et al.[61] reported IVF pregnancy rate of 8.5% in women with hydrosalpinges and 38.6% in women without hydrosalpinges. Several other authors have suggested to perform salp-ingectomy before IVF treatment to overcome the negative effects of hydrosalpinges on pregnancy, implantation, and miscarriage rates.[53,62–64]

Shelton et al.[65] were the first to conduct a prospective study that demon-strated a positive impact on pregnancy rates in patients with repeated IVF fail-ures by removing the hydrosalpinges. The pregnancy rate rose to 25%. Dechaud et al.[66] performed a prospective randomized trial examining the effect of sur-gical intervention before IVF and showed a positive effect of salpingectomy on implantation rates. There were trends toward increased pregnancy rates per cycle and per embryo transfer in salpingectomized patients as compared with control patients, although the size of the study was small to reach statistical significance. It was the multicenter prospective randomized study of Stran-dell et al.[67] which proved that in patients with bilateral hydrosalpinges, salp-ingectomies significantly improved the implantation rate. In the same study in patients with visible hydrosalpinges on ultrasonographic examination the preg-nancy and delivery rates also improved after salpingectomy (45.7 vs. 22.5% and 40 vs. 17%, respectively). The benefit was major if hydrosalpinx was both bilateral and visible in ultrasound (60 vs. 15.8%; $P = 0.008$).

Johnson et al.[68] in a Cohrane review of all randomized controlled studies state that laparoscopic surgical treatment for hydrosalpinges versus nonsurgi-cal management significantly increased the odds of pregnancy (OR = 1.75, 95% CI 1.07–2.86) and the live birth plus ongoing viable pregnancy (OR = 2.13, 95% CI 1.24–3.65). No significant differences were seen in the odds of implantation per embryo transferred, ectopic pregnancy, miscarriage per preg-nancy, or treatment complications related to pre-IVF intervention. The authors conclude that laparoscopic salpingectomy should be considered for all women with hydrosalpinges due to undergo IVF.[68]

The risk of ovarian function disturbance after salpingectomy is a point of concern.[69] Lass et al.[70] demonstrated a significant reduction in the number of developed follicles and the number of retrieved oocytes from the ovary ipsilateral to which a unilateral salpingectomy was previously performed, al-though there were no differences in total numbers when considering both sides. Other retrospective studies do not show any differences in ovulation stimula-tion variables.[60–63] Whether salpingectomy harms the blood and nerve supply of the ovary, which are important parameters of follicle and hormonal produc-tion, needs further evaluation. In cases of surgical intervention salpingectomy should be performed very close to tube to avoid disturbance of blood flow to the ovary.[71]

Puttemans and Brosens,[72] after a debate, agreed that salpingectomy should be performed only in those tubes with severe, extensive, and inflammatory tubal disease that are without hope of surgical repair. Salpingoscopy should be the first choice for surgical intervention if the hydrosalpinx is thin-walled and free from ampullary adhesions. If the tubal damage is not severe salpingostomy should be the method of choice.

OTHER SURGICAL METHODS

Other surgical, but not so invasive techniques, which have also been proposed before IVF in patients with hydrosalpinx include needle aspiration of the hydrosalpinx fluid before or at the time of oocyte retrieval, cautery, or mechanical occlusion of the tube proximal to the uterus and salpingoplasty.[73,74]

Aboulghar et al.[43] reported that aspiration of the hydrosalpinges fluid before beginning IVF stimulation produced a better ovarian response and a higher number of embryos available for transfer but without pregnancy rate improvement. In another small study an improved pregnancy rate was found in patients that had drainage of the hydrosalpinx immediately following oocyte retrieval.[75] On the contrary, no improvement in pregnancy rate was found following hydrosalpinx drainage in a series of 56 women.[76] These conflicting results do not prove the efficacy of the procedure.

Proximal tubal ligation prior to IVF was evaluated as another treatment option.[61,64] Murray et al.[61] reported pregnancy rates of 39%, 43%, and 60% in salpingectomy, neosalpingostomy, and proximal tubal occlusion groups, respectively. In another study, cautery of the proximal tubal end was performed and the pregnancy rates were higher in this group of patients than in the group of women that had IVF without any treatment.[77] The size of these studies is small to reach statistically significant difference and the method needs further evaluation. Others have reported that the efficacy of laparoscopic proximal occlusion of the affected fallopian tube with bipolar diathermy was equal to laparoscopic salpingectomy, and the response to ovarian stimulation was not altered by either surgical modality.[78] Recently, successful proximal occlusion of hydrosalpinx by hysteroscopic placement of microinert before IVF embryo transfer was reported.[79] The procedure was performed under local anesthesia and intravenous sedation, and whether it might be an alternative to laparoscopic tubal occlusion or salpingectomy will need further studies to be proven.

Reports of pregnancy rates after laparoscopic salpingoplasty showed encouraging results but no prospective randomized trials are at present available.[6,11,80] Operative laparoscopy may be effective for the correction of hydrosalpinges in selected patients. The probability of achieving an intrauterine or an ectopic pregnancy can be predicted based on combinations of significant variables.[81]

The issue whether all hydrosalpinges have to be removed prior to IVF or whether reconstructive surgery and other less invasive methods have priority over salpingectomy still needs further evaluation with prospective randomized trials.

Our own strategy toward patients with hydrosalpinges includes at first an estimation of other infertility factors as well (age of women, ovarian function, male factor) and laparoscopic and salpingoscopic evaluation when possible. If stage I or II hydrosalpinx is diagnosed, salpingostomy at the same time is performed and a period of 18 months is allowed for pregnancy to occur without any further intervention. If hydrosalpinx stage III or IV is diagnosed, salpingectomy is performed followed by IVF. The preliminary results of our ongoing randomized study comparing the IVF outcome in two groups of women with hydrosalpinges are in favor of the salpingectomy prior to IVF group. The pregnancy rates in women with hydrosalpinges who had salpingectomy prior to IVF and in women who did not have salpingectomy prior to IVF are 24.13% and 13.3%, respectively, in a total of 59 women that were included in the study so far.

CONCLUSION

Hydrosalpinx impairs *in vitro* fertilization outcome. Lower implantation and pregnancy rates have been reported in women with hydrosalpinges. Mechanical factors, toxicity of the hydrosalpingeal fluid, and receptivity dysfunction may explain the impaired IVF outcome in the presence of hydrosalpinx. Patients should be counseled about the negative effect of hydrosalpinx on IVF outcome and the available treatment options prior to IVF. Adequate patient selection is the key to finding the best therapeutic approach. IVF and endoscopic tubal surgery must be considered complementary rather than competitive procedures. Laparoscopic surgery has a place in the diagnosis and a positive role in the management of hydrosalpinx as there is strong evidence that laparoscopic salpingectomy should be offered in those women that have bilateral disease or in cases where hydrosalpinges are large enough to be visible on ultrasound. Laparoscopic salpingostomy, laparoscopic or hysteroscopic tubal occlusion, and drainage of hydrosalpinx before or during oocyte retrieval should be evaluated in a randomized manner.

REFERENCES

1. STRANDELL, A., U. WALDERNSTROM, L. NILSSON, *et al*. 1994. Hydrosalpinx reduces *in vitro* fertilisation/embryo transfer pregnancy rates. Hum. Reprod. **9:** 861–863.
2. ANDERSEN, A., Z. YUE, F. MENG, *et al*. 1994. Low implantation rate after *in vitro* fertilisation in patients with hydrosalpinges diagnosed by ultrasonography. Hum. Reprod. **9:** 1935–1938.
3. VANDROMME, J., B. CHASSE, B. LEJEUNE, *et al*. 1995. Hydrosalpinges in *in vitro* fertilisation: an unfavorable prognostic feature. Hum. Reprod. **10:** 576–579.
4. STRANDELL, A., J. THORBURN, L. HAMBERGER. 1999. Risk factors for ectopic pregnancy in assisted reproduction. Fertil. Steril. **71:** 282–286.
5. BOER-MEISEL, M.E., E.R. TE VELDE, J.D.F. HABBEMA & J.W.F.P. KARDAUN. 1986. Predicting the pregnancy outcome in patients treated for hydrosalpinx: a prospective study. Fertil. Steril. **45:** 23–29.
6. BONTIS, J., B.V. TARLATZIS, G. GRIMBIZIS, *et al*. 1996. Microsurgical and laparoscopic management of tubal fertility: report of 763 cases. Middle East Fertil. Soc. J. **1:** 17–29.

7. BONTIS, J. & K. DINAS. 2000. Management of hydrosalpinx: reconstructive surgery or IVF? Ann. N.Y. Acad. Sci. **900:** 260–271.
8. MARANA, R. & J. QUAGLIARELLO. 1988. Distal tubal occlusion: microsurgery versus *in vitro* fertilization. A review. Int. J. Fertil. **33:** 107–115.
9. WINSTON, R.M.L. & R.A. MARGARA. 1991. Microsurgical salpingostomy is not an obsolete procedure. Br. J. Obstet. Gynaecol. **98:** 637–642.
10. TARLATZIS, B.C. & G. GRIMBIZIS. 1997. Tubal factor infertility: treatment in the era of *in vitro* fertilization. Middle East Fertil. Soc. J. **2:** 177–184.
11. MILINGOS, S.D., G.K. KALLIPOLITIS, K.D. LOUTRADIS, *et al.* 2000. Laparoscopic treatment of hydrosalpinx: factors affecting pregnancy rate. J. Am. Assoc. Gynecol. Laparosc. **7:** 355–361.
12. ROCK, J.A., P. KATAYAMA, E.J. MARTIN, *et al.* 1978. Factors influencing the success of salpingostomy techniques for distal fimbrial obstruction. Obstet. Gynecol. **52:** 591–596.
13. DONNEZ, J. & F. CASANAS-ROUX. 1986. Prognostic factors of fimbrial microsurgery. Fertil. Steril. **46:** 1089–1092.
14. JEANTY, P., S. BESNARD, A. ARNOLD, *et al.* 2000. Air-contrast sonohysterography as a first step assessment of tubal patency. J. Ultrasound Med. **19:** 519–527.
15. HOLZ, K., R. BECKER & R. SCHURMANN. 1997. Ultrasound in the investigation of tubal patency. A meta-analysis of three comparative studies of Echovist-200 including 1007 women. Zentralb. Gynakol. **119:** 366–373.
16. KODAMAN, P.H., A. ARICI & E. SELI. 2004. Evidenced-based diagnosis and management of tubal factor infertility. Curr. Opin. Obstet. Gynecol. **16:** 221–229.
17. BERKER, B., A. MAHDAVI, B. SHAHMOHAMADY & C. NEZHAT. 2005. Role of laparoscopic surgery in infertility. Middle East Fertil. Soc. J. **10:** 94–104.
18. SWART, P., B.W.J. MOL, F. VAN DER VEEN, *et al.* 1995. The accuracy of hysterosalpingography in the diagnosis of tubal pathology, a meta-analysis. Fertil. Steril. **64:** 486–491.
19. MOL, B.W.J., P. SWART, P.M.M. BOSSUYT, *et al.* 1996. Reproducibility of the interpretation of hysterosalpingography in the diagnosis of tubal pathology. Hum. Reprod. **11:** 1204–1208.
20. DE BRUYNE, F., P. PUTTEMANS, W. BOECK & I. BROSENS. 1989. The clinical value of salpingoscopy in tubal infertility. Fertil. Steril. **51:** 339–340.
21. MARANA, R., G.F. CATALANO, L. MUZII, *et al.* 1999. The prognostic role of salpingoscopy in laparoscopic tubal surgery. Hum. Reprod. **14:** 2991–2995.
22. MARCHINO, G.L., V. GIGANTE, G. GENNARELLI, *et al.* 2001. Salpingoscopic and laparoscopic investigations in relation to infertility outcomes. J. Am. Assoc. Gynecol. Laparosc. **8:** 218–221.
23. MAGE, G., J. POULY, J. BOUQUET DE JOLINIERE, *et al.* 1984. A preoperative classification to predict the intrauterine and ectopic pregnancy rates after distal tubal microsurgery. Fertil. Steril. **46:** 807–810.
24. CANIS, M., G. MAGE, J. POULY, *et al.* 1991. Laparoscopic distal tuboplasty: report of 87 cases and a 4-year experience. Fertil. Steril. **56:** 616–621.
25. DUBUISSON, J., P. MORICE, C. CHAPRON, *et al.* 1994. Laparoscopic salpingostomy: fertility results according to the tubal mucosal appearance. Hum. Reprod. **9:** 334–339.
26. VASQUEZ, G., W. BOECKX & I. BROSENS. 1995. Prospective study of tubal mucosal lesions and fertility in hydrosalpinges. Hum. Reprod. **10:** 1075–1078.
27. GORTS, S., R. CAMPO, L. ROMBAUTS & I. BROSENS. 1998. Transvaginal salpingoscopy: an office procedure for infertility investigation. Fertil. Steril. **70:** 523–526.

28. VEJTROP, M., K. PETERSEN, A.N. ANDERSEN, et al. 1995. Fertilisation in vitro in the presence of hydrosalpinx and in advanced age. Ugeskr. Laeger **157:** 4131–4134.
29. FLEMING, C. & M.J.R. HULL. 1996. Impaired implantation after in vitro fertilization treatment associated with hydrosalpinx. Br. J. Obstet. Gynaecol. **103:** 268–272.
30. KATZ, E., M.A. AKMAN, M.D. DAMEWOOD, et al. 1996. Deleterious effect of the presence of hydrosalpinx on implantation and pregnancy rates with in vitro fertilisation. Fertil. Steril. **66:** 122–125.
31. FREEMAN, M.R., C.M. WHITWORTH & A.H. GEORGE. 1998. Permanent impairment of embryo development by hydrosalpinges. Hum. Reprod. **13:** 983–986.
32. AKMAN, M.A., J.E. GARCIA, M.D. DAMEWOOD, et al. 1996. Hydrosalpinx affects the implantation of previously cryopreserved embryos. Hum. Reprod. **1:** 1013–1014.
33. DEWIT, W., C.J. GOWRISING, D.J. KUIK, et al. 1998. Only hydrosalpinges visible on ultrasound are associated with reduced implantation and pregnancy rates after in vitro fertilization. Hum. Reprod. **13:** 1696–1701.
34. NG, E.H., W.S. YEUNG & P.C. HO. 1997. The presence of hydrosalpinx may not adversely affect the implantation and pregnancy rates in in vitro fertilization treatment. J. Assist. Reprod. Genet. **14:** 508–512.
35. ZEYNOGLOU, H.B., A. ARICI & D.L. OLIVE. 1998. Adverse effects of hydrosalpinx on pregnancy rates after in vitro fertilization-embryo transfer. Fertil. Steril. **70:** 492–499.
36. CAMUS, E., C. PONCELET, F. GOFFINET, et al. 1999. Pregnancy rates after in vitro fertilization in cases of tubal infertility with or without hydrosalpinx: a meta-analysis of published comparative studies. Hum. Reprod. **14:** 1243–1249.
37. MANSOUR, R.T., M.A. ABOULGAR, G.I. SEROUR, et al. 1991. Fluid accumulation of the uterine cavity before embryo transfer: a possible hindrance for implantation. J. In Vitro Fertil. Embryo Transf. **8:** 157–159.
38. BLOECHLE, M., T.H. SCHREINER & K. LISSE. 1997. Recurrence of hydrosalpinges after transvaginal aspiration of tubal fluid in an IVF cycle with development of serometra. Hum. Reprod. **12:** 703–705.
39. SHARARA, F.I. 1999. What effect does hydrosalpinx have on assisted reproduction? The role of hydrosalpinx in IVF: simply mechanical? Hum. Reprod. **14:** 101–102.
40. ANDERSEN, A.N., A. LINDHARD, A. LOFT, et al. 1996. The infertile patient with hydrosalpinges-IVF with or without salpingectomy? Hum. Reprod. **11:** 2081–2084.
41. LEVI, A.J., J.H. SEGARS, B.T. MILLER & M.P. LEONDIRES. 2001. Endometrial cavity fluid is associated with poor ovarian response and increased cancellation rates in ART cycles. Hum. Reprod. **16:** 2610–2615.
42. HILL, G.A., C.M. HERBERT, A.S. FLEISCER, et al. 1986. Enlargement of hydrosalpinges during ovarian stimulation protocols for in vitro fertilization and embryo replacement. Fertil. Steril. **45:** 883–885.
43. ABOULGHAR, M.A., R.T. MANSOUR, G.I. SESOUR, et al. 1990. Transvaginal ultrasonic needle guided aspiration of pelvic inflammatory masses before ovulation induction for in vitro fertilisation. Fertil. Steril. **53:** 311–314.
44. EYTAN, O., F. AZEM, I. GULL, et al. 2001. The mechanism of hydrosalpinx in embryo implantation. Hum. Reprod. **16:** 2662–2667.
45. IJLAND, M.M., H.J. HOOGLAND & G.A. DUNSELMAN. 1999. Endometrial wave direction switch and the outcome of in vitro fertilization. Fertil. Steril. **71:** 476–481.
46. MUKHERJEE, T., A.B. COPPERMAN, C. MCCAFFREY, et al. 1996. Hydrosalpinx fluid has embryotoxic effects on murine embryogenesis: a case for prophylactic salpingectomy. Fertil. Steril. **66:** 851–853.

47. STRANDELL, A. 2000. The influence of hydrosalpinx on IVF and embryo transfer: a review. Hum. Reprod. Update **6:** 387–395.
48. STRANDELL, A., A. SJOGREN, U. BENTIN-LEY, *et al.* 1998. Hydrosalpinx fluid does not adversely affect the normal development of human embryos and implantation *in vitro.* Hum. Reprod. **13:** 2921–2925.
49. GRANOT, I., N. DEKEL, I. SEGAL, *et al.* 1998. Is hydrosalpinx fluid cytotoxic? Hum. Reprod. **13:** 1620–1624.
50. MURRAY, C.A., H.J. CLARKE, T. TULANDI & S.L. TAN. 1997. Inhibitory effect of human hydrosalpingeal fluid on mouse preimplantation embryonic development is significantly reduced by the addition of lactate. Hum. Reprod. **11:** 2504–2507.
51. BROOKS, P.C., S. STROMBALD, L.C. SANDERS, *et al.* 1996. Localization of matrix metalloproteinase MMP-2 to the surface of invasive cells by interaction with integrin alpha v beta 3. Cell **85:** 683–693.
52. LESSEY, B.A., A.O. ILESANMI, M.A. LESSEY, *et al.* 1996. Luminal and glandular endometrial epithelium express integrins differentially throughout the menstrual cycle: implications for implantation, contraception and infertility. Am. J. Reprod. Immunol. **35:** 195–204.
53. MEYER, W.R., A.J. CASTELBAOUM, S. SOMKUTI, *et al.* 1997. Hydrosalpinges adversely affect markers of endometrial receptivity. Hum. Reprod. **12:** 1393–1398.
54. BEN-RAFAEL, Z. & R. ORVIETO. 1992. Cytokines-involvement in reproduction. Fertil. Steril. **58:** 1093–1099.
55. LA VERDA, D., M.V. KALAYOGLU & G.I. BRYNE. 1999. Chlamydial heat shock proteins and disease pathology: new paradigms for old problem? Infect. Dis. Obstet. Gynecol. **7:** 64–71.
56. WITKIN, S.S., K.M. SULTAN, G.S. NEAL, *et al.* 1994. Unsuspected chlamydia trachomatis infection and *in vitro* fertilization outcome. Am. J. Obstet. Gynecol. **171:** 1208–1214.
57. NEUER, A., S.D. SPANDORFER, P. GIRALDO, *et al.* 2000. The role of heat shock proteins in reproduction. Hum. Reprod. Update **6:** 149–159.
58. AJONUMA, L.C., E.H.Y. NG & H.C. CHAN. 2002. New insights into the mechanisms underlying hydrosalpinx fluid formation and its adverse effect on IVF outcome. Hum. Reprod. Update **8:** 255–264.
59. STRANDELL, A. & A. LINDHARD. 2002. Why does hydrosalpinx reduce fertility? The importance of hydrosalpinx fluid. Hum. Reprod. **17:** 1141–1145.
60. KASSABJI, M., J. SIMS, L. BUTLER & S. MUASHER. 1994. Reduced pregnancy outcome in patients with unilateral or bilateral hydrosalpinx after *in vitro* fertilization. Eur. J. Obstet. Gynaecol. Reprod. Biol. **56:** 129–132.
61. MURRAY, D.L., A.W. SAGOSKIN, E.A. WIDRA, *et al.* 1998. The adverse effect of hydrosalpinges on *in vitro* fertilization pregnancy rates and the benefit of surgical correction. Fertil. Steril. **69:** 41–45.
62. EJDRUP BREDKJAER, H., S. ZIEBE, B. HAMID, *et al.* 1999. Delivery rates after *in vitro* fertilization following bilateral salpingectomy due to hydrosalpinges: a case control study. Hum. Reprod. **14:** 101–105.
63. VERLHURST, G., N. VANDERSTEEN, A.C. VAN STEIRTEGHEM, *et al.* 1994. Bilateral salpingectomy does not compromise ovarian stimulation in an *in vitro* fertilization/embryo transfer programme. Hum. Reprod. **9:** 624–628.
64. SAGOSKIN, A.W., B.A. LESSEY, G.L. MOLTA, *et al.* 2003. Salpingectomy or proximal tubal occlusion of unilateral hydrosalpinx increases the potential for spontaneous pregnancy. Hum. Reprod. **18:** 2634–2637.

65. SHELTON, K.E., L. BUTLER, J.P. TONER, *et al.* 1996. Salpingectomy improves the pregnancy rate *in vitro* fertilisation with hydrosalpinx. Hum. Reprod. **11:** 523–525.
66. DECHAUD, H., J.P. DAURES, F. ARNAL, *et al.* 1998. Does previous salpingectomy improve implantation and pregnancy rates in patients with severe tubal factor infertility who are undergoing *in vitro* fertilisation? A pilot prospective randomized study. Fertil. Steril. **69:** 1020–1025.
67. STRANDELL, A., A. LINDHARD, U. WALDERNSTROM, *et al.* 1999. Hydrosalpinx and IVF outcome: a prospective, randomized multicentre trial in Scandinavia on salpingectomy prior to IVF. Hum. Reprod. **14:** 2762–2769.
68. JOHNSON, N.P., W. MAK & M.C. SOWTER. 2002. Laparoscopic salpingectomy for women with hydrosalpinges enhances the success of IVF: a Cochrane review. Hum. Reprod. **17:** 543–548.
69. DAR, P., G.S. SACHS, D. STRASSBURGER, *et al.* 2000. Ovarian function before and after salpingectomy in artificial technology patients. Hum. Reprod. **15:** 142–144.
70. LASS, A., A. ELLENBOGEN, R.C. CROUCHE, *et al.* 1998. The effect of salpingectomy on ovarian response to superovulation in an *in vitro* fertilization-embryo transfer programme. Fertil. Steril. **70:** 1035–1038.
71. DECHAUD, H. & B. HEDON. 2000. What effect does hydrosalpinx have on assisted reproduction? The role of salpingectomy remains controversial. Hum. Reprod. **15:** 234–235.
72. PUTTEMANS, P. & I.A. BROSENS. 1996. Salpingectomy improves *in vitro* fertilization outcome in patients with hydrosalpinx: blind victimization of the fallopian tube? Hum. Reprod. **11:** 2079–2081.
73. MANSOUR, R., M. ABOULGHAR & G.I. SEROUR. 2000. Controversies in the surgical management of hydrosalpinx. Curr. Opin. Obstet. Gynecol. **12:** 297–301.
74. ZEYNELOGLOU, H.B. 2001. Hydrosalpinx and assisted reproduction: options and rationale for treatment. Curr. Opin. Obstet. Gynecol **13:** 281–286.
75. VAN VOORHIS, B.J., A.E.T. SPARKS, C.H. SYROP, *et al.* 1998. Ultrasound guided aspiration of hydrosalpinges is associated with improved pregnancy and implantation rates after *in vitro* fertilisation cycles. Hum. Reprod. **13:** 736–739.
76. SOWTER, M.C., V.A. AKANDE, J.A. WILLIAMS, *et al.* 1997. Is the outcome of *in vitro* fertilization and embryo transfer treatment improved by spontaneous or surgical drainage of a hydrosalpinx? Hum. Reprod. **12:** 2147–2150.
77. STADTMAUER, L.A., R.M. RIEHL, S.K. TOMA, *et al.* 2000. Cauterisation of hydrosalpinges before *in vitro* fertilization is an effective surgical treatment associated with improved pregnancy rates. Am. J. Obstet. Gynecol. **183:** 367–371.
78. SURREY, E.S. & W.B. SCHOOLCRAFT. 2001. Laparoscopic management of hydrosalpinges before *in vitro* fertilization-embryo transfer: salpingectomy versus proximal tubal occlusion. Fertil. Steril. **75:** 612–617.
79. ROSENFIELD, R.B., R.E. STONES, A. COATES, *et al.* 2005. Proximal occlusion of hydrosalpinx by hysteroscopic placement of microinert before *in vitro* fertilization-embryo transfer. Fertil. Steril. **83:** 1547–1550.
80. AUDEBERT, A.J., J.L. POULY & P. VON THEOBALD. 1998. Laparoscopic fimbrioplasty: an evaluation of 35 cases. Hum. Reprod. **13:** 1496–1499.
81. TAYLOR, R.C., J. BERKOWITZ & P.F. MCCOMB. 2001. Role of laparoscopic salpingectomy in the treatment of hydrosalpinx. Fertil. Steril. **75:** 594–600.

Laparoscopic Management of the Adnexal Mass

GEORGE PADOS, DIMITRIS TSOLAKIDIS, AND JOHN BONTIS

First Department of OB-GYN, Aristotle University of Thessaloniki and "Diavalkaniko" Hospital, Thessaloniki, Greece

ABSTRACT: In the past few years the contribution of operative laparoscopy in all fields of gynecological surgery has been revolutionary.
Nowadays laparoscopic management of adnexal masses is the most frequently performed laparoscopic intervention. Laparoscopy in comparison to laparotomy has the advantages of lower morbidity, shorter length
of hospital stay, decreased postoperative pain, lesser *de novo* adhesion formation, better cosmetic results, faster recovery, and reduced overall cost
of care. However, careful preoperative evaluation is important for the appropriate and successful use of laparoscopy for removal of adnexal masses
and the advantages of the laparoscopic approach should, in no way, compromise the clinical outcome in women with malignancy. Patient's age,
history, findings of physical examination, and the results of serum markers in combination with the imaging assessment, such as Doppler sono-
grapy, CT, or MRI, should be considered to reach the diagnosis preoperatively. However, only pathology of the adnexal mass can provide the
definitive diagnosis. The specific characteristics of the adnexal masses
in childhood, adolescent, reproductive, and postmenopausal age represent the essential parameters that will determine the therapeutic strategy
to be followed. Furthermore, the clinician has to determine whether an
adnexal mass requires surgery or expectant management as well as to
estimate the possibility of malignancy.

KEYWORDS: laparoscopy; adnexal masses; cyst; laparoscopic surgery

INTRODUCTION

In the past few years operative laparoscopy has been applied in almost all
fields of gynecological surgery and nowadays laparoscopic management of
adnexal masses is one of the most frequently performed laparoscopic interventions in gynecology.[1–5] It has been estimated that approximately 5–10% of
women in the United States will undergo a surgical procedure for a suspected
ovarian neoplasm during their lifetime and 13–21% of these women will be

Address for correspondence: George Pados, Mitropoleos 40 Str., 54623, Thessaloniki, Greece. Voice:
+30-2310-263212; fax: +30-2310-241133.
e-mail: padosgyn@hol.gr

Ann. N.Y. Acad. Sci. 1092: 211–228 (2006). © 2006 New York Academy of Sciences.
doi: 10.1196/annals.1365.018

found to suffer from ovarian malignancy.[6] There is growing body of evidence in the literature to support the advantages of laparoscopy over laparotomy, as it is associated with decreased febrile morbidity, less postoperative pain and analgesic requirements, shorter length of hospital stay, less *de novo* adhesion formation, faster recovery, better cosmetic results, and reduced overall cost on the gynecologic health care of women.[7–9] The advances in accurate preoperative diagnosis and in minimally invasive techniques of suspicious adnexal masses have expanded the indications of operative laparoscopy and reduced the unnecessary laparotomies without sacrificing the principles of oncologic surgery in cases of unexpected malignancy.

PREOPERATIVE INVESTIGATION OF ADNEXAL MASSES

Careful patient selection for the appropriate use of laparoscopy in the management of adnexal masses is a critical issue. It is of utmost importance to determine preoperatively whether a patient with an adnexal mass is at a high risk of malignancy taking into consideration the patient's age, menopausal status, family history, symptoms, ultrasonographic features, and level of tumor markers. Nevertheless, even if intraoperative diagnosis based on frozen sections for suspicious adnexal masses is a crucial step for adequate surgical management, only postoperative histology can provide the definite diagnosis.

The age of the patient should always be taken into consideration in the differential diagnosis of adnexal masses, since the incidence of ovarian cancer increases from 15.7/100.000 at the age of 40 years to 54/100.000 at the age of 65 years.[10] Fewer than 5% of all ovarian malignancies occur in children and adolescents. Ovarian tumors account for approximately 1% of all tumors in these age groups. In newborns, under the influence of maternal and placental hormones, small functional cysts less than 2–4 cm can be observed. In children 65% of adnexal masses are functional cysts (follicular or corpus luteum cysts), 28% benign ovarian tumors, and 8% malignant ovarian neoplasms (dysgerminomas and immature teratomas). Dermoid cysts originate from germ cells and represent 65% of benign tumors in this age group.[11] In the reproductive age group, the majority of adnexal masses are benign with malignancy found in only 7% to 13%.[11] Functional cysts remain the most common type of adnexal mass found in this age group and benign cystic teratomas are the most common neoplastic adnexal masses. Of course, ectopic pregnancy, pelvic inflammatory disease, hydrosalpinx, pelvic kidney, and a leiomyoma in the broad ligament should always be included in the differential diagnosis of adnexal masses. In postmenopausal women the risk of malignancy in ovarian neoplasms increases from 8% to 45%.[12]

A family history of ovarian cancer should alert the clinician in the management of adnexal masses of women aged between 35 and 45 years because inherited forms of ovarian cancer represent 5% of all ovarian malignancies.[13]

In this age group, ultrasound screening may be justified and should be commenced at a young age. Women with a first-degree relative with ovarian cancer have a 5% risk of developing it themselves. Furthermore, there is a 30% lifetime risk for women with two affected close relatives.[14]

The majority of adnexal masses are asymptomatic unless they have been subjected to rupture or torsion with acute onset of symptoms, such as pelvic pain. Large adnexal masses represent a common cause of chronic pelvic pain and dyspareunia. Unfortunately, there are no specific symptoms indicative of ovarian mass presence that lead women to seek medical care. Dissemination of ovarian cancer in the peritoneal cavity may be asymptomatic at early stages of disease, until ascites causes abdominal distention. Consequently, only one-third of women with ovarian cancer are diagnosed at an early stage, when the disease is confined to the ovary.[15] Olson *et al.* reported that among 168 cases of ovarian cancer, 93% manifested at least one symptom, compared to 42% of controls. The most common symptoms among these cases were unusual bloating, fullness, and pressure of recent onset compared to control, as well as abdominal or back pain and lack of energy.[16]

Palpation of an asymptomatic adnexal mass during routine pelvic examination is still the most common method for the detection of ovarian neoplasm. Pelvic examination is mandatory to identify an adnexal mass and is greatly facilitated by a rectovaginal examination, which allows better evaluation through deeper penetration of the Douglas pouch.[7] Benign tumors are commonly smooth, cystic, mobile, and unilateral. On the other hand, malignant adnexal masses are usually solid irregular, fixed, accompanied by ascites, and grow with a rapid rate.[17] Women with bilateral neoplasms have a 2.6-fold increased risk of malignancy when compared to women who had unilateral neoplasms.[18] However cul-de-sac nodularity, fixed adnexa, and ascites may also occur with benign adnexal masses, such as endometriosis.

Pelvic ultrasonography remains the first choice modality in the differentiation between benign and malignant adnexal mass because it is inexpensive, noninvasive, and accompanied by excellent diagnostic accuracy. Both transvaginal and transabdominal ultrasound, as complementary examinations, should be performed at the same time, especially in large adnexal masses. Adnexal masses should fit the sonographic criteria listed in TABLE 1 to ensure the increased probability of benign pathology. The sensitivity of transvaginal ultrasound varies between 48–100% and the specificity 65–98%. On the contrary, sensitivity of transabdominal ultrasound varies between 60–93% and the specificity between 42–95%. This discrepancy is related to the operator's experience and what criteria indicative of malignancy have been used.[19] However, the diagnostic accuracy of ultrasound is limited by the cyclic changes caused in ovulating premenopausal women. Granberg *et al.* found malignancy rates for multilocular cysts, defined as cysts with at least one septum, of 8% compared to 0.3% for unilocular cysts.[20] Other studies found that the risk of malignancy in simple cysts, defined as unilocular with smooth inner wall, rises from

TABLE 1. Ultrasonographic evaluation of adnexal masses

	Benign	Suspicious
Size	≤5 cm	>10 cm
	<10 cm	>10 cm
Septum thickness	≤3 mm	>3 mm
Cyst wall thickness	≤3 mm	≥ 3mm
Papillary excrescences height	≤3 mm	>3 mm
Solid part	Absent	Present
Free fluid	Absent	Present
Doppler RI	>0.42	<0.42
Doppler PI	>1	<1

0.8% in premenopausal women to 9.6% in postmenopausal women.[21,22] Bailey *et al.* found in 7,705 asymptomatic postmenopausal women 256 unilocular cysts, all of which were < 10 cm in diameter, and 90% were < 5 cm and were associated with minimal risk for ovarian cancer.[23] Solid parts, semi-solid, and mixed tumors seem to be malignant in 2–17% in premenopausal and 66–74% in postmenopausal women.[24] The risk for malignancy in unilocular cysts with papillary formations or solid parts rises from 2.1% in premenopausal to 10% in postmenopausal.[25] In a prospective study the positive predictive value of the sonographic evidence of malignancy was 73%, whereas benign tumors were predicted correctly in 95.6%.[26] In other words, ultrasonography is more accurate in predicting which masses are benign than which ones are malignant. The presence of papillary excrescence into the cyst cavity defined as a solid tissue projection 1–15 mm in height or 1–10 mm in width into the cyst cavity from the cyst wall is the most frequent sonographic feature in 48–63% of borderline ovarian masses. On the other hand, it should not be considered a highly sensitive sonographic marker as it may be found positive in 4% of benign as well as in 4% of invasive tumors.[27]

There is no consensus among investigators about the sensitivity and specificity of Doppler ultrasound in the assessment of vascularity of adnexal masses because it varies from 50% to 100%.[28] It has been reported that 82.7% of benign adnexal masses may have peripherally and pericystically located vessels, which originate from host vessels with resistance and pulsatility index moderate to high (RI > 0.42 and PI > 1, respectively). On the contrary, malignant adnexal masses usually have centrally located vessels, which lack smooth muscle in their walls with low resistance and pulsatility index (RI < 0.42 and PI < 1, respectively).[29] In 1994, a review of 14 published studies about the usefulness of color Doppler in the evaluation and discrimination between benign and malignant adnexal masses concluded that 51% of the studies were in favor, 19% against, and 30% found its usefulness limited in the assessment of adnexal masses.[30] These discrepant results are due to the lack of standard criteria and varying threshold values. The color Doppler indexes have a lower specificity and sensitivity in premenopausal women (63% and 80%, respectively) due to physiologic alterations of ovarian vascularity in different phases of the menstrual cycle. On the contrary, in postmenopausal women the sensitivity of color Doppler was 93% and the specificity 88%.[31] Of course, benign conditions, such as acute inflammatory adnexal disease and endometriosis, are associated with increased neovascularization with low blood vessel resistance mimicking malignancy. The application of color Doppler in venous flow in the differentiation of malignant from benign adnexal lesions is being investigated with promising results. Venous flow velocity was found significantly higher in malignant than in benign masses (18.1 cm/sec vs. 8.9 cm/sec, $P = 0.0006$). Sensitivity, specificity, and positive and negative predictive value for the combination of both arterial and venous Doppler were 88%, 91%, 79%, and 95%, respectively.[32]

More recently 3D power Doppler depicts the morphology of tumor vessels and with the use of contrast-enhanced imaging, it reaches sensitivity and specificity values of 100% and 93.3%, respectively. The positive and negative predictive value of this method was found 85.7% and 100%, respectively reaching diagnostic accuracy of 95.6% in discriminating benign from malignant adnexal lesions.[33]

It is proved that MRI allows better evaluation of internal architecture of adnexal masses because it can distinguish the fibrinous debris, adherent clot, or fat in the cyst wall, which mimicks the appearance of papillary projections. Several studies have proved that MRI is superior to CT and Doppler ultrasound in diagnosis of malignant ovarian masses, as it has a sensitivity of 98% and a specificity of 88%.[34] In addition, the gadolinium-enhanced MRI increased the sensitivity to 100% and specificity to 98%, achieving an accuracy of 99%.[35] However, the high cost of MR imaging is a disadvantage of applying this diagnostic modality in the evaluation of all adnexal masses. It seems that MRI has an important value in most sonographically indeterminate lesions to distinguish benign from malignant adnexal masses.[36]

CA-125 is the most often used tumor marker to differentiate benign from malignant neoplasms, but using 35 U/mL as the upper limit of normal range, the sensitivity and false-positive rate of the CA-125 range between 50–83% and 14–36%, respectively.[24] Bast *et al.* reported that only 1% of 888 apparently healthy women and 6% of 143 patients with nonmalignant disease had serum CA-125 levels above 35 U/mL.[37] In symptomatic premenopausal women, a CA-125 measurement has not been shown to be useful in most circumstances because elevated levels of CA-125 are associated with a variety of common benign conditions, including uterine leiomyomata, pelvic inflammatory disease, endometriosis, adenomyosis, pregnancy, and even menstruation. However, a normal CA-125 measurement alone does not rule out ovarian cancer because up to 50% of early stage cancers and 20–25% of advanced cancers are associated with normal values. The sensitivity of the CA-125 serum concentration test at a cut-off level of 65 IU/mL was 72.7%, the specificity 90.2%, the positive predictive value 90.7%, and the negative predictive value 71.6%. In other words, the sensitivity is low at both cutoff levels, but the specificity is higher at the cutoff level of 65 IU/mL and in those patients only a few unnecessary tests and interventions can be undertaken.[38]

Sassone *et al.*, in an attempt to maximize the discrimination between benign and malignant adnexal masses, proposed a scoring system based on morphologic criteria (papillary protrusions, solid parts, thick septa, wall thickness, and echogenicity), many of which are given a numeric value to produce a summated score. A score > 8/15 indicates that a malignancy is likely and when this score is used as a cutoff value, the sensitivity, specificity, and positive and negative predictive value are 100%, 83%, 37%, and 100%, respectively.[39] Later, Ferrazzi *et al.* developed a "multicenter" scoring systems to identify malignant adnexal masses and prospectively compared it with four previously reported scoring systems of Grandeber, Sassone, De Priest, and Lerner. The area under the receiver operating characteristic (ROC) curve for the multicenter score was 0.84 and this was significantly better than the areas of the other four scoring systems. It seems that 9 is the best cutoff value of Ferrazzi's multicenter scoring system, achieving a sensitivity of 87%, specificity of 67%, and diagnostic accuracy of 72%. This scoring system improved the specificity because it allowed correction for typical dermoid cysts and enhemorrhagic corpora lutea. By lowering the cutoff value from 9 to 8 for lesions ≤ 5 cm the sensitivity rose to 93% and the specificity fell to 56%.[40] Berlanda *et al.* evaluated masses as low, moderate, and high risk according to Ferrazzi's sonographic morphological score taking into consideration additional risk factors, such as ascites, diameter ≥ 10 cm, bilaterality, immobility, resistance index ≤ 0.6, and serum level of CA-125 > 35 IU/mL. Masses with abnormal morphological score and any of these additional risk factors were considered as high risk and treated by laparotomy. The accuracy of this new algorithm was better than the sonographic morphological score alone with a sensitivity of 90%, specificity 97%, positive predictive value of 82%, and negative predictive value of 99%. This approach allowed treatment of 96% of benign adnexal masses by laparoscopy without mismanagement of any cases of ovarian cancer.[41] Poznan index is a newly created ultrasonographic scale and it was proved to be superior to other applied morphological indices. Employing score 8 as the cutoff level, the new index has a specificity of 77% and sensitivity of 86% with a negative and positive predictive value of 90.7% and 69.1%, respectively, achieving a diagnostic accuracy of 80.6%.[42] It was found retrospectively that the combination of Sassone's scoring system (4–8) in benign range and serum CA-125 with a cutoff level 65 IU/mL can distinguish malignant from benign adnexal masses 3–10 cm in postmenopausal women. Employing this algorithm Lee *et al.* accurately predicted benign cystic masses. Subsequently, operative laparoscopy was proven a safe procedure in 99.5% of cases with failure in only one patient who had a borderline ovarian malignancy.[43] According to the latest prospective multicenter study of assessing the diagnostic accuracy of transvaginal sonographic examination in the differentiation of small, < 5 cm adnexal masses, by simple descriptive sonographic scoring, the sensitivity was 92% and the specificity 76.9% with a score 8 or higher. This study concluded that morphologic scoring systems may overcome the subjectivity of interpretation of morphologic characteristics in small masses and at the same time it can incorporate criteria to avoid simplistic description of a complex mass.[44]

In many hospitals the risk malignancy index (RMI) is employed, simply calculated by multiplying the serum CA-125 level, the menopausal status (1 if premenopausal and 3 if postmenopausal), and the ultrasound scan result (expressed as a score of 0 for ultrasound score of 0, 1 for ultrasound score of 1, and 3 for ultrasound score of 2–5). Ultrasound scans are given 1 point for each of the following characteristics: multilocular cyst, evidence of solid areas, evidence of metastases, and presence of ascites and bilateral lesions. Using a cutoff level of 200, the sensitivity was 70.6–85% and the specificity was 89.3–97% for the discrimination of malignant from benign lesions. High-risk patients are referred to cancer units with specialized oncologists, as the best prognosis for women with ovarian cancer is given when a laparotomy and full staging procedure is carried out by a trained gynecological oncologist.[45,46] However, none of the above available modalities can offer 100% specificity and sensitivity in differentiation between malignant from benign adnexal masses, but help to minimize the incidence of unsuspected malignancy at laparoscopy to 0.04% (TABLE 2).[47–58]

Laparoscopic Approach of Adnexal Masses in Childhood and Adolescent Age

Although the application of operative laparoscopy is more frequent in recent years, this increase is confined to postmenarchal young women, on whom

TABLE 2. Unsuspected borderline and malignant tumors during laparoscopic management of adnexal masses

Authors	Year	Patients–Cysts	Borderline (B) Cancer (Ca)	Percentage (%)
Lehmann *et al.*	1991	969/1,016	36 (Ca + B)	2.0
Nezhat *et al.*	1992	1,011/1,209	4Ca	0.04
Cristalli *et al.*	1992	100	3B	3.0
Canis *et al.*	1992	652	6Ca + 4B	1.8
Audebert	1994	700	17Ca + 8B	3.57
Nicoloso *et al.*	1995	5,307	60B + 18Ca	1.47
Wallwiener *et al.*	1996	100	2B + 1Ca	3.0
Sadik *et al.*	1996	220	1B + 1Ca	0.9
Guglielmina	1997	803	9Ca + 25B	4.2
Malik *et al.*	1998	292/316	11 (Ca + B)	3.5
Mettler *et al.*	2005	493	4Ca + 2B	1.2
Pados *et al.*	2005	655/972	5B	0.5

gynecologists are more likely to operate. The malignancy potential of lesions in this age group is rare in comparison to younger premenarchal patients.

Patients older than 15 years are more likely to have benign adnexal masses than younger patients. Occasionally, these masses may undergo torsion due to their volume, shape, or elongation of ovarian ligament. Abdominal pain and palpable mass with abdominal distention and vomiting are usually the presenting symptoms in these patients.

Functional cysts will resolve or decrease in size in 70% usually in 2–8 weeks. Unilocular cysts can be serous cystadenomas, which do not resolve and need laparoscopic cystectomy and not oophorectomy, as child bearing is an important consideration in these young patients.

In twisted ischemic functional or benign cysts with persistent pain, laparoscopic detorsion with cystectomy seems to be an effective adnexa-sparing approach in place of traditional salpingoophorectomy, without any risk of thromboembolism, when the diagnosis of torsion is not delayed. This conservative approach is safe with minimal postoperative morbidity and quick recovery of normal ovarian function.[59]

Other nonneoplastic adnexal masses in adolescents that may need laparoscopic intervention include endometriomas, tuboovarian abscesses, and ectopic pregnancies.

Laparoscopic Approach of Adnexal Masses in Reproductive Age

In reproductive age, functional cysts remain the most common adnexal masses, which are usually, smaller than 10 cm with a normal CA-125 value. Usually, they resolve in 73% spontaneously, with or without the suppressive effect of oral contraceptives, in 4–6 weeks.[60] Persistence, increase of the unilocular mobile anechoic mass, torsion, recurrence after aspiration of its content, or presence of symptoms calls for laparoscopic evaluation and cystectomy. In large unilocular thin-walled cysts with diameter > 10 cm, after drainage of the serous content of the cyst, its capsule is removed. Sometimes when the aspirated fluid is suspicious, it is sent for cytology and the inner cyst wall is inspected. This procedure is called cystoscopy. If any sign of malignancy is present, a frozen section is requested.[5]

Corpus luteum cysts may mimic complex adnexal masses, but proper clinical, laboratory, and ultrasound with Doppler assessment prevent unnecessary laparoscopic explorations. Usually, after a 4-week follow-up period, corpus luteum cysts decrease in size or disappear. In case of rupture causing hemodynamic instability, laparoscopic control of hemorrhage with the use of bipolar diathermy is the treatment of choice.

Dermoid cysts or benign cystic teratomas are the most common neoplastic adnexal masses in reproductive age, which are bilateral in 15–25% of cases. The incidence of malignancy associated with ovarian teratomas is 1–3%.[61]

Furthermore, the incidence of torsion of dermoid cyst is as high as 12–16%, while the tumor may rupture occasionally, resulting in acute peritonitis. The first step of laparoscopic management of any adnexal mass is purely diagnostic. Inspection of the abdominal cavity and the cyst's surface is mandatory to identify suspicious lesions that are biopsied for frozen section. Of course, any free fluid in the pouch of Douglas or peritoneal washings is sent, if necessary, for cytological examination. The next step of laparoscopic management of dermoid cysts depends on its size. If the diameter of the dermoid cyst is smaller than 5 cm, it can be removed intact without rupture and spillage of its content with the use of endoscopic bag or via colpotomy. In case of a dermoid cyst larger than 5 cm, it is better to aspirate its sebaceous content through a small opening on its surface and to flash it copiously. Then the capsule of the cyst is hydrodissected from the surrounding normal ovarian tissue and is extracted from the abdomen with the use of an endoscopic bag via 12 mm trocar or with the use of a morcellator instrument. Furthermore, aspiration of the cyst content may also be done inside the bag, preventing spillage into the peritoneal cavity. Finally, the abdominal cavity is rinsed with abundant lactated Ringer solution (4–6 L) to remove all debris from the peritoneal cavity to prevent chemical peritonitis, granulomas, extensive adhesions, or fistula formation. The ovarian edges are approximated by superficially lasering or low power bipolar coagulation. The fewer sutures applied, the fewer adhesions are formed.[62–64]

Ovarian endometriomas are often associated with endometriotic implants in other areas of the pelvic cavity. They may or may not be symptomatic and their size varies from 2 cm to 10 cm. Endometriomas less than 2 cm are biopsed to confirm the diagnosis and coagulated, vaporized, or excised completely. When their diameter is 3–5 cm, the ovary is opened at the invagination site after adhesiolysis and resection of the fibrotic ring. After aspiration of its chocolate content, the cyst and the abdominal cavity are subsequently flushed abundantly with sterile saline until the fluid becomes clear using the suction irrigator device. If the pseudocapsule of the endometrioma is distinguished from the surrounding normal ovarian tissue it is stripped completely and is sent for complete histologic examination. Sometimes, usually after the preoperative administration of GnRH-analog, the capsule is adhered by fibrotic tissue to the surrounding ovarian cortex. So stripping as well as hydrodissection are not feasible because of the absence of cleavage plane. In these cases, bipolar coagulation or laser CO_2 vaporization of the inner lining of the cyst pseudocapsule and the superficial endometriotic lesions are performed instead of stripping, thus causing minimal damage to the ovarian cortex.[63,65]

In large endometriomas exceeding 5 cm in diameter, the stripping technique can take longer due to hemorrhage especially in the hilar region and difficulty in slight reapproximation of the ovarian edges. Complete removal of these large cysts results in sacrificing normal ovarian cortex tissue with follicles and postoperative adhesion formation affecting woman's reproductive potential. Donnez proposed the two-staged procedure with a recurrence rate of 8%.[10] The initial step involves drainage of the large endometrioma, followed by a 12-week course of GnRH-analog. Then the patients undergo a second laparoscopy to vaporize the capsule wall with CO_2 laser. No tissue should be left in the peritoneal cavity or within the abdominal wall because of the risk of implantation that can cause ovarian remnant syndrome, endometriosis, or metastasis in case of malignancy at the site of trocar.

Most adnexal masses are benign, with malignancy found in only 7–13% of premenopausal women.[12] Any adnexal mass less than 8–10 cm with solid content should be considered suspicious and laparoscopy is used initially only for inspection of the abdominal cavity (ovaries, omentum, peritoneum, stomach, diaphragm, and liver) and peritoneal cytology. If there are no signs of extraovarian dissemination, which of course would require immediate midline laparotomy, laparoscopic adnexectomy can be carried out. In this case, adnexa should be extracted intact in an endoscopic bag. Then a frozen section will indicate if midline laparotomy is necessary during the same procedure provided the patient has signed an informed consent for an immediate radical surgery or later within 7 days.[66] Fibroadenomas are most common benign solid masses in this age group and tend to be unilateral. Ascites and a right hydrothorax (Meigs syndrome) can be associated with this ovarian mass and resolve with its removal.

LAPAROSCOPIC APPROACH OF ADNEXAL MASSES IN POSTMENOPAUSAL AGE

In postmenopausal women the incidence of malignant adnexal masses is 8–45%.[12] The finding of an adnexal mass in a postmenopausal woman needs careful evaluation and the gynecologist has to exclude malignancy. According to the "risk malignancy index" patients are divided in low (< 25), moderate (25–250), and high risk (> 250) of malignancy. By employing a cutoff point of 250, a sensitivity of 70% and a specificity of 90% can be achieved.[62]

Patients with unilocular, unilateral, thin-walled cysts smaller than 3–5 cm without ascites, with no solid component and a normal serum CA-125 value, should be considered at low risk. The risk of malignancy in such patients is less than 1%. Conservative management can be applied in this situation. After 1-year follow-ups at 4-month intervals with serial ultrasounds, laparoscopic management is indicated if the cyst will not resolve. Following this strategy we avoid unnecessary operations, because 50% of these simple cysts will resolve spontaneously. In these selected postmenopausal patients, after inspection of the pelvis and the upper abdomen, intraoperative evaluation includes peritoneal washings and possible frozen section from suspected extraovarian areas. If there is no indication of malignancy, the gynecologist proceeds to bilateral oophorectomy with removal of the ovaries intact in a bag without cyst rupture into the peritoneal cavity. Frozen sections of both ovaries are sent to search for an early carcinoma that may escape gross detection. If malignancy is detected, immediate surgical staging by a midline laparotomy should be performed.[24] Otherwise, the woman is referred to a cancer center for further management as soon as possible. At laparotomy the staging procedure and treatment of ovarian cancer should include cytology of peritoneal washings or ascites, biopsies from adhesions and suspicious areas, total abdominal hysterectomy with bilateral oophorectomy, and infracolic omentectomy as well as selective pelvic and paraaortic lymphadenectomy.[19]

In few selective cancer centers, laparoscopic management of highly suspicious adnexal masses is attempted by surgeons trained in advanced laparoscopic techniques. This approach seems to be safe and effective with less morbidity compared to open techniques.

THE SIGNIFICANCE OF RUPTURE OF THE OVARIAN CAPSULE

Another critical issue is the worsening of prognosis after inadvertent laparoscopic management due to spillage of the content of an unsuspected ovarian cancer. In the absence of prospective clinical trials, the prognostic value of intraoperative rupture of cysts in stage Ia ovarian cancer is a controversial topic.[67–69] According to multivariate analysis of a large in size but retrospective international study in 1,545 patients from six different countries with epithelial ovarian cancer stage I, the degree of differentiation, rupture before surgery, rupture during surgery, International Federation of Obstetricians-Gynecologists (FIGO) stage, and age were strong and independent powerful prognostic variables of disease-free survival.[67] However, this study was criticized for its weak points, which included the fact that the study was retrospective, the endoscopists did not follow the same steps during laparoscopic surgery, and routine peritoneal washings and scraping of the diaphragm as well as pelvic lymphadenectomy were done in only 277 of 1,545 patients. These data were essential to assess the prognostic value of cyst rupture during surgery.[70] Furthermore, it was not possible from surgical reports to distinguish between accidental intraoperative rupture and leakage due to needle aspiration intraoperatively. Finally, in the presence of dense adhesions, all adjacent organs were not routinely biopsied, except in cases of an invasion.[71] All these notifications justified the fact that 20–30% of patients with malignant adnexal masses, managed by laparoscopy or laparotomy, were upstaged due to inadequate staging procedures.[72,73] Laparoscopic staging in early ovarian cancer should involve one- or two-sided salpingoophorectomy with laparoscopic-assisted vaginal hysterectomy, infrarenal lymphadenectomy, complete resection of infundibu-lopelvic ligament, appendectomy, and partial omentectomy.[74]

However, the issue of laparoscopy safety has not yet been established. It was found that abdominal wall wound metastases in rats were more frequent during laparoscopy in comparison to laparotomy. Furthermore, a negative effect although not significant, was noticed in the survival rates of patients, who developed wound metastases after laparoscopic management of unsuspected malignant adnexal masses. But this occurred only in stages III and IV cases with ascites and it was possibly related to the biology of tumor rather than to the previous laparoscopic procedure.[75] Canis et al. in 1,600 patients with laparoscopically treated adnexal masses, reported 32 invasive cancers and 34 borderline tumors.[71] Only 16 of the invasive adnexal masses were stage I and most of them were suspected without puncture as a result of extracystic signs of malignancy, although the risk of preoperative rupture of a stage Ia tumor is fairly low.

To reduce the unnecessary laparotomies for suspicious but benign adnexal masses according to preoperative evaluation, Canis suggested the following algorithm, despite the absence of prospective studies.[71] Preoperative evaluation of adnexal masses is accomplished by using ultrasonography, Doppler, and tumor markers, while MRI should be applied only in the suspicious ones, since it provides additional information about the specific characteristics of the tumor. Then the adnexal masses diagnosed as benign at ultrasound can be managed effectively laparoscopically in any gynecologic department. The remaining suspicious masses can be managed laparoscopically, only by experienced laparoscopic surgeons, thus resulting in 40% reduction of laparotomies for benign adnexal masses according to permanent histological results. After careful inspection of the upper abdomen, ovaries, and peritoneum, peritoneal washings are obtained for immediate cytologic examination. In low suspicious masses, especially in young women less than 40 years old, puncture followed by endocystic examination is performed with the use of a strong aspiration system and meticulous peritoneal lavage to minimize spillage. Then any suspicious mass is sent for frozen section. By this approach, the ultrasound suspicious masses from 35.6% were reduced to 12.1% at diagnostic laparoscopy. In women with highly suspicious adnexal masses, laparoscopic adnexectomy without puncture is performed. Adnexal mass is extracted in an endoscopic bag to prevent spillage into the peritoneal cavity. In the case of malignant masses, immediate staging procedure is performed by laparoscopy whenever possible if the frozen section confirms the laparoscopic diagnosis.[71] A restaging procedure is planned within 1–3 weeks after laparoscopy, if permanent section establishes the diagnosis of malignancy later, because frozen section might give false-negative results due to inadequate sampling. In TABLE 3 the protocol of laparoscopic management of adnexal masses followed in our department is depicted. By following this approach, there is a trend to limit laparotomies to the suspicious adnexal masses at laparoscopy.

TABLE 3. Laparoscopic management of adnexal mass in our department

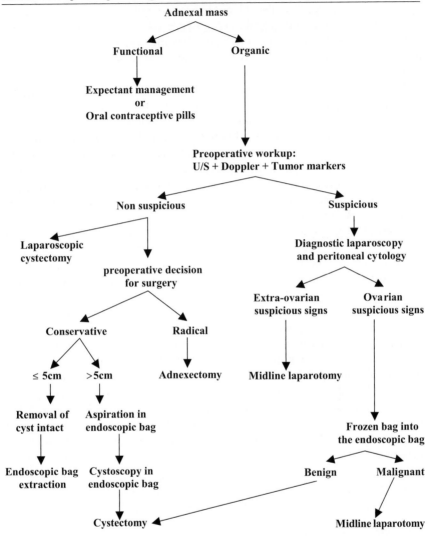

LAPAROSCOPIC MANAGEMENT OF ADNEXAL MASSES IN PREGNANCY

The "technological boom" of operative laparoscopy and also the adequate experience and training gained have revolutionized the surgical approach to many conditions previously considered indications for traditional laparotomy. Laparoscopy has not been widely used in pregnancy, especially after the first trimester, and this is probably due to the limited surgical field at the time of operation, risk of injury to the enlarged uterus, possible impact of teratogenic anesthetic drugs on fetal growth, and possible risk of fetal loss.[76] Also, the potential risk of decreased uterine blood flow due to increased intraabdominal pressure and the possible threat of carbon dioxide to the fetus should be considered.

The most commonly reported laparoscopic intervention during the first trimester of pregnancy is cholecystectomy, while other procedures include diagnosis and management of extrauterine pregnancy and appendicitis, as well as management of the adnexal mass. In this case, the indications are symptomatic adnexal mass, acute abdomen due to torsion or rupture of ovarian cyst, and sonographically abnormal adnexal mass. Most of these interventions are considered for laparoscopy mainly during the first trimester of pregnancy, while the second and third trimesters have been considered a relative contraindication for endoscopic surgery.[77]

To avoid perforation of the enlarged uterus it is advised to insert the Verres needle and the trocars through the upper left quadrant of the abdominal wall, or the open technique as described by Hasson.[78] Increase of the visibility of the otherwise limited surgical field can be obtained by rotation of the operative table toward the opposite direction of the lesion. The theoretic problem of fetal hypercarbia due to absorption of CO_2 may be overcome by the use of gasless laparoscopy, although in this case the visibility is further worsened. Postoperatively patients are treated with a tocolytic agent intravenously for 24 h to avoid uterine contractions and preterm labor, although it seems that the possible impact of increased intraabdominal pressure due to insufflation of CO_2 is outweighed by the reduction of intraoperative uterine manipulations.

It has been shown[79,80] that laparoscopic management of adnexal mass can be performed safely during pregnancy, even in the second and third trimesters, although more studies are needed to draw conclusions on its safety and exact complication rates.

CONCLUSION

Laparoscopic management of the adnexal mass offers the potential for safe and effective minimal invasive surgery. Proper preoperative evaluation, and adequate training and experience of the laparoscopist are the most crucial parameters, which will determine the long-term success of the endoscopic approach. Adequate intraoperative assessment and reasonable use of rapid frozen section are also important for optimal clinical outcome. Finally, well-designed research must continue to evaluate the eventual role of treating adnexal masses by laparoscopy and especially the potential harm caused by dissemination due to inadvertent management of ovarian cancer. In this case, sound surgical and oncological principles must always be applied.

REFERENCES

1. MAIS, V. *et al.* 1995. Treatment of nonendometriotic benign adnexal cysts: a randomised comparison of laparoscopy and laparotomy. Obstet. Gynecol. **86:** 770–774.
2. YUEN, P.M. *et al.* 1997. A randomised prospective study of laparoscopy and laparotomy in the management of benign ovarian masses. Am. J. Obstet. Gynecol. **177:** 109–113.
3. PADOS, G. *et al.* 1997. Video-laparoscopic treatment of adnexal masses in women of reproductive age: analysis of 116 cases. Hellen. Obstet. Gynecol. **9:** 137–142.
4. YINKA, O. *et al.* 2002. Asymptomatic postmenopausal simple ovarian cyst. Obstet Gynecol. Survey **12:** 803–809.
5. PETERSON, H.B., J.F. HULKA & J.M. PHILLIPS. 1990. American Association of Gynecologic Laparoscopists' 1988 membership survey on operative laparoscopy. J. Reprod. Med. **35:** 587–589.
6. PEJOVIC, T. & F. NEZHAT. 2001. Laparoscopic management of adnexal masses the opportunities and the risks. Ann. N.Y. Acad. Sci. **943:** 255–268.
7. MEDEIROS, L.R. *et al.* 2005. Laparoscopy versus laparotomy for benign ovarian tumours. Cochrane Database Syst. Rev. **20**(3): CD004751.
8. PADOS, G. & P. DEVROEY. 1992. Adhesions. Curr. Opin. Obstet. Gynecol. **4:** 412–418.
9. DECKARDT, R. *et al.* 1994. Comparison of minimally invasive surgery and laparotomy in the treatment of adnexal masses. J. Am. Assoc. Gynecol. Laparosc. **1:** 338–339.
10. DONNEZ, J. *et al.* 1996. Large ovarian endometriomas. Hum. Reprod. **11**(3): 641–646.
11. DISAIA, P.J. & W.T. CREASMAN. 1997. The adnexal mass and early ovarian cancer. *In* Clinical Gynecologic Oncology. Fifth edition. 253–281. Mosby. St. Louis.
12. MAHDAVI, A. *et al.* 2004. Laparoscopic management of ovarian cysts. *In* Obstetrics and Gynecological Clinics of North America. Vol. 31: 581–592. Elsevier Saunders. Philadelphia.
13. LYNCH, H.T. *et al.* 1982. Surveillance and management of patients at high genetic risk for ovarian carcinoma. Obstet. Gynecol. **59:** 589–596.
14. WEBB, M. 1993. Screening for ovarian cancer. Still a long way to go. Br. Med. Centre **306:** 1015–1016.
15. BENEDET, J.L. *et al.* 2000. FIGO staging classifications and clinical practice guidelines in the management of gynecologic cancers. FIGO Committee on Gynecologic Oncology. Int. J. Gynaecol. Obstet. **70:** 209–262.
16. OLSON, S.H. *et al.* 2001. Symptoms of ovarian cancer. Obstet. Gynecol. **98:** 212–217.
17. PAULA, J.A.H. 2002. Benign diseases of the female reproductive tract: symptoms and signs. *In* Novak's Gynecology. Thirteenth edition. S.B. Jonathan, Ed.: 351–420. Lippincott Williams & Wilkins. Philadelphia.
18. KOONINGS, P.P. *et al.* 1990. Bilateral ovarian neoplasms and the risk of malignancy. Am. J. Obstet. Gynecol. **162:** 167–169.
19. CHAPRON, C. *et al.* 1996. Diagnosis and management of organic ovarian cysts: indications and procedures for laparoscopy. Hum. Reprod. Update **2:** 435–446.
20. GRANBERG, S., M.WIKLAND, & I.JANSSON. 1989. Macroscopic characterization of ovarian tumours and the relation to the histological diagnosis: criteria to be used for ultrasound evaluation. Gynecol. Oncol. **35:** 139–144.

21. OSMERS, R.G. *et al*. 1996. Preoperative evaluation of ovarian tumors in the premenopause by transvaginosonography. Am. J. Obstet. Gynecol. **175:** 428–434.
22. OSMERS, R.G. *et al*. 1998. Evaluation of ovarian tumors in postmenopausal women by transvaginal sonography. Eur. J. Obstet. Gynecol. Reprod. Biol. **77:** 81–88.
23. BAILEY, C.L. *et al*. 1998. The malignant potential of small cystic ovarian tumours in women over 50 years of age. Gynecol. Oncol. **69:** 3–7.
24. KNUDSEN, U.L. *et al*. 2004. Management of ovarian cysts. Acta Obstet. Gynecol. Scand. **83:** 1012–1021.
25. EKERHOVD, E. *et al*. 2001. Preoperative assessment of unilocular adnexal cysts by transvaginal ultrasonography: a comparison between ultrasonographic morphologic imaging and histopathologic diagnosis. Am. J. Obstet. Gynecol. **184:** 48–54.
26. HERRMANN, U.J., JR., G.W. LOCHER, & A., GOLDHIRSCH. 1987. Sonographic patterns of ovarian tumors: prediction of malignancy. Obstet. Gynecol. **69:** 777–781.
27. EXACOUSTOS, C. *et al*. 2004. Preoperative sonographic features of borderline ovarian tumors. Ultrasound Obstet. Gynecol. **25:** 50–59.
28. YONG-YEON, J. *et al*. 2000. Imaging evaluation of ovarian masses. Radiographics **20:** 1445–1470.
29. KURJAK, A. *et al*. 1998. Malignant adnexal masses. *In* Doppler Ultrasound in Gynecology. A. Kurjak & A.C. Fleischer, Eds.: 47–60. The Parthenon Publishing Group. Lancashire, UK.
30. KURJAK, A., I. BEKAVAC, & S. KUPESIC. 2003. Color Doppler in Adnexal Masses. *In* Textbook of Ultrasound in Obstetrics and Gynecology. A. Kurjak & F.A. Chervenak, Eds.: 639–657. Parthenon Publishing. Lancashire, UK.
31. RELES, A., U. WEIN, & W. LICHTENEGGER. 1997. Transvaginal color Doppler sonography and conventional sonography in the preoperative assessment of adnexal masses. J. Clin. Ultrasound **25:** 217–225.
32. ALCAZAR, J.L. & G. LOPEZ-GARCIA. 2001. Transvaginal color Doppler assessment of venous flow in adnexal masses. Ultrasound Obstet. Gynecol. **17:** 434–438.
33. KUPESIC, S. & A. KURJAK. 2000. Contrast enhanced three-dimensional power Doppler sonography for the differentiation of adnexal masses. Obstet. Gynecol. **96:** 452–458.
34. KURTZ, A.B. *et al*. 1999. Diagnosis and staging of ovarian cancer: comparative values of Doppler and conventional US, CT, and MR imaging correlated with surgery and histopathologic analysis-report of the Radiology Diagnostic Oncology Group. Radiology **212:** 19–27.
35. KOMATSU, T. *et al*. 1996. Adnexal masses: transvaginal US and gadolinium-enhanced MR imaging assessment of intratumoral structure. Radiology **198:** 109–115.
36. YAMASHITA, Y. *et al*. 1997. Characterization of sonographically indeterminate ovarian tumors with MR imaging. A logistic regression analysis. Acta Radiol. **38:** 572–577.
37. BAST, R.C. *et al*. 1983. A radioimmunoassay using a monoclonal antibody to monitor the course of epithelial ovarian cancer. N. Engl. J. Med. **309:** 883–887.
38. MILOJKOVIC, M. *et al*. 2004. Significance of CA 125 serum level in discrimination between benign and malignant masses in the pelvis. Arch. Gynecol. Obstet. **269:** 176–180.
39. SASSONE, A.M. *et al*. 1991. Transvaginal sonographic characterization of ovarian disease: evaluation of a new scoring system to predict ovarian malignancy. Obstet. Gynecol. **78:** 70–76.

40. FERRAZZI, E. *et al*. 1997. Transvaginal ultrasonographic characterization of ovarian masses: comparison of five scoring systems in a multicenter study. Ultrasound Obstet. Gynecol. **10:** 192–197.
41. BERLANDA, N. *et al*. 2002. Impact of a multiparameter, ultrasound-based triage on surgical management of adnexal masses. Ultrasound Obstet. Gynecol. **20:** 181–185.
42. SZPUREK, D. *et al*. 2005. An ultrasonographic morphological index for prediction of ovarian tumor malignancy. Eur. J. Gynaecol. Oncol. **26:** 51–54.
43. LEE, J.W. *et al*. 2005. Selected adnexal cystic masses in postmenopausal women can be safely managed by laparoscopy. J. Korean Med. Sci. **20:** 468–472.
44. FERRAZZI, E. *et al*. 2005. Differentiation of small adnexal masses based on morphologic characteristics of transvaginal sonographic imaging: a multicenter study. J. Ultrasound Med. **24:** 1467–1473.
45. JACOBS, I. *et al*. 1990. A risk of malignancy index incorporating CA 125, ultrasound and menopausal status for the accurate preoperative diagnosis of ovarian cancer. Br. J. Obstet. Gynaecol. **97:** 922–929.
46. ANDERSEN, E.S. *et al*. 2003. Risk of malignancy index in the preoperative evaluation of patients with adnexal masses. Gynecol. Oncol. **90:** 109–112.
47. NEZHAT, F. *et al*. 1992. Four ovarian cancers diagnosed during laparoscopic management of 1011 women with adnexal masses. Am. J. Obstet. Gynecol. **167:** 790–796.
48. LEHMANN, E. *et al*. 1991. Pelviscopic ovarian surgery–a retrospective study of 1016 operated cysts. Geburtshilfe Frauenheilkd **51:** 280–287.
49. CRISTALLI, B. *et al*. 1992. Benefit of operative laparoscopy for ovarian tumors suspected of benignity. Laparoendosc. Surg. **2:** 69–73.
50. AUDEBERT, A. 1998. Laparoscopic ovarian surgery and ovarian torsion. *In* Endoscopic Surgery for Gynecologists. Sutton & Diamond. Second edition. 212–220. Saunders. London.
51. NICOLOSO, E. *et al*. 1995. Borderline tumors and cancers of the ovary. Laparoscopic-surgical evaluation. Presse Med. **24:** 1421–1422.
52. WALLWIENER, D. *et al*. 1996. Laparoscopy in (apparently) benign ovarian tumors between benefit and catastrophy and the deceptive safety of laparoscopic lapsacs. Zentralbl Gynakol. **118:** 53–61.
53. SADIK, S. *et al*. 1999. Laparoscopic management of selected adnexal masses. J. Am. Assoc. Gynecol. Laparosc. **6:** 313–316.
54. GUGLIELMINA, J.N. *et al*. 1997. Treatment of ovarian cysts by laparoscopy. Contracept. Fertil. Sex. **25:** 218–229.
55. MALIK, E. *et al*. 1998. Laparoscopic management of ovarian tumors. Surg. Endosc. **12:** 1326–1333.
56. METTLER, L. *et al*. 2001. Laparoscopic management of 641 adnexal tumors in Kiel, Germany. J. Am. Assoc. Gynecol. Laparosc. **8:** 74–82.
57. CANIS, M. *et al*. 1992. Fertility following laparoscopic management of benign adnexal cysts. Hum. Reprod. **7:** 529–531.
58. PADOS, G. *et al*. 2005. Laparoscopic management of borderline ovarian tumors in women of reproductive age and preoperative diagnosis of benign adnexal masses. Gynecol. Surg. **2**(Suppl 1)**:** Abstract S46.
59. GABRIEL, O. *et al*. 2003. Minimal surgery for the twisted ischaemic adnexa can preserve ovarian function. Hum. Reprod. **18:** 2599–2602.
60. DRAKE, J. 1998. Diagnosis and management of the adnexal mass. Am. Fam. Physician **57:** 2471–2476, 2479–2480.

61. PADOS, G. *et al.* 1996. Laparoscopic removal of dermoid cysts. Hum. Reprod. **11**(Suppl 1): 146, Abstract I124.
62. ROYAL COLLEGE OF OBSTETRICIANS AND GYNECOLOGISTS. 2003. Ovarian cysts in postmenopausal women: Guideline No. 34.
63. DEVROEY, P. & G. PADOS. 1992. Laparoscopic treatment of ovarian cysts: technique and long term results. *In* Year book of the Flemish Society of Obstetricians-Gynecologists. J. Amy, Ed.: 102–107. Brussels.
64. PADOS, G. 1996. Laparoscopic treatment of dermoid cysts. Presented at the Proceedings—Operative Video-Laser Laparoscory and Hysteroscopy. ESHRE Workshop Campus. "Hippocratio" General Hospital. Thessaloniki, Greece. Nov 22–24.
65. MARTIN, D.C. & D.T. O'CONNER. 2003. Surgical management of endometriosis-associated pain. *In* Obstetrics and Gynecology Clinics of North America. Vol. 30. T. Tulandi, Ed.: 151–162. Elsevier Saunders. Philadelphia.
66. CHILDERS, J.M., A. NASSERI, & E.A. SURWIT. 1996. Laparoscopic management of suspicious adnexal masses. Am. J. Obstet. Gynecol. **175**: 1451–1459.
67. VERGOTE, I. *et al.* 2001. Prognostic importance of degree of differentiation and cyst rupture in stage I invasive epithelial ovarian carcinoma. Lancet **357**: 176–182.
68. SEVELDA, P. *et al.* 1990. Prognostic factors for survival in stage I epithelial ovarian carcinoma. Cancer **65**: 2349–2352.
69. DEMBO, A.J. *et al.* 1990. Prognostic factors in patients with stage I epithelial ovarian cancer. Obstet. Gynecol. **75**: 263–273.
70. ALON, B.A. & O. LAVIE. 2001. Cyst rupture during surgery. Lancet **358**: 72–73.
71. CANIS, M. *et al.* 2002. Laparoscopic management of adnexal masses: a gold standard? Curr. Opin. Obstet. Gynecol. **14**: 423–428.
72. HOPKINS, M.P., V. VON GRUENIGEN, & S. GAICH. 2000. Laparoscopic port site implantation with ovarian cancer. Am. J. Obstet. Gynecol. **182**: 735–736.
73. HELAWA, M.E., G.V. KREPART, & R. LOTOCKI, 1986. Staging laparotomy in early epithelial ovarian carcinoma. Am. J. Obstet. Gynecol. **154**: 282–286.
74. ROUZIER, R. & C. POMEL. 2005. Update on the role of laparoscopy in the treatment of gynaecological malignancy. Curr. Opin. Obstet. Gynecol. **17**: 77–82.
75. CANIS, M. *et al.* 1997. Laparoscopic management of adnexal masses suspicious at ultrasound. Obstet. Gynecol. **89**: 679–683.
76. MARURI, F. & R. AZZIZ. 1993. Laparoscopic surgery for ectopic pregnancies: technology assessment and public health implications. Fertil. Steril. **59**: 487–498.
77. SORIANO, D. *et al.* 1999. Laparoscopy versus laparotomy in the management of adnexal mass during pregnancy. Fertil. Steril. **71**: 955–960.
78. HASSON, H. 1974. Open laparoscopy: a report of 150 cases. J. Reprod. Med. **12**: 234–238.
79. FATUM, M. & N. ROJANSKY. 2001. Laparoscopic surgery during pregnancy. Obstet. Gynecol. Surv. **56**: 50–59.
80. MATHEVET, P. *et al.* 2002. Laparoscopic management of adnexal masses in pregnancy: a case series. Eur. J. Obstet. Gynecol. Reprod. Biol. **108**: 217–222.

Safety Issues of Hysteroscopic Surgery

MINAS PASCHOPOULOS, NIKOLAOS P. POLYZOS,
LAZAROS G. LAVASIDIS, THOMAS VREKOUSSIS,
NIKOLAOS DALKALITSIS, AND EVANGELOS PARASKEVAIDIS

Department of Obstetrics and Gynaecology, Endoscopic Unit, University of Ioannina School of Medicine, Ioannina, Greece

ABSTRACT: The term *hysteroscopy* is used to determine the procedure during which an endoscopic view of the endometrial cavity is achieved with the help of a type of endoscopic device called "the hysteroscope." Hysteroscopy is used to assist the diagnosis for a series of female pathology. Apart from its diagnostic value, hysteroscopy can also be used for operative procedures including ablation and resection. Both diagnostic and operative hysteroscopy have been used for a number of years and various studies have been published to describe their success and complication rates throughout this period. Diagnostic hysteroscopy is relatively safe, whereas complications occur more frequently when operative hysteroscopy is used. These complications include uterine perforation, hemorrhage, fluid overload, gas embolization, and hyponatremia. The rate in the appearance of these complications is dependent on the type of the hysteroscopic procedure, the distending medium, and the experience of the hysteroscopist. To avoid any problems concerning the application of hysteroscopic procedures, it is important to take the necessary precautions both preoperatively and intraoperatively. For example, the preoperative use of thinning agents of the endometrium and the reduction of the operating time, or the avoidance of cutting too deeply into the myometrium, are some of the parameters to be considered when hysteroscopy is in argument.

KEYWORDS: hysteroscopy; complications; perforation; hemorrhage; gas embolization; fluid overload; hyponatremia; review

INTRODUCTION

Hysteroscopy is the procedure during which a view of the endometrial cavity can be achieved with the use of especially designed instrumentation. The endoscopists can identify focal uterine lesion or assess the severity of an expanded pathology. At the same time, there can also be a therapeutic intervention; in this way, hysteroscopy is considered to be a modern method for the

Address for correspondence: Minas Paschopoulos, M.D., Department of Obstetrics and Gynaecology, University of Ioannina School of Medicine, Ioannina 45110-Greece. Voice: +30-26510-99302; fax: +30-26510-99224.
e-mail: mpasxop@cc.uoi.gr

Ann. N.Y. Acad. Sci. 1092: 229–234 (2006). © 2006 New York Academy of Sciences.
doi: 10.1196/annals.1365.019

assessment and treatment of endometrial abnormalities such as dysfunctional uterine bleeding, polyps, myomas, septae, and adhesions. It can also be used for guided biopsies of the uterine cavity, for the removal of intrauterine devices (IUDs) and other foreign bodies, or during the investigation of infertility. However, hysteroscopy may be accompanied by complications, some of which are life-threatening. Complications are either procedure related (dependent on the technical skills of the hysteroscopist and the instrumentation) or media related (dependent on the distending medium used). The latter are usually more severe and potentially lethal; therefore, they should be identified and treated immediately.

PROCEDURE-RELATED COMPLICATIONS

Uterine Perforation

According to the American Association of Gynecologic Laparoscopists (AAGL), the rate of uterine perforation during the hysteroscopic procedures accounted for 1.1% in 1991.[1] Almost 50% of these perforations occurred during the dilatation of the cervix, while the other 50% of them were closely related to the technique used and to the improper use of the operating probe; the perforation of the uterus due to the insertion of the hysteroscope is also reported in one case.[2] Since uterine perforation is directly related to the type of procedure performed, the perforation rate is considerably lower in diagnostic rather than in operative hysteroscopy.[3] The uterine perforation seems to be directly associated with the surgeon's experience and technical skills during the insertion of the hysteroscope.[2,3] It is shown that 55% of the perforations were entry related, whereas 45% were technique related,[3] with no statistical difference reported between the incidence of the two groups of complications.[3]

The highest risk of uterine perforation occurs during transcervical resection of adhesions (TCRA), transcervical removal of foreign bodies (TCRF), and transcervical resection of the endometrium (TCRE).[3] The rate of perforation in cases of TCRE is considerably higher in women with repeated resections of the endometrium compared to those with a single resection.[4] The rates are significantly lower in transcervical resection of myomas (TCRM), transcervical resection of endometrial polyps (TCRP), and transcervical resection of uterine septae (TCRS).[3]

Dilatation of the cervix and insertion of the hysteroscope need attention to avoid perforation, while ultrasound or laparoscopic monitoring, during hysteroscopy seem to lower the risk for possible uterine perforation.[2,3]

Hemorrhage

Hemorrhage during hysteroscopy can occur at a general rate of 0.16%[2] and is related to the type of the operating procedure.[5] The risk for hemorrhage is reported higher during hysteroscopic adhesiolysis (2.51%) in comparison to other procedures like endometrial ablation (0.48%), polyp resection (0.47%), myoma resection (0.37%), and uterine septae ablation (0%).[5] With the exception of hysteroscopic adhesiolysis, the risk for hemorrhage during the other procedures mentioned above revealed no difference compared to the general expected rate of hemorrhage.[5]

To avoid the danger of intraoperative hemorrhage, many parameters have been studied but the evidence is still inadequate. Preoperative intracervical administration of vasopressin reduced the incidence of hemorrhage;[6] therefore, it is suggested before any operative hysteroscopic procedures. Microhemorrhages during hysteroscopy are likely to be controlled with the use of electrocoagulation;[5] if this fails, the procedure must be terminated and a Foley catheter, instilled with 10–30 mL of liquid, should be placed for 24 h to tamponate the site of bleeding.[5] If the blood loss is not controlled, a hysterectomy is always a radical treatment of choice.

MEDIA-RELATED COMPLICATIONS

Gas Embolism

Gas embolism is the most catastrophic complication to occur during a hysteroscopy, which is performed with the use of carbon dioxide (CO_2) as a distending medium. It appears in 0.017% of hysteroscopies with the use of CO_2;[1] CO_2 may not be the major cause for the emboli since the gas itself may not be responsible for this complication. In a trial published in 1999, the gas supply tube was deaerated before each procedure. The reported difference between the study and the control group was statistically significant since no emboli occurred.[7] This confirms the theory that emboli, which occur during hysteroscopy with CO_2, are caused by room air. Regarding operative hysteroscopy, it is suggested that the use of carbon dioxide is contraindicated since intravasation of CO_2 may lead to gas embolism. The mean pressure of CO_2 and the endometrial pressure during the procedure are leading causes for this complication in cases of endometrial resection and other procedures that cause endometrial injury. The gas pressure should be strictly below 100 mm Hg, its flow below 100 mL/min, and the pressure inside the endometrial cavity below 80 mm Hg.[8]

Precaution measures include careful monitoring of mean arterial pressure, heart rate, blood gases, and pressures of supplied CO_2 and endometrial cavity, throughout the procedure. In patients without previously known heart valve disease or heart failure, the occurrence of the characteristic metallic heart sound during the heart contractions, caused by the intracardiac presence of free CO_2, is an absolute indication for immediate termination of the hysteroscopic procedure until improvement.[9]

In cases of affected vital signs, immediate transfer to the intensive care unit, intubation, heparin administration and, if necessary, cardiopulmonary resuscitation, may be needed.

Fluid Overload

According to the AAGL, the rate of fluid overload during hysteroscopic procedures was 0.14% in 1991.[1] The responsible factors for any intravasation of liquid distending media and fluid overload are the following: type and duration of the procedure, depth of the resection, and level of pressure inside the endometrial cavity during a hysteroscopic procedure.[1] No evidence regarding the type and duration of the hysteroscopic procedure and the depth of the resection performed is available. When the endometrium is seriously injured, procedures such as myoma resection, endometrial ablation, and septum resection are more likely to cause intravasation. The possibility of intravasation is significantly enhanced when the procedure lasts more than 60 min.[1]

Increased intrauterine pressure (IUP) seems to affect the onset of the fluid-overload syndrome. It seems when IUP exceeds the mean arterial pressure, the relative risk for fluid overload increases significantly.[10] This finding is not consistent with a previous study that supports that an IUP below 200 mm Hg is unlikely to lead to fluid intravasation.[11] Nevertheless, maintaining the pressure of the endometrial cavity at a level of 80 mm Hg may diminish the rate of fluid overload.[12]

To identify any fluid overload as soon as possible, several methods were proposed. By detecting breath alcohol after addition of a 2% alcohol solution to the distending medium purisole, fluid absorption over 400 mL may be prevented.[13] Alcohol extravasation at this extent was proved harmless for the patient and of clinical importance for major hysteroscopic procedures such as myoma resection, endometrial ablation, and septum resection.[13] Also, the use of a 1% alcohol/1.5% glycine solution was reported as insufficient to assess the overall fluid balance.[14] On the contrary, GnRH analogues administered preoperatively were of benefit by lowering the risk of distending media intravasation.[15]

One of the main priorities during a hysteroscopic procedure should always be to monitor the arterial pressure, the hematocrit, the proteins of plasma, the plasma volume, and the deficit of the distending medium. Any deficit greater than 1,000 mL should lead to the termination of the hysteroscopic procedure, administration of diuretics and oxygen, and monitoring of blood and central venous pressure. Cardiovascular disease further restricts fluid deficits due to increased risk for pulmonary edema and high morbidity.

Electrolytic Disorders (Hyponatremia)

The rate of hyponatremia is considerably higher in operative hysteroscopy[3] depending both on the type of operative procedure[16] as well as on the type of the solution used. Procedures that cause extended endometrial injury such as myomectomy or hysteroscopic endometrial ablation are more likely to trigger hyposmolarity and hyponatremia.[16,17] The amount of the tissue resected is related to the severity of the disorders. Isotonic solutions (i.e., manitol 5%) rather than nonisotonic solutions (glycine 1.5%) are related to hyponatremia without hyposmolarity, thus presenting lower risk for encephalopathy.[18] Finally, sorbitol 2.5%-mannitol 0.54% irrigation solution, commonly used in hysteroscopic endometrial ablation, is not associated with hyponatremia and hyposmolarity.[19]

The existing risk for hyponatremia demands close monitoring of blood electrolyte concentrations, especially in extended or prolonged hysteroscopic procedures.

CONCLUSION

Hysteroscopic complications remain a relatively rare event. Nevertheless, their occurrence may become fatal for the patient. The present review summarizes the most important potential dangers for hysteroscopists to have in mind and underlines that physician's awareness may be life saving for the patient. Preoperative evaluation, excellent training in the use of instrumentation, and close monitoring of the patient during and after the hysteroscopic procedure can both predict and prevent a complication from happening.

REFERENCES

1. HULKA, J.F., H.B. PETERSON, J.M. PHILLIPS, *et al.* 1993. Operative hysteroscopy. American Association of Gynecologic Laparoscopists 1991 membership survey. J. Reprod. Med. **38:** 572–573.
2. XIA, E.L., H. DUAN, J. ZHANG, *et al.* 2003. Analysis of 16 cases of uterine perforation during hysteroscopic electro-surgeries. Zhonghua Fu Chan Ke Za Zhi. **38:** 280–283.
3. JANSEN, F.W., C.B. VREDEVOOGD, K. VAN ULZEN, *et al.* 2000. Complications of hysteroscopy: a prospective, multicenter study. Obstet. Gynecol. **96:** 266–270.
4. McLEAN-FRASER, E., D. PENAVA & G.A. VILOS. 2002. Perioperative complication rates of primary and repeat hysteroscopic endometrial ablations. J. Am. Assoc. Gynecol. Laparosc. **9:** 175–177.
5. AGOSTINI, A., L. CRAVELLO, R. DESBRIERE, *et al.* 2002. Hemorrhage risk during operative hysteroscopy. Acta Obstet. Gynecol. Scand. **81:** 878–879.
6. PHILLIPS, D.R., H.G. NATHANSON, S.J. MILIM, *et al.* 1996. The effect of dilute vasopressin solution on blood loss during operative hysteroscopy: a randomized controlled trial. Obstet. Gynecol. **88:** 761–766.
7. BRANDNER, P., K.J. NEIS & C. EHMER. 1999. The etiology, frequency, and prevention of gas embolism during CO_2 hysteroscopy. J. Am. Assoc. Gynecol. Laparosc. **6:** 421–428.

8. NATHANSON, M.H. & U. EZEH. 1995. Carbon dioxide embolism following diagnostic hysteroscopy. Br. J. Obstet. Gynaecol. **102:** 505.
9. BRUNDIN, J. & K. THOMASON. 1989. Cardiac gas embolism during carbon dioxide hysteroscopy: risk and management. Eur. J. Obstet. Gynecol. R.B. **33:** 241–245.
10. BENNETT, K.L., C. OHRMUNDT & J.A. MALONI. 1996. Preventing intravasation in women undergoing hysteroscopic procedures. AORN J. **64:** 792–799.
11. VULGAROPULOS, S.P., L.C. HALEY & J.F. HULKA. 1992. Intrauterine pressure and fluid absorption during continuous flow hysteroscopy. Am. J. Obstet. Gynecol. **167:** 386–390; discussion 390–391.
12. SHIRK, G.J. & J. KAIGH. 1994. The use of low-viscosity fluids for hysteroscopy. J. Am. Assoc. Gynecol. Laparosc. **2:** 11–21.
13. WALLWIENER, D., B. AYDENIZ, S. RIMBACH, et al. 1996. Addition of ethanol to the distension medium in surgical hysteroscopy as screening to prevent "fluid overload." A prospective randomized comparative study of ablative versus non-ablative surgical hysteroscopy and different ethanol concentration. Geburtshilfe Frauenheilkd **56:** 462–469.
14. MOLNAR, B.G., A.L. MGOS & J. KAY. 1997. Monitoring fluid absorption using 1% ethanol-tagged glycine during operative hysteroscopy. J. Am. Assoc. Gynecol. Laparosc. **4:** 357–362.
15. TASKIN, O., A. YALCINOGLOU, S. KUCUK, et al. 1996. The degree of fluid absorption during hysteroscopic surgery in patients pretreated with goserelin. J. Am. Assoc. Gynecol. Laparosc. **3:** 555–559.
16. KIM, A.H., M.D. KELTZ, A. ARICI, et al. 1995. Dilutional hyponatremia during hysteroscopic myomectomy with sorbitol-mannitol distention medium. J. Am. Assoc. Gynecol. Laprosc. **2:** 237–242.
17. AGRAHARKAR, M. & A. AGRAHARKAR. 1997. Posthysteroscopic hyponatremia: evidence for a multifactorial cause. Am. J. Kidney Dis. **30:** 717–719.
18. PHILLIPS, D.R., S.J. MILIM, H.G. NATHANSON, et al. 1997. Preventing hyponatremic encephalopathy: comparison of serum sodium and osmolality during operative hysteroscopy with 5% mannitol and 1.5% glycine distention media. J. Am. Assoc. Gynecol. Laparosc. **4:** 567–576.
19. MOIR, C.L., H. MANDIN & R. BRANT. 1997. Sorbitol 2.5% mannitol 0.54% irrigation solution for hysteroscopic endometrial ablation surgery. Can. J. Anaesth. **44:** 473–478.

Oocyte Maturation in Assisted Reproductive Techniques

DIMITRIS LOUTRADIS,[a] ERASMIA KIAPEKOU,[a]
EVANGELIA ZAPANTI,[b] AND ARISTIDIS ANTSAKLIS[a]

[a] 1st Department of Obstetrics and Gynecology, Alexandra Hospital,
University of Athens, Athens, Greece

[b] 1st Endocrine Section, Alexandra Hospital, Athens, Athens, Greece

ABSTRACT: Human oocyte maturation is a long process during which nuclear maturation occurs resulting in germinal vesicle breakdown (transition from prophase I to metaphase II) and extrusion of the first polar body. During oocyte maturation, in parallel with nuclear maturation, a number of events take place in the oocyte cytoplasm that assist fertilization and early embryonic development. So far several attempts have been made to mature human oocytes *in vitro*. The main patient group to which *in vitro* maturation (IVM) has been applied is polycystic ovarian syndrome. In a concise review we present the techniques used for the IVM of oocytes and the role of hormones and growth factors in IVM and subsequent fertilization and early embryonic development.

KEYWORDS: *in vitro* maturation; folliculogenesis; fertilization; cryopreservation

INTRODUCTION

Since the first live birth after *in vitro* fertilization (IVF) was reported a lot of progress has been made in assisted reproduction techniques. Thousands of women with infertility problems were helped, even though many disadvantages of this treatment emerged. Although the first successful IVF attempt was performed in a normally cycling woman without prior hormonal treatment,[1] modern IVF protocols utilize daily gonadotropin injections with several side effects and high cost. Medication used in IVF protocols stimulates the ovaries leading to multiple follicles production. Some of the treated women are tremendously perceptive to IVF treatment, especially those with polycystic ovaries, and are at increased risk to develop ovarian hyperstimulation syndrome (OHSS).[2] The side effects and high cost of medication employed made research for other assistant reproductive techniques imperative.

Address for correspondence: Erasmia Kiapekou, 25 Karaiskaki St., 15 772 Athens, Greece. Voice: 0030-6977252111; fax: 0030-210-7470460.
e-mail: ekiapek@otenet.gr

Ann. N.Y. Acad. Sci. 1092: 235–246 (2006). © 2006 New York Academy of Sciences.
doi: 10.1196/annals.1365.020

In 1935, Pincus and Enzmann,[3] demonstrated for the first time the ability of immature oocytes to resume meiosis spontaneously, and in 1965 Edwards[4,5] confirmed this observation. The same author described 4 years later the successful fertilization of human oocytes matured *in vitro*.[6] Since then, several researchers have announced successful attempts of maturing oocytes *in vitro*. So far, women with polycystic ovary syndrome (PCOS) are the main patient group to which *in vitro* maturation (IVM) has been applied for clinical use.[7,8]

ELEMENTS OF OVARIAN ONTOGENY AND PHYSIOLOGY

Folliculogenesis

The basic reproductive unit of the ovary is the primordial follicle. Primordial follicles are derived from oogonia, which are the precursor forms of oocytes and are divided by mitosis. Oogonia arrive at the genital ridge by the 5th week of gestation.[9] By about 8 weeks of gestation oogonia increase their number to 600,000 by mitotic division.[10] Since the 16th week of gestation, the oogonial endowment is subject to three processes: mitosis, meiosis, and oogonial atresia.[10] The combination of these three processes results in an increase of the number of oogonia, which at mid-gestation number seven million in both ovaries of the female fetus. Between weeks 8 and 13 of fetal life, some of the oogonia enter the prophase of the first meiotic division. This change marks the conversion of oogonia to primary oocytes that remain arrested in prophase I at dictyate phase (germinal vesicle stage oocytes, GV). At this stage the oocyte is surrounded by one layer of poorly differentiated, flattened elongation of granulosa cells (pregranulosa cells) and the functional unit created represents the primordial follicle. Oogonia that persist beyond the 7th month of gestation and have not divided by meiosis are subject to atresia.[11] Consequently, no oogonia are present in ovaries at birth. The majority of follicles in women's ovaries of all ages are primordial. Approximately one million primordial follicles are present in the ovaries at birth, and only 400,000 at the onset of puberty.[12] Of this cohort of follicles about 400 will ovulate during a woman's reproductive life, while all others will be destroyed by atresia.

Primordial follicles ($\sim$30 μM in diameter) are located in the ovarian cortex and form a thick stroma beneath germinal epithelium, which constitutes a source (pool) of follicles. Primordial follicles enter to a growth phase continuously throughout a woman's life, even during pregnancy, anovulation periods, lactation, and perimenopause period, until the end of the reproductive period.[13] The number of primordial follicles that initiate growth depends on the total number of ovarian follicles and decreases with age.

Folliculogenesis is a long process during which recruitment of primordial follicles, follicular growth, and selection and maturation of the preovulatory follicles occur. In humans, the time for primordial follicles to attain the preantral stage is probably several months.[14] Even though gonadotropins play an important role on fullicogenesis,[15] it seems that they do not suffice to initiate and complete the growing process.[16,17]

A number of factors may act synergically with gonadotropins to trigger the initiation of follicular growth and to modulate early follicular development. These factors include pituitary hormones, such as growth hormone (GH), pro-lactin (PRL), and thyroid stimulation hormone (TSH), which affect follicular growth and maturation. Kit ligand is another factor that may be involved in the initiation of follicular growth. It is expressed in granulosa cells of primordial follicles both in human and mouse[18,19] and acts via c-kit receptor. Some other factors like growth differentiation factor 9 (GDF-9), insulin-like growth factors (IGFs), and transforming growth factor (TGF) have been detected in human follicular tissues at early stages of follicular development.[14,20-23]

After their recruitment from the follicle pool, primordial follicles grow in size and they transform into primary follicles ($\sim$100 μM in diameter). When the follicle becomes 200 μM in diameter and the surrounding oocyte granulosa cells are stratified in two or more layers, the follicle is called secondary. At this stage of development several stromal cells differentiate into theca cells constituting a layer that surrounds the follicles, and the oocyte begins to form its zona pellucida.[24] At the next stage of follicle development antrum formation occurs with accumulation of fluid between granulosa cells. During antrum formation the oocyte and a portion of granulosa cells, called cumulus cells, gradually display on one side of the follicular cavity (antral follicle, 2–5mm in diameter). The complex constituted by the oocyte and the surrounded cumulus cells is called cumulus oocyte complex (COC). Further enlargement of the antral follicle forms the preovulatory follicle ($\sim$20 mm in diameter).[14] From early antral stage to the preovulatory stage, follicular development is under the influence of pituitary follicle stimulating hormone (FSH).

Follicles that reach 2–5 mm in diameter in late luteal phase will be selected for further development, composing the group from which the dominant follicle will be destined to ovulate during the following menstrual cycle.[14] These are about 6–11 per ovary and this number decreases with age. The size of the dominant follicle increases significantly during follicular phase until the middle of the menstrual cycle, when luteinizing hormone (LH) surge induces reinitiation of meiosis (breakdown of the oocyte nucleus: germinal vesicle breakdown (GVBD). At this time, oocytes complete the first meiotic division that is characterized by the appearance of the first polar body. Subsequently, they start the second meiotic division and they reach metaphase II prior to ovulation.[14]

Oocyte Maturation

Oocyte maturation is a long and enigmatic process during which nuclear and cytoplasmic changes happen, resulting in transition from GV stage to the metaphase II stage and the extrusion of the first polar body. During oocyte maturation several products are synthesized and stored. These products support embryonic development until embryonic genome becomes capable to support embryogenesis. Cumulus cells also contribute to substance production during oocyte maturation. They secrete products in response to gonadotropins that control nuclear and cytoplasmic maturation.

Nuclear maturation refers to the acquisition of oocyte to reinitiate meiosis and progress to metaphase II. Germinal vesicle breakdown begins with the middle-cycle surge of LH.[25] However, COCs can spontaneously resume meiosis when they are cultured *in vitro*.[26] The exact molecular mechanisms that participate in this process are not fully understood. Many factors seems to be involved in the modulation of GVBD, such as cyclic adenosine monophosphate (cAMP), purines, steroids, inositol 1,4,5-triphosphate (IP3), Ca^{2+}, and many others. Modulator factors pass freely between the oocyte and cumulus cells through gap junctions. High levels of cyclic adenosine monophosphate and purine hypoxanthine in culture medium prevent GVBD.[27] Additionally, it has been suggested that the gap junction-mediated transmission of follicular cell cAMP to the oocyte inhibits oocyte maturation.[28] Conversely, LH addition to culture medium induces GVBD. Protein synthesis is essential for GVBD and for the progression of oocytes to metaphase II.[29–31] In absence of protein synthesis maturation-promoting factor (MPF), a cytoplasmic protein, is unable to be activated.[32,33]

MPF is composed of two proteins, a cyclin and a cyclin-dependent kinase (cyclin B and p34^{cac2} serine/threonin kinase, respectively). Cyclins form a complex by binding cyclin-dependent kinases, activating them and thus they control the cell cycle. MPF stimulates cell cycle progression by phosphorylating specific proteins in the cell, necessitated for the transition from G2 to M-cell cycle phase. Its action is so strong that it can induce the initiation of mitosis even in nonreplicating cells. When oocytes are in the interphase (interval between divisions), inactive cyclin-kinase complex levels are high. Cyclin-kinase complex when activated induces GVBD. However, p34^{cac2} serine/threonin kinase concentration is high just before fertilization when oocytes are arrested in metaphase II. Cytostatic factor (CSF), which also regulates oocyte nuclear maturation, is suggested to be responsible for the arrest.[34] In addition, Mos protein (product of *c-mos* gene) seems to participate in this arrest by acting like CSF. MPF is activated either via Mos protein or via mitogen-activated protein kinase (MAPK). In conclusion, GVBD, metaphase II arrest, and subsequently the passage from MII to anaphase II depend on activation and inactivation of proteins that control the cell cycle, such as p34^{cac2} serine/threonin kinase.

Cytoplasmic maturation is a process during which a number of phenomena occur in the oocyte cytoplasm that in parallel to nuclear maturation prepare the oocyte for fertilization and support early embryonic development. The quality of oocyte depends on cytoplasmic maturation. Oocytes with insufficient or defective cytoplasmic maturation are unable to be fertilized and develop further. Among the events that take place during the cytoplasmic maturation are RNA synthesis and protein production.[35] Most of the RNA present in oocytes is synthesized during folliculogenesis. However, RNA synthesis decreases before GVBD, so that embryonic development depends on mRNA and proteins already stored in the cytoplasm during the period before ovulation.

IN VITRO MATURATION OF HUMAN OOCYTES

Two techniques have been used to mature human oocytes *in vitro*. In the first, called IVM, oocytes at the germinal vesicle stage are assembled from unstimulated antral follicles, cultured for 24–48 h until they resume meiosis and reach metaphase II.[25] Because of the fact that not all oocytes collected are at the same stage of development and a considerable number of oocytes reach MII after 23–25 h of culture, culture time has been limited to 28–36 h.[36] In the second technique, called *in vitro* follicular growth, follicles at primordial or early preantral stage are cultured for widen intervals, until they are capable of undergoing IVM and subsequently to be fertilized.

Culture of primary and secondary follicles in humans and several animal species has also been performed with varying results.[37–39]

The *in vitro* growth of primordial follicles is achieved by culturing small pieces of ovarian cortex for approximately a 2-week period. The follicles reach secondary follicle stage[37] and rarely early antral stage,[40] before their degeneration. The only live offspring after long-term primordial follicles culture has been demonstrated in mouse by Eppig *et al.* in 1996.[38]

Oocytes from Unstimulated Ovaries

The first live birth from IVM of immature oocytes was accomplished by Cha *et al.* in 1991.[41] Oocytes were collected from unstimulated ovaries during Caesarean section in a donation program. A few years later Hwang *et al.* confirmed the ability of immature oocytes derived from Caesarean section to mature and develop *in vitro*.[42] Further research is required to clarify the capacity of oocytes obtained from a Caesarean section for early embryonic development. In 1994, Trounson *et al.* demonstrated for the first time pregnancy and live birth after IVM of immature oocytes acquired from a woman with PCOS followed by IVF.[8] In this study, authors showed that oocytes from anovulatory PCOS patients have similar capacity to mature, fertilize, and develop as the oocytes from ovulatory PCOS and non-PCOS patients. The following year, Barnes *et al.* presented another successful pregnancy after IVM of immature oocytes, combined with intracytoplasmic sperm injection (ICSI) in a PCOS patient.[43] In 2000, Cha *et al.* demonstrated high pregnancy rate after IVM (27.1%).[44] Nevertheless, even though the number of embryos transferred was very high, (approximately six embryos per patient) the implantation rate was as low as 6.9%.

In conclusion, even if immature oocytes obtained from unstimulated ovaries either of PCOS or regularly menstruating women have the capacity to mature, to be fertilized and develop *in vitro*, the implantation rate is extremely low.[44-46] However, recently Soderstrom-Anttila *et al.* presented both high pregnancy and implantation rates after IVM, both in patients with regular cycles and with PCOS, while the mean number of embryos transferred was 1.6.[47]

Oocytes from Stimulated Ovaries

As the implantation rate after IVM of immature oocytes remains low, mild ovarian stimulation with FSH or human chorionic gonadotropin (hCG), prior to immature oocyte retrieval, may represent an alternative approach.[48] Wynn *et al.* demonstrated that FSH pretreatment increases recovery and IVM of immature oocytes.[49] Furthermore, it has been reported that low-dose FSH priming (37.5 IU) not only promotes efficient immature oocytes recovery and IVM rates but also fertilization rates.[48] Nevertheless, Mikkelsen *et al.* showed that FSH priming has no beneficial effect on *in vitro* oocyte maturation, fertilization rate, cleavage rate, or embryonic development in regularly menstruating women.[46] In contrast, the same authors, soon after, presented that FSH priming during follicular phase enhances oocyte maturation potential, pregnancy, and implantation rates.[50]

Chian *et al.* reported that priming with 10,000 IU hCG 36 h before immature oocyte retrieval from PCOS women increases IVM rate of immature oocytes.[51] In addition, hCG priming may increase pregnancy rates and the number of oocytes retrieved.[52,53] In a multicenter study of 1,000 IVM cycles hCG priming showed to increase pregnancy and implantation rates in women with polycystic ovaries and PCOS.[7] On the other hand, Lin *et al.* reported that pretreatment with 75 IU FSH did not improve maturation, fertilization, and pregnancy rates in PCOS women, when 10,000 IU hCG were given 36 h before oocyte retrieval.[53]

OVARIAN TISSUE CRYOPRESERVATION

Currently, the number of cancer survivors is high. More women in reproductive age undergo treatment against malignant diseases that are potentially gonadotoxic. This group of patients necessitates to preserve their fertility before such treatment. This is especially important for survivors from pediatric cancer.

Ovarian tissue cryopreservation and transplantation is a very promising method in preserving female fertility. More than 40 years ago, Parrott *et al.* reported live births in mice after autografting (reimplantation) of frozen-thawed ovarian tissue.[54] The lack of effective cryoprotectants and cryopreservation devices delayed the progression of this technique for a few decades. In the

1990s and afterward live births have been reported in several species after reimplantation of frozen-thawed ovarian tissue.[55,56] Recently, Lee *et al.* described the first live birth of a female monkey after successful transplantation of fresh ovarian tissue,[57] while Donnez *et al.* illustrated the first live birth of a baby after orthotopic transplantation of cryopreserved ovarian tissue.[58] Despite successful results, ovarian tissue cryopreservation is still experimental and not a totally effective treatment.

Since most of the ovarian cortex follicles are primordial, *in vitro* culture of primordial follicles contained in cryopreserved ovarian tissue represents another potential method for restoring female fertility. So far, various culture systems and protocols investigating *in vitro* follicular growth in humans have been developed.[37,40,59] The results of these studies underline the necessity of further improvement in culture techniques.

THE ROLE OF HORMONES AND GROWTH FACTORS ON *IN VITRO* OOCYTE MATURATION

Numerous hormones and growth factors are involved in folliculogenesis and in oocyte maturation *in vivo*. Gonadotropins are essential for the follicular development of preantral, antral, and preovulatory follicles *in vivo*. Under the control of FSH, the small antral follicles reach the preovulatory stage, while the LH surge triggers the reinitiation of meiosis *in vivo*. FSH is also important for induction of LH receptors in granulosa cells. However, it is crucial to identify whether gonadotropins can promote *in vitro* oocyte maturation as well as *in vivo*. Their *in vitro* effects in oocyte maturation are controversial, although most IVM protocols use recombinant FSH and LH or hCG in the culture medium. In *in vitro* conditions it was believed that LH induces GVBD through cumulus cells as the presence of LH receptors (R) in oocytes had not been demonstrated.[60] However, we have recently demonstrated the mRNA expression of LH-R and FSH-R in mouse and human oocytes, zygotes, and preimplantation embryos. These results indicate the important role of gonadotropins in the modulation of meiosis and in early embryonic development.[61,62]

GDF-9, TGFs, basic fibroblast growth factor, and several others are suggested to take part in the initiation of follicular growth. Epidermal growth factor appears to have a very effective stimulatory action on cumulus cells expansion and meiotic resumption (GVBD) in mouse and rat COCs.[63,64] The combination of EGF (in doses ≥ 5 ng/mL) with hCG during *in vitro* culture of mouse COCs significantly increases the transition of oocytes from MI to MII,[65] while the combination of EGF with IGF-1 induces cumulus expansion and increases nuclear maturation rates in cultures of bovine COCs.[66] IGFs enhance the response of follicles to gonadotropins.[67,68] IGF-1 receptors are present in follicles throughout all stages of development in humans (from primordial to preovulatory stage).[69] Follicles of IGF-1 knockout mice are unable to reach the antral stage of development and these mice are infertile due to the lack of ovulation.[70] The addition of IGF-1 to the culture medium increases the *in vitro* nuclear maturation rate of oocytes.[21,71,72]

Growth hormone is another hormone involved in oocyte maturation. Studies in many species have shown that GH-R is present in various stages of follicular development and that GH accelerates the *in vitro* oocyte maturation.[20,21,73–75] Growth hormone affects oocyte maturation either through GH-R or through the action of IGF-1.[73,75]

PRL controls numerous physiological processes. The role of PRL in oocyte maturation is controversial. Studies in rabbits, mice, and rats have shown a direct stimulatory effect of PRL in *in vitro* oocyte maturation and in embryo development.[76–79] Recently, we demonstrated the expression of PRL-R mRNA in mouse oocytes and preimlantation embryos.[80] Furthermore, we showed that the addition of PRL to the culture medium during long-term cultures of mouse preantral follicles increases nuclear maturation rate and subsequently fertilization and early embryonic development rates (Kiapekou *et al.,* unpublished data).

CONCLUSIONS

Folliculogenesis is a long and complicated process, initiation and completion of which involve many factors that act either on the oocyte or the surrounding cells. IVM of human oocytes has been achieved to a certain degree. *In vitro* maturation protocols used are simple and ovarian stimulation, when necessary, has to be applied for a short period of time with the minimum dose of drugs and the less possible side effects and cost. In the future, the combination of *in vitro* follicular growth with IVM and the improvement of follicular and ovarian tissue freezing methods will help more groups of infertile patients to preserve their fertility such as young patients with cancer.

REFERENCES

1. STEPTOE, P.C. & R.G. EDWARDS. 1978. Birth after the reimplantation of a human embryo. Lancet **2:** 366.
2. BEERENDONK, C.C. *et al.* 1998. Ovarian hyperstimulation syndrome: facts and fallacies. Obstet. Gynecol. Surv. **53:** 439–449.
3. PINCUS, G. & E.V. ENZMANN. 1935. The comparative behavior of mammalian eggs *in vivo* and *in vitro*: I. The activation of ovarian eggs. J. Exp. Med. **62:** 665–675.
4. EDWARDS, R.G. 1965. Maturation *in vitro* of human ovarian oocytes. Lancet **2:** 926–929.
5. EDWARDS, R.G. 1965. Maturation *in vitro* of mouse, sheep, cow, pig, rhesus monkey and human ovarian oocytes. Nature **208:** 349–351.
6. EDWARDS, R.G., B.D. BAVISTER & P.C. STEPTOE. 1969. Early stages of fertilization *in vitro* of human oocytes matured *in vitro*. Nature **221:** 632–635.

7. CHIAN, R.C. 2004. In-vitro maturation of immature oocytes for infertile women with PCOS. Reprod. Biomed. Online **8:** 547–552.

8. TROUNSON, A., C. WOOD & A. KAUSCHE. 1994. *In vitro* maturation and the fertilization and developmental competence of oocytes recovered from untreated polycystic ovarian patients. Fertil. Steril. **62:** 353–362.

9. BAKER, T.G. & L.L. FRANCHI. 1967. The fine structure of oogonia and oocytes in human ovaries. J. Cell Sci. **2:** 213–224.

10. MOTTA, P.M., S. MAKABE & S.A. NOTTOLA. 1997. The ultrastructure of human reproduction. I. The natural history of the female germ cell: origin, migration and differentiation inside the developing ovary. Hum. Reprod. Update **3:** 281–295.

11. BULUM, S.E. & E.Y. ADASHI. 2003. The physiology and pathology of the female reproductive axis. *In* Williams textbook of endocrinology. R.H. Williams, J.D. Wilson & D.W. Foster, Eds.: 587–664. Saunders. Philadelphia, PA.

12. BAKER, T.G. 1963. A quantitative and cytological study of germ cells in human ovaries. Proc. R. Soc. Lond. B. Biol. Sci. **158:** 417–433.

13. PETERS, H. 1969. The development of the mouse ovary from birth to maturity. Acta. Endocrinol. (Copenh) **62:** 98–116.

14. GOUGEON, A. 1996. Regulation of ovarian follicular development in primates: facts and hypotheses. Endocr. Rev. **17:** 121–155.

15. LINTERN-MOORE, S. 1977. Initiation of follicular growth in the infant mouse ovary by exogenous gonadotrophin. Biol. Reprod. **17:** 635–639.

16. HALPIN, D.M. *et al.* 1986. Postnatal ovarian follicle development in hypogonadal (hpg) and normal mice and associated changes in the hypothalamic-pituitary ovarian axis. J. Reprod. Fertil. **77:** 287–296.

17. HOWE, E. *et al.* 1978. Ovarian development in hypopituitary Snell dwarf mice. The size and composition of the follicle population. Biol. Reprod. **19:** 959–964.

18. MOTRO, B. & A. BERNSTEIN. 1993. Dynamic changes in ovarian c-kit and steel expression during the estrous reproductive cycle. Dev. Dyn. **197:** 69–79.

19. TANIKAWA, M. *et al.* 1998. Expression of c-kit messenger ribonucleic acid in human oocyte and presence of soluble c-kit in follicular fluid. J. Clin. Endocrinol. Metab. **83:** 1239–1242.

20. LIU, X. *et al.* 1998. Effects of growth hormone, activin, and follistatin on the development of preantral follicle from immature female mice. Endocrinology **139:** 2342–2347.

21. KIAPEKOU, E. *et al.* 2005. Effects of GH and IGF-I on the *in vitro* maturation of mouse oocytes. Hormones (Athens) **4:** 155–160.

22. ZHAO, J. *et al.* 2001. Insulin-like growth factor-I (IGF-I) stimulates the development of cultured rat pre-antral follicles. Mol. Reprod. Dev. **58:** 287–296.

23. PICTON, H., D. BRIGGS & R. GOSDEN. 1998. The molecular basis of oocyte growth and development. Mol. Cell. Endocrinol. **145:** 27–37.

24. FORTUNE, J.E. 2003. The early stages of follicular development: activation of primordial follicles and growth of preantral follicles. Anim. Reprod. Sci. **78:** 135–163.

25. CHA, K.Y. & R.C. CHIAN. 1998. Maturation *in vitro* of immature human oocytes for clinical use. Hum. Reprod. Update **4:** 103–120.

26. CHIAN, R.C., J.H. LIM & S.L. TAN. 2004. State of the art in in-vitro oocyte maturation. Curr. Opin. Obstet. Gynecol. **16:** 211–219.

27. EPPIG, J.J., P.F. WARD-BAILEY & D.L. COLEMAN. 1985. Hypoxanthine and adenosine in murine ovarian follicular fluid: concentrations and activity in maintaining oocyte meiotic arrest. Biol. Reprod. **33:** 1041–1049.

68. ADASHI, E.Y. 1993. The intraovarian insulin-like growth factor system. *In* The Ovary. E.Y. Adashi & P.C.K. Leing, Eds.: 319–335. Raven Press. New York, NY.
69. ZHOU, J. & C. BONDY. 1993. Anatomy of the human ovarian insulin-like growth factor system. Biol. Reprod. **48:** 467–482.
70. BAKER, J. *et al.* 1996. Effects of an Igf1 gene null mutation on mouse reproduction. Mol. Endocrinol. **10:** 903–918.
71. YOSHIMURA, Y. *et al.* 1996. Effects of insulin-like growth factor-I on follicle growth, oocyte maturation, and ovarian steroidogenesis and plasminogen activator activity in the rabbit. Biol. Reprod. **55:** 152–160.
72. GOMEZ, E., J.J. TARIN & A. PELLICER. 1993. Oocyte maturation in humans: the role of gonadotropins and growth factors. Fertil. Steril. **60:** 40–46.
73. SIROTKIN, A.V. *et al.* 1998. Effect of follicular cells, IGF-I and tyrosine kinase blockers on oocyte maturation. Anim. Reprod. Sci. **51:** 333–344.
74. IZADYAR, F. *et al.* 1999. Messenger RNA expression and protein localization of growth hormone in bovine ovarian tissue and in cumulus oocyte complexes (COCs) during *in vitro* maturation. Mol. Reprod. Dev. **53:** 398–406.
75. ZHAO, J. *et al.* 2000. The effect of growth hormone on rat pre-antral follicles *in vitro*. Zygote **8:** 275–283.
76. YOHKAICHIYA, T. *et al.* 1988. Improvement of mouse embryo development *in vitro* by prolactin. Tohoku J. Exp. Med. **155:** 241–246.
77. YOSHIMURA, Y. *et al.* 1989. Developmental potential of rabbit oocyte matured *in vitro*: the possible contribution of prolactin. Biol. Reprod. **41:** 26–33.
78. YOSHIMURA, Y. *et al.* 1991. Possible contribution of prolactin in the process of ovulation and oocyte maturation. Horm. Res. **35**(Suppl. 1): 22–32.
79. KARABULUT, A.K., R. LAYFIELD & M.K. PRATTEN. 1999. The mechanism of growth-promoting effects of prolactin in embryogenesis-links to growth factors. Cells Tissues Organs **164:** 2–13.
80. KIAPEKOU, E. *et al.* 2005. Prolactin receptor mRNA expression in oocytes and preimplantation mouse embryos. Reprod. Biomed. Online **10:** 339–346.

Prevention and Management of Ovarian Hyperstimulation Syndrome

NIKOS F. VLAHOS AND ODYSSEAS GREGORIOU

Second Department of Obstetrics and Gynecology, Aretaieion Hospital, National Kapodestrian University of Athens, School of Medicine, Greece

ABSTRACT: The Ovarian Hyperstimulation Syndrome (OHSS) represents one of the biggest nightmares of all physicians involved in Assisted Reproductive Technologies (ART). Every year, several hundreds of women are hospitalized and to date several deaths have been reported. The pivotal event in the development of OHSS is the disruption of capillary integrity that results in leakage of intravascular fluid and proteins into third space. On the molecular level, human chorionic godadotropin (HCG) either exogenous or endogenous, functions as the triggering point for the production of vascular endothelial growth factor (VEGF) that is the main mediator to increase permeability on the vascular bed. Spontaneous OHSS has also been reported, either due to inappropriate activation of a mutant FSH receptor or due to very high levels of HCG during pregnancy. The available evidence on the several preventive and therapeutic approaches with special attention to level 1 evidence when available is also presented. OHSS is a self-resolving condition and the main role of the physician is to correct and maintain the intravascular volume, to support renal function and respiration and prevent thrombotic events. An algorithm on the management of OHSS on an outpatient basis and in the hospital is based on the previous mentioned principles.

KEYWORDS: gonadotropins; ovarian hyperstimulation syndrome (OHSS); oocytes, pregnancy

DEFINITIONS

The term Ovarian Hyperstimulation Syndrome (OHSS) refers to an exacerbated response to medications used for ovarian stimulation such as clomiphene citrate and gonadotropins.[1–5] While the syndrome has been reported occasionally with the use of clomiphene citrate, the vast majority of the cases have been associated with the use of gonadotropins either for ovulation induction in anovulatory women or in the process of superovulation for *in vitro* fertilization. Cases of spontaneous OHSS have also been reported in pregnancy and

Address for correspondence: Nikos F. Vlahos, 28 Dorileou Street, Athens 11521, Greece. Voice: 210-6429-334; fax: 210-748-5591.
e-mail: nvlahos@jhmi.edu

Ann. N.Y. Acad. Sci. 1092: 247–264 (2006). © 2006 New York Academy of Sciences.
doi: 10.1196/annals.1365.021

they are invariably associated with the levels of endogenous human chorionic godadotropin (HCG).[6–11]

CLINICAL PRESENTATION

The use of ovulation stimulating drugs, especially gonadotropins, has been associated with some degree of ovarian hyperstimulation to all women that respond to treatment. The development of more than two or three follicles in intrauterine insemination (IUI) cycles or the development of 10–12 mature follicles with estradiol levels 2000–3000 pg/mL in IVF cycles is supraphysiologic and often associated with mild abdominal discomfort easily tolerated by most of the patients. What, however, distinguishes this common and often desired response to gonadotropins (often called controlled ovarian hyperstimulation) from a potentially life-threatening condition such as OHSS is the severity of the symptoms and signs and the changes in homodynamic variables and fluid balance. Mild and moderate forms of OHSS may occur in 15–20% of all ovarian stimulation cycles, however, the severe form of the syndrome has been reported as frequently as 1–3%.[4] Often there are two phases in the clinical course of the syndrome. The first one follows by 1–2 days the administration of HCG for final follicular maturation the second one may occur 2–3 weeks later at the establishment of a pregnancy and the production of endogenous HCG from the trophoblast.[12]

CLASSIFICATION

There have been several attempts to describe the severity of the syndrome not only to compare the incidence between different types of gonadotropin stimulation but also to evaluate methods of prevention and establish guidelines for the treatment. One of the first methods introduced in 1967 by Rabau et al.[13] combined both clinical and laboratory parameters (24-h urinary levels of estradiol and pregnanediol) to separate six grades of severity followed by Schenker & Weinstein[14] that reclassified the syndrome into three categories and six grades. With the widespread of ultrasonography Golan et al.[15] included the sonographic evaluation of the ovarian size and the presence of ascites as a criterion for OHSS and omitted 24-h urinary measurements of estradiol and pregnanediol as obsolete. In 1992 Navot et al.[16] used specific laboratory cut-off points to define severe and critical OHSS and argued that the ovarian size is not necessarily related to the severity of the syndrome. In 1999 Rizk and Aboulghar[17] proposed their own classification of the syndrome further describing three grades of severe OHSS. Grade A required admission to the hospital and supportive care, grade B required an intensive care unit, and grade C included severe complications of the syndrome (thromboembolic phenomena, renal failure, respiratory distress syndrome, etc.) that required directed treatment. In 2003 the Practice Committee of the American Society for Reproductive Medicine proposed a simplified classification of the syndrome into mild, worsening, and serious.[4] It also defined criteria for outpatient or inpatient management. Serious illness was defined by the presence of abdominal pain plus one or more of the following signs: rapid weight gain, tense ascites, hemodynamic instability, respiratory distress, progressive oliguria, and laboratory abnormalities. Laboratory criteria for women with serious illness include: hematocrit of more than 45%, white cell count of more that 15,000 mm³, sodium less than 135 meq/mL, potassium of more that 5.0 meq/ml, elevated liver enzymes, and serum creatinine of more than 1.2 mg/dL.

According to the Practice Committee most patients with serious illness require hospitalization.[4]

RISK FACTORS

Recognizing risk factors and early signs of impending OHSS is the key to prevention. Young age, low body weight, history of polycystic ovarian syndrome, and previous history of OHSS are some of the factors associated with increased risk of developing OHSS in a subsequent stimulation. Historically high estradiol levels in conjunction to increased numbers of follicles and increased numbers of oocytes retrieved are associated with the development of the syndrome.[18] Nevertheless these variables are not independent from each other and merely reflect increased ovarian response to gonadotropins that eventually leads to the formation of multiple corpora lutea after the retrieval of the oocytes. Needless to say, high levels of estradiol as well as an increased number of follicles are factors that may indicate increased risk of OHSS late in the course of the stimulation. Furthermore, the number of oocytes retrieved may be associated with OHSS but adds nothing to the prevention of the syndrome, since the patient has already received HCG and there is little to be done to prevent the cascade of events. The pivotal role of HCG in the development of OHSS cannot be overemphasized and will be discussed later.

PATHOPHYSIOLOGY AND INVOLVED FACTORS

The key element for the development of the syndrome is increased vascular permeability that leads to fluid shifts from the intravascular to the interstitial or third space compartments. The clinical manifestations originate from the combination of decreased intravascular space and the accumulation of protein-rich fluid into body cavities and interstitial space. Loss of intravascular volume leads to hemodynamic changes manifested as hypotension severe tachycardia, and decreased renal perfusion as well as hemoconcentration. Hemoconcentration with increase in blood coagulability is responsible for arterial and venous thrombotic phenomena in patients with OHSS. Loss of intravascular volume combined with decreased renal perfusion results in electrolyte abnormalities (hyperkalemia, hyponatremia), increase in hematocrit and white cell count, and decrease in creatinine clearance. The most common symptom of OHSS (abdominal discomfort) is due to the development of ascites. Accumulation of protein-rich fluid in the peritoneal cavity leads to abdominal distention and increased intra-abdominal pressure. Compression of the retroperitoneal renal vessel can further compromise renal function and acts synergistically to decrease renal blood flow. The same is true for all the intra-abdominal low-pressure vessels that supply the intestines. Initial venous compression results in parenchyma edema that may further aggravate the one resulting from loss of capillary integrity. Intestinal edema is responsible for the nausea and the diarrhea, which often occur in patients with OHSS. Liver edema is manifested with an increase in liver function tests. Pulmonary function may be compromised in cases of severe OHSS by several mechanisms that act synergistically: elevation of the diaphragm, accumulation of fluid in the pleura, and interstitial edema.

On the molecular levels a variety of factors have been investigated including the ovarian rennin–angiotensin system, prostaglandins, histamine, prolactin, and vascular endothelial factor.[19–26] Estradiol levels have been correlated with the development of OHSS but administration of high doses of estradiol cannot induce the syndrome in an animal model.[27] In addition, a severe form of OHSS has been reported in a patient with 17–20 desmolase deficiency and very low estradiol levels.[28,29] Out of all those factors, the pivotal role of VEGF has been recognized. VEGF is produced from mature follicles under the effect of HCG.[21,30,31] VEGF stimulates mitotic activity of endothelial cells and increases capillary permeability to high molecular weight proteins.[32–35] VEGF is also produced by luteinized granulosa cells[21] and is released into the systemic circulation as well as directly into the peritoneum to induce systemic as well as localized effects.

SPONTANEOUS OHSS

The presence of HCG is the absolute requirement for the development of OHSS. In artificially stimulated cycles the action of HCG on the hyperstimulated ovaries with multiple corpora lutea triggers the cascade of a series of other factors with the end result the disruption of the capillary barrier and the leakage of intravascular fluid.

There are, however, several reports of OHSS not associated with ovarian stimulation that occurred during the course of a normal spontaneous conception. In 1992 severe OHSS occurred in a women with history of Polycystic Ovary Syndrome (PCOS) who conceived spontaneously.[36] Prior to that there were reports on spontaneous OHSS in two women with untreated hypothyroidism.[37,38] There are also reports on recurrent spontaneous OHSS.[25,39,40] Mutations in the FSH receptor have been implicated to the pathophysiology of the spontaneous OHSS.[41–45] It has been shown that promiscuous activation of a mutant FSH receptor is responsible for the development of spontaneous OHSS in women with normal thyroid function and normal levels of HCG. Nevertheless, spontaneous OHSS may also occur due to natural promiscuous activation of a wild-type FSH receptor from abnormally high levels of HCG or TSH.[41] Spontaneous OHSS typically occurs between the 8th and 14th weeks of gestation[46] but second trimester cases have also been reported.[47] Clinically, the syndrome is indistinguishable from the iatrogenic OHSS and the treatment is directed to the underlying cause (i.e., hypothyroidism) and supportive measurements.

STRATEGIES FOR PREVENTION

Once risk factors have been identified a series of strategies has been described to reduce the incidence of OHSS. The most common and reasonable approach is to reduce the initial dose of gonadotropins used for the stimulation. While this is probably the safest approach it is associated with the possibility of a decreased ovarian response that may result either in cycle cancellation or in reduced numbers of oocyte retrieved. The selection of the appropriate gonadotropin dose that can achieve optimal ovarian response yet without leading to OHSS is the art in Assisted Reproductive Technologies (ART).

Coasting is the most popular approach for patients at risk for OHSS followed by administration of human albumin or starch or cryopreservation of all embryos.[48] Coasting is defined as the discontinuation of gonadotrophin once the estradiol levels reach a certain critical level (i.e., >3,000 pg/mL) for 2–3 days and withholding HCG until estradiol levels reach a safer level. Estradiol has been used as a surrogate marker of ovarian activity and a good predicting factor for OHSS. While estradiol by itself does not seem to play any significant role in the development of the syndrome, it can offer a good prediction on the subsequent development of multiple corpora lutea, which release VEGF, the key element in the pathophysiology of OHSS. Hence the reduction of estradiol levels is not the objective of coasting but it is used as a marker of functional granulosa.[49] A possible explanation why acute gonadotropin withdrawal (coasting) may be of benefit relates to the fact that it may lead to apoptosis of small and intermediate size follicles that are more dependent on gonadotropins than the large follicles. The observed reduction of serum estradiol at the end of the coasting period results from the demise of these follicles and subsequent reduction of VEGF.[50,51] Coasting has been used in ovarian stimulation cycles long before in IVF. In a review of 12 studies that included 493 patients at risk for OHSS (E2 > 3,000 pg/mL, 2500–6000 and or number of follicles > 20–30)[52] the observed incidence of severe OHSS in the coasted group was 2.5%. The authors concluded that there was a reduction in the incidence of severe OHSS in high-risk patients. In contrast, in a Cochrane review of evidence on the efficacy of coasting for OHSS prevention, 13 RCT were identified but only 1 met inclusion criteria. According to that study,[53] there was no difference in the incidence of moderate and severe OHSS ($n = 30$, OR $= 0.76$, 95% CI $= 0.18$, 3.24) and in the clinical pregnancy rate ($n = 30$, OR $= 0.75$, 95% CI $= 0.17$, 3.33) between the groups. The authors also concluded that there is a lack of good quality evidence to determine if coasting is an effective method to prevent OHSS. Similarly, there was no difference in the incidence of OHSS in a group of 30 women at risk for OHSS who were randomly allocated into coasting and early follicular aspiration (12 h after HCG).[54] In another study from the same group involving 30 women, unilateral follicular aspiration (6–8 h) prior to HCG did not seem to prevent the development of OHSS.[55]

Administration of human albumin is another popular approach in the prevention as well as in the treatment[5] of OHSS. Albumin has a low molecular weight and is the main contributor to the plasma oncotic pressure. Use of human albumin has been reported in the treatment of conditions associated with capillary leakage and third space accumulation of fluid. Whereas there is widespread belief that human albumin is nontoxic and safe from viral contamination,[56,57] others have argued that albumin is a human product and the possibility of transmission of blood-borne viral or prion infection cannot be excluded entirely.[58–62] There is also no universal agreement on the time of administration or the total dose required.[63,64] In a Cochrane review[65] evaluating randomized controlled trials on the use of albumin five studies were included with 193 patients in the treatment group and 185 controls. The odds ratio for developing OHSS was 0.28 (95% CI 0.11–0.73) in the treated group. According to their findings 18 women at risk for OHSS should have been treated to prevent one case of OHSS. In another prospective randomized placebo controlled clinical trial[66] including 250 patients (cycles) at risk of developing OHSS (estradiol value of more than 3,000 pg/mL or the presence of more than 20 follicles on the day of HCG administration) patients were randomized to receive either 20% human albumin 50 mL ($n = 82$); 6% hydroxyethyl starch (HES) (200/0.5) 500 mL ($n = 85$), or a placebo of 500 mL 0.9% NaCl solution ($n = 83$) over 30 min during oocyte collection. There was no severe OHSS in patients who received albumin and HES while four patients who received placebo developed severe OHSS. On the other hand, moderate OHSS was encountered in four patients in the albumin group; 5 patients receiving HES and 12 patients receiving placebo. There was a significant reduction in the incidence of moderate, severe, and overall OHSS between the HES and albumin treated groups as compared to the 0.9% NaCl group. The authors concluded that HES is a cheaper and safer alternative to human albumin in OHSS prevention.[66] In contrast, in a randomized controlled trial from one center,[64] including 988 patients at risk for OHSS, no benefit was shown from the administration of human albumin. In that study patients were randomized into a treatment group that received 40 g of human albumin and into a control group. Women were monitored on an outpatient basis until menstruation, or until fetal heart activity was detected. From the 977 patients that completed the study there was no difference in blood parameters in terms of hemoconcentration liver and renal dysfunction at 7 days after oocyte retrieval between the two groups. Moderate/severe OHSS was diagnosed in 66 patients and only severe in 46 patients. There was no difference in the incidence of OHSS between the two groups. Furthermore, in women who developed OHSS, there was no difference in the number of patients with paracentesis, hospital admissions, complications, and days of OHSS until resolution between the two groups. The authors concluded that intravenous albumin administration on the day of oocyte retrieval is not a useful means of preventing the development of moderate–severe OHSS. Other agents such as HES[66] and low molecular-weight dextran[67] have been reported to be even more efficacious than human albumin.

Since the initiation of the cascade for the development of OHSS is due to the effect of HCG on the mature follicles and corpora lutea it would make sense that the reduction of the triggering dose of HCG could possibly prevent the development of the syndrome. While in most protocols the usual dose for triggering ovulation is 10,000 IU of HCG it has been shown that a single dose of 5,000 IU or even lower is equally effective in inducing oocyte maturity.[68] There are no randomized controlled trials comparing head to head the two different doses in terms of subsequent development of OHSS. In a retrospective report,[68] however, the use of a lower dose (3,300) of HCG in high responders seems to offer some protection without compromising cycle outcome even if there was no statistical difference documented in the incidence of OHSS. Eliminating completely the administration of HCG could theoretically abolish the risk of OHSS. Alternative methods for inducing oocyte maturation prior to retrieval include the administration of a GnRH agonist that can trigger an endogenous LH surge or recently the administration of recombinant LH instead of HCG.

Inducing oocyte maturation with a GnRH agonist has been used in the past in gonadotropin only stimulated cycles with some success.[69–71] Recently, with the development of stimulation protocols with GnRH antagonist, it became of favor again and several reports have appeared in the literature.[69] Unfortunately, there are also reports associating the use of GnRH agonists for triggering with significantly lower pregnancy rates as compared to conventional triggering with HCG.[72]

The recent development of recombinant LH allowed investigators to evaluate the efficacy of this agent to induce oocyte maturation without the need of exogenous HCG. In a prospective randomized trial, several doses of recombinant LH were compared head to head with 5,000 IU of HCG. It was shown that a single dose 15–30,000 IU of recombinant LH can achieve adequate follicular maturation and can significantly decrease the incidence of moderate OHSS.[73] The cost of such an approach, however, is currently prohibitory.

In the context of OHSS prevention, if a patient has met the criteria for any stage of OHSS in the course of a stimulation cycle consideration should be given to the possibility of canceling the cycle if it is early in the stimulation, or withholding HCG injection if the cycle is at culmination. If HCG has already been administered, the patient and her partner need to be counseled about the potential risks of proceeding with IUI or embryo transfer and she should be aware that her condition may worsen if pregnancy ensues. Withholding transfer and cryopreserving of the resulting embryos for transfer at a later time cannot, of course, prevent the early phase of OHSS but may prevent the late second phase.

MANAGEMENT OF OHSS

Depending on the severity of the condition inpatient or outpatient management includes careful monitoring and supportive measurements. OHSS is a self-resolving condition and there is no specific treatment. Generally the decision to admit a patient to the hospital is based on the severity of the symptoms and the hemodynamic changes.

OUTPATIENT MANAGEMENT OF PATIENTS WITH OHSS

Management of a patient at home involves adequate oral fluid and electrolyte replacement, daily weight monitoring, and measurement of urine output. Since fluid replacement is of paramount importance patients who cannot tolerate fluids should be admitted. The same is true for patients with respiratory distress and severe abdominal discomfort. Patients should engage in light physical activity as tolerated. Hyperstimulated ovaries are markedly enlarged and therefore prone to ovarian torsion. While restriction of physical activity is recommended, strict bed rest is not advisable since these patients are in a hypercoagulable state that may result in thromboembolic episodes. Animal data have supported the use of prostaglandin inhibitors as treatment[74,75] for OHSS. Borenstein *et al.*, however, demonstrated that for patients with severe OHSS, paracentesis alone was superior to a medical regimen that included indomethacin, in bringing about resolution of the disease.[74]

Patients should record the volume of their 24-h fluid intake and urine output. These records are reviewed with the patient on a daily basis, usually over the phone. Fluid intake of less than 1,000 mL/day, urine output of less than 1,000 mL/day, or a fluid balance discrepancy of more than a 1,000 mL/day are matters of concern. Many popular "sports drinks" are electrolyte balanced to correct for dehydration conditions. These would seem to be optimal in the outpatient management of OHSS patients who require hydration but must minimize "free water," which will probably contribute to third space fluid and ascites. Weight changes should also be monitored daily, and patients should be queried about symptoms and appetite. If symptoms are worsening, appetite is decreasing, or if there is a weight gain of more than 2 lbs/day, the patient should be reevaluated to determine if admission is required.

IN-HOUSE MANAGEMENT OF PATIENTS WITH OHSS

Any patient with serious illness should be admitted.[4] In addition to daily physical examination, checking of vital signs every 4 h, and tabulation of fluid balance every 4 h, the following parameters are monitored on a daily basis:

- Leukocyte count.
- Hemoglobin concentration and hematocrit.
- Full electrolyte panel.
- Liver function tests.
- Daily weights and abdominal girth.
- Prothrombin time (PT) and partial tromboplastin time (PTT) are initially measured to obtain a baseline value in case therapeutic anticoagulation is later necessary.

If liver function tests are initially normal, these only need to be repeated periodically if the patient's hospital stay becomes prolonged. A chest X-ray and pulse oximetry are mandatory for any patient with shortness of breath or any other signs of pulmonary compromise. Repeated abdominal ultrasonography should be reserved for situations in which the findings may direct clinical management or as needed for paracentesis. Leukocyte count, hemoglobin level, and hematocrit should be measured on at least a daily basis, since the degree of hemoconcentration and blood viscosity have been shown to closely correlate with the severity of OHSS.[74] It is not uncommon for OHSS patients to have a leukocyte count in the range of 20,000–30,000 cells/mm^3. The patient's overall stress response to her discomfort, as well as hemoconcentration, accounts for this finding. Although leukocytosis is commonly found, a leukocyte count of 22,000 cells/mm^3 or more has been reported as an ominous sign of imminent thromboembolism. Daily assessment of electrolytes is necessary since the hyperpermeability of the vasculature in OHSS can result in rapid dynamic changes of both sodium and potassium levels. Information should also be available on a daily basis to be used for calculation of creatinine clearance. Weight loss and reversal of abdominal girth seem to correlate well with reversal of OHSS. With the above parameters serving as a framework for daily clinical assessment, the clinical management of the OHSS patient is threefold: fluid management, prevention of thrombosis, and treatment of ascites.[5]

Fluid and Electrolyte Management

Typically, the patients with severe OHSS are hypovolemic due to decreased oral intake, third space fluid retention, and vomiting or diarrhea. A hematocrit of 45% or more at the time of admission to the hospital is not unusual. A fluid bolus of 1 L of normal saline intravenously over 1 h should restore an adequate urine output of at least 50 cc/h. An IV fluid "maintenance" protocol of 5% dextrose in normal saline (D5NS) at 125–150 mL/h should follow with urine output and hematocrit assessed every 4–6 h to evaluate the reversal of hemoconcentration. Theoretically, intravenous fluid hydration to correct hemoconcentration may exacerbate the patient's ascites and possibly lead to pulmonary edema and respiratory distress. As long as pulmonary status is closely monitored, and the patient has adequate urine output this possibility is remote. If there is inadequate response in urine output from the initial fluid bolus, crystalloid fluids are stopped and a regimen of low-volume, hyperosmolar therapy is begun. An IV infusion of 200 mL of 25% human albumin solution is given over 4 h for a total of 50 g of albumin per 4-h interval, with a recheck of hematocrit approximately 1 h after the infusion. This protocol is repeated in a serial fashion until the hematocrit is brought within 36–38%. The relatively low total IV input of a hyperosmotic agent at this point should help to increase intravascular oncotic pressure to draw third space fluid back into the intravascular space. It is important to infuse intravenous albumin slowly, since a bolus may reverse hemoconcentration so quickly that hemodilution actually develops, with subsequent leakage of free water back into third spaces (e.g., pulmonary edema) before renal filtration occurs. Once a hematocrit of 36–38% has been achieved, but oliguria persists, furosemide (20 mg IV) may be given to assess renal response. It is important to document a correction in hemoconcentration before diuretics are initiated. Use of diuretics in an intravascularly depleted patient will only worsen hemoconcentration, increase the risk for a thrombotic event, and cause vascular collapse. Human albumin for hospital use in the United States has been subjected to alcohol fractionation and heat inactivation so that it is free of both enveloped and nonenveloped viruses; nevertheless, the possibility of prion transmission, as mentioned previously, cannot be completely eliminated.

Other "plasma expanders" have been used to increase intravascular oncotic pressure and thus bring third space fluid back into the intravascular space, including mannitol,[16] dextran,[76] and fresh frozen plasma.[74] In these studies, dextran was associated with development of ARDS, and neither mannitol nor fresh frozen plasma has been shown to be superior to albumin in treating OHSS.

Intravenous albumin administered to the OHSS patient as a single therapeutic agent has been shown to normalize hematocrit and induce diuresis.[77] In cases of severe oliguria or anuria despite adequate fluid replacement and treatment with human albumin and diuretics, paracentesis of the ascetic fluid should be performed without delay. Most of the patients, however, will respond to this supportive management within 24–48 h. As soon as the intravascular volume and electrolyte changes have been corrected, and the patient has adequate urine output with relatively benign physical examination, she can be switched to oral hydration and feeding. Once the patient can tolerate oral intake she could be discharged to home. She should be monitored continuously, however, in an outpatient basis until all signs and symptoms of OHSS have completely resolved. The patients should be warned that if the subsequent pregnancy testing is positive, the possibility of re-exacerbation of OHSS is quite possible.

Thrombosis Prevention

Patients with severe OHSS are treated with subcutaneous heparin (5,000 U twice daily) or with low molecular weight heparin (LMWH) immediately on admission to the hospital. This regimen is continued throughout the hospital stay. Since these patients are likely to be very inactive, we also place thigh-high venous support stockings for the duration of hospitalization. Otherwise, the patient is encouraged to ambulate frequently and avoid prolonged sedentary positions. The use of intermittent pneumatic compression hose for the legs is advisable for the patient who is so uncomfortable that she is essentially confined to bed. These measures, together with prompt correction of the intravascular volume should be adequate for thrombosis prevention. The physician should be well aware of the signs and symptoms of acute thrombosis and have a ready plan for diagnostic testing, therapeutic anticoagulation, and appropriate care in the event of thrombosis.

Ascites Management

Some degree of abdominal ascites will usually already be present in most cases of OHSS requiring hospitalization. The previously discussed protocol of fluid management will hopefully halt and reverse the process of ascites accumulation or, at worst, only contribute a small amount of additional fluid to the existing ascites. Once euvolemia is maintained and the syndrome begins to subside, the ascites fluid will shift back to the intravascular space, thus initiating spontaneous, sometimes massive, diuresis. Such cases usually do not require surgical intervention for drainage of ascites. In our experience,[5] the following three situations serve as indications for paracentesis to relieve abdominal ascites:

- Severe discomfort or pain
- Respiratory compromise (as assessed by persistent tachypnea, shortness of breath, etc.)

- Low-pulse oximetry, or evidence of hydrothorax
- Evidence of renal compromise that does not respond to other measures

Often, despite adequate fluid replacement of the intravascular volume, there is persistent or worsening oliguria and renal compromise in patients with severe OHSS. This is due to the increased intra-abdominal pressure resulting from massive ascites that may initially compress the retroperitoneal renal veins and subsequently the renal arteries leading to decreased renal perfusion and renal failure. This condition should be recognized promptly and requires immediate paracentesis of the ascitic fluid to correct renal dysfunction.[78] Paracentesis can be accomplished either abdominally or under sonographic visualization in a similar manner to the oocyte retrieval. In case of massive ovarian enlargement, abdominal paracentesis may be particularly difficult. During the transvaginal approach a slightly reverse Trendeleburg position during the procedure seems to cause less pulmonary compromise and may allow a more efficient fluid evacuation.[79,80]

MANAGEMENT OF THE OHSS PATIENT
IN THE INTENSIVE CARE UNIT

With early recognition of OHSS and prompt, aggressive, and vigilant attention to fluid management, thrombosis prevention, and treatment of ascites, most cases should not result in critical sequelae. OHSS can, however, be unpredictable in severity and course. Renal failure, hepatic damage, thromboembolic phenomena, and ARDS are known to occur despite attentive care. Intensive care unit monitoring is required for any patient with renal failure that is not responding to previously mentioned treatments, thrombotic events that require therapeutic anticoagulation, or pulmonary compromise resulting in persistent hypoxia or abnormal arterial blood gas indices despite paracentesis.

Renal failure should be treated initially with a "renal dose" dopamine drip but may also require hemodialysis. Treatment of oliguric severe OHSS patients using an intravenous dopamine regimen of 0.18 mg/kg/h has been shown to dilate renal vessels and increase renal blood flow without affecting blood pressure or heart rate.[81] A central venous catheter should be placed so that central venous pressure (CVP) and pulmonary capillary wedge pressure (PCWP) monitoring can assist in fluid management. Thrombotic events should be treated aggressively with therapeutic anticoagulation and reversal of hemoconcentration. Pulmonary compromise should be treated initially with high-percentage inspired oxygen supplementation, and intubation and assisted ventilation if needed. Thoracocentesis may be necessary for significant hydrothorax. Serial arterial blood gas measurements should be monitored, and a ventilation-perfusion scan should be obtained if pulmonary embolus is suspected. The abdomen and pelvis should be appropriately shielded during diagnostic radiology procedures to prevent radiation exposure to an early pregnancy. If, however, an early pregnancy has been diagnosed in the patient with critical complications of OHSS, elective termination should be considered to prevent further deterioration of her condition.

ADDITIONAL TREATMENT OPTIONS

The variety of factors that have been implicated in the pathophysiology of OHSS has led to the development of several other therapeutic approaches. None of those, however, has gained wide acceptance. Prostaglandin inhibitors, mainly indomethacin, have been used as a preventive and/or therapeutic agent with conflicting results.[74,82] Glucocorticoids have been shown to be ineffective in preventing OHSS.[83] Despite evidence of angiotensin II as a potential ovarian mediator in OHSS, it is unclear whether angiotensin-converting enzyme inhibitors or angiotensin receptor inhibitors may be an effective or appropriate treatment for OHSS in humans. Furthermore, these drugs are relatively contraindicated in pregnancy, thus limiting their applicability in patients with a potential pregnancy. Case reports have described replacing intravascular volume with protein-rich ascites fluid with favorable results.[84,85]

OHSS represents one of the most important complications of ovarian stimulation. Only recently its pathophysiology has been investigated further mainly implicating the secretion of VEGF from corpora lutea under the effect of HCG. Current management is focused on supportive care until the spontaneous resolution of the condition. Target-specific drugs (i.e., VEGF blocking agents) could offer theoretical advantages but are still remote from clinical applications in humans. Prevention cannot be overemphasized and fine tuning of the gonadotropin dose combined to close surveillance for early signs of exacerbated response could theoretically prevent at least some of these cases.

REFERENCES

1. ENGEL, T. *et al*. 1972. Ovarian hyperstimulation syndrome. Report of a case with notes on pathogenesis and treatment. Am. J. Obstet. Gynecol. **112:** 1052–1060.
2. GAYRAL, M.N., D. MILLET & A. NETTER. 1975. Ovarian hyperstimulation syndrome. Notes on the physiopathology and treatment apropos of 3 cases. J. Gynecol. Obstet. Biol. Reprod. (Paris) **4:** 255–266.
3. BORENSTEIN, R. *et al*. 1981. Ovarian hyperstimulation syndrome after different treatment schedules. Int. J. Fertil. **26:** 279–282.
4. OVARIAN HYPERSTIMULATION SYNDROME. 2004. Fertil. Steril. **82**(Suppl. 1): S81–S86.
5. WHELAN, J.G., III & N.F. VLAHOS. 2000. The ovarian hyperstimulation syndrome. Fertil. Steril. **73:** 883–896.
6. ABU-LOUZ, S.K., A.A. AHMED & R.W. SWAN. 1997. Spontaneous ovarian hyperstimulation syndrome with pregnancy. Am. J. Obstet. Gynecol. **177:** 476–477.

7. AKERMAN, F.M. *et al.* 2000. A case of spontaneous ovarian hyperstimulation syndrome with a potential mutation in the hCG/LH receptor gene. Fertil. Steril. **74:** 403–404.

8. AYHAN, A., Z.S. TUNCER & A.T. AKSU. 1996. Ovarian hyperstimulation syndrome associated with spontaneous pregnancy. Hum. Reprod. **11:** 1600–1601.

9. CEPNI, I. *et al.* 2006. Spontaneous ovarian hyperstimulation syndrome presenting with acute abdomen. J. Postgrad. Med. **52:** 154–155.

10. CHAE, H.D. *et al.* 2001. Ovarian hyperstimulation syndrome complicating a spontaneous singleton pregnancy: a case report. J. Assist. Reprod. Genet. **18:** 120–123.

11. CHEN, C.P., C.W. CHEN & K.G. WANG. 1996. Spontaneous ovarian hyperstimulation syndrome and hyperprolactinemia in primary hypothyroidism. Acta. Obstet. Gynecol. Scand. **75:** 70–71.

12. LYONS, C.A. *et al.* 1994. Early and late presentation of the ovarian hyperstimulation syndrome: two distinct entities with different risk factors. Hum. Reprod. **9:** 792–799.

13. RABAU, E. *et al.* 1967. Human menopausal gonadotropins for anovulation and sterility. Results of 7 years of treatment. Am. J. Obstet. Gynecol. **98:** 92–98.

14. SCHENKER, J.G. & D. WEINSTEIN. 1978. Ovarian hyperstimulation syndrome: a current survey. Fertil. Steril. **30:** 255–268.

15. GOLAN, A. *et al.* 1989. Ovarian hyperstimulation syndrome: an update review. Obstet. Gynecol. Surv. **44:** 430–440.

16. NAVOT, D., P.A. BERGH & N. LAUFER. 1992. Ovarian hyperstimulation syndrome in novel reproductive technologies: prevention and treatment. Fertil. Steril. **58:** 249–261.

17. RIZK, B. & M. ABOULGHAR. 1999. Classification, pathophysiology and management of the ovarian hyperstimulation syndrome. *In In vitro* Fertilization and Assisted Reproduction. P. Brisden, Ed.: 131–155. The Parthenon Publishing Group. New York. London.

18. ASCH, R.H. *et al.* 1991. Severe ovarian hyperstimulation syndrome in assisted reproductive technology: definition of high risk groups. Hum. Reprod. **6:** 1395–1399.

19. AGRAWAL, R. 2000. What's new in the pathogenesis and prevention of ovarian hyperstimulation syndrome? Hum. Fertil. (Camb) **3:** 112–115.

20. DOURRON, N.E. & D.B. WILLIAMS. 1996. Prevention and treatment of ovarian hyperstimulation syndrome. Semin. Reprod. Endocrinol. **14:** 355–365.

21. NEULEN, J. *et al.* 1995. Human chorionic gonadotropin-dependent expression of vascular endothelial growth factor/vascular permeability factor in human granulosa cells: importance in ovarian hyperstimulation syndrome. J. Clin. Endocrinol. Metab. **80:** 1967–1971.

22. PAU, E. *et al.* 2006. Plasma levels of soluble vascular endothelial growth factor receptor-1 may determine the onset of early and late ovarian hyperstimulation syndrome. Hum. Reprod. **21:** 1453–1460.

23. RIZK, B. *et al.* 1997. The role of vascular endothelial growth factor and interleukins in the pathogenesis of severe ovarian hyperstimulation syndrome. Hum. Reprod. Update **3:** 255–266.

24. DELBAERE, A. *et al.* 1994. Angiotensin II immunoreactivity is elevated in ascites during severe ovarian hyperstimulation syndrome: implications for pathophysiology and clinical management. Fertil. Steril. **62:** 731–737.

25. DI CARLO, C. *et al.* 1997. Increased concentrations of renin, aldosterone and Ca125 in a case of spontaneous, recurrent, familial, severe ovarian hyperstimulation syndrome. Hum. Reprod. **12:** 2115–2117.

26. GUL, T.G., C. POSACI & S. CALISKAN. 2001. The role of enalapril in the prevention of ovarian hyperstimulation syndrome: a rabbit model. Hum. Reprod. **16:** 2253–2257.

27. PRIDE, S.M., C. JAMES & B.H. HO YUEN. 1990. The ovarian hyperstimulation syndrome. Semin. Reprod. Endocrinol. **8:** 247–260.

28. BAUMANN, P. & K. DIEDRICH. 2000. Thromboembolic complications associated with reproductive endocrinologic procedures. Hematol. Oncol. Clin. North. Am. **14:** 431–443.

29. PELLICER, A. *et al*. 1991. *In vitro* fertilization as a diagnostic and therapeutic tool in a patient with partial 17,20-desmolase deficiency. Fertil. Steril. **55:** 970–975.

30. WANG, T.H. *et al*. 2002. Human chorionic gonadotropin-induced ovarian hyperstimulation syndrome is associated with up-regulation of vascular endothelial growth factor. J. Clin. Endocrinol. Metab. **87:** 3300–3308.

31. PELLICER, A. *et al*. 1999. The pathogenesis of ovarian hyperstimulation syndrome: *in vivo* studies investigating the role of interleukin-1beta, interleukin-6, and vascular endothelial growth factor. Fertil. Steril. **71:** 482–489.

32. ELBJEIRAMI, W.M., & J.L. WEST. 2006. Angiogenesis-like activity of endothelial cells co-cultured with VEGF-producing smooth muscle cells. Tissue Eng. **12:** 381–390.

33. BIANCO, F. *et al*. 2005. Angiogenic activity of swine granulosa cells: effects of hypoxia and the role of VEGF. Vet. Res. Commun. **29**(Suppl. 2): 157–159.

34. VALABLE, S. *et al*. 2005. VEGF-induced BBB permeability is associated with an MMP-9 activity increase in cerebral ischemia: both effects decreased by Ang-1. J. Cereb. Blood Flow Metab. **25:** 1491–1504.

35. WEIS, S. *et al*. 2004. Endothelial barrier disruption by VEGF-mediated Src activity potentiates tumor cell extravasation and metastasis. J. Cell Biol. **167:** 223–229.

36. ZALEL, Y. *et al*. 1992. Spontaneous ovarian hyperstimulation syndrome concomitant with spontaneous pregnancy in a woman with polycystic ovary disease. Am. J. Obstet. Gynecol. **167:** 122–124.

37. ROTMENSCH, S. & A. SCOMMEGNA. 1989. Spontaneous ovarian hyperstimulation syndrome associated with hypothyroidism. Am. J. Obstet. Gynecol. **160:** 1220–1222.

38. NAPPI, R.G. *et al*. 1998. Natural pregnancy in hypothyroid woman complicated by spontaneous ovarian hyperstimulation syndrome. Am. J. Obstet. Gynecol. **178:** 610–611.

39. ZALEL, Y. *et al*. 1995. Recurrent spontaneous ovarian hyperstimulation syndrome associated with polycystic ovary syndrome. Gynecol. Endocrinol. **9:** 313–315.

40. OLATUNBOSUN, O.A. *et al*. 1996. Spontaneous ovarian hyperstimulation syndrome in four consecutive pregnancies. Clin. Exp. Obstet. Gynecol. **23:** 127–132.

41. DE LEENER, A. *et al*. 2006. Presence and absence of follicle-stimulating hormone receptor mutations provide some insights into spontaneous ovarian hyperstimulation syndrome physiopathology. J. Clin. Endocrinol. Metab. **91:** 555–562.

42. DAELEMANS, C. *et al*. 2004. Prediction of severity of symptoms in iatrogenic ovarian hyperstimulation syndrome by follicle-stimulating hormone receptor Ser680Asn polymorphism. J. Clin. Endocrinol. Metab. **89:** 6310–6315.

43. MONTANELLI, L. *et al*. 2004. Modulation of ligand selectivity associated with activation of the transmembrane region of the human follitropin receptor. Mol. Endocrinol. **18:** 2061–2073.

44. MONTANELLI, L. *et al*. 2004. A mutation in the follicle-stimulating hormone receptor as a cause of familial spontaneous ovarian hyperstimulation syndrome. J. Clin. Endocrinol. Metab. **89:** 1255–1258.

81. FERRARETTI, A.P. *et al.* 1992. Dopamine treatment for severe ovarian hyperstimu-
    lation syndrome. Hum. Reprod. **7:** 180–183.
82. PRIDE, S.M., B. HO YUEN & Y.S. MOON. 1984. Clinical, endocrinologic, and in-
    traovarian prostaglandin F responses to H-1 receptor blockade in the ovarian
    hyperstimulation syndrome: studies in the rabbit model. Am. J. Obstet. Gynecol.
    148: 670–674.
83. TAN, S.L. *et al.* 1992. The administration of glucocorticoids for the prevention of
    ovarian hyperstimulation syndrome in *in vitro* fertilization: a prospective ran-
    domized study. Fertil. Steril. **58:** 378–383.
84. BECK, D.H. *et al.* 1995. Continuous ascitic recirculation in severe ovarian hyper-
    stimulation syndrome. Intensive Care Med. **21:** 590–593.
85. FUKAYA, T. *et al.* 1994. Treatment of severe ovarian hyperstimulation syndrome
    by ultrafiltration and reinfusion of ascitic fluid. Fertil. Steril. **61:** 561–564.

Fertility Drugs and Gynecologic Cancer

NIKOS KANAKAS AND THEMIS MANTZAVINOS

In Vitro *Fertilization Unit, Euromedica, Athens, Greece*

ABSTRACT: Fertility drugs (FD) are spreading worldwide fast and therefore many studies have reviewed the possible association between the use of these drugs and cancer. Since the drugs used for ovulation induction during *in vitro* fertilization (IVF) like hCG, hMG, rFSH increase the levels of gonadal hormones, concerns have grown regarding the risk of developing cancer in breast, ovary, endometrium, and other target organs. In this review, we discuss a number of different studies published in recent years that show no association between the use of these drugs and most cancers.

KEYWORDS: fertility drugs; cancer; *in vitro* fertilization; ovulation induction

INTRODUCTION

In the past three decades follow-up studies and multiple case reports have discussed the safety of ovulation-inducing drugs and the risks associated with their use. Ovulation-inducing drugs are widely used for ovarian follicular stimulation during *in vitro* fertilization (IVF) cycles. IVF treatment programs were initially designed to treat women with mechanical infertility and no evidence of ovulation disturbances. Currently, IVF treatment programs are used to treat all types of infertility.

CANCER INCIDENCE FOLLOWING TREATMENT FOR INFERTILITY

A Dutch study estimated that between 14% and 16.5% of couples seek medical care for infertility problems during their reproductive life.[1,2] In the United States, it is estimated that almost 2.5% of live births per year result from assisted reproductive technologies. In the United States, the number of women treated annually with fertility drugs (FD) has nearly doubled between 1973 and 1991. Further increase in rates of use can be expected given recent

Address for correspondence: Dr. N. Kanakas, Kifisias Ave. 11526 Athens, Greece. Voice and fax: 0030210 777 99 20.
e-mail: nkanakas@hol.gr

Ann. N.Y. Acad. Sci. 1092: 265–278 (2006). © 2006 New York Academy of Sciences.
doi: 10.1196/annals.1365.022

projections that by the year 2015 between 5.4 and 7.7 million women aged 15–44 years will be diagnosed with some form of infertility.[3,4]

In the past years, much attention has been focused on the possible association between the use of FD and the development of malignancies of the ovary, breast, endometrium, and thyroid gland as well as of melanoma.

A number of investigations have attempted to address the long-term effects of ovulation-inducing drugs on cancer risk, but most have had shortcomings. These include small number of study subjects, short follow-up, imprecise information on drug exposures and indications for usage, and absence of information on other correlates of drug exposure that could influence cancer risk.[5–8]

Since hormonal and reproductive factors are known to be involved in the etiology of cancers of the female reproductive system, a stimulating effect of FD on the risk of these cancers is theoretically possible. The precise mechanisms involved in the pathogenesis of hormone-related cancers remain unclear, and thus, it is difficult to predict how and to which extent FD may affect the risk of various cancers.

Ovarian cancer is the fifth most common malignancy in women in developed countries and accounts for approximately 4% of all malignancies in females. In general, the highest incidence rates of ovarian cancer are seen in North America and Scandinavia whereas the lowest rates are seen in Asia.[9]

The large majority of ovarian malignancies originates from the ovarian epithelium (80–90%). Nonepithelial tumors of the ovary, such as germ cell tumors and sex-cord tumors, originate from the ovarian stroma and account for only 4–6% of all ovarian neoplasms.

To explain the epidemiology of epithelial ovarian cancer, three main hypotheses have been developed. First, ovarian cancer might be caused by repeated ovulations disrupting the ovarian epithelium and leading to malignant transformation of the epithelial cells.[10] The second hypothesis proposes a model in which persistent stimulation of the ovary by gonadotrophins increases the risk of malignant changes.[11] The third hypothesis proposes a carcinogenic role for exposure of the ovarian epithelium to environmental agents, such as talcum powder, that may enter the pelvic cavity through the vaginal canal. Talcum powder can be contaminated with asbestos minerals known to be associated with excess mortality from various cancers.[12]

Recently, another two new hypotheses have been postulated. One is the "endometriosis hypothesis" where endometriosis may act to promote the development of ovarian cancer if endometriotic implants cause irritation and subsequently an inflammatory reaction.[13] The other hypothesis is that ovarian cancer may be increased by factors associated with excess androgenic stimulation of ovarian epithelial cells and may be decreased by factors related to greater progesterone stimulation.

Three lines of evidence raise concern regarding potential effects of ovulation-inducing drugs on cancer risk. First the most commonly used medications,

TABLE 1. Review of major cohorts reporting association between fertility drugs and ovarian cancer risk (Brinton et al.).[15]

Location	No.	Years	Follow-up
Israel (Ron et al.)[39]	2,575	1964–1974	12.3
USA (Rossing et al.)[18]	3,837	1974–1985	12.3
Australia (Venn et al.)[22]	10,358	1978–1992	6.5
Israel (Modan et al.)[37]	2,496	1964–1974	21.4
Israel (Potashnik et al.)[26]	1,197	1960–1984	17.9
USA (Croughan-Minihane et al.)[19]	51,371	1965–1998	5.6
Netherlands (Klip et al.)[23]	25,152	1980–1995	5.6
UK (Doyle et al.)[24]	5,556	1975–1989	7.9
USA (Brinton et al.)[20]	12,193	1965–1988	18.8
Israel (Dor et al.)[27]	5,026	1981–1992	3.6
Israel (Lerner-Geva et al.)[48]	1,082	1984–1992	6.5

clomiphene citrate and gonadotropins, are effective for stimulating ovulation, a factor implicated in the etiology of both breast and ovarian cancers. Second, these drugs raise both E_2 and P levels, hormones that are recognized as affecting the development and growth of breast and gynecology cancers as well as some other cancers. Finally, some clinical and epidemiological studies have linked use of these drugs with an increased incidence of various cancers.

Epidemiological studies were carefully reviewed with respect to methodological strengths and weaknesses.[14–16] Many cohort studies have had short follow-up periods and thus effects that require long latency intervals may remain undetectable. Participants in these studies are often still young and have not yet reached the age of peak cancer incidence (TABLE 1).

The availability of appropriate comparison groups is also problematic for cohort studies. In many of these studies, the disease experience of cohorts of infertile women is compared with the experience of the general population through the calculation of standardized incidence ratios (SIRs). SIRs compare the number of observed cancers in the cohort of interest to the number expected based on incidence rates in the general population.

The general population incidence rates take into account age, race, and calendar time but have no information about the likely differences in other cancer predictors between infertile women and the rest of the population. Of notable concern is the inability to adjust for parity, a recognized risk factor for breast, endometrical, and ovarian cancers. Additionally, anovulation, a major indication for drug usage, has been linked in a number of endometrial and possibly breast cancers. Other causes of infertility have also been related to the risks of subsequent cancers: endometriosis to ovarian and breast cancers and tubal factor to ovarian cancers. Thus, comparisons of cancer rates among infertile women (with or without ovulation induction) with cancer rates in the general population can be difficult to interpret.

OVARIAN CANCER

Numerous clinical reports have expressed concern about a potential link between the use of ovulation-inducing drugs and ovarian cancer risk. Klip *et al.* published an extensive review of this subject using as methodology: identification of papers published between 1966 and 1999, examination of FD, and specific causes of subfertility in relation to the risk of cancers of the ovary, breast, endometrium, thyroid, and melanoma.[17] The results showed no difference in cancer risk between treated and untreated patients.

Rossing *et al.* from Seattle studied the long-time use of clomiphene citrate in 3,837 women between 1974 and 1985. There were 11 invasive ovarian tumors as compared with an expected number of 4.4. The relative risk (RR) of ovarian cancer associated with long-term use (12 cycles) of clomiphene citrate was 9.1 among women without ovulatory abnormalities and 7.4 among women with ovulatory abnormalities. Thus, both among women with and without ovulatory abnormalities, an extended period of subfertility treatment with clomiphene citrate was associated with an increased risk of ovarian malignancies (2.3-fold increased risk). Use of clomiphene for less than 1 year was not associated with an increased risk, but five of the nine women with cancer had taken the drug for 12 or more monthly cycles resulting in a RR of 11.1.[18]

In the industrial world, 10 new cases of ovarian cancer develop per 100,000 women (all ages) per year corresponding to a life risk of 2%. The etiology of ovarian cancer of multifactorial several studies is that infertility implies an increased risk, although less pronounced than in nulliparity.

In another United States published abstract, it was also found no effect of ovulation-inducing drugs on ovarian cancer risk by Croughan-Minihane *et al.*[19] After 5.6 years of follow-up of 51,371 patients seen for conception difficulties or ovum donation in 15 California clinics between 1965 and 1998, 50 ovarian cancers were diagnosed. Several recent cohort studies have failed to provide confirmatory evidence for a large increase in ovarian cancer risk associated with use of FD. The most recent of these published studies by Brinton *et al.* was a multicenter retrospective cohort study conducted in five U.S. areas.[20] This study followed 12,193 infertile women for a median of 18.8 years and had detailed information on drug exposures and causes of infertility from medical records as well as questionnaire data on potential cancer risk factors for a substantial proportion of the patients. This study was unique in being able to identify subjects who underwent a bilateral oophorectomy and were thus no longer at risk for developing ovarian cancer. The results were largely reassuring, showing no increase in risk associated with every use of either clomiphene or gonadotrophins followed for the longest period of time, that is, 15 or more years.[21]

Most malignant ovarian tumors arise from the epithelial cells that are present around the ovary or in underlying inclusion cysts. The risk of epithelial ovarian cancer is decreased by factors that suppress ovulation (e.g., pregnancy, breast feeding, oral contraceptive pill) whereas uninterrupted ovulation (nulliparity) and more recently hyperovulation (infertility drugs) have been associated with increased risk. Ovulation may encourage the development of ovarian cancer by increasing exposure of epithelial cells to gonadotropins and other growth factors or by stimulating formation of possible premalignant epithelial inclusion cysts. Alternatively, ovulation may lead to increased proliferation of ovarian epithelial cells to repair the ovulatory defect in the ovarian surface, which may increase the frequency of spontaneous mutations.

Epithelial ovarian cancer is exceedingly rare in women with Turner syndrome, who are anovulatory. In addition, epithelial ovarian cancer is rare in other animal species, such as rats and mice, which ovulate infrequently; whereas it is common in hens, which like humans are frequent ovulators.

Several other observations that are somewhat inconsistent with the gonadotropin hypothesis would predict that breast feeding should increase the risk of ovarian cancer due to increase in pituitary secretion of FSH, whereas breast feeding has been shown to be protective in most studies. In addition, the gonadotropin hypothesis would predict that estrogen replacement therapy after menopause should decrease risk due to suppression of pituitary gonadotropin secretion, whereas no protective effect has been demonstrated. However, gonadotropin levels in postmenopausal women receiving hormone replacement remain higher than those of premenopausal women. Therefore, it is not clear whether the lack of protective effect of hormone replacement is because levels remain above a critical threshold or because gonadotropins do not influence the carcinogenic process.

Ovarian tumor risk observed in studies was associated with length of time in infertility treatment and nullgravid. However, no associations of risk were found for ovulation-inducing drugs and risk, even when dose, formulation, and number of treatment cycles were considered.

While these studies focused primarily on woman exposed to ovulation-inducing agents at earlier times, a number of other studies have concentrated on exposures received during IVF. From 29,666 women referred to 10 Australian IVF clinics, 13 ovarian cancers were observed during a follow-up period of 7–8 years.[22] The investigators had detailed information on indications for FD use, but only limited information on patient characteristics. The standardized incidence ratio (SIR) overall was 0.99, with no higher risk for the women who underwent at least one IVF treatment cycle (0.88) as compared with those who received no drug treatment (1.16). Women with unexplained infertility were at a significantly increased risk compared with the general population, but within this subgroup there was no difference in risk between treated and untreated women.

In a cohort of 25,152 women treated for subfertility in the Netherlands, Klip et al. observed 17 ovarian cancers during 5.6 years of following up. The strength of this study included detailed information on causes of infertility and drug exposures from medical records, as well as on cancer risk predictors, obtained through completed questionnaires from many of the study subjects. The results showed no difference in risk between treated and untreated subjects, even when the number of cycles or ampoules received were considered.[23]

Selected cohort studies and case-control studies reporting associations between FD and ovarian cancer risk have been published by Rossing et al., Brinton et al., Venn et al., Doyle et al., Kashyap et al., Potashnik et al., and Dor et al.[12,18,22,24–27]

It has also been questioned whether fertility medications might have a preferential effect on certain ovarian tumor types. Clear cell, malignant germ cell, and granulosa cell tumors of ovulation linked by case reports to the use of ovulation-inducing drugs. Granulosa cell tumors appear to be of particular interest given existing evidence that gonadotropins can induce these tumors in rodents and stimulate cells in human in vitro models.

However, arguing against a specific relationship for granulosa cell tumors, descriptive data from Finland show decreases in the incidence of this tumor concomitant with increasing use of ovulation inducers.[28]

Based on the evidence to date, there is no conclusive link between FD use and ovarian cancer. However, most of the studies had relatively small numbers and/or short follow-up. Because of the lack of large studies with sufficient follow-up time since FD use, the discussion about a possible association is mostly inspired by theories concerning the pathogenesis of ovarian cancer. In contrast, multiple punctures as needed for IVF may, through repeated ruptures of the ovarian epithelium, cause increased mitotic activity in the ovary. The etiology of ovarian cancer is probably multifactorial with genetic, environmental, and endocrinological factors interacting in various causal pathways.

It must be kept in mind that most subfertile women use FD for a period that is rather limited as compared to the total length of their reproductive lives. Even if ovulation-inducing agents do exert a stimulatory effect on ovarian cancer risk, it is questionable whether such an effect would be detectable.

In summary, uninterrupted ovulation is the strongest predisposing risk factor for ovarian cancer development in several ways, including increased hormone and growth factor exposure that leads to proliferation and inclusion cyst formation in the epithelium. In addition to other studies that have suggested a role for dietary factors, such as galactose consumption, the precise causative pathways may vary and it appears that alteration of several causing genes occurs in all ovarian cancers. Specific genetic alterations have been described in some ovarian cancers, but other unknown genes also are likely affected. In addition to defining the full spectrum of genes involved in ovarian carcinogenesis, studies are needed to define molecular mechanisms by which ovulation contributes to this process.

BREAST CANCER

Breast cancer is the most common malignancy in women in developed countries and accounts for 30–35% of all malignancies in females. In the

United States, recent estimates of approximately 178,700 new cases and more than 43,500 breast cancer deaths per year have been published.

One in eight women has the probability of developing breast cancer during her lifetime. Breast cancer is the leading cause of death among women aged 20–59 years. One of the earliest reports of a relationship between breast cancer and ovarian hormones appeared in Lancet in the year 1896. A young woman with advanced breast cancer had a cancerous growth on her thorax. Eight months after removal of the ovaries, her tumor had regressed. Subsequent studies showed, however, that only one in three women would respond to oopheroctomy. The reason for this was to remain unknown until the discovery of the estrogen receptors (ER) and the subsequent development of the ER assay to predict the hormonal responsiveness of breast cancer. Breast cancers can be divided into two groups: those whose growth is hormone-dependent and those that are not responsive to hormones. In general, the hormone-responsive tumors are estrogen receptor positive and these ER-positive tumors represent 60–75% of all breast cancer incidents. Of the ER-positive tumors, 60% do not respond. With time, many breast cancers progress from a hormone-responsive to a hormone-resistant state. However, because a large proportion of breast cancers are ER positive, intensive study focused on the estrogen receptor.

For the most part, both cohort and case-control studies that have assessed the relationship of fertility medications to breast cancer risk have not found any remarkable associations.[29–33] Other epidemiological investigations that had sufficient power to assess relationships with breast cancer, according to detailed parameters of FD use, are the Australian and Dutch follow-up studies of IVF patients.[22,23]

However, several other studies that have assessed detailed timing effects of last drug use found no support for a promoting effect by either clomiphene or gonadotropins. In the Australian study of 2004, Venn and others also assessed causes of death among their cohort of infertile women.[22] The breast cancer-related included deaths and showed no appreciable differences between those who did and did not undergo IVF.

Given that breast cancer is widely recognized as having a hormonal etiology, further assessment of the effects of ovulation-inducing drugs should be undertaken. Studies to date have shown both decreases as well as possible increases in risk. Additional studies that can account for effects of other recognized risk factors (including delays in fertility) should be undertaken.

In a study from Israel published in Fertility Sterility in 2002 in a cohort of women treated with IVF from 1981 to 1992 in three medical centers, no excess risk for cancer was noted.[27] The same paper showed that although a 40% increase in the risk of breast cancer was found among women with anovulatory infertility as compared to the general population, there were no differences between women who were treated by ovulation-inducing drugs and those who were not.

ENDOMETRIAL CANCER

Endometrial cancer ranks fourth among diagnosed cancers, behind breast, lung, and bronchus and colon and rectum cancers. In most industrialized countries, cancer of the corpus uteri is about as frequent as ovarian cancer accounting for 6% of all new cancers. Recognized risk factors for endometrial cancer are nulliparity, late age menopause, obesity, polycystic ovary syndrome, and presence of estrogen-secreting malignancies. Anovulation, infrequent ovulations, and various progesterone deficiencies mostly characterize hormonal subfertility. Irregular menstrual cycles are often anovulatory or have a prolonged follicular phase. Both features result in prolonged exposure to estrogen or progesterone and this might raise the risk of endometrial cancer.

Throughout her lifetime, a woman has a 1 in 37 chance of developing endometrial cancer. In general, two types of endometrial cancer have been described. Type I is associated with hyperestrogenic states and expresses estrogen and progesterone receptors. Type II is not associated with hyperestrogenic states and functional ERs are rarely expressed.

Much like hormone-dependent breast cancer, the theory behind hormone-dependent endometrial cancer is that estrogen stimulates the mitotic activity of the endometrium, whereas it induces differentiation. Increased cell division increases the probability of random mutations, leading to cancer.

Most cohort studies have not observed an association between endometrial cancer and use of FD, but the majority had follow-up times of less than 10 years and few associated cases of uterine cancer.[34-36]

The two larger cohort studies raise some concern regarding effects of ovulation-inducing agents on the endometrium. In one of the Israeli cohorts by Modan *et al.* in which 21 uterine cancers were diagnosed during an average of more than 20 years of follow-up, a significant twofold increase in risk was associated with FD use.[37] Similarly, the multicenter U.S. cohort study by Althuis *et al.*, which detected 39 cases of endometrial cancer among cohort members, found clomiphene use associated with a nonsignificant increase in risk. Further increases in risk were found among subjects with higher dosages of exposure or longer follow-up periods, with trends in risk for the latter variable being statistically significant. Drug effects were also more apparent among nulligravid and obese women RR of 3.5 and 6, respectively.[38]

Use of FD in relation to the risk of endometrial cancer has been studied as well in two papers by Ron *et al.* and Venn *et al.*[39,22] Ron *et al.* showed after 12 years of follow-up no significant increase in risk. A SIR of 6.8 only after 21 years of follow-up was demonstrated. In the study by Venn *et al.*, the cancer of the uterus was not associated with IVF treatment or any of the specific FD examined, but the risk estimate was based on very small numbers ($n = 5$).

In conclusion, all published studies show an increased risk of endometrial cancer in subfertile women. This increase is largely restricted to women with hormonal disorders. Increased risk of endometrial cancer associated with hormonal subfertility is compatible with current insights into the pathogenesis of endometrial cancer.

The relation between FD use and endometrial cancer is suffering from short follow-up and lack of information on important confounders, such as the cause of subfertility and/or parity. In future studies, it is crucial to disentangle the effects of different types of medication and the cause of infertility.

MELANOMA

The potential role for hormones in the etiology of melanomas has received increasing attention and this raises the question of possible effects of fertility medications. Although several clinical reports suggest a relationship, a small number of epidemiological studies have addressed the question. The biological mechanism underlying an effect of FD on the development of cutaneous melanoma is unclear. Some epidemiologic studies suggest a possible increase in melanoma risk in relation to hormonal subfertility and/or its treatment.

The larger study assessing the effects of FD on the risk of melanoma has been the Dutch IVF follow-up study by Klip *et al.*[17,23] A total of 34 melanomas were observed during follow-up, but there was no difference in risk between the exposed and unexposed patients.

The other three cohort investigations that assessed the effects of FD on the occurrence of melanoma included limited numbers of women who developed melanomas. These include the Rossing study in Seattle (12 cases) and two investigations in Australia (12 and 14 cases, respectively).

In the Seattle study,[18] no overall association was found with drug use, but nonsignificant increase in melanoma risk was associated with 12 or more cycles of clomiphene (RR = 2.2; 95% cl, 0.5 – 10.2) and hCG (1.7, 0.5–6.2). However, it was unclear whether these increases were due to effects of the drugs or some underlying hormonal abnormalities among the women.

The Australian study of Venn[22,40] and others found no overall risk associated with drug usage but would not evaluate effects of specific FD. The other Australian study, which focused on 3,186 women attending an infertility clinic, 14 of whom developed melanoma, is difficult to interpret.[41] All cases were exposed to fertility medications, but women who developed melanoma had fewer cycles of exposure to fertility medications than other cohort members. Further study may be warranted.

Data regarding the relationship of ovulation-inducing drugs to the risk of other cancers are sparse, but limited data exist with respect to cervical, thyroid, and trophopblastic tumors.

CERVICAL

Although cervical cancer is not generally viewed as a hormonally related tumor, supported relationships of the disease with parity and use of oral contraceptives have raised concerns regarding the effects of the other hormonal agents. The most informative data derive from the Seattle study in which 36 *in situ* and invasive cervical cancers were detected.[34] In line with other studies, which have shown that parity is a risk factor for this cancer, infertile women were at a decreased risk of developing cervical cancer as compared with the general population.[42]

The risk among women who had taken clomiphene was reduced in regard to nonusers (RR = 0.4; 95% cl, 0.2–0.8) but there was no apparent relation according to duration of use. The investigations recommended further assessment of the hypothesis that the use of antiestrogenic agents leads to a reduced risk of cervical neoplasia.

THYROID

Since incidence rates of thyroid cancer are much higher in females than in males, a role of hormonal factors has long been suspected. In summary, studies published to date do not show convincing evidence of an association between thyroid cancer risk and subfertility (treatment).[43,44]

In a pooled analysis of 13 case-control studies from North America, Asia, and Europe, use of FD was found to be associated with a 60% increase in thyroid cancer risk (95% cl, 0.9–2.9). One of the studies included in this meta-analysis individually reported a significant fourfold excess risk associated with the use of FD. It was not possible either in this study or the meta-analysis to determine if the treatment itself or other correlates of infertility were responsible for the observed risk.

TROPHOBLASTIC TUMORS

Given that ovulation-inducing drugs cause ovulation of more than one oocyte, it has been questioned whether the increase in the production of immature or anucleated oocytes might increase the risk of developing gestational trophoblastic tumors, particularly persistent ones. Several instances of gestational trophoblastic tumors, often occurring with a coexisting fetus, have been found among women exposed to ovulation-inducing agents. Cohort studies were difficult to undertake given the rarity of the condition. Hydatidiform moles were reported to occur at a rate of 1/659 among 2,369 clomiphene-induced pregnancies, a rate considerably higher than the natural incidence of 0.5–1.1/1,000.

A recent comprehensive review of the literature concluded that women having a singleton pregnancy after exposure to ovulation inducers had no additional risk of persistent trophoblastic tumors compared with those who conceive without drugs.[45]

CONCLUSION

Given that clomiphene was first approved for clinical use in 1967 and gonadotropins in 1969, the women who first used these drugs during their late 20s and early 30s have only recently reached the age when hormonally related cancers are common.

Most studies are reassuring in not showing a strong association between use of these medications and risks of most cancers. A consistent observation is the increased risk of endometrial cancer for women with infertility due to hormonal disorders.

An association between ovulation induction and ovarian cancer does not necessarily mean a causal effect. Infertility alone is an independent risk factor for the development of ovarian cancer. Nulliparous women with refractory infertility may harbor a particularly high risk of ovarian cancer, irrespective of their use of infertility drugs.

There has been little attention focused on the long-term effects of assisted reproductive technologies, which often involve much higher exposures to gonadotropins than those received by women in previous eras.

In addition, most IVF protocols include luteal phase support for several weeks with supplemental progestogens, which raises concern since these agents have been linked to increases in breast cancer risk.

There are other issues of interest that have not been widely pursued. First is the question of whether women at particularly high risk of cancer, including those with a genetic predisposition, experience unusual risks from the use of fertility medications. Second, it is of interest whether FD have unusual effects among women who have used other hormones. This includes oral contraceptives, which have been shown to be associated with reduced risks of endometrial and ovarian cancer creations and somewhat increased risks of breast cancers.

The shortcomings of most of the data on cancer risk and the use of FD are: retrospective study designs, relatively small numbers of cancer cases, inconsistent reporting of FD use, and inconsistent reporting of type of fertility. For these reasons no convincing relation exists between FD and risks for ovarian, breast, endometrial, and thyroid cancer. Also, the risk for cutaneous melanoma is not amplified by FD.

From the majority of the literature data, it can be concluded that FD and IVF do not increase the risk of breast and ovarian cancer.[46–49] There is, however, concern about the risk of endometrial cancer. The small increased risk of endometrial cancer in these women is apparently not correlated with hormone use but rather with the polycystic ovary syndrome, and this with subfertility.

REFERENCES

1. BEURSKENS, M.P., J.W. MAAS & J.L. EVERS. 1995. Subfertility in South Limburg: calculation of incidence and appeal for specialist care. Ned. Tijdschr. Geneeskd. **139:** 235–238.
2. DE JONG VAN DEN BERG, L.T.W, M.C. CORNEL, P.B. VAN DEN BERG, et al. 1992. Ovulation inducing drugs: a drug utilization and risk study in the Dutch population. Int. J. Risk Safety Med. **3:** 99–112.
3. STEPHEN, E. & A. CHANDRA. 1998. Updated projections of infertility in the United States: 1995–2025. Fertil. Steril. **70:** 30–34.
4. WYSOWSKI, D.K. 1993. Use of fertility drugs in the United States, 1973 through 1991. Fertil. Steril. **60:** 1096–1098.
5. PARAZZINI, F., E. NEGRI, C. LA VECCHIA, et al. 1997. Treatment for infertility and risk of invasive epithelial ovarian cancer. Hum. Reprod. **12:** 2159–2161.
6. MOSGAARD, B.J., O. LIDEGAARD, S.K. KJAER, et al. 1997. Infertility, fertility drugs and invasive ovarian cancer: a case control study. Fertil. Steril. **67:** 1005–1012.
7. VENN, A., L. WATSON, J. LUMLEY, et al. 1995. Breast and ovarian cancer incidence after infertility and in vitro fertilisation. Lancet **346:** 995–1000.
8. AKHMEDKHANOV, A., A. ZELENIUCH-JACQUOTTE & P. TONIOLO. 2001. Role of exogenous and endogenous hormones in endometrial cancer: review of the evidence and research perspectives. Ann. N. Y. Acad. Sci. **943:** 296–315.
9. RIES, L.A.G., C.L. KOSARY, B.F. HANKEY, et al. 1998. SEER Cancer Statistics Review 1973–1995. National Cancer Institute. Bethesda, MD.
10. FATHALLA, M.F. 1971. Incessant ovulation—a factor in ovarian neoplasia? Lancet. **2:** 163.
11. RISCH, H.A. 1998. Hormonal etiology of epithelial ovarian cancer, with a hypothesis concerning the role of androgens and progesterone. J. Natl. Cancer Inst. **90:** 1774–1786.
12. COOK, L.S., M.L. KAMB & N.S. WEISS. 1997. Perineal powder exposure and the risk of ovarian cancer. Am. J. Epidemiol. **145:** 459–465.
13. PAULSON, R.J. 1997. Fertility drugs and ovarian epithelial cancer: the endometriosis hypothesis. J. Assist. Reprod. Genet. **14:** 228–230.
14. NESS, R., D. CRAMER, M. GOODMAN, et al. 2002. Infertility, fertility drugs and ovarian cancer. A pooled analysis of case-control studies. Am. J. Epidemiol. **155:** 217–224.
15. BRINTON, L.A., K.S. MOGHISSI, B. SCOCCIA, et al. 2005. Ovulation induction and cancer risk. Fertil. Steril. **83:** 261–274.
16. ROSSING, M.A., M.T. TANG, E.W. FLAGG, et al. 2004. A case control study of ovarian cancer in relation to infertility and the use of ovulation-inducing drugs. Am. J. Epidemiol. **160:** 1070–1078.
17. KLIP, H., C.W. BURGER, P. KENEMANS & F.A. VAN LEEUWEN. 2000. Cancer risk associated with subfertility and ovulation induction. Cancer Causes Control **11:** 319–344.
18. ROSSING, M.A., J.R. DALING, N.S. WEISS, et al. 1994. Ovarian tumors in a cohort of infertile women. N. Engl. J. Med. **331:** 771–776.
19. CROUGHAN-MINIHANE, M.S., L. CAMARANO, S. FEIGENBAUM, et al. 2001. The risk of ovarian cancer associated with infertility and infertility treatments. Fertil. Steril. **76**(Suppl 1): 68.
20. BRINTON, L.A., E.J. LAMB, K.S. MOGHISSI, et al. 2004. Ovarian cancer risk after the use of ovulation stimulating drugs. Obst. Gynecol. **103:** 1194–1203.

21. BRINTON, L.A., E.J. LAMB, K.S. MOGHISSI, et al. 2004. Ovarian cancer risk associated with varying causes of infertility. Fertil. Steril. **82**: 405–414.
22. VENN, A., L. WATSON, F. BRUINSMA, et al. 1999. Risk cancer after use of fertility drugs with in-vitro fertilization. Lancet **354**: 1586–1590.
23. KLIP, H., C.W. BURGER, F.E. VAN LEEUWEN & THE OMEGA PROJECT GROUP. 2002. Risk of hormone-related cancers after ovarian stimulation for *in-vitro* fertilization in a cohort of 25152 women. *In* Long-term Health Effects of Subfertility Treatment. H. Klip, Ed.: 55–82. PrintPartners Ipskamp B.V. Enschede, the Netherlands.
24. DOYLE, P., N. MACONOCHIE, V. BERAL, et al. 2002. Cancer incidence following treatment for infertility at a clinic in the UK. Hum. Reprod. **17**: 2209–2213.
25. KASHYAP, S., D. MOHER, F.M. FUNG & Z. ROSENWAKS. 2004. Assisted reproductive technology and the incidence of ovarian cancer: a meta analysis. Obstet. Gynecol. **103**: 785–794.
26. POTASHNIK, G., L. LERNER-GEVA, L. GENKIN, et al. 1999. Fertility drugs and the risk of breast and ovarian cancers: results of a long-term follow-up study. Fertil. Steril. **71**: 853–859.
27. DOR, J., L. LERNER-GEVA, J. RABINOVICI, et al. 2002. Cancer incidence in a cohort of infertile women who underwent *in vitro* fertilization. Fertil. Steril. **77**: 324–327.
28. UNKILA-KALLIO, L., A. LEMINEN, A. TIITINEN & O. YLIKORKALA. 1998. Nationwide data on falling incidence of ovarian granulose cell tumours concominant with increasing use of ovulation inducers. Hum. Reprod. **13**: 2828–2830.
29. BURKMAN, R., M. TANG, K. MALONE, et al. 2003. Infertility drugs and the risk of breast cancer: findings from the National Institute of Child Health and Human Development Women's Contraceptive and Reproductive Experience Study. Fertil. Steril. **79**: 844–851.
30. GAUTHIER, E., X. PAOLETTI, F. CLAVEL-CHAPELON, E3N Group. 2004. Breast cancer risk associated with being treated for infertility: results from the French E3N cohort study. Hum. Reprod. **19**: 2216–2221.
31. HEALY, D. & A. VENN. 2003. Infertility medications and the risk of breast cancer. Fertil. Steril. **79**: 852–854.
32. SALHAB, M., W. AL SARAKBI & K. MOKBEL. 2005. *In vitro* ferilization and breast cancer risk: a review. Int. J. Fertil. Womens Health **50**: 259–266.
33. KASHYAP, S., D. MOHER, F.M. FUNG, Z. ROSENWAKS. 2004. Impact of assisted reproduction on the incidence of breast cancer. Fertil. Steril. **82**(Suppl 16). 60th AFS meeting of ASRM. Philadelphia.
34. ROSSING, M.A., J.R. DALING, N.S. WEISS, et al. 1996. *In situ* and invasive cervical carcinoma in a cohort of infertile women. Fertil. Steril. **65**: 19–22.
35. BENSHUSHAN, A., O. PALTIEL, A. BRZEZINSKI, et al. 2001. Ovulation induction and risk of endometrial cancer: a pilot study. Eur. J. Obstet. Gynecol. Reprod. Biol. **98**: 53–57.
36. ALTHUIS, M.D., K.S. MOGHISSI, C.L. WESTHOFF, et al. 2005. Uterine cancer after use of clomiphene citrate to induce ovulation. Am. J. Epidemiol. **161**: 607–615.
37. MODAN, B., E. RON, L. LERNER-GEVA, et al. 1998. Cancer incidence in a cohort of infertile women. Am. J. Epidemiol. **147**: 1038–1042.
38. ALTHUIS, M.D., K.S. MOGHISSI, C.L. WESTHOFF, et al. 2005. Uterine cancer after use of clomiphene citrate to induce ovulation. Am. J. Epidemiol. **161**: 607–615.
39. RON, E., B. LUNENFELD, J. MENCZER, et al. 1987. Cancer incidence in a cohort of infertile women. Am. J. Epidemiol. **125**: 780–790.

40. VENN, A., E. HEMMINKI, L. WATSON, et al. 2001. Mortality in a cohort of IVF patients. Hum. Reprod. **16:** 2691–2696.
41. YOUNG, P., D. PURDIE, L. JACKMAN, et al. 2001. A study of infertile treatment and melanoma. Melanoma Res. **11:** 535–541.
42. MUNOZ, N., S. FRANCESCHI, C. BOSETTI, et al. 2002. Role of parity and human papillomavirus in cervical cancer: the IARC multicentric case-control study. Lancet **359:** 1093–1101.
43. KOLONEL, L.N., J.H. HANKIN, L.R. WILKENS, et al. 1990. An epidemiologic study of thyroid cancer in Hawaii. Cancer Causes Control **1:** 223–234.
44. LA VECCHIA, C., E. RON, S. FRANCESCHI, et al. 1999. A pooled analysis of case control studies of thyroid cancer III, oral contraceptives, menopausal replacement therapy and other female hormones. Cancer Causes Control **10:** 157–166.
45. PETIGNAT, P., P. VASSILAKOS & A. CAMPANA. 2002. Are fertility drugs a risk factor for persistent trophoblastic tumour? Hum. Reprod. **17:** 1610–1615.
46. PARAZZINI, F., C. PELUCCHI, E. NEGRI, et al. 2001. Use of fertility drugs and risk of ovarian cancer. Hum. Reprod. **16:** 1372–1375.
47. BRINTON, L.A., B. SCOCCIA, K.S. MOGHISSI, et al. 2004. Breast cancer risk associated with ovulation-stimulating drugs. Hum. Reprod. **19:** 2005–2013.
48. LERNER-GEVA, L., E. GEVA,, J. LESSING, et al. 2003. The possible association between *in vitro* fertilization treatments and cancer development. Int. J. Gynecol. Cancer **13:** 23–27.
49. MAHDAVI, A., T. PEJOVIC & F. NEZHAT. 2006. Induction of ovulation and ovarian cancer: a critical review of the literature. Fertil. Steril. **85:** 819–826.

Preimplantation Genetic Diagnosis

GEORGE B. MAROULIS AND NIKOLETTA KOUTLAKI

Department of Obstetrics and Gynecology Democritus University of Thrace, Greece

ABSTRACT: Preimplantion genetic diagnosis (PGD) is now used for iden-tification of gene and chromosomal defects in embryos. In this article we describe its use primarily for identification of chromosomal defects in women with recurrent abortions, repeated *in vitro* fertilization (IVF) fail-ure, and advanced maternal age. In all these situations there is increase in chromosomal defects. The identification of normal embryos and the elimination of abnormal embryos are argued to be helpful in increasing implantation and pregnancy rates in these women.

KEYWORDS: preimplantation; embryos; pregnancy; blastomere; PGD; IVF

INTRODUCTION

Prenatal diagnosis can be accomplished by a number of methods, which include chorionic villi biopsy, amniocentesis, cordocentesis, and now preim-plantation genetic diagnosis (PGD). With the use of PGD, embryo defects related to chromosomal abnormalities of single gene defects can be detected even before the embryo implants.[1,2]

Preimplantation genetic diagnosis was introduced some 14 years ago and since then it is being used for the identification of embryos carrying defects that are single gene (i.e., Thalassemia) or chromosome related (either sex chromosome-linked, such as Duchene muscular dyshtrophy (male has it), or autosomal chromosome-linked, such as 21 trisomy. The identification of these embryos permits the transfer of those without the defects, so if pregnancy occurs the birth of an abnormal child is avoided. Today PGD is used for the indications shown in TABLE 1.

METHODOLOGY

Following IVF PGD is performed either on polar body biopsy[3] or on the blastomere or blastomeres removed from embryos usually on day 3 after

Address for correspondence: Prof. G.B. Maroulis, Department of Obstetrics and Gynecology, Dem-ocritus University of Thrace, University Hospital of Alexandroupolis, Dragana, Alexandroupolis 68100, Greece

e-mail: gbmaroul@yahoo.com

Ann. N.Y. Acad. Sci. 1092: 279–284 (2006). © 2006 New York Academy of Sciences.
doi: 10.1196/annals.1365.023

TABLE 1. Indications of prenatal genetic diagnosis[a]

Problem	Method
A. Identification of abnormal embryos	
a. Single gene defects	
Autosomal recessive: Cystic fibrosis	PCR
Autosomal dominant: Huntington's chorea	
b. Sex chromosome-linked: Duchene muscular dystrophy	FISH
B. Recurrent abortion	FISH
Chromosomal abnormalities in embryo	Identifying chromosomal abnormalities
C. Recurrent IVF failure	FISH
Chromosomal abnormalities in embryo	Identifying chromosomal abnormalities
D. To improve IVF outcome in older women (>40 years)	FISH
Chromosomal abnormalities in embryo	Identifying chromosomal abnormalities

[a] Ref. 21.

fertilization when the embryos are on the 6–8 cell stage.[4] The following techniques are used for the identification of defects on the embryo: polymerase chain reaction (PCR)[5] and fluorescent *in situ* hybridization (FISH).[6]

PCR

Polymerase chain reaction is used primarily for the identification of single gene defects and its application has been very effective in eliminating the birth of children whose parents are carrying defective genes (i.e., Thalassemia, Huntington's chorea).[7]

FISH

This method involves the use of probes that are labeled with fluorescent material, which bind to the chromosomes that need to be analyzed. Today we can identify the following chromosomes by FISH: 1,13,15,16,17,18,21, 22, X, Y.

The blastomere is removed from the embryo on day 3, is examined by FISH on day 4, and the "normal" embryos are replaced on day 5. The defective embryos are allowed to grow until they die *in vitro*. This method today is primarily used for the sex and abnormal chromosome identification in embryos to improve the term pregnancy rate in women with recurrent abortion, recurrent implantation failure, and advanced maternal age where the outcome is anticipated to be poor due to the presence of an abnormally high number of chromosomally abnormal embryos.

RECURRENT ABORTION

Pregnancy loss in the first trimester has been associated with a more than 50% incidence of abnormal embryos most of which are aneuploid.[8–10] The other causes of recurrent abortion are cervical incompetence, uterine abnormalities, hormonal inadequacy, poor endometrium, immunological dysfunction (auto- or alloimmune). The treatment of these conditions includes the correction of cervical incompetence, uterine abnormalities (diaphragm, polyp, leiomyomata), correction of hormonal secretion or aspirin, and anticoagulant therapy in case of autoimmune problems. However, since the cause in many abortions is embryonal, the latest addition to the treatment is PGD of embryos. The evaluation of the embryos before implantation may help reduce the number of abnormal embryos to be implanted thus reducing the abortion rate. As a result, a number of centers have used this method to cure repeated pregnancy abortion.

In a recent study by Munné et al., 58 women with repeated abortions were subjected to PGD. The pregnancy rate following PGD was 50% and the abortion rate only 17%.[11] In another study by Rubio et al.[12] it was found that women aged 35 years or younger with recurrent abortions had a higher incidence of abnormal embryos than those who did not (70.7% vs. 33.3%, respectively) and following PGD the abortion rate decreased to 13%.

In a recently published study Munné et al.[13] retrospectively compared the spontaneous abortion rate after 2,279 cycles of PGD to that after non-PGD cycles. They showed that PGD significantly reduces pregnancy loss in infertile couples. The patients underwent PGD to improve pregnancy outcome and were 35 years or older. Chromosomes 13,15,16,18,21,22,X,Y and either 1 or 17 were evaluated. The pregnancy rate per retrieval was 26.7%. In 393 of 2,279 (17.2%) cycles there was no replacement due to lack of chromosomally normal embryos. The mean pregnancy loss for the PGD group was significantly lower than that of the non-PGD group (16.6% vs. 21.5%, respectively) ($P < 0.01$). In the 35–40 years age group the difference between the PGD and the non-PGD group was 14.1% versus 19.4% and for the ones of age 40 years or older was 14% to 22.2%, respectively ($P < 0.001$). In patients with recurrent abortion the pregnancy loss was 13.7%.

Staessen et al. did not find a decrease in spontaneous abortion[14] but in that study two cells were removed from each embryo, which may reduce implantation rate by 30%. It is therefore thought that the removal of two blastomeres is detrimental to the overall outcome. Platteau et al. also used a two-cell biopsy technique with poor results in pregnancy rate (3%) in women 40 years and older,[15] which also is highly suggestive that the two-cell biopsy is very traumatic to the embryo.

The PGD technique does not seem to improve the success rates in recurrent abortions due to Robertsonian Translocation.[16] In these situations fortunately the natural success rate is relatively good so that eventually parents can hope for a normal child to be born, which is much more difficult to accomplish when the problem is due to aneuploides where PGD does help.

RECURRENT IVF FAILURE AND RECURRENT IMPLANTATION FAILURE

Recurrent implantation failure, which leads to repeated IVF failure, is a very distressing problem, since the ultimate treatment of infertility that is, IVF, proves to be unsuccessful. We consider a couple to have repeated failure when three or more attempts with completed embryo transfer have been fruitless. The most commonly considered causes are (*a*) poor endometrium, (*b*) old age, (*c*) presence of hydrosaplinges, fibroids (debatable), endometriomata (debatable), endometrial polyps, and finally the embryo itself. It has been recognized for some time that the decrease of implantation with increasing age is associated with an increase in chromosomally abnormal embryos in abortions as well as in the fetuses of women of older age.[17,18] So it was expected to use PGD to evaluate chromosomal constitution of embryos in women with repeated implantation failure.

Gianaroli *et al.* reported on the use of PGD in patients with IVF failure. The abnormal embryos were 64% of the total embryos examined. Following PGD the implantation rate was 17.3% and pregnancy rate was 25% as opposed to implantation rate of 9.5% ($P < 0.01$) in those who did not use PGD.[19]

In a study by Pellicer the implantation rate after PGD was 19.8% and pregnancy rate 34%. Women under the age of 37 years had implantation rate 24.6% and pregnancy rate 40.7%, compared to 12.2% and 25%, respectively for women 38 years or older.[20] Munné *et al.* showed that the percentage of abnormal embryos increased with age and that the use of PGD increased pregnancy rate by 6–9% in these women with recurrent implantation failure.[18] We have reported[21] that in women with recurrent implantation failure (RIF, Group B) chromosomal abnormalities were increased, which was also observed in women with recurrent abortions (RA, Group A), when compared to women who were normal and had PGD done for sex preselection (C, Group C) (TABLE 2).

TABLE 2. Incidence of abnormal embryos according to age

Age	Abnormal embryos (%)		
	Group A (RA)	Group B (RIF)	Group C (C)
<35	58	53	19
35–40	67	58	22
>40	80	88	37

ADVANCED MATERNAL AGE

Finally, PGD has been used for women undergoing IVF with advanced maternal age in whom as already mentioned aneuploidy increases[12,21] and implantation rate decreases.[17,20] In one study by Munné et al. the PGD group in such women with advanced maternal age had a higher implantation rate than controls (17.6% vs. 10.6% $P < 0.05$).[22]

Gianaroli et al. similarly showed an increase in implantation rate in patients undergoing PGD when compared to those who did not have PGD (25.8% vs. 14.3%, respectively) ($P < 0.05$).[19] Staessen et al. reported that in the PGD group the implantation rate was 17.1% versus 11.5% in controls ($P = 0.09$) and pregnancy rate 16.5% versus 10.4%, respectively ($P = 0.06$), which although not being statistically significant at the 0.05 level is very close to it suggesting that PGD does help.[14]

From the above studies in women with recurrent abortion, repeated implantation failure, and advanced maternal age, what emerges is that the common underlying factor is an increase in incidence of chromosomally abnormal embryos. In such conditions the use of PGD seems to improve the pregnancy outcome.

REFERENCES

1. DELHANTY, J.D., D.K. GRIFFIN, A.H. HANDYSIDE, et al. 1993. Detection of aneuploidy and chromosomal mosaicism in human embryos during preimplantation sex determination by fluorescent in situ hybridization (FISH). Hum. Mol. Genet. **2:** 1183–1185.
2. MUNNÉ, S., H. WEIER, J. GRIFO & J. COHEN. 1994. Chromosome mosaicism in human embryos. Bio. Reprod. **51:** 373–379.
3. VERLINSKY, Y., N. GINSBERG, A. LIFCHEZ, et al. 1990. Analysis of the first polar body: preconception genetic diagnosis. Hum. Reprod. **5:** 826–829.
4. MUNNÉ, S., A. LEE, Z. ROSENWAKS, et al. 1993. Diagnosis of major chromosome aneuploidies in human preimplantation embryos. Hum. Reprod. **8:** 2185–2191.
5. MOUTOU, C., N. GARDES & S. VIVILLE. 2004. Duplex, triplex and quadruplex PCR for the preimplantation genetic diagnosis (PGD) of cystic fibrosis (CF), an exhaustive approach. Prenat. Diagn. **24:** 562–569.
6. VERLINSKY, Y., J. GIESLAK, M. FRIEIDINE, et al. 1995. Pregnancies following preconception diagnosis of common aneuploidies by fluorescence in situ hybridization. Hum. Reprod. **10:** 1923–1927.
7. ESHRE PGD CONSORTIUM STEERING COMMITTEE. 1999. ESHRE Preimplantation Genetic Diagnosis (PGD) Consortium: preliminary assessment of data from January 1997 to September 1998. Hum. Reprod. **14:** 3138–3148.
8. STEPHENSON, M.D., K.A. AWARTANI & W.P. ROBINSON. 2002. Cytogenetic analysis of miscarriages from couples with recurrent miscarriage: a case-control study. Hum. Reprod. **17:** 446–451.

9. STERN, J.J., A.D. DORFMAN & M.D. GUTIERREZ-NAJAR. 1996. Frequency of abnormal karyotype among abortuses from women with and without a history of recurrent spontaneous abortions. Fertil. Steril. **65:** 250–253.

10. WARBURTON, D., J. KLINE, Z. STEIN & B. STROBINO. 1986. Cytogenetic abnormalities is spontaneous abortions of recognized conceptions. *In* Perinatal Genetics: Diagnosis and Treatment. I.H. Porter & A. Willey, Eds.: 133–148. Academic Press. New York.

11. MUNNÉ, S., S. CHEN, J. FISCHER, *et al.* 2005. Preimplantation genetic diagnosis reduces pregnancy loss in women 35 and older with a history of recurrent miscarriages. Fertil. Steril. **84:** 331–335.

12. RUBIO, C., C. SIMON, F. VIDAL, *et al.* 2003. Chromosomal abnormalities and embryo development in recurrent miscarriage couples. Hum. Reprod. **18:** 182–188.

13. MUNNÉ, S., J. FISCHER, A. WARNER, *et al.* 2006. Preimplantation genetic diagnosis significantly reduces pregnancy loss in infertile couples: a multicenter study. Fertil. Steril. **85:** 326–332.

14. STAESSEN, C., P. PLATTEAU, E. VAN ASSCHE, *et al.* 2004. Comparison of blastocyst transfer with or without preimplantation genetic diagnosis for aneuploidy screening in couples with advanced maternal age: a prospective randomized controlled trial. Hum. Reprod. **19:** 2849–2858.

15. PLATTEAU, P., C. STAESSEN, A. MICHIELS, *et al.* 2005. Preimplantation genetic diagnosis for aneuploidy screening in patients with unexplained recurrent miscarriages. Fertil. Steril. **83:** 393–397.

16. SUGIURA OGASAWARA, M. & K. SUZUMORI. 2005. Can preimplantation genetic diagnosis improve success rates in recurrent aborters with translocations? Hum Reprod **20:** 3267–3270.

17. SANDALINAS, M., S. SADOWY, M. ALIKANI, *et al.* 2001. Developmental ability of chromosomally abnormal human embryos to develop to blastocyst stage. Hum. Reprod. **16:** 1954–1958.

18. MUNNÉ, S., J. COHEN & D. SABLE. 2002. Preimplantation genetic diagnosis for advanced maternal age and other indications. Fertil. Steril. **78:** 234–236.

19. GIANAROLI, L., CH. MAGLI, A.P. FERRARETTI & S. MUNNÉ. 1999. Preimplantation diagnosis for aneuploidies in patients undergoing *in vitro* fertilization with a poor prognosis: identification of the categories for which it should be proposed. Fertil. Steril. **72:** 837–844.

20. PELLICER, A., C. RUBIO, F. VIDAL, *et al.* 1999. *In vitro* fertilization plus preimplantation genetic diagnosis in patients with recurrent miscarriage: an analysis of chromosome abnormalities in human preimplantation embryos. Fertil. Steril. **71:** 1033–1039.

21. KAPETANAKIS, E., T. DAMIANAKIS, E. LEVVEKI, *et al.* 2005. The significance of eliminating chromosomally abnormal embryos in recurrent abortions vs in recurrent implantation failures. Fertil. Steril. **84:** S101.

22. MUNNÉ, S., M. SANDALINAS, T. ESCUDERO, *et al.* 2003. Improved implantation after preimplantation genetic diagnosis of aneymploidy. Reprod. Biomed. Online **7:** 91–97.

Recent Developments in the Detection of Fetal Single Gene Differences in Maternal Plasma and the Role of Size Fractionation

YING LI, SINUHE HAHN, AND WOLFGANG HOLZGREVE

University Women's Hospital/Department of Research, University Hospital, CH Basel, Switzerland

ABSTRACT: The presence of cell-free fetal DNA in maternal plasma allowed noninvasive prenatal diagnosis of fetal loci completely absent from the maternal genome, such as SRY gene and RhD gene. However, the detection of fetal point mutations is hindered by the predominance of maternal DNA sequences. Recent studies have shown that cell-free fetal DNA exists in maternal plasma in small fragments. Thus, cell-free fetal DNA can be enriched by size fractionation, which improves detection of fetal gene mutations. Furthermore, it has been shown that Matrix Assisted Laser Desorption Ionization Time-of-Flight (MALDI-TOF) mass spectrometry also permits the detection of fetal SNPs from maternal plasma. These two new developments are discussed.

KEYWORDS: point mutation; size fractionation; cell-free DNA; MALDI-TOF mass spectrometry

INTRODUCTION

Hereditary disorders caused by point mutations, such as β-thalassemia, are a major issue in prenatal diagnosis, as it is important to detect their presence early in pregnancy. Thus an affected pregnancy can be terminated. Currently, prenatal diagnosis of the disorder is mainly based on invasive procedures, such as amniocentesis or chorionic villous sampling, which present a small but significant risk for fetus and mother.[1]

There are two fetal materials that can be considered for noninvasive prenatal diagnosis: fetal cells in maternal circulation and cell-free fetal DNA in maternal plasma. Cheung *et al.* examined two pregnancies at risk for sickle cell anemia and β-thalassemia by isolation of fetal erythroblasts from maternal

Address for correspondence: Wolfgang Holzgreve, M.D., Laboratory for Prenatal Medicine, University Women's Hospital, Spitalstrasse 21, CH 4031 Basel, Switzerland. Voice: +41-61-265-9018; fax: +41-61-265-9399.
  e-mail: wholzgreve@uhbs.ch

Ann. N.Y. Acad. Sci. 1092: 285–292 (2006). © 2006 New York Academy of Sciences.
doi: 10.1196/annals.1365.024

blood, and successfully identified the fetal genotypes.[2] Later, Di Naro et al. also correctly determined β-thalassemia mutations using fetal erythroblasts in maternal circulation.[3] Subsequent studies have shown that this approach is not suitable for clinical diagnosis due to the rarity of fetal cells in maternal circulation, difficult enrichment procedures, and complex PCR analysis.[1] The presence of cell-free fetal DNA in maternal plasma has been reliably used for the noninvasive analysis of fetal genetic loci, which are absent from maternal genome, such as SRY gene and fetal RhD gene.[4]

The detection, however, of fetal single gene mutations using maternal plasma from pregnant women is challenging because of the low amount of cell-free fetal DNA as compared to the high amount of maternal DNA background. The first detection of a paternally inherited disease—causing mutation in maternal plasma—was reported by Amicucci et al., who were able to detect a trinucleotide repeat expansion in the dystrophia myotonic protein kinase gene in maternal plasma DNA.[5] Since then, several reports have shown that paternally inherited single gene mutations in maternal plasma could be detected by using PCR or nested PCR combined with restriction enzyme digestion (TABLE 1). Saito et al. reported the detection of a single point mutation in the plasma of a pregnant woman carrying a fetus suspected for having achondroplasia.[6] Gonzalez-Gonzalez et al. identified a cystic fibrosis mutation in fetal DNA from maternal plasma.[7] Fucharoen et al. identified a fetal hemoglobin E gene mutation in the plasma of Thai pregnant women.[8] However, this method, involving PCR combined with restriction digestion, is relatively insensitive. Another caveat is that all these reports were based on one or only a few cases.

Chiu et al. employed mutation-specific real-time PCR analysis to exclude β-thalassemia major caused by a four-base deletion in the β-globin gene.[9] The deletion of the four bases of the codon 41/42 mutation (-CTTT) made the detection possible. When, however, the authors tried to detect three other point mutations in the β-globin gene using the same method for discrimination of the fetal mutant alleles from the background maternal DNA they were unsuccessful.[10]

Subsequently, advances in the detection of fetal single gene point mutations in maternal plasma and the role of size fractionation will be discussed.

DETECTION OF FETAL POINT MUTATIONS USING SIZE FRACTIONATED MATERNAL PLASMA DNA

Recent studies have shown that cell-free fetal DNA in maternal plasma is of smaller size than comparable maternal DNA.[11,12] Therefore, enrichment of cell-free fetal DNA by size fractionation is possible. Using such an enrichment procedure permits the detection of fetal STR sequences in maternal plasma.[12] We were interested in applying this technique for the detection of paternally inherited single gene point mutations. This method is hindered, however, by

TABLE 1. Studies reporting the detection of paternally inherited fetal gene mutations in maternal plasma

Authors	Gene	Disorder	Cases	Method	Ref
Amicucci *et al.*	DMPK	Myotonic Dystrophy	1	FQ-PCR	5
Saito *et al.*	FGFR3	Achondroplasia	1	PCR+Restriction enzyme	6
Gonzalez-Gonzalez *et al.*	Q890X	Cystic Fibrosis	1	PCR+Restriction enzyme	7
Fucharoen *et al.*	Hemoglobin E	Hemoglobin E/ β-thalassemia	5	PCR+Restriction enzyme	8
Chiu *et al.*	β-globin gene	β-thalassemia	8	Allele specific real-time PCR	9
Li *et al.*	FGFR3	Achondroplasia	1	Size fractionation + PCR + Restriction enzyme	13
Ding *et al.*	β-globin gene	β-thalassemia	11	MS	20
Li *et al.*	β-globin gene	β-thalassemia	32	Size fractionation + PNA-clamping PCR	14

the large excess of maternal DNA sequences in the circulation. In this regard, we first examined in maternal plasma a paternally inherited mutation in the Fibroblast Growth Factor Receptor 3 (FGFR3) gene, which causes achondroplasia. Due to a G-A mutation at nucleotide 1138, a unique SfcI restriction site is created. We used touchdown PCR to amplify the enriched fetal DNA, followed by digestion of the amplicon with SfcI enzyme. The digested fragments were visualized on a 6% polyacrylamide gel with SYBR Green staining. We found that this approach allowed improved detection of the fetal mutation allele, compared with conventional analysis of total plasma circulating DNA.[13]

We next examined in maternal plasma paternally inherited fetal point mutations in the β-globin gene, which cause β-thalassemia.[14] The examination of paternally inherited mutant alleles in maternal plasma can exclude the risk for compound heterozygous pregnancies. In our study, four different β-thalassemia point mutations, commonly occurring in individuals of Mediterranean descent: IVSI-1, IVSI-6, IVSI-110, and codon39, were identified from 32 maternal plasma samples taken at 10–12 weeks of pregnancy. For all samples, it was known that the father was a carrier for one of the four mutations described above, and that the mother carried another β-globin gene mutation. However, whether or not the fetus carried the mutations was unknown at the time of analysis. Circulating fetal DNA was enriched by size fractionation and subjected to PCR with peptide nucleic acid (PNA) clamping. PNA sequences for maternal alleles block the amplification of normal maternal sequences, resulting in amplification of only mutant alleles. The paternal mutant alleles were then identified by allele-specific real-time PCR using SYBR Green Dye. We compared our results with results from CVS tests performed in an independent diagnostic laboratory in Bari, Italy. The presence or absence of paternal mutant alleles was correctly determined with greater than 94% accuracy. In comparison, the simultaneous assessment of total plasma DNA samples, without size fractionation, resulted in incorrect evaluation of almost 50% of the cases of paternally inherited allele.

MS-BASED TECHNOLOGY AND ITS APPLICATION IN THE DETECTION OF FETAL POINT MUTATIONS IN MATERNAL PLASMA

Matrix Assisted Laser Desorption Ionization Time-of-Flight (MALDI-TOF) mass spectrometry (MS) has emerged as an important tool for SNP genotyping. Several strategies have been developed for SNP genotyping.[15] One of these is homogenous MassEXTEND® (hME) assay from Sequenom, Inc. (San Diego, California). This assay is based on an allele-specific primer extension reaction that allows the differentiation of homozygous normal, heterozygous mutant, and homozygous mutant samples. Briefly, the target DNA sequence is amplified by PCR after which nonincorporated dNTPs are removed from the reaction using Shrimp Alkaline Phosphatase (SAP) incubation. The hME primer is annealed to the target DNA adjacent to the SNP of interest. The addition of a DNA polymerase along with a mixture of terminator nucleotides allows extension of the hME primer through the polymorphic site and generates allele-specific extension products, each having a unique molecular mass. The resulting masses of the extension products are then analyzed by MALDI-TOF MassArray® software (www.sequenom.com).

The advantages of MS-based assay for the detection of cell-free fetal DNA are numerous. It can examine a large number of genetic markers simultaneously, which cannot be done by conventional PCR-based methods.[16] For example, more than 200 different point mutations in the β-globin gene have been identified to cause β-thalassemia. However, only a relatively small number of mutations account for the majority of β-thalassemia cases in any given ethnic population. Thus, the most common mutations could be simultaneously examined by MS in a single-run setup. Another advantage is that MS-based assay is very sensitive. Ding and Cantor showed that they could achieve multiplex genotyping and haplotyping using 3 pg of genomic DNA template (equivalent to one copy of genomic template).[17] This feature makes MS suitable for the detection of the small amounts of cell-free fetal DNA in maternal plasma. Finally, the MS-based assay system is extremely accurate and highly reproducible.[18] Recently, Trisomy 21 has been successfully detected in amniotic fluid, CVS, and placental tissue, by quantitative analysis of SNPs using the MALDI-TOF MS assay.[19] Moreover, the direct detection of analytes based on molecular weight eliminates the need for any labeling or separation steps.

Ding *et al.* have used MALDI-TOF MS assay to detect fetal single gene differences in maternal plasma. Their assay, known as Single Allele Base Extension Reaction (SABER), was developed to increase the sensitivity of detection. Compared to the hME assay, which involves base extension of both the mutant fetal allele and the background maternal allele, SABER assay only extends the fetal-specific mutant allele.[20] They correctly determined the mutations present or absent in 11 β-thalassemia samples by analysis for four common mutations in Southeast Asia. This, however, was based on a small number of samples: only five cases were single gene point mutations and the rest presented CD41/42 (-CTTT) 4 bases deletion.

THE ROLE OF SIZE FRACTIONATION IN THE DETECTION OF FETAL POINT MUTATIONS

Our studies so far have indicated that the size fractionation approach improved the detection of fetal single gene point mutations in maternal plasma. However, Ding *et al.* showed that fetal single gene differences could be correctly discriminated in maternal plasma by MALDI-TOF MS combined with SABER assay without size fractionation approach.[20] But then, if SABER can

achieve 100% accuracy for the analysis of single gene point mutations, do we
need size fractionation at all?

To answer this question, we evaluated the size fractionation approach for
the detection of single gene point mutations by MALDI-TOF MS assay using
both the SABER approach and the standard hME assay. We examined 41 SNP
markers in 18 maternal plasma samples, in which both the genotypes of mothers
and fetuses were known. The samples were taken from early pregnancy to close
to term. Our results indicated that the SABER assay did improve the detection
of fetal SNPs in maternal plasma. Moreover, the size fractionated cell-free
DNA approach afforded a much greater distinction of the detection signals,
compared with the examination of total plasma DNA by either SABER assay or
hME assay.[21] FIGURE 1A showed that in the examination of total plasma DNA

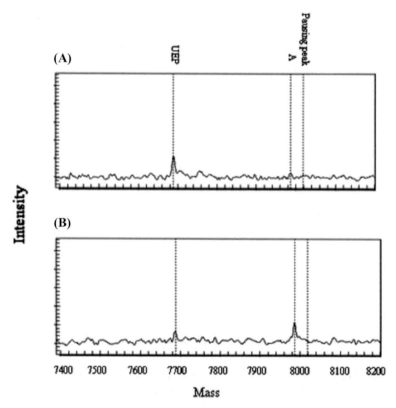

FIGURE 1. (**A**) Detection of SNP rs 1475840 allele in total maternal plasma DNA by
MALDI-TOF mass spectroscopy combined with the SABER assay. The paternally inherited
allele (**A**) was slightly detected. (**B**) Detection of SNP rs 1475840 allele in size fractionated
maternal plasma DNA by MALDI-TOF mass spectroscopy combined with the SABER
assay. Compared to the analysis of total plasma DNA, the signal of the paternally inherited
allele (**A**) is significantly greater. UEP: Unexpected primer.

by SABER assay, the detection signal (A allele) is so close to the detection limit that it is difficult to give correct diagnosis. In fact, analysis by the MassArray software identified this peak as "low probability," suggesting that that could also be a potassium ion peak. However, in the analysis of size fractionated cell-free DNA by SABER assay, the signal is much more clearly distinguishable (FIG. 1B). Our results indicated that using the size fractionation approach combined with the SABER assay could provide additional security for making an accurate clinical diagnosis.

CONCLUSIONS AND FUTURE DIRECTIONS

Mutation detection has become an important part of routine clinical prenatal diagnosis, especially in populations where diseases are caused by commonly occurring single gene mutations. To develop noninvasive tests with simple and accurate strategies is the long-term goal. The greatest hope for this lies with cell-free fetal DNA in maternal plasma.

The discovery of size distribution of cell-free fetal DNA in maternal plasma opened up the possibility to enrich cell-free fetal DNA by size fractionation. Such enriched fetal DNA improves the detection of fetal single gene point mutations in maternal plasma. This approach may be useful for clinical diagnosis of diseases caused by fetal single gene point mutations from maternal plasma in the future.

MALDI-TOF mass spectrometry appears to be a valuable tool for the detection of SNPs. Its highly sensitive and robust features make it suitable for noninvasive prenatal diagnosis.

Currently, it is technologically difficult to detect the maternally inherited fetal allele due to the predominant maternal DNA background. However, the size fractionation approach, combined with accurate quantitative analysis, may eventually overcome this problem.

ACKNOWLEDGMENTS

We thank Dr. D. J. Huang for her helpful comments and proofreading.

REFERENCES

1. HAHN, S. & W. HOLZGREVE. 2002. Prenatal diagnosis using fetal cells and cell-free fetal DNA in maternal blood: what is currently feasible? Clin. Obstet. Gynecol. **45:** 649–656.
2. CHEUNG, M.C., J.D. GOLDBERG & Y.W. KAN. 1996. Prenatal diagnosis of sickle cell anaemia and thalassaemia by analysis of fetal cells in maternal blood. Nat. Genet. **14:** 264–268.

3. Di Naro, E., F. Ghezzi, A. Vitucci, *et al.* 2000. Prenatal diagnosis of beta-thalassaemia using fetal erythroblasts enriched from maternal blood by a novel gradient. Mol. Hum. Reprod. **6:** 571–574.
4. Bianchi, D.W., N.D. Avent, J.M. Costa & C.E. van der Schoot. 2005. Noninvasive prenatal diagnosis of fetal Rhesus D: ready for Prime(r) Time. Obstet. Gynecol. **106:** 841–844.
5. Amicucci, P., M. Gennarelli, G. Novelli & B. Dallapiccola. 2000. Prenatal diagnosis of myotonic dystrophy using fetal DNA obtained from maternal plasma. Clin. Chem. **46:** 301–302.
6. Saito, H., A. Sekizawa, T. Morimoto, M. Suzuki & T. Yanaihara. 2000. Prenatal DNA diagnosis of a single-gene disorder from maternal plasma. Lancet **356:** 1170.
7. Gonzalez-Gonzalez, M.C., M. Garcia-Hoyos, M.J. Trujillo, *et al.* 2002. Prenatal detection of a cystic fibrosis mutation in fetal DNA from maternal plasma. Prenat. Diagn. **22:** 946–948.
8. Fucharoen, G., W. Tungwiwat, T. Ratanasiri, *et al.* 2003. Prenatal detection of fetal hemoglobin E gene from maternal plasma. Prenat. Diagn. **23:** 393–396.
9. Chiu, R.W., T.K. Lau, T.N. Leung, *et al.* 2002. Prenatal exclusion of beta thalassaemia major by examination of maternal plasma. Lancet **360:** 998–1000.
10. Chiu, R.W. & Y.M. Lo. 2004. Recent developments in fetal DNA in maternal plasma. Ann. N. Y. Acad. Sci. **1022:** 100–104.
11. Chan, K.C., J. Zhang, A.B. Hui, *et al.* 2004. Size distributions of maternal and fetal DNA in maternal plasma. Clin. Chem. **50:** 88–92.
12. Li, Y., B. Zimmermann, C. Rusterholz, *et al.* 2004. Size separation of circulatory DNA in maternal plasma permits ready detection of fetal DNA polymorphisms. Clin. Chem. **50:** 1002–1011.
13. Li, Y., W. Holzgreve, G.C. Page-Christiaens, *et al.* 2004. Improved prenatal detection of a fetal point mutation for achondroplasia by the use of size-fractionated circulatory DNA in maternal plasma—case report. Prenat. Diagn. **24:** 896–898.
14. Li, Y., E. Di Naro, A. Vitucci, *et al.* 2005. Detection of paternally inherited fetal point mutations for beta-thalassemia using size-fractionated cell-free DNA in maternal plasma. JAMA **293:** 843–849.
15. Gut, I.G. 2004. DNA analysis by MALDI-TOF mass spectrometry. Hum. Mutat. **23:** 437–441.
16. Tost, J. & I.G. Gut. 2005. Genotyping single nucleotide polymorphisms by MALDI mass spectrometry in clinical applications. Clin. Biochem. **38:** 335–350.
17. Ding, C. & C.R. Cantor. 2003. Direct molecular haplotyping of long-range genomic DNA with M1-PCR. Proc. Natl. Acad. Sci. USA **100:** 7449–7453.
18. Braun, A., R. Roth & M.J. McGinniss. 2003. Technology challenges in screening single gene disorders. Eur. J. Pediatr. **162**(Suppl. 1): S13–S16.
19. Tsui, N.B., R.W. Chiu, C. Ding, *et al.* 2005. Detection of trisomy 21 by quantitative mass spectrometric analysis of single-nucleotide polymorphisms. Clin. Chem. **51:** 2358–2362.
20. Ding, C., R.W. Chiu, T.K. Lau, *et al.* 2004. MS analysis of single-nucleotide differences in circulating nucleic acids: application to noninvasive prenatal diagnosis. Proc. Natl. Acad. Sci. USA **101:** 10762–10767.
21. Li, Y., F. Wenzel, W. Holzgreve, *et al.* 2006. Genotyping fetal paternally inherited SNPs by MALDI-TOF MS using cell-free fetal DNA in maternal plasma: influence of size fractionation. Electrophoresis **27:** 3889–3896.

Intrauterine Growth Restriction, Brain-Sparing Effect, and Neurotrophins

ARIADNE MALAMITSI-PUCHNER, K.E. NIKOLAOU,
AND K-P. PUCHNER

*Neonatal Division, Second Department of Obstetrics and Gynecology,
University of Athens, Athens, Greece*

ABSTRACT: Intrauterine growth restriction (IUGR) is failure of the fetus to achieve his or her intrinsic growth potential, due to anatomi-
cal/functional diseases or disorders in the feto–placental–maternal unit.
Growth restriction successfully balances reduced oxygen delivery and
consumption; however, chronic hypoxia is responsible for fetal blood
flow redistribution to cardinal organs (brain, myocardium, and adrenal
glands), the so-called brain-sparing effect. The neurotrophin family comprises four structurally related molecules: the nerve growth factor (NGF),
the brain-derived neurotrophic factor (BDNF), the neurotrophin-3
(NT-3), and the neurotrophin-4 (NT-4). By exerting neuroprotection, neurotrophins are critical for pre- and postnatal brain development. Based
on the assumption that the brain-sparing effect might be activated in full-
term IUGR infants, we hypothesized that circulating neurotrophin levels
should not differ between IUGR and appropriate for gestational age
(AGA) infants. Indeed, we found that in both groups, circulating NT-3,
NT-4, and BDNF levels do not differ, and this finding could possibly be
attributed to the activation of the brain-sparing effect. In contrast, NGF
levels were higher in the AGA compared to the IUGR group. However,
only NGF levels positively correlated with the customized centile and the
birth weight of the infants, and both of them were lower in the IUGR
group.

KEYWORDS: intrauterine growth restriction; neurotrophins; brain-
derived neurotrophic factor

INTRAUTERINE GROWTH RESTRICTION

Intrauterine growth restriction (IUGR) is the failure of the fetus to achieve
his or her intrinsic growth potential. Factors determining the intrinsic growth

Address for correspondence: A. Malamitsi-Puchner, M.D., Neonatal Division, Second Department
of Obstetrics and Gynecology, University of Athens, 19, Soultani Str., GR-10682 Athens, Greece.
Voice: +30-6944-443815; fax: +30-210-7233330.
e-mail: malamitsi@aias.gr

Ann. N.Y. Acad. Sci. 1092: 293–296 (2006). © 2006 New York Academy of Sciences.
doi: 10.1196/annals.1365.026

potential include maternal height and booking weight, ethnicity, parity, gender of the infant, number of *in utero* coexisting fetuses, and altitude at which pregnancy evolves.[1–3] IUGR is usually the consequence of anatomical and or functional diseases or disorders in the feto–placental–maternal unit, depriving the fetus of sufficient nutrient and oxygen supplies[4] and resulting in increased risk for pre-, peri-, and postnatal morbidity and mortality.[5,6] Therefore, IUGR fetuses are those with an estimated weight below the 10th customized centile,[2] that is, fetuses that are not constitutionally (symmetrically) small, but display signs of chronic malnutrition and hypoxia[7] (asymmetrical pattern) due to pathological conditions during pregnancy.

Growth restriction is the major mechanism for balancing reduced oxygen delivery and consumption.[8] Due to growth restriction arterial oxygen concentration is maintained normal or minimally decreased until substrate delivery is severely reduced.[9] Nevertheless, chronic hypoxia is responsible for fetal blood flow redistribution[8] to the most important organs: the brain, the myocardium, and the adrenal glands, while other organs (e.g., the kidneys) are hypoperfused. This phenomenon has been called the brain-sparing effect, resulting on one hand to preservation of cerebral metabolism and on the other to oligohydramnios[8,10,11] and diminished amniotic fluid.[12]

Previous studies have shown that IUGR infants may present increased risk for major intracranial injury,[13] cerebral palsy,[14] and cognitive deficits,[15,16] while school-age children may demonstrate learning and behavioral problems.[16]

NEUROTROPHINS

The neurotrophin family comprises four structurally related molecules: the nerve growth factor (NGF), the brain-derived neurotrophic factor (BDNF), the neurotrophin-3 (NT-3), and the neurotrophin-4 (NT-4). Neurotrophins share a greater than 80% identity of the aminoacid structure and act via two types of receptors; the high-affinity tyrosine kinase (Trk) receptors A (NGF), B (BDNF and NT-4), and C (NT-3)[17] and the low-affinity p75 receptor, the latter being a member of the tumor necrosis factor receptor family.[18]

The main role of neurotrophins is neuroprotection by reducing apoptosis and by promoting survival and maintenance of specific populations of neurons in the peripheral (sympathetic and sensory neurons) and central nervous system (cholinergic, dopaminergic, adrenergic neurons).[17,19–21] Neurotrophins are implicated in axon growth during development,[22] in higher neuronal functions,[23] in developmental maturity of the cortex and synaptic plasticity, leading to refinement of connections,[24] and in morphologic differentiation and neurotransmitter expression.[25] Therefore, their role is critical for prenatal and postnatal brain development.[26]

INTRAUTERINE GROWTH RESTRICTION AND NEUROTROPHINS

Based on the assumption that the brain-sparing effect might be activated in full-term IUGR infants, and that circulating levels of neurotrophins would reflect central nervous system levels due to the immature blood–brain barrier,[27] we hypothesized that blood neurotrophin levels should not differ between IUGR and appropriate for gestational age (AGA) infants. Therefore, we conducted a study, investigating the blood levels of NGF, BDNF, NT-3, and NT-4 and including mothers before delivery, as well as their AGA or IUGR full-term fetuses and neonates.

In both groups fetuses presented with Doppler studies of the umbilical and middle cerebral artery within normal limits, and neonates at the transition (first day postpartum) and stabilization (fourth day postpartum) period did not show any pathological signs. Additionally, cerebral ultrasounds performed on the third and tenth day postpartum were normal.

We found that in IUGR and AGA full-term fetuses and neonates, circulating neurotrophin NT-3, NT-4, and BDNF levels did not differ, and this finding could possibly be attributed to the activation of the brain-sparing effect. In contrast, NGF levels were found higher in the AGA compared to the IUGR group. However, only NGF levels positively correlated with the customized centile and the birth weight of the infants, and both of them were lower in the IUGR group. Furthermore, maternal neurotrophin levels were in both groups higher than fetal and neonatal ones, most likely due to the mature adult nervous system. Lastly, no gender differentiation in neurotrophin levels of both IUGR and AGA groups was observed, indirectly implying similar neural development between both genders.

Future studies should focus on preterm IUGR infants and on those with impaired either prenatal Doppler studies or postnatal brain ultrasounds. The determination of circulating neurotrophin levels in these cases could possibly indicate the activation or not of the brain-sparing effect.

REFERENCES

1. GARDOSI, J., A. CHANG, B. KALYAN, *et al.* 1992. Customised antenatal growth charts. Lancet **339:** 283–287.
2. GARDOSI, J., M. MONGELLI, M. WILCOX, *et al.* 1995. An adjustable fetal weight standard. Ultrasound Obstet. Gynecol. **6:** 168–174.
3. MOORE, L.G., M. SHRIVER, L. BEMIS, *et al.* 2004. Maternal adaptation to high-altitude pregnancy: an experiment of nature—a review. Placenta **25**(Suppl A): S60–S71.
4. SOOTHILL, P.W., R.A. AJAYI & K.N. NICOLAIDES. 1992. Fetal biochemistry in growth retardation. Early Hum. Dev. **29:** 91–97.
5. BARDE, Y.A. 1990. The nerve growth factor family. Prog. Growth Factor Res. **2:** 237–248.

6. RESNIK, R. 2002. Intrauterine growth restriction. Obstet. Gynecol. **99:** 490–496.
7. VILLE, Y. & D.A. NYBERG. 2003. Growth, Doppler and fetal assessment. *In* Diagnostic Imaging of Fetal Anomalies. D.A. Nyberg, J.P. McGahan, D.H. Pretorius & G. Pilu, Eds.: 31–58. Lippincott, Williams and Wilkins. Philadelphia.
8. PEEBLES, D.M. 2004. Fetal consequences of chronic substrate deprivation. Semin. Fetal Neonatal Med. **9:** 379–386.
9. RICHARDSON, B.S. & A.D. BOCKING. 1998. Metabolic and circulatory adaptations to chronic hypoxia in the fetus. Comp. Biochem. Physiol. **119A:** 717–723.
10. DUBIEL, M., A. SEREMAK-MROZIKIEWICZ, G.H. BREBOROWICZ, *et al.* 2005. Fetal and maternal Doppler velocimetry and cytokines in high-risk pregnancy. J. Perinat. Med. **33:** 17–21.
11. HARKNESS, U.F. & G. MARI. 2004. Diagnosis and management of intrauterine growth restriction. Clin. Perinatol. **31:** 743–764.
12. BRAEMS, G. & A. JENSEN. 1991. Hypoxia reduces oxygen consumption of fetal skeletal muscle cells in monolayer culture. J. Dev. Physiol. **16:** 209–215.
13. ZAW, W., R. GAGNON & O. SILVA. 2003. The risks of adverse neonatal outcome among preterm small for gestational age infants according to neonatal versus fetal growth standards. Pediatrics **111:** 1273–1277.
14. THORNTON, J.G., J. HORNBUCKLE, A. VAIL, *et al.* 2004. Infant wellbeing at 2 years of age in the Growth Restriction Intervention Trial (GRIT): multicentred randomised controlled trial. Lancet **364:** 513–520.
15. SCHERJON, S., J. BRIET, H. OOSTING, *et al.* 2000. The discrepancy between maturation of visual-evoked potentials and cognitive outcome at five years in very preterm infants with and without hemodynamic signs of fetal brain-sparing. Pediatrics **105:** 385–391.
16. PAZ, I., R. GALE, A. LAOR, *et al.* 1995. The cognitive outcome of full-term small for gestational age infants at late adolescence. Obstet. Gynecol. **85:** 452–456.
17. LEWIN, G. & Y.A. BARDE. 1996. Physiology of the neurotrophins. Annu. Rev. Neurosci. **19:** 289–317.
18. BARBACID, M. 1995. Neurotrophic factors and their receptors. Curr. Opin. Cell. Biol. **7:** 148–155.
19. ARENAS, E. & H. PERSSON. 1994. Neurotrophin-3 prevents the death of adult central noradrenergic neurons in vivo. Nature **367:** 368–371.
20. HEFTI, F. 1986. Nerve growth factor promotes survival of septal cholinergic neurons after fimbrial transections. J. Neurosci. **6:** 2155–2162.
21. HYMAN, C., M. HOFER, Y.A. BARDE, *et al.* 1991. BDNF is a neurotrophic factor for dopaminergic neurons of the substantia nigra. Nature **350:** 230–232.
22. TUCKER, K.L., M. MEYER & Y.A. BARDE. 2001. Neurotrophins are required for nerve growth during development. Nat. Neurosci. **4:** 29–37.
23. CHAO, M.V. 2001. Trophic factors: an evolutionary cul-de-sac or door into higher neuronal function? J. Neurosci. Res. **59:** 353–355.
24. LU, B. & A. FIGUROV. 1997. Role of neurotrophins in synapse development and plasticity. Rev. Neurosci. **8:** 1–12.
25. TAKEI, N. & H. NAWA. 1998. Roles of neurotrophins on synaptic development and functions in the central nervous system. Hum. Cell **11:** 157–165.
26. CHOUTHAI, N.S., J. SAMPERS, N. DESAI, *et al.* 2003. Changes in neurotrophin levels in umbilical cord blood from infants with different gestational ages and clinical conditions. Pediatr. Res. **53:** 965–969.
27. POLIN, R.A. & W.W. FOX. 1998. Fetal and Neonatal Physiology. WB Saunders. Philadelphia.

Doppler Assessment of the Intrauterine Growth-Restricted Fetus

D. BOTSIS, N. VRACHNIS, AND G. CHRISTODOULAKOS

Second Department of Obstetrics and Gynecology, University of Athens, Aretaieio Hospital, Greece

ABSTRACT: The evaluation of fetal well-being by Doppler velocimetry in cases of intrauterine growth restriction (IUGR) is of great importance as it is very useful in detecting those IUGR fetuses that are at high risk because of hypoxemia. Several Doppler studies initially on fetal arteries and recently on the fetal venous system provide valuable information for the clinicians concerning the optimal time to deliver. Doppler sonography in combination with the other biophysical methods such as cardiotocogram and biophysical profile score should be used in everyday practice for the monitoring and appropriate management of the growth-restricted fetuses. The purpose of this review is to describe the current approaches in Doppler assessment of IUGR fetal circulation.

KEYWORDS: intrauterine growth restriction (IUGR); hypoxemia; Doppler velocimetry

INTRODUCTION

The term intrauterine growth restriction (IUGR) refers to a condition in which a fetus is unable to achieve its genetically determined potential size. Of all fetuses below the 10th percentile for growth only approximately 40% are at high risk of potentially preventable perinatal death. Another 40% of these fetuses are constitutionally small but healthy and the remaining 20% are intrinsically small secondary to a chromosomal or environmental abnormality.

The identification of IUGR fetuses with hypoxia, whose health is at risk because of a hostile intrauterine environment, has always been a challenge for the clinicians to monitor and intervene appropriately.

It is generally accepted that IUGR and fetal hypoxia are currently related to placental insufficiency. Hypoxia induces a hemodynamic adaptation that can be detected and quantified by Doppler analysis.

Nowadays, by the use of routine ultrasonography we can detect IUGR fetuses, which represent about 15% of all pregnancies and with the assistance

Address for correspondence: Prof. D. Botsis, 76 Vas. Sofias Avenue, Athens 115-28, Greece. Voice: 0030-210-7286353; fax: 0030-210-7233330.
e-mail: nvrachnis@med.uoa.gr

Ann. N.Y. Acad. Sci. 1092: 297–303 (2006). © 2006 New York Academy of Sciences.
doi: 10.1196/annals.1365.027

of the Doppler analysis we can identify those IUGR fetuses at risk, which correspond approximately to 40% of all IUGR fetuses.

Doppler assessment of the IUGR fetus mainly concerns three groups of vessels:

- The Uterine artery Doppler for the prediction of IUGR.
- The Arterial Doppler: the umbilical Doppler, useful in the evaluation of placental insufficiency and the cerebral Doppler for the estimation of "brain-sparing effect."
- The Venous Doppler mainly used for the evaluation of the decompensation of fetal circulation.

UTERINE ARTERY DOPPLER

Flow patterns of uterine arteries reflect the impact of placentation on maternal circulation. It is usually performed as a screening test at 23 weeks that is effective in identifying pregnancies with poor perinatal outcomes prior to 34 weeks related to uteroplacental insufficiency. This test has sensitivity of up to 75% for false positive rate of 5%.[1,2] The same screening test at 11–14 weeks can also identify a woman at risk of developing IUGR but has lower sensitivity (60%) compared to that carried out at 23 weeks.[1]

After 23 weeks of gestation the screening test can identify a woman at risk for uterine artery Doppler abnormalities such as high mean resistance estimated on pulsatility index (PI) or resistance index (RI) (the average of left and right uterine artery resistance) with persistence of either a unilateral or bilateral notch. We should keep in mind that even if the notches disappear later in the pregnancy, the risk of complication remains. The likelihood ratio for severe adverse outcome (as preeclampsia, IUGR, fetal death) related to mean uterine artery PI at 23 weeks is represented in FIGURE 1.[2]

The prevention of IUGR-based uterine artery Doppler findings is highly desirable. Despite the theoretical benefit of aspirin in many studies, the role of prophylactic treatment with low-dose aspirin or vitamins C, E, and nitric oxide donors in pregnancies with abnormal uterine artery Doppler screening test at 23 weeks is still unclear.[3,4]

ARTERIAL DOPPLER

The arterial Doppler mainly concerns the evaluation of the blood flow in umbilical artery (UA) and in the middle cerebral artery (MCA). In specific indications and especially during scientific research we can also examine the aorta, splenic artery, the renal, coronary, and adrenal arteries.

UA Doppler reflects placental vascular resistance and is strongly correlated with IUGR and the multisystem effects of placental insufficiency. In normal pregnancy UA resistance shows a continuous decline. In placental insufficiency

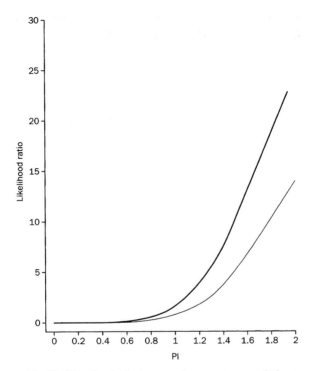

FIGURE 1. The likelihood ratio for severe adverse outcome relating to mean uterine artery PI at 23 weeks.[2]

three major and progressive abnormalities of UA Doppler are described: raised resistance (PI), absent end-diastolic flow (EDF), and reversed EDF.

UA Doppler only gives information on placental blood flow. This information does not reflect the adaptation to hypoxia or the consequences of this adaptation.[5] Absent and reversed EDF in the UA are commonly associated with severe IUGR and oligohydramnios.[6]

There is a significant difference in perinatal mortality for absent EDF (20%) versus reversed EDF (68%) in the UA.[7]

The MCA, which is a main branch of the circle of Willis, is the most accessible to sonographic imaging fetal cerebral vessel and carries more than 80% of cerebral blood. In normal pregnancy MCA has high impedance up to 34 weeks. The cerebral/umbilical ratio is more than 1 (MCA/UA >1). After 34 weeks of gestation, the resistance in MCA decreases as a "physiological redistribution of fetal blood flow." For this reason, several investigators propose the estimation of the aorta/UA ratio after the 34th week.

CENTRALIZATION OF FETAL BLOOD FLOW IN IUGR

The redistribution of fetal blood to the vital organs represents a compensatory mechanism to prevent fetal damage by hypoxemia. In fetal hypoxemia, there

TABLE 1. Hemodynamic changes in fetal arterial vessels during hypoxemia induced by uteroplacental insufficiency[8]

Vessel	Impedance to flow
Descending aorta	increased
Renal artery	increased
Femoral artery	increased
Peripheral pulmonary artery	increased
Mesenteric arteries	increased
Cerebral arteries	increased
Adrenal artery	increased
Splenic artery	increased
Coronary arteries	increased

is an increase in the blood supply to the brain, myocardium, and to the adrenal glands and reduction in the perfusion of the kidneys, gastrointestinal tract, and the lower extremities (TABLE 1).

Although knowledge of the factors governing circulatory readjustments and their mechanism of action is incomplete, it appears that partial pressures of oxygen and carbon dioxide play a role presumably through their action on chemoreceptors. The early stage of fetal blood redistribution shows an increase of the resistance of the UA with a decrease of the resistance of the MCA. The cerebral/umbical ratio becomes less than 1 (MCA/UA <1). This condition is widely known as "brain-sparing effect." The advanced stage of fetal redistribution is characterized by further increase in the resistance of UA and further decrease in the resistance of the MCA.[8]

Deterioration of fetal hypoxemia leads to the decompensatory stage. This stage is characterized by the incipient heart failure leading to the reverse flow in UA and MCA and disappearance of the "brain-sparing effect." This hemodynamic pattern is associated with severe abnormalities involving several fetal organ systems.[9–11]

FETAL VENOUS DOPPLER

Venous Doppler provides information about fetal cardiovascular and respiratory responses to each intrauterine environment. Changes in the fetal venous circulation are associated with an advanced stage of fetal hypoxemia leading to Doppler abnormalities of the ductus venosus (DV), inferior vena cava (IVC), and umbilical vein (UV). When a fetus is severely compromised, venous Doppler analysis provides evidence in support of an expedited delivery. It has been reported[15] that only the DV measurements consistently predicted adverse perinatal outcomes up to 7 days prior to delivery.

Ductus venosus is the short, narrow vascular connection between UV and the right atrium. It carries oxygenated blood from the UV into the fetal circulation toward the foramen ovale. The typical DV waveform has two peaks. The first peak appears during the ventricular systole (*s*) and the second peak during the ventricular diastole (*d*). The notch between the two cycles represents the atrial (*a*) contraction. The DV Doppler abnormalities concern several conditions, such as raised resistance, "a" wave approaching the baseline or reversed "a" wave. Many recent studies present a strong association between these abnormalities and adverse perinatal outcome.[12–15]

The Inferior Vena Cava (IVC) waveform is clearly distinguishable from that of DV and also has three phases: S, D, and reversed A. The pulsation observed at the IVC and DV reflects the normal heart function and it is not transmitted to the UV because of the existence of DV sphincter.

The Umbilical Vein in severe fetal heart failure can give important information (pulsations) especially if the DV cannot be visualized. These pulsations should not be confused with the physiological pulsations due to fetal breathing.

Resuming the Venous Doppler changes in IUGR after the decompensatory stage, we can observe decrease or reverse flow at the DV, increase at the reverse flow at the IVC, and UV pulsations. These alterations are presented when there is a severe deterioration of hypoxemia and may be of great clinical significance in deciding the timing of delivery.[11]

MANAGEMENT

In the absence of effective fetal therapy, timing of delivery is of high importance, given that the risk of intrauterine fetal damage has to be balanced against the potential risk of prematurity. The goal in the management of IUGR is to deliver the most mature fetus in the best physiological condition possible while minimizing the risk to the mother. Such a goal requires the use of antenatal testing with the hope of identifying the fetus with IUGR before it becomes acidotic.

The most frequently used clinical tools to time delivery are fetal heart rate (FHR) or biophysical profile score (BPP), which reflects central nervous system involvement and their changes are a late sign of fetal compromise. Recently, many clinicians have turned their attention to fetal venous Doppler analysis with the hope that this would allow delivery during the early phase of decompensation.[15–18]

The evolution of fetal hypoxemia leads to abnormal fetal growth, abnormal arterial Doppler, abnormal venous Doppler resulting in abnormal FHR/BPP score. The interval between abnormal arterial and venous Doppler is approximately 2 weeks and the time between abnormal venous Doppler and abnormal FHR/BPP score is up to 7 days. Apart from this sequence, there are several recent studies that consider that FHR abnormalities may precede an abnormal venous Doppler in about 50% of the cases.[18,19]

The analysis of the available current data cannot reach a conclusion about the relative merits of using FHR and BPP score, the arterial and venous fetal Doppler analysis or a specific combination of these tests.[20]

We believe that in daily practice delivery is undertaken when the fetus shows signs of decompensation, but the choice of the appropriate test to identify decompensation is difficult and it is better to be based on the experience of each unit.

REFERENCES

1. MARTIN, A., R. BINDRA, P. CURCIO, et al. 2001. Screening for pre-clampsia and fetal growth restriction by uterine artery Doppler at 11–14 weeks of gestation. Ultrasound Obstet. Gynecol. **18:** 583–586.
2. LEES, C., M. PARRA, H. MISSFELDER-LOBOS, et al. 2001. Individualized risk assessment for adverse pregnancy outcome by uterine artery Doppler at 23 weeks. Obstet. Gynecol. **98:** 369–373.
3. LEITICH, H., C. EGARTER, P. HUSSEIN. 1997. A meta analysis of low dose aspirin for the prevention of intrauterine growth retardation. Br. J. Obstet. Gynecol. **104:** 450–459.
4. HARRINGTON, K.F. 2000. Making best and appropriate use of fetal biophysical and Doppler ultrasound data in the management of the growth-restricted fetus. Ultrasound Obstet. Gynecol. **16:** 399–401.
5. TOBAL, N., M. CHEVILLOT, J. HIMILY, et al. 2002. Doppler monitoring of fetal circulation from multiple arteries over several days to improve evaluation of fetal prognosis. J. Radiol. **83:** 1943–1951.
6. FARINE, D., S GRANOVSKY-GRISARU, G. RYAN, et al. 1998. Umbilical artery blood flow velocity in pregnancies complicated by systemic lupus erythematosus. J. Clin. Ultrasound **26:** 379–382.
7. MANDRUZZATO, G.P., P. BOGATTI, L. FISCHER & C. GIGLI. 1991. The clinical significance of absent or reverse end-diastolic flow in the fetal aorta and umbilical artery. Ultrasound Obstet. Gynecol. **1:** 192–196.
8. NICOLAIDES, K.H., G. RIZZO & K. HECHER. 2000. Doppler Studies in Fetal Hypoxemic Hypoxia in Placental and Fetal Doppler. The Parthenon Publishing Group New York. London. 67–87.
9. CLERICI & G., R. LUZIETTI, P. NARDUCCI, G. DIRENZO. 2003. Fetal cerebral blood flow. Ultrasound Rev. Obstet. Gynecol. **3:** 111–116.
10. ABUHAMAD, A. 2003. Color and pulsed Doppler ultrasonography of the fetal coronary arteries: has the time come for its clinical application? Ultrasound Obstet. Gynecol. **21:** 423–425.
11. PRADO VASQUES, F.A., A. MORON, C. MURTA, et al. 2004. The assessment of fetal well-being by venous Doppler velocimetry. Ultrasound Rev. Obstet. Gynecol. **4:** 121–125.
12. MULLER, J., R. NANAH, M. ROHN, P. KRISTEN & J. DIETI. 2002. Arterial and ductus venosus Doppler in fetuses with absent or reversed and diastolic flow in the umbilical artery: correlation with short term perinatal outcome. Acta Obstet. Gynecol. Scan. **81:** 860–866.
13. FIGUERAS, F., J. MARTINEZ, B. PUERTO, et al. 2003. Contraction stress test versus ductus venosus Doppler evaluation for the prediction of adverse perinatal

outcome in growth-restricted fetuses with non-reassuring, non-stressed test. Ultrasound Obstet. Gynecol. **21:** 250–255.

14. BASCHAT, A.A. 2003. Relationship between placental blood flow resistance and precordial venous Doppler indices. Ultrasound Obstet. Gynecol. **22:** 561–566.

15. BILARDO, C., H. WOLF, R. STIGTER, *et al.* 2004. Relationship between monitoring parameters and perinatal outcome in severe early intrauterine growth restriction. Ultrasound Obstet. Gynecol. **23:** 119–125.

16. HECHER, K. & B.J. HACKELOER. 1997. Cardiotocogram compared to Doppler investigation of the fetal circulation in the premature growth-retarded fetus: longitudinal observations. Ultrasound Obstet. Gynecol. **9:** 152–161.

17. BASCHAT, A.A., U. GEMBRUSH & C.R. HARMAN. 2001. The sequence of changes in Doppler and biophysical parameters as severe fetal growth restriction worsens. Ultrasound Obstet. Gynecol. **18:** 571–577.

18. FERRAZZI, E., M. BOZZO, S. RIGANO, *et al.* 2002. Temporal sequence of abnormal Doppler changes in the peripheral and central circulatory systems of the severely growth-restricted fetus. Ultrasound Obstet. Gynecol. **19:** 140–146.

19. HECHER, K., H. BILARDO, R. STIGTER, *et al.* 2001. Monitoring of fetuses with intrauterine growth restriction: a longitudinal study. Ultrasound Obstet. Gynecol. **18:** 564–570.

20. ROMERO, R., K. KALACHE & N. KADAR. 2002. Timing of delivery of the preterm severely growth restricted fetus: venous Doppler, Cardiotocography or the biophysical profile? Ultrasound Obstet. Gynecol. **19:** 118–121.

The Fetus That Is Small for Gestational Age

NIKOLAOS VRACHNIS, DIMITRIOS BOTSIS, AND ZOE ILIODROMITI

Second Department of Obstetrics and Gynecology, University of Athens Medical School, Aretaieion Hospital, Athens, Greece

ABSTRACT: The symmetric small for gestational age (SGA) fetus presents a complex management problem for the obstetrician, but the growth restriction affects morbidity and mortality at all stages of life. The differential diagnosis in symmetric growth aberration includes the constitutionally small fetus, the fetus with pathology, and the cases with incorrect dating of pregnancy. The ultrasonographic examination focuses in the detection of anomalies, signs of intrauterine infection, and serial assessment of fetal growth. Accuracy of fetal biometry may be improved by using individualized fetal growth curves. From the available surveillance tools, the uterine artery Doppler has a value in predicting poor perinatal outcome. Magnetic resonance imaging is also useful in the evaluation of anomalies. Cesarean section is not justified for all symmetric SGA fetuses that may carry a guarded prognosis.

KEYWORDS: symmetric; small for gestational age (SGA); intrauterine growth restriction (IUGR); screening; ultrasonography; diagnosis; delivery

INTRODUCTION

The small for gestational age (SGA) fetus has failed to achieve its growth potential by a specific gestational age and this poses a significantly increased risk of poor prognosis. The growth restriction affects morbidity and mortality at all stages of life. Thus in perinatal life these fetuses are at greater risk of stillbirth, neonatal mortality, prematurity, perinatal depression, hypoglycemia, hypothermia, and infection, while in childhood they are at increased risk for poor growth, sudden infant death syndrome, and impaired neurodevelopment. Finally, in adult life they are at greater risk for hypertension, coronary heart disease, and type 2 diabetes.[1–3]

As by definition 10% of all pregnancies will be "too small." The differential diagnosis of a symmetric SGA fetus (20-30% of SGA cases) will include

Address for correspondence: Dr. N. Vrachnis, Second Department of Obstetrics and Gynecology, University of Athens Medical School, Aretaieion Hospital, 124B Vas. Sofias Av., 115-26, Athens, Greece. Voice: 00302107777442; fax: 00302107777390.
e-mail: nvrachnis@med.uoa.gr

Ann. N.Y. Acad. Sci. 1092: 304–309 (2006). © 2006 New York Academy of Sciences.
doi: 10.1196/annals.1365.028

the constitutionally small fetus, the fetus with pathology, and the fetus with infection. The characteristics and particularly the height of the parents, the fetal growth on the same low centile throughout pregnancy, and the obstetric history of prior healthy deliveries on a low centile are helpful clues to the direction of a constitutionally small fetus. An SGA fetus with pathology may be seen as a result of fetal factors such as trisomies or triploidy, nonaneuploid syndromes, structural abnormalities, or intrauterine fetal infection. Finally, the differential diagnosis will include cases with incorrect dating of pregnancy where the accurate menstrual history in the presence of normal fetal anatomy plays a vital role. Our initial diagnosis of incorrect dating will be later boosted by the normal interval growth on follow-up exams.

The SGA fetus presents a complex management problem for the obstetrician who must diagnose inadequate fetal growth and recognize the SGA.[4] The earliest scan is the most accurate and in cases that an early scan was missed, the presence of distal femoral epiphysis and the proximal tibial epiphysis in a fetus declares that the fetus is more than 32 or 35 weeks, respectively. As accurate dating is the key for making the diagnosis, the application of individualized fetal growth ultrasound curves results in a further increased detection rate of true growth restriction and a reduction in false-positive diagnoses for SGA.[5] The individualized ultrasound growth curves take into account characteristics such as maternal booking height and weight, ethnic origin, parity, and fetal sex.[6–9] However, more studies are required to show if their widespread use is going to improve further the detection of a fetus at risk for stillbirth in comparison with the standard (population-based) curves.

The abdominal circumference (AC) and the estimated fetal weight (EFW) are the most accurate measurements to predict an SGA fetus, whereas from all the biometric measurements the AC is the most sensitive one.[10] The AC mainly reflects the fetal liver size, which is dependent on glycogen storage in it and consequently the AC mirrors fetal nutrition. As growth is a dynamic procedure, serial measurements of AC and EFW are superior to single ones for prediction of SGA and adverse perinatal outcome.[11] FIGURE 1 shows serial measurements in a symmetric SGA fetus.

The various formulas for estimating birth weight *in utero* (EFW) present various methodological or analytical faults.[12] The best formulas for EFW for fetuses between 2,080 g and 4,430 g are the Shepard and Aoki formulas as these have the least decline from the actual birth weight.[12] However, for very low birth weights, the Hadlock formula is more appropriate to use.

The decision if the SGA fetus is symmetric or asymmetric is arbitrary with considerable overlap.[13,14] The symmetric SGA usually reflects a fetal problem with early onset even in the first trimester as growth restriction is usually the same for all parameters (biometry). In contrast, the asymmetric SGA usually reflects a placental problem with onset in the late second or the third trimester, while growth restriction is discordant with the abdominal circumference most

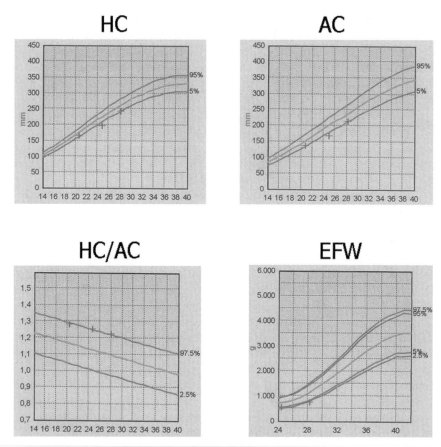

FIGURE 1. Example of growth charts showing the head circumference (HC), the abdominal circumference (AC), the head/abdominal circumference ratio (HC/AC), and the estimated fetal weight (EFW) in a symmetric SGA fetus.

affected. Differences in pathophysiology and etiology in both groups are shown in TABLE 1.

The ultrasound findings in a SGA symmetric fetus vary from normal to multiple abnormalities if aneuploidy, structural anomaly, or infection is present. The combination of SGA with polyhydramnios is an ominous one with high risk for trisomy 18, while the association of SGA with oligohydramnios increases the risk of perinatal mortality. Cardiac and renal structural anomalies are common fetal conditions associated with SGA.[15] Infection may be due to cytomegalovirus, malaria, HIV, herpes virus, parvovirus, rubella, or toxoplasmosis.[14,16] A careful search for anomalies and signs of intrauterine infection (venticulomegaly, hydrops, intracranial, or liver calcifications) is required.[17] The AIDS embryopathy results in characteristic craniofacial abnormalities.

TABLE 1. Differences in symmetric and asymmetric SGA fetuses

	Symmetric SGA	Asymmetric SGA
Pathophysiology	Reduced cell number	Reduced cell size
	Impaired cell hyperplasia	Impaired cell hypertrophy
Etiology	Abnormal karyotype	Placental vascular factors
	Congenital malformations	Hypertension
	Infections	Diabetes mellitus
	Drugs	Renal disease
	Early onset preeclampsia	Collagen vascular disease
		Thrombophilia

Maternal dental disease or infection by *Helicobacter pylori* have also been associated with SGA.[18,19]

The magnetic resonance imaging (MRI) has a possible application in the evaluation of anomalies, being most valuable in the assessment of the central nervous system. It is particularly useful in the confirmation of destructive intracranial processes as a result of infection. Thus, MRI documentation can affect the mode of delivery as Cesarean section for fetal distress is not indicated if the fetal brain is damaged.[20]

The presence of fetal anomalies will affect karyotype assessment and infection screen for viral DNA in the amniotic fluid.[21] It may be appropriate to discuss karyotyping with parents even in cases with normal anatomical survey, as up to 19% of fetuses with an AC and EFW below the fifth centile may have abnormal karyotype. If termination is offered in the presence of abnormalities, this should be accompanied by autopsy for achievement of specific diagnosis.

From all surveillance tools (cardiotocography, biophysical profile [BPP], umbilical artery Doppler [UA Doppler], and estimation of liquor volume), the uterine artery Doppler has a value in predicting poor perinatal outcome particularly in the high-risk cases.[22,23] Nevertheless, if a woman is screened and uterine artery Doppler is positive (presence of bilateral notches, increased resistance index), this is expected to increase the frequency of antenatal visits. For the constitutionally small fetus the BPP and the UA Doppler are usually normal, while in a fetus with structural abnormality, abnormal karyotype, or fetal infection the BPP may be variable with a normal UA Doppler. The cardiotocography has not been shown to improve the perinatal morbidity and mortality.

There are no sufficient data to justify an elective Cesarean section for all SGA fetuses.[24] A trial of labor may be considered if the UA Doppler is normal.[25] Especially in pregnancies with constitutionally small fetus a term delivery may be anticipated. On the contrary, in a fetus with abnormality or infection, the surveillance and the time of delivery are dependent on the etiology or the fetal well-being. In cases with known poor prognosis, that is, trisomy 18 that the parents elect to continue in pregnancy there is no need for intervention due to fetal indication during labor. However, if the pregnancy progresses with ambiguous diagnosis, the intrapartum cardiotocography can reduce perinatal death rates and the neonatal resuscitation is appropriate. Delivery should take place in a unit with relevant facilities and neonatal expertise.

The symmetric SGA fetuses carry a guarded prognosis.[26] Outcome is less likely to improve due to aggressive monitoring and use of Doppler compared with the asymmetric SGA fetus in which they play an important role in the evaluation of fetal condition and decision making.[27] The recurrence risk for SGA is 29% if a previous pregnancy was affected and 44% if two previous pregnancies were affected.[28]

REFERENCES

1. McINTIRE, D.D., S.L. BLOOM, B.M. CASEY, et al. 1999. Birthweight in relation to morbidity and mortality among newborn infants. N. Engl. J. Med. **340:** 1234–1238.
2. BARKER, D.J., P.D. GLUCKMAN, K.M. GODFREY, et al. 1993. Fetal nutrition and cardiovascular disease in adult life. Lancet **341:** 938–941.
3. BARKER, D.J. 1997. The long-term outcome of retarded fetal growth. Clin. Obstet. Gynecol. **40:** 853–863.
4. BAMBERG, C. & K.D. KALACHE. 2004. Prenatal diagnosis of fetal growth restriction. Semin. Fetal Neonatal. Med. **9:** 387–394.
5. GARDOSI, J. 1998. The application of individualised fetal growth curves. J. Perinat Med. **26:** 137–142.
6. PANG, M.W., T.N. LEUNG, D.S. SAHOTA, et al. 2003. Customizing fetal biometric charts. Ultrasound Obstet. Gynecol. **22:** 271–276.
7. CLAUSSON, B., J. GARDOSI, A. FRANCIS, et al. 2001. Perinatal outcome in SGA births defined by customised versus population-based birth weight standards. BJOG **108:** 830–834.
8. OWEN, P., J. OGAH, L.M. BACHMANN, et al. 2003. Prediction of intrauterine growth restriction with customised estimated fetal weight centiles. BJOG **110:** 411–415.
9. LYON, V., A. HOWATSON, K.S. KHAN, et al. 2004. Unadjusted and customised weight centiles in the identification of growth restriction among stillborn infants. BJOG **111:** 1460–1463.
10. CHANG, T.C., S.C. ROBSON, R.J. BOYS, et al. 1992. Prediction of the small for gestational age infant: which ultrasonic measurement is best? Obstet. Gynecol. **80:** 1030–1038.
11. CHANG, T.C., S.C. ROBSON, J.A. SPENCER, et al. 1993. Identification of fetal growth retardation: comparison of Doppler waveform indices and serial ultrasound measurements of abdominal circumference and fetal weight. Obstet. Gynecol. **82:** 230–236.
12. CHIEN, P.F., P. OWEN & K.S. KHAN. 2000. Validity of ultrasound estimation of fetal weight. Obstet. Gynecol. **95:** 856–860.
13. LIN, C.C., S.J. SU & L.P. RIVER. 1991. Comparison of associated high-risk factors and perinatal outcome between symmetric and asymmetric fetal intrauterine growth retardation. Am. J. Obstet. Gynecol. **164:** 1535–1541.

14. LIN, C.-C & J. SANTOLAYA-FORGAS. 1998. Current concepts of fetal growth restriction: part I. Causes, classification, and pathophysiology. Obstet. Gynecol. **92:** 1044–1055.

15. DE JONG, C.L.D. 2000. Optimal antenatal care by the application of individualised standards. Eur. J. Obstet. Gynaecol. Reprod. Biol. **92:** 185–187.

16. GULMEZOGLU, M., O.M. DE & J. VILLAR. 1997. Effectiveness of interventions to prevent or treat impaired fetal growth. Obstet. Gynecol. Surv. **52:** 139–149.

17. BASCHAT, A.A. 2004. Pathophysiology of fetal growth restriction: implications for diagnosis and surveillance. Obstet. Gynecol. Surv. **59:** 617–627.

18. OFFENBACHER, S., S. LIEFF, K.A. BOGGESS, *et al.* 2001. Maternal periodontitis and prematurity. Part I. Obstetric outcome of prematurity and growth restriction. Ann. Periodontol. **6:** 164–174.

19. ESLICK, G.D., P. YAN, H.H. XIA, *et al.* 2002. Foetal intrauterine growth restrictions with Helicobacter pylori infection. Aliment Pharmacol. Ther. **16:** 1677–1682.

20. GOLJA, A.M., J.A. ASTROFF & R.L. ROBERTSON. 2004. Fetal imaging of central nervous system abnormalities. **14:** 293–306.

21. SNIJDERS, R.J., C. SHERROD, C.M. GOSDEN, *et al.* 1993. Fetal growth retardation: associated malformations and chromosomal abnormalities. Am. J. Obstet. Gynecol. **168:** 547–555.

22. ALFIREVIC, Z. & J.P. NEILSON. 1995. Doppler ultrasonography in high-risk pregnancies: systematic review with meta-analysis. Am. J. Obstet. Gynecol. **172:** 1379–1387.

23. SOOTHILL, P.W., R.A. AJAYI, S. CAMPBELL, *et al.* 1993. Prediction of morbidity in small and normally grown fetuses by fetal heart rate variability, biophysical profile score and umbilical artery Doppler studies. Br. J. Obstet. Gynaecol. **100:** 742–745.

24. GRANT, A. & C.M., GLAZENER. 2001. Elective versus selective caesarean section for delivery of the small baby. Cochrane Database Syst. Rev. **1:** CD000078.

25. WILLIAMS, K.P., D.F. FARQUAHARSON, M. BEBBINGTON, *et al.* 2003. Screening for fetal well-being in a high-risk pregnant population comparing the nonstress test with umbilical artery Doppler velocimetry: a randomized controlled clinical trial. Am. J. Obstet. Gynecol. **188:** 1366–1371.

26. ILLANES, S. & P. SOOTHILL. 2004. Management of fetal growth restriction. Semin. Fetal Neonatal Med. **9:** 395–401.

27. RESNIK, R. 2002. Intrauterine growth restriction. Obstet. Gynecol. **99:** 490–496.

28. ABUZZAHAB, M.J., M.D. SCHNEIDER, A. GODDARD, *et al.* 2003. IGF-I receptor mutations resulting in intrauterine and postnatal growth retardation. N. Engl. J. Med. **349:** 2211–2222.

"Reproductive" Corticotropin-Releasing Hormone

NIKOLAOS VITORATOS,[a] DIMITRIOS C. PAPATHEODOROU,[b]
SOPHIA N. KALANTARIDOU,[c] AND GEORGE MASTORAKOS[d]

[a]Second Department of Obstetrics and Gynecology, Aretaieion Hospital,
Medical School, University of Athens, Athens, Greece

[b]Department of Obstetrics and Gynecology, Nikaia General Hospital, Athens,
Greece

[c]Division of Reproductive Endocrinology, Department of Obstetrics and
Gynecology, University of Ioannina Medical School, Ioannina, Greece

[d]Endocrine Unit, Second Department of Obstetrics and Gynecology, Aretaieion
Hospital, Medical School, University of Athens, Athens, Greece

ABSTRACT: Corticotropin-releasing hormone (CRH), a 41 amino acid
peptide, is an important regulatory molecule synthesized by neurons of
the parvocellular and magnocellular hypothalamic paraventricular nuclei. It acts as the major physiologic corticotropin (ACTH) secretagogue.
The CRH gene is located in humans on chromosome 8. The CRH hormone family has at least four ligands, two receptors (CRH-R1 and CRH-
R2), and a binding protein (CRHbp). CRH is the principal regulator of
the hypothalamic-pituitary-adrenal axis. Furthermore, CRH has been
identified in most female reproductive tissues including the uterus, the
placenta, and the ovary. CRH produced in the endometrium may participate in decidualization, implantation, and early maternal tolerance to
semiallograft embryo. Placental CRH may participate in the physiology
of pregnancy, in late pregnancy complications such as preterm labor and
preeclampsia, and also in the onset of parturition. Ovarian CRH is involved in follicular maturation, ovulation, and luteolysis. Increased levels
of unbound placental CRH may be responsible for the hypercortisolism
of the second half of pregnancy. This hypercortisolism is followed by a
transient suppression of hypothalamic CRH secretion in the postpartum
period. This may explain the depressive states frequently observed in the
postpartum period.

KEYWORDS: corticotropin-releasing hormone; CRH; hypothalamic paraventricular nuclei; hypothalamic-pituitary-adrenal axis; HPA

Address for correspondence: Dr. G. Mastorakos, 3 Neofytou Vamva Street, Athens, Greece, 10674.
Voice: +30-6977698009; fax: +302103636229.
e-mail: mastorak@mail.kapatel.gr

Ann. N.Y. Acad. Sci. 1092: 310–318 (2006). © 2006 New York Academy of Sciences.
doi: 10.1196/annals.1365.029

INTRODUCTION

Corticotropin-releasing hormone (CRH), the principal regulator of the hypothalamic-pituitary-adrenal axis as well as its receptors, has been identified in most female reproductive tissues including the endometrial glands, decidualized endometrial stroma, placental trophoblast, decidua, and ovaries.[1–4] In addition, CRH and its receptors have also been identified in Leydig cells of the testis, where CRH exerts autocrine inhibitory actions on testosterone biosynthesis.[5] "Reproductive" CRH is a form of "tissue" CRH (CRH found in peripheral tissues) and is analogous to the "immune" CRH found in peripheral inflammatory sites.[6] "Reproductive" CRH seems to regulate key reproductive functions with an inflammatory component (aseptic inflammation) such as ovulation, luteolysis, implantation, and parturition.

ROLE OF CRH ON OVARIAN FUNCTION

CRH and its receptors are present in rat and human ovaries.[7,8] Ovarian CRH may participate in the "aseptic" inflammatory processes of the ovary including ovulation and luteolysis. CRH has been found in the cytoplasm of thecal cells surrounding the ovarian follicles, in luteinized cells of the stroma, in large granulose-derived luteinized cells of developing corpora lutea, and in human follicular fluid.[7,8] Corticotropin-releasing hormone type 1 receptors (CRH-R1) are also found in the stroma and theca and in the cumulus oophorus.

In normal human ovaries, there is no CRH present in oocytes of primordial follicles, whereas there is abundant expression of the gene encoding CRH and its CRH-R1 in mature follicles, suggesting that CRH may play auto/paracrine roles in follicular maturation.[8,9] CRH receptor type 1 mRNA signal has been found exclusively in thecal cells of mature follicles and moderately in small antral follicles,[9] while granulosa cells are devoid of CRH and CRH-R1 mRNA. Furthermore, the concentration of CRH is higher in the premenopausal than the postmenopausal ovaries, suggesting that ovarian CRH is related to normal ovarian function during the reproductive life span.[10] Interestingly, in women with polycystic ovarian syndrome, CRH is present in the theca; however, it is less prominent in the stroma or the corpora lutea, whereas it is detected in oocytes of primordial follicles.[8]

In vitro experiments have shown that CRH exerts an inhibitory effect on ovarian steroidogenesis in a dose-dependent, interleukin (IL)-1-mediated manner,[11,12] suggesting that ovarian CRH may also have antireproductive actions. Thus, ovarian CRH may play a role in the ovary through auto/paracrine inhibitions of steroid biosynthesis and it may also participate in follicular maturation, ovulation, and luteolysis.[13]

ROLE OF CRH ON DECIDUALIZATION

Human and rat uterus express the CRH gene. The epithelial cells of human and rodent endometrium produce CRH throughout the menstrual cycle, while the stroma needs to undergo decidualization to produce CRH.[1,14–16] CRH-R1 is present on the human endometrium[17] and the human myometrium.[18]

Estrogens and glucocorticoids inhibit and prostaglandin E2 stimulates the promoter of human CRH gene transfected to human endometrial cells, suggesting that the endometrial CRH gene is under the control of these hormones.[19]

The endometrial glands are full of CRH during both the proliferative and the secretory phases of the cycle.[1] However, the concentration of CRH is significantly higher in the secretory phase, associating endometrial CRH with intrauterine phenomena of the secretory phase of the menstrual cycle such as decidualization and implantation.[10] Indeed, endometrial CRH is under the positive control of progesterone, participating in the decidualization process of endometrial stroma, by regulating the production of local modulators of decidualization such as prostaglandin E2, IL-1, and IL-6.[1,20,21]

ROLE OF CRH ON IMPLANTATION

During blastocyst implantation, the maternal endometrial response to the invading semiallograft embryo has the characteristics of an acute, aseptic inflammatory response. However, once implanted the embryo suppresses this response and prevents rejection. At the same time, the mother's immune system inhibits a graft versus host reaction that might ensue from the fetal immune system.[22]

The Fas molecule and its ligand (FasL) play an important role in the regulation of immune tolerance mainly by inducing apoptosis in activated leukocytes carrying FasL.[23,24] Embryonic trophoblast and maternal decidua produce CRH and express FasL. Similarly, the gene encoding the CRH-R1 is expressed in human endometrial stromal cells.[17]

Early in pregnancy, the implantation sites in rat endometrium contain 3.5-fold higher concentrations of CRH compared to the interimplantation regions,[16] indicating that CRH might participate in implantation. Antalarmin, a CRH-R1 antagonist, decreased FasL expression and promoted apoptosis of activated T lymphocytes, an effect that was potentiated by CRH and inhibited by antalarmin.[25] Female rats treated with antalarmin showed a marked decrease in implantation sites and live embryos and diminished FasL expression.[25] Thus, locally produced CRH promotes implantation and maintenance of early pregnancy primarily by killing activated T cells. In the past, we had also described this phenomenon in experimental autoimmune uveoretinitis in rodents. We had shown that retinal cells during experimental autoimmune uveoretinitis undergo apoptosis with concurrent upregulation of Fas and FasL. The local presence of CRH appears to be of pivotal importance in this process.[26,27] Recent studies reveal that CRH inhibits trophoblast invasion by decreasing the expression of carcinoembryonic antigen-related cell adhesion molecule 1 (CEACAM1), which is expressed in extravillous trophoblasts (EVTs) of normal human placenta. This effect might be involved in the pathophysiology of clinical conditions such as preeclampsia and placenta accreta.[28] A 40 amino acid peptide that is closely related to CRH and binds with high affinity to both CRH type 1 and type 2 receptors, urocortin (UCN), seems to be expressed in EVT. The functional significance of urocortin for the physiology of EVT requires further investigation.[29]

ROLE OF CRH ON PARTURITION

Placental CRH is produced in syncytiotrophoblast cells[30] as well as in placental decidua and fetal membranes,[31] and its expression increases as much as 100 times during the last 6 to 8 weeks of pregnancy.[32] Placental CRH drives the fetal pituitary-adrenal axis to produce increased amounts of cortisol secretion during the latter half of pregnancy.[33] The increased production of cortisol in the third trimester is a result of increased activity of the hypothalamic-pituitary-adrenal (HPA) axis that acts in a noncircadian, nonpulsatile fashion.[34] Most circulating CRH is neutralized by CRH-binding protein produced by the liver. By 28 to 30 weeks of gestation, CRH levels in plasma are similar of those in the portal system, whereas the levels of CRH-binding protein are similar to those in nonpregnant women.[33,35,36] However, between weeks 34 and 35 of gestation, the concentrations of CRH-binding protein fall by about 60%, leading to increase of unbound CRH. Subsequently, plasma-free CRH levels rise further, to peak at labor and delivery. CRH seems to increase local matrix metalloproteinase[37] (MMP) activity in the placenta and fetal membranes, thereby contributing to membrane rupture with the onset and progression of human labor.

The hypercortisolism of pregnancy is followed by a transient inertia of hypothalamic CRH secretion in the postpartum period, which may explain the blues or depression and autoimmune phenomena seen during this period.[33,38,39]

Because the human placenta cannot synthesize estrogens directly, the fetal adrenal zone is the predominant source of their precursor, dehydroepiandrosterone. Placental CRH stimulates fetal adrenocorticotropic hormone (ACTH) release and fetal adrenal steroidogenesis both via ACTH secretion as well as by direct action on adrenals, satisfying the high demand for synthesis of dehydroepiandrosterone.[40] In addition, newer data suggest that placental CRH exerts a tonic stimulatory effect on estrogen production as shown by cultures of human placental trophoblast cells.[41] It should be noted that via stimulation of fetal cortisol secretion, placental CRH contributes to fetal organ maturation.[40]

Placental CRH induces vasodilation of the fetoplacental circulation by activating nitric oxide synthase and participates in labor by stimulating secretion of prostaglandin $F_{2alpha,}$ and E2 by the fetal membranes and by promoting constriction of myometrial cells.[31,42] Furthermore, CRH-R1 is significantly upregulated at the time of labor in the human myometrium and the fetal membranes.[43] Placental CRH secretion is stimulated by glucocorticoids, inflammatory cytokines, and anoxic conditions, including the stress of preeclampsia or eclampsia,[33,44,45] whereas it is repressed by estrogens.[46]

CRH may be the placental clock determining the onset of parturition.[47] The highest levels of CRH are achieved as labor approaches and subsequently they fall to prepartum values within 24 h after delivery.[33,40] Inappropriately high CRH levels have been described in pregnancies complicated by preterm labor.[48] Indeed, a prospective longitudinal study showed that CRH levels measured at 16 to 20 weeks' gestation could predict term, preterm, or postterm birth.[47] Thus, plasma levels of CRH are markedly elevated in preeclamptic or eclamptic mothers, mothers with intrauterine infections, and in healthy pregnant women during normal labor. Elevated CRH levels at 33 weeks' gestation[49] were significantly associated with a 3.3-fold increase in the relative risk (RR) for spontaneous preterm birth and with a 3.6-fold increase in the RR for fetal growth restriction. Women who delivered post term had significantly lower CRH levels in the early third trimester than those who delivered at term.

Recently, we found[50] that women with preterm labor show significantly higher maternal IL-1β levels as compared to women of same gestational age with normal pregnancy. It is known that proinflammatory cytokines such as tumor necrosis factor-α, IL-1β, and IL-6 play a role in the onset of labor.[51] Interestingly, a positive correlation was found between IL-1β and CRH levels in women with preterm labor and women with normal pregnancy of the same gestational age, although it was statistically significant only in the former group of women. The coefficient of correlation was clearly stronger in the preterm labor group. This is probably due to the fact that the increased levels of CRH and IL-1β during preterm labor reflect better the intensity of the quantitative relationship of these two substances and thus correlate in a more statistically obvious way. IL-1β may act in synergy with other factors inducing, in combination with them, the production and release of biologically significant amounts of prostaglandins resulting in the initiation of preterm labor. Our findings support the hypothesis that IL-1β acts directly and/or indirectly as a biological effector on placental CRH release in women with preterm labor. It seems, however, that critical levels of CRH should be achieved for the initiation of labor. Further investigation is necessary to confirm this hypothesis. Of note, in sheep, administration of antalarmin, a CRH receptor type 1 antagonist, can delay the onset of parturition.[52]

CONCLUSIONS

CRH, the principal regulator of the HPA axis as well as its receptors, have been identified in most female reproductive tissues including the uterus, placenta, and ovary. "Reproductive" CRH is a form of tissue CRH (CRH found in peripheral tissues) and is analogous to the "immune" CRH found in peripheral inflammatory sites. These include endometrial, placental, and ovarian CRH that may participate in decidualization, implantation, physiology of pregnancy, parturition, ovulation, and luteolysis. The hypercortisolism of the latter half of pregnancy can be explained by high levels of placental CRH in plasma. This hypercortisolism causes a transient adrenal suppression in the postpartum period, which may explain the blues or depression and autoimmune phenomena frequently observed during this period.[53] Antalarmin (a pyrrolopyrimidine antagonist) is a specific CRH-R1 antagonist, which has been used in investigations of the physiologic central and peripheral roles of CRH, in the immune/inflammatory response, and the reproductive function. In recent experiments,[25] antalarmin prevented implantation in rats by reducing the inflammatory-like reaction of the endometrium to the invading blastocyst. Consequently, antalarmin and analogous compounds might represent a new class of nonsteroidal inhibitors of pregnancy at its very early stages.

REFERENCES

1. MASTORAKOS, G., C.D. SCOPA, L.C. KAO, *et al*. 1996. Presence of immunoreactive corticotropin releasing hormone in human endometrium. J. Clin. Endocrinol. Metab. **81:** 1046–1050.
2. GRAMMATOPOULOS, D. & G.P. CHROUSOS. 2002. Structural and signaling diversity of corticotropin-releasing hormone (CRH) and related peptides and their receptors: potential clinical applications of CRH receptor antagonists. Trends Endocrinol. Metab. **13:** 436–444.
3. MASTORAKOS, G., M.G. PAVLATOU & M. MIZAMTSIDI. 2006. The hypothalamic-pituitary-adrenal and the hypothalamic- pituitary-gonadal axes interplay. Review. Pediatr. Endocrinol. Rev. **3**(Suppl 1): 172–181.
4. KALANTARIDOU, S.N., A. MAKRIGIANNAKIS, G. MASTORAKOS & G.P. CHROUSOS. 2003. Roles of reproductive corticotropin-releasing hormone. Review. Ann. N.Y. Acad. Sci. **997:** 129–135.
5. FABRI, A., J.C. TINAJERO & M.L. DUFAU. 1990. Corticotropin-releasing factor is produced by rat Leydig cells and has a major local antireproductive role in the testis. Endocrinology **127:** 1541–1543.
6. CHROUSOS, G.P. 1995. The hypothalamic-pituitary-adrenal axis and immune-mediated inflammation. N. Engl. J. Med. **332:** 1351–1362.
7. MASTORAKOS, G., C.D. SKOPA, A. VRYONIDOU, *et al*. 1994. Presence of immunoreactive corticotropin-releasing hormone in normal and polycystic ovaries. J. Clin. Endocrinol. Metabol. **79:** 934–939.

8. MASTORAKOS, G., E.L. WEBSTER, T.C. FRIEDMAN & G.P. CHROUSOS. 1993. Immunoreactive corticotropin-releasing hormone and its binding sites in the rat ovary. J. Clin. Invest. **92:** 961–968.

9. ASAKURA, H., I.H. ZWAIN & S.S.C. YEN. 1997. Expression of genes encoding corticotropin-releasing factor (CRF), type 1 receptor and CRF- binding protein and localization of the gene products in the human ovary. J. Clin. Endocrinol. Metabol. **82:** 2720–2725.

10. ZOUMAKIS, E., E. CHATZAKI, I. CHARALAMBOPOULOS, et al. 2001. Cycle and age-related changes in corticotropin-releasing hormone levels in human endometrium and ovaries. Gynecol. Endocrinol. **15:** 98–102.

11. CALOGERO, A.E., N. BURELLO, P. NEGRI-CESI, et al. 1996. Effects of corticotropin-releasing hormone on ovarian estrogen production in vitro. Endocrinology **137:** 4161–4166.

12. GHIZZONI, L., G. MASTORAKOS, A. VOTTERO, et al. 1997. Corticotropin-releasing hormone (CRH) inhibits steroid biosynthesis and interleukin-1 receptor mediated fashion. Endocrinology **138:** 4806–4811.

13. MASTORAKOS, G. & I. ILIAS. 2003. Maternal and fetal hypothalamic-pituitary-adrenal axes during pregnancy and postpartum. Review. Ann. N.Y. Acad. Sci. **997:** 136–149.

14. MAKRIGIANNAKIS, A., E. ZOUMAKIS, A.N. MARGIORIS, et al. 1995. The corticotropin-releasing hormone in normal and tumoral epithelial cells of human endometrium. J. Clin. Endocrinol. Metab. **80:** 185–193.

15. PETRAGLIA, F.S., S. TABANELLI, M.C. GALASSI, et al. 1992. Human decidua and in vitro decidualized endometrial stromal cells at term contain immunoreactive corticotropin-releasing factor (CRF) and CRF-messenger ribonucleic acid. J. Clin. Endocrinol. Metabol. **74:** 1427–1431.

16. MAKRIGIANNAKIS, A., A.N. MARGIORIS, C. LEGOASCOGNE, et al. 1995. Corticotropin-releasing hormone (CRH) is expressed at the implantation sites of early pregnant rat uterus. Life Sci. **57:** 1869–1875.

17. DIBLASIO, A., F. PEROCI-GIRALDI, P. VIGANO, et al. 1997. Expression of corticotropin-releasing hormone and its R1 receptor in human endometrial stromal cells. J. Clin. Endocrinol. Metabol. **82:** 1594–1597.

18. HILLHOUSE, E.W., D. GRAMMATOPOULOS, N.G. MILTON & H.W. QUARTERO. 1993. The identification of a human myometrial corticotropin-releasing hormone receptor that increases in affinity during pregnancy. J. Clin. Endocrinol. Metabol. **76:** 736–741.

19. MAKRIGIANNAKIS, A., E. ZOUMAKIS, A.N. MARGIORIS, et al. 1996. Regulation of the promoter of the human corticotropin-releasing hormone gene in transfected human endometrial cells. Neuroendocrinology **64:** 85–93.

20. FERRARI, A., F. PETRAGLIA & E. GURPIDE. 1995. Corticotropin-releasing factor decidualizes human endometrial stromal cells in vitro. Interaction with progestin. J. Steroid. Biochem. Mol. Biol. **54:** 251–255.

21. ZOUMAKIS, E., A.N. MARGIORIS, C. STOURNARAS, et al. 2000. Corticotropin-releasing hormone (CRH) interacts with inflammatory prostaglandins and interleukins and affects the decidualization of human endometrial stroma. Mol. Hum. Reprod. **6:** 344–351.

22. GILL, T.J. 1986. Immunological and genetic factors influencing pregnancy and development. Am. J. Reprod. Immunol. Microbiol. **10:** 116–120.

23. NAGATA, S. 1997. Apoptosis by death factor. Cell **88:** 355–365.

24. HUANG, D.C., M. HAHNE, M. SCHROETER, *et al.* 1999. Activation of Fas by FasL induces apoptosis by a mechanism that cannot be blocked by Bcl-2 or Bcl-x(L). Proc. Natl. Acad. Sci. USA **96:** 14871–14876.
25. MAKRIGIANNAKIS, A., E. ZOUMAKIS, S. KALANTARIDOU, *et al.* 2001. Corticotropin-releasing hormone promotes blastocyst implantation and early maternal tolerance. Nat. Immunol. **2:** 1018–1024.
26. POULAKI, V., N. MITSIADES, G. MASTORAKOS, *et al.* 2001. Fas/Fas ligand-associated apoptosis in experimental autoimmune uveoretinitis in rodents: role of proinflammatory corticotropin-releasing hormone. Exp. Eye Res. **72:** 623–629.
27. MASTORAKOS, G., E.A. BOUZAS, P.B. SILVER, *et al.* 1995. Immune corticotropin-releasing hormone is present in the eyes of and promotes experimental autoimmune uveoretinitis in rodents. Endocrinology **136:** 4650–4658.
28. BAMBERGER, A.M., V. MINAS, S.N. KALANTARIDOU, *et al.* 2006. Corticotropin-releasing hormone modulates human trophoblast invasion through carcinoembryonic antigen-related cell adhesion molecule-1 regulation. Am. J. Pathol. **168:** 141–150.
29. BAMBERGER, C.M., V. MINAS, A.M. BAMBERGER, *et al.* 2006. Expression of urocortin in the extravillous human trophoblast at the implantation site. Placenta Epub ahead of print.
30. RILEY, S.C., J.C. WALTON, J.M. HERLICK & J.R. CHALLIS. 1991. The localization and distribution of corticotropin-releasing hormone in the human placenta and fetal membranes throughout gestation. J. Clin. Endocinol. Metabol. **72:** 1001–1007.
31. JONES, S.A., A.N. BROOKS & J.R. CHALLIS. 1989. Steroids modulate corticotropin-releasing hormone production in human fetal membranes and placenta. J. Clin. Endocrinol. Metabol. **68:** 825–830.
32. FRIM, D.M., R.L. EMANUEL, B.G. ROBINSON, *et al.* 1988. Characterization and gestational regulation of corticotropin-releasing hormone messenger RNA in human placenta. J. Clin. Invest. **82:** 287–292.
33. CHROUSOS, G.P., D.J. TORPY & P.W. GOLD. 1998. Interactions between the hypothalamic-pituitary-adrenal axis and the female reproductive system: clinical implications. Ann. Intern. Med. **129:** 229–240.
34. MAGIAKOU, M.A., G. MASTORAKOS, D. RABIN, *et al.* 1996. The maternal hypothalamic-pituitary-adrenal axis in the third trimester of human pregnancy. Clin. Endocrinol. (Oxf). **44:** 419–428.
35. CHALLIS, J.R., S.G. MATTHEWS, C. VAN MEIR & M.M. RAMIREZ. 1995. Current topic: the placental corticotropin-releasing hormone-adrenocorticotrophin axis. Placenta **16:** 481–502.
36. LINTON, E.A., A.V. PERKINS, R.J. WOODS, *et al.* 1993. Corticotropin releasing hormone binding protein (CRH-BP): plasma levels during the third trimester of normal human pregnancy. J. Clin. Endocrinol. Metabol. **76:** 260–262.
37. LI, W. & J.R. CHALLIS. 2006. Corticotropin-releasing hormone and urocortin induce secretion of matrix metalloproteinase-9 (MMP-9) without change in tissue inhibitors of MMP-1 by cultured cells from human placenta and fetal membranes. J. Clin. Endocrinol. Metabol. **90:** 6569–6574.
38. MAGIAKOU, M.A., G. MASTORAKOS, D. RABIN, *et al.* 1996. Hypothalamic corticotropin releasing hormone suppression during the postpartum period: implications for the increase of psychiatric manifestations during this time. J. Clin. Endocrinol. Metabol. **81:** 1912–1917.

39. ELENKOV, I.J., R.L. WILDER, V.K. BAKALOV, et al. 2001. Interleukin 12, tumor necrosis factor-alpha and hormonal changes during late pregnancy and early postpartum: implications for autoimmune disease activity during these times. J. Clin. Endocrinol. Metabol. **86:** 4933–4938.
40. MAJZOUB, J.A. & K.P. KARALIS. 1999. Placental corticotropin-releasing hormone: function and regulation. Am. J. Obstet. Gynecol. 180(Suppl): 242–246.
41. YOU, X., R. YANG, X. TANG, et al. 2006. Corticotropin-releasing hormone stimulates estrogen biosynthesis in cultured human placental trophoblasts. Biol. Reprod. **74:** 1067–1072.
42. GRAMMATOPOULOS, D.K. & E.W. HILLHOUSE. 1999. Role of corticotropin releasing hormone in onset of labor. Lancet **354:** 1546–1549.
43. STEVENS, M.Y., J.R. CHALLIS & S.J. LYE. 1998. Corticotropin-releasing hormone subtype 1 is upregulated at the time of labor in human myometrium. J. Clin. Endocrinol. Metabol. **83:** 4107–4115.
44. ROBINSON, B.G., R.L. EMANUEL, D.M. FRIM & J.A. MAJZOUB. 1998. Glucocorticoids stimulate expression of corticotropin-releasing hormone gene in human placenta. Proc. Natl. Acad. Sci. USA **85:** 5244–5248.
45. GOLAND, R.S., I.M. CONWELL & S. JOZAK. 1995. The effect of preeclampsia on human placental corticotropin-releasing hormone content and processing. Placenta **16:** 375–382.
46. NI, X., R.C. NICHOLSON, B.R. KING, et al. 2002. Estrogen represses whereas the estrogen-antagonist ICI 182780 stimulates placental CRH gene expression. J. Clin. Endocrinol. Metabol. **87:** 3774–3778.
47. MCLEAN M., A. BITSIS, J. DAVIES, et al. 1995. A placental clock controlling the length of human pregnancy. Nat. Med. **1:** 460–463.
48. ERICKSON, K., P. THORSEN, G. CHROUSOS, et al. 2001. Preterm birth: associated neuroendocrine, medical, and behavioral risk factors. J. Clin. Endocrinol. Metabol. **86:** 2544–2552.
49. WADHWA, P.D., T.J. GARITE, M. PORTO, et al. 2004. Placental corticotropin-releasing hormone (CRH), spontaneous preterm birth, and fetal growth restriction: a prospective investigation. Am. J. Obstet. Gynecol. **191:** 1063–1069.
50. VITORATOS, N., G. MASTORAKOS, A. KOUNTOURIS, et al. 2006. Positive association of serum interleukin-1 beta and corticotropin releasing hormone levels in women with preterm labor. J. Endocrinol. Invest. In press.
51. CHALLIS, J.R.G., S.G. MATTHEWS, W. GIBB & S.J. LYE. 2000. Endocrine and paracrine regulation of birth at term and preterm. Endocr. Rev. **21:** 514–550.
52. CHENG-CHAN, E., J. FALKONER, G. MADSEN, et al. 1998. A corticotropin-releasing hormone type 1 receptor antagonist delays parturition in sheep. Endocrinology **139:** 3357–3360.
53. MASTORAKOS, G. & I. ILIAS. 2000. Maternal hypothalamic-pituitary-adrenal axis in pregnancy and the postpartum period. Postpartum-related disorders. Review. Ann. N. Y. Acad. Sci. **900:** 95–106.

Fetal Growth Restriction and Postnatal Development

MAKARIOS ELEFTHERIADES,[a,b] GEORGE CREATSAS,[b]
AND KYPROS NICOLAIDES[a]

[a]Harris Birthright Research Centre for Fetal Medicine, King's College Hospital,
University of London, London, United Kingdom

[b]Second Department of Obstetrics and Gynecology, Aretaieio Hospital,
University of Athens School of Medicine, Athens, Greece

ABSTRACT: The interaction between genetic constitution and *in utero*
environment determines fetal growth and development and influences
the susceptibility to certain disorders in adulthood. Data from both animal and human studies indicate that prenatal and early postnatal malnutrition can program the hypothalamus-pituitary-adrenal axis (HPA
axis), altering neuroendocrine response to stressors throughout lifetime.
Impaired uteroplacental perfusion results in fetal growth restriction
(FGR). In FGR there is evidence of chronic hypoxemia and alterations in
metabolic, endocrine, and hematological parameters, compatible with
starvation. Furthermore, FGR is associated with increased perinatal
mortality and in the survivors there is increased susceptibility to diabetes and cardiovascular disease in adulthood. There is evidence that
early postnatal growth acceleration, which would normally be considered desirable, may exacerbate metabolic dysfunction in later life.

KEYWORDS: fetal growth restriction; stress system; postnatal growth
acceleration; metabolic syndrome

DEVELOPMENTAL ORIGINS OF ADULT DISEASE

Both human and animal studies suggest that prenatal and early postnatal
environment and their interaction can modify developmental, physiological,
and endocrine mechanisms determining the risk of disease in adulthood.[1]

Birth weight is inversely related to the mortality rate due to adult cardiovascular disease. This finding led to the hypothesis that impaired fetal nutrition has
long-term adverse impact on adult health, by permanently altering or programming the structure, physiology, and metabolism of the developing organism.[2,3]

Address for correspondence: Makarios Eleftheriades, 26 Haravgis Street, Halandri, 152 32 Athens,
Greece. Voice: 0030-210-6833936; fax: 0030-210-6525013.
e-mail: makarios.eleftheriadis@kcl.ac.uk

Ann. N.Y. Acad. Sci. 1092: 319–330 (2006). © 2006 New York Academy of Sciences.
doi: 10.1196/annals.1365.047

Subsequently, in an attempt to clarify the relationship between low birth weight and cardiovascular disease, hypertension, insulin resistance, and dyslipidemia later in life, the "thrifty phenotype hypothesis" was proposed, which integrates the effect of prenatal and postnatal environment on susceptibility of adult disease.[4]

Thus, impaired *in utero* nutrition triggers an adaptive energy-sparing response by the fetus in which the growth of the brain, heart, and adrenals is preserved at the expense of other organs, such as the pancreas, with subsequent development of insulin resistance. This metabolic alteration would be beneficial in the presence of a deprived postnatal environment but maladaptive in an abundant environment. Consequently, a single genotype can produce more than one phenotype depending on both prenatal and postnatal environmental influences.[5]

An extension to the "thrifty phenotype hypothesis" proposes that fetal phenotypic responses to a hostile environment can either have immediate or long-term selective advantages for the individual (Predictive Adaptive Responses [PARs]).[6] In response to a predicted adverse postnatal environment, there are adaptive changes in body and organ size and composition as well as in neurohormonal and behavioral activity. Such adjustments would be beneficial if the environment turns out to be as predicted but disadvantageous if not.

Environmental factors can induce programming by producing epigenetic changes in DNA affecting gene expression. Altered gene expression of various hormones, enzymes, and/or their receptors can have a direct impact on certain metabolic pathways affecting fetal homeostasis.[7] Fetal tissue growth and differentiation can also be induced by suboptimal intrauterine conditions during critical developmental stages, permanently modifying the number or proportion of cells and consequently the physiology of the affected organ.[8,9] Furthermore, nutritional intrauterine adversities may induce endothelial dysfunction, impairing fetal cardiovascular circulation, endocrine function, and growth.[10]

THE STRESS SYSTEM AS MEDIATOR OF FETAL PAR

The fetal adaptive response to stressors is mediated largely by the stress system.[11] Exposure to a stressor activates the hypothalamus-pituitary-adrenal axis (HPA axis) and the locus caeruleus/norepinephrine-sympathetic nervous system (LC/NE-SNS). The HPA axis, the LC/NE-SNS and their mediators, corticotrophin-releasing hormone (CRH), arginine vasopressin (AVP), cortisol, norepinephrine (NE), and epinephrine (E) are responsible for both the immediate response to the stressor and for inducing long-term organizational changes in the central and peripheral nervous system that constitute the PAR. It has been shown that both CRH and cortisol have strong kindling and organizational impact on the developing organism.[12]

There is evidence that HPA axis programming can be induced by a wide range of stressors such as nursing conditions, maternal behavior, prenatal and postnatal malnutrition, or prenatal administration of glucocorticoids.[13]

Animal Studies

It is well documented that adversities during prenatal and early postnatal life can program rodent HPA axis, leading to inappropriate neuroendocrine responsiveness to stessors throughout lifetime.[14] In rats, prenatal stress has been associated with adrenal hypertrophy and elevated basal plasma corticosterone in the offspring.[15]

Prenatal stress may even sensitize rat offspring to postnatal stressors. Thus, CRH levels in the median eminence are significantly increased following postnatal handling of prenatally stressed rats compared to offspring whose mothers had not been stressed.[16] Furthermore, adult female rats exposed to stress *in utero* exhibited spatial learning impairment, providing evidence that prenatal stress can be associated with cognitive disorders in adulthood.[17]

Repeated maternal restraint during the last week of pregnancy has been associated with reduced hippocampal corticosteroid receptors, increased poststress corticosterone concentrations and prolonged corticosterone response to stress in the adult offspring.[18]

Prenatal nutritional stress (50% maternal caloric restriction) during the last week of pregnancy is associated with elevation in both maternal plasma corticosterone concentrations and relative adrenal weight at term. In addition, nutritional stress during pregnancy can induce epigenetic changes such as altered placental 11βHSD2 gene expression.[19] Moreover, postnatal overfeeding has been associated with permanent upregulation of the HPA axis exposing adult rats to elevated circulating adrenocorticotropic hormone (ACTH) and corticosterone concentrations.[20]

Administration of glucocorticoids during pregnancy impairs fetal renal development and induces hypertension, glucose intolerance, and insulin resistance programming the development of metabolic syndrome postnatally.[21,22]

Studies in primates have also shown that *in utero* adversities can modify HPA function in the offspring. In rhesus monkeys, juvenile offspring whose mothers were repeatedly exposed to unpredictable noise during mid to late gestation exhibited higher plasma ACTH concentrations under both basal and stressed conditions and significantly elevated basal plasma cortisol concentrations.[23]

Human Studies

Accumulating data in humans suggest that intrauterine adversities are associated with alterations in the HPA axis. A study in which fetal blood samples were obtained by cordocentesis at 18–38 weeks gestation reported that in small for gestational age (SGA) fetuses, plasma cortisol concentration was higher and ACTH lower than in appropriate for gestational age (AGA) fetuses and plasma cortisol was inversely correlated to fetal hypoglycemia, suggesting that in the chronically hypoglycemic SGA fetus the fetal pituitary is under negative inhibition.[24]

A birth cohort study in Finland reported that basal cortisol concentrations in adulthood were inversely related to birth weight in subjects born before 39 weeks. On the contrary, positive correlation was documented after 40 weeks of gestation, indicating that the relationship between birth weight and cortisol later in life depends on gestational age at birth. It is further proposed that adult elevated or decreased cortisol concentrations may occur as a consequence of *in utero* programming of the HPA axis.[25]

The association between low birth weight and elevated plasma cortisol concentrations, high blood pressure and obesity in adulthood, has been documented by epidemiological studies. It is suggested that plasma concentrations of cortisol could have an important effect on blood pressure and glucose tolerance, providing evidence that intrauterine programming of the HPA axis may be a mechanism underlying the association between low birth weight and detrimental health consequences in adulthood.[26]

In a prospective cohort study, blood pressure levels and heart rate responses to psychological stressors in women were inversely related to their birth weight, indicating that stress system response can be programmed *in utero* impairing adult cardiovascular physiology.[27]

Furthermore, a South African cohort study involving young disadvantaged, urbanized adults, has demonstrated an inverse relationship between both cortisol concentrations and cortisol response to ACTH and birth weight. Individuals who were born small (below the 10th centile) exhibited also glucose intolerance and high blood pressure suggesting that neuroendocrine programming by *in utero* adversities could induce development of cardiovascular and metabolic disorders in adult life.[28]

FETAL GROWTH RESTRICTION

SGA fetuses, defined by estimated weight below the 10th or 5th centile, can be constitutionally small (normal small), FGR due to impaired placentation (starved small), or FGR due to congenital abnormalities or intrauterine infection (abnormal small).

The normal small group, which constitute about 80% of the SGA, are symmetrically small with normal amniotic fluid and normal activity and are not at increased risk of perinatal death.

The starved small, accounting for about 15% of the total, are asymmetrically small with sparing in the growth of the head and brain at the expense of the rest of the body. The amniotic fluid and fetal activity are reduced. These fetuses are at substantially increased risk of perinatal mortality and long-term morbidity, including neurodevelopment delay.[29,30] In addition, FGR is associated with increased risk of carbohydrate intolerance or type 2 diabetes mellitus, hypertension, dyslipidemia, obesity, and cardiovascular disease in adulthood.[31] The clustering of these conditions is known as metabolic syndrome or dysmetabolic syndrome.[32]

Diagnostic Approach to FGR

The diagnosis of fetal SGA is based on the ultrasonographic demonstration that the abdominal circumference (AC) is below the 10th or 5th centile of the normal range for gestation. In placental insufficiency the fetal femur length is also commonly reduced but the head circumference (HC) is often within the normal range. The measurements of AC, HC, and femur length can be used to estimate the fetal weight (EFW). The assessment of fetal growth velocity by serial ultrasound evaluation of AC and EFW are superior to single estimates of AC and EFW in the prediction of FGR.

Ultrasound is also important in excluding major fetal abnormalities or features of chromosomal defects as the underlying cause of FGR. In addition, it is important to assess the amniotic fluid volume. Placental insufficiency and fetal hypoxemia cause fetal oliguria and consequently oligohydramnios, which is considered to be present when the largest vertical pocket of amniotic fluid is less than 2 cm or the amniotic fluid index (AFI) is less than 5 cm.

Doppler ultrasound assessment of the uterine and umbilical arteries helps distinguish FGR due to impaired placentation from constitutionally small fetuses. In FGR, Doppler studies of the fetal middle cerebral artery and ductus venosus are used to assess the degree of fetal hypoxemia and compromise.

In cases of unexplained FGR, viral infection assessment (TORCH—toxoplasma, rubella, cytomegalovirus, or herpes simplex virus) and fetal karyotyping could be offered based on the ultrasound findings.[33]

Fetal Cardiovascular Changes

In FGR due to impaired placentation, Doppler ultrasound studies have demonstrated increased impedance to flow (pulsatility index [PI]) in the maternal uterine arteries and/or umbilical arteries. In fetal hypoxemia there is increased PI in the umbilical artery and in acidemia there is absence or even reversed end diastolic flow.

In response to the associated fetal hypoxemia there is redistribution in the fetal circulation with increase in the blood supply to the brain, myocardium, and the adrenal glands and reduction in the perfusion of the kidneys, gastrointestinal tract, and extremities. During this phase of compensation decreased PI in the fetal middle cerebral artery is documented by Doppler assessment.[34–36]

Decompensation due to exhaustion of fetal physiologic adaptation to hypoxemia is manifested by cardiac compromise and increased impedance to flow in ductus venosus, with absence or reversal of forward flow during atrial contraction.[34–36]

Fetal Biophysical Changes

In FGR fetuses there is delayed maturation of biophysical parameters. Fetal behavioral responses to placental vascular dysfunction include delayed decline of the average baseline heart rate with advancing gestational age, decreased short- and long-term variability, delayed reactivity maturation, or even heart rate decelerations indicating metabolic compromise.

Hypoxemic FGR is associated with abnormal heart rate patterns.[37] A significant linear correlation has been documented between biophysical profile score and umbilical venous pH both at delivery and prenatally in samples obtained by cordocentesis.[38,39] With increasing hypoxemia there is progressive decrease in breathing movements, followed by reduction in amniotic fluid volume and, finally, loss of movements and fetal tone.[40]

Fetal Metabolic Changes

Studies investigating the metabolic status of growth restricted fetuses by cordocentesis have documented fetal compromise by hypoxemia, hypercapnicemia, hyperlacticemia, and acidocemia.[41]

In hypoxemic FGR fetuses the plasma ratio of nonessential to essential amino acids is increased suggesting intrauterine starvation. Moreover, these fetuses are hypoglycemic and hypoinsulinemic and their degree of hypoinsulinemia is disproportional to the degree of hypoglycemia, suggesting pancreatic dysfunction.[42–45]

In FGR fetuses, triglyceride levels are increased secondary to enhanced lipolysis and impaired utilization with hypertriglyceridemia being most pronounced in cases of fetal hypoxia.[45]

In normal pregnancy fetal blood thyroid-stimulating hormone (TSH), thyroid hormones (T3 and T4), and thyroid-binding globulin increase with advancing gestation demonstrating functional maturation of the pituitary, thyroid, and liver, respectively. In FGR the concentrations of TSH are higher, whereas thyroid hormone concentrations are decreased. These alterations may manifest a downregulated metabolism, and their occurrence is a sign of reduced substrate availability, as well as of an adaptation to a reduction of caloric expenditure that enables the fetus to survive in an adverse intrauterine environment.[46]

In normal fetuses, the insulin-like growth factor 1 (IGF-1) concentration is positively correlated and growth hormone (GH) negatively correlated to gestational age. In FGR, GH levels are higher and IGF-1 levels are lower compared to AGA fetuses. These data suggest that fetal GH production is under hypothalamic control and that the physiological decrease in serum GH concentration during pregnancy is mediated by a negative feedback mechanism due to elevated IGF-1 levels. Furthermore, liver IGF-1 production seems to be primarily controlled by fetal energy resources and only partly by GH secretion.[47]

FGR AND POSTNATAL GROWTH ACCELERATION

Catch-up growth is determined as height velocity above the limits of normal for a given postnatal age lasting more than 1 year, following a transient period of growth arrest. It is considered more appropriate to define catch-up growth or postnatal growth acceleration as change in standard deviation score for weight or height at a specific age that produces significant percentile crossing on standard growth charts.[48]

Significant catch-up growth mainly occurs during the first 2 years of life when infants compensate for intrauterine growth restriction, and their genetically determined growth trajectory tends to be restored.[49,50] About 30% of all infants show catch-up growth and mainly those that have lower birth weight whereas about 90% of SGA infants exhibit growth acceleration during the first 6 months postnatally.[51,52]

It is suggested that postnatal growth acceleration of the SGA infant could be an evolutionary phenomenon because infant survival rates are positively related to postnatal size.[53] Although restoration of the previously impaired growth velocity to normal is regarded advantageous, it is becoming increasingly apparent that there may be a long-term cost.[54]

Animal Studies

Animal studies focusing on the interaction between prenatal and postnatal nutritional environment suggest that prenatal starvation combined with rich postnatal diet increases the risk of developing obesity, hypertension, and insulin resistance.[55] There is evidence that accelerated growth based on early postnatal nutrition determines susceptibility to the metabolic syndrome.[56]

A study in which FGR offspring were nursed by normally fed mothers showed that there was rapid catch-up growth at 3 weeks and continued accelerated growth, resulting in increased body weight, percentage of body fat, and plasma leptin levels.[57] Furthermore, growth acceleration during early postnatal life in rats has been associated with impaired glucose tolerance and lifespan, whereas it is suggested that postnatal nutritional restriction has improved longevity.[58–60]

Studies in primates suggest that nutritional restriction early in life could prevent or delay the onset of cardiovascular disease and diabetes.[61]

Human Studies

The association of impaired fetal development and obesity has been demonstrated in the Dutch Famine Study where poor maternal diet in early gestation followed by adequate nutrition during the rest of pregnancy and postnatal period resulted in higher body weight, BMI, and waist circumference in middle-aged women.[62]

A Finish cohort study demonstrated that men who were born small and then showed accelerated childhood growth exhibited the highest rates of cardiovascular disease.[63] According to the Avon longitudinal study of pregnancy and childhood, early postnatal growth acceleration constitutes a risk factor for childhood obesity associating FGR and risk of disease in adulthood.[51] Another study reported that Indian children with the most adverse cardiovascular risk profiles had the lowest birth weight complicated with accelerated childhood growth.[64] Furthermore, low birth weight followed by accelerated childhood growth has been associated with glucose intolerance in 7-year-old children, making them susceptible to the development of type 2 diabetes later in life.[65]

Flow-mediated endothelium-dependent dilation (FMD) was 4% lower in adolescents with the highest rates of growth acceleration during the first 2 weeks postnatal, indicating endothelial dysfunction similar to that caused by insulin-dependent diabetes (4%) or smoking (6%) in adults.[66]

Randomized intervention trials of neonatal nutrition found that development of insulin resistance was greatest in adolescents born preterm with accelerated growth in the first 2 weeks postnatally. These results suggest that early high-nutrient diet programs the development of metabolic syndrome by promoting catch-up growth. Moreover, it is proposed that a slower postnatal growth velocity, induced by relative undernutrition, may improve future cardiovascular health.[67]

CONCLUSIONS

The fetal adaptive response to environmental stressors, which is mainly mediated by the stress system, programs the structure and function of organs, their physiology and metabolism. The FGR phenotype reflects fetal metabolic dysfunction and the evolutionary aim of this fetal phenotypic alteration is to ensure survival, reproduction enhancement, and thus genome preservation.

Antenatal surveillance of FGR pregnancies is currently based on longitudinal monitoring of fetal growth and assessment of oxygenation. Because there is no effective intrauterine therapy for FGR, the management is directed toward the appropriate timing of delivery to avoid fetal death due to delayed delivery or neonatal death due to premature delivery.

FGR is associated with increased risk of dysmetabolic syndrome in adulthood. There is evidence that early postnatal growth acceleration, which would normally be considered desirable, may exacerbate metabolic dysfunction in later life. Regular developmental and growth follow-up of FGR infants may be required to assess patterns of postnatal intervention that would optimize future health and longevity.

REFERENCES

1. GLUCKMAN, P.D. & M.A. HANSON. 2004. Developmental origins of disease paradigm: a mechanistic and evolutionary perspective. Pediatr. Res. **56:** 311–317.
2. BARKER, D.J., C. OSMOND, J. GOLDING, *et al.* 1989. Growth *in utero*, blood pressure in childhood and adult life, and mortality from cardiovascular disease. Br. Med. J. **298:** 564–567.
3. LUCAS, A. 1991. Programming by early nutrition in man. *In* The Childhood Environment and Adult Disease. G.R. Bock, J. Whelan, Eds.: 38–55. Wiley, CIBA Foundation Symposium 156. Chichester, West Sussex, UK.
4. HALES, C.N. & D.J. BARKER. 1992. Type 2 (non-insulin-dependent) diabetes mellitus: the thrifty phenotype hypothesis. Diabetologia **35:** 595–601.
5. BARKER, D.J. 2004. Developmental origins of adult health and disease. J. Epidemiol. Community Health **58:** 114–115.
6. GLUCKMAN, P.D. & M.A. HANSON. 2004. The developmental origins of the metabolic syndrome. Trends Endocrinol. Metab. **15:** 183–187.
7. EINSTEIN, F., G. ATZMON, X. YANG, *et al.* 2005. Differential responses of visceral and subcutaneous fat depots to nutrients. Diabetes **54:** 672–678.
8. LANGLEY-EVANS, S.C., S.J.M. WELHAM & A.A. JACKSON. 1999. Fetal exposure to a maternal low protein diet impairs nephrogenesis and promotes hypertension in the rat. Life Sci. **64:** 965–974.
9. BERTRAM, C.E. & M.A. HANSON. 2002. Prenatal programming of postnatal endocrine responses by glucocorticoids. Reproduction **124:** 459–467.
10. BRAWLEY, L., C. TORRENS, F.W. ANTHONY, *et al.* 2004. Glycine rectifies vascular dysfunction induced by dietary protein imbalance during pregnancy. J. Physiol. **554:** 497–504.
11. CHROUSOS, G.P. & P.W. GOLD. 1992. The concepts of stress system disorders: overview of behavioral and physical homeostasis. JAMA **267:** 1244–1252.
12. CHARMANDARI, E., C. TSIGOS & G. CHROUSOS. 2005. Endocrinology of the stress response. Annu. Rev. Physiol. **67:** 259–284.
13. MATTHEWS, S.G. 2002. Early programming of the hypothalamo-pituitary-adrenal axis. Trends Endocrinol. Metab. **13:** 373–380.
14. MEANEY, M.J., D.H. AITKEN, S. SHARMA, *et al.* 1992. Basal ACTH, corticosterone and corticosterone binding globulin levels over the diurnal cycle, and age-related changes in hippocampal type I and type II corticosteroid receptor binding capacity in young and aged, handled and nonhandled rats. Neuroendocrinology **55:** 204–213.
15. WARD, H.E., E.A. JOHNSON, A.K. SALM, *et al.* 2000. Effects of prenatal stress on defensive withdrawal behavior and corticotrophin releasing factor systems in rat brain. Physiol. Behav. **70:** 359–366.
16. SMYTHE, J.W., C.M. MCCORMICK & M.J. MEANEY. 1996. Median eminence corticotrophin-releasing hormone content following prenatal stress and neonatal handling. Brain Res. Bull. **40:** 195–199.

17. DARNAUDERY, M., M. PEREZ-MARTIN, G. BELIZAIRE, *et al.* 2006. Insulin-like growth factor 1 reduces age-related disorders induced by prenatal stress in female rats. Neurobiol. Aging **27:** 119–127.

18. BARBAZANGES, A., P.V. PIAZZA, M. LE MOAL & S. MACCARI. 1996. Maternal glucocorticoid secretion mediates long-term effects of prenatal stress. J. Neurosci. **16:** 3943–3949.

19. LESAGE, J., B. BLONDEAU, M. GRINO, *et al.* 2001. Maternal undernutrition during late gestation induces fetal overexposure to glucocorticoids and intrauterine growth retardation, and disturbs the hypothalamo-pituitary adrenal axis in the newborn rat. Endocrinology **142:** 1692–1702.

20. BOULLU-CIOCCA, S., A. DUTOUR, V. GUILLAUME, *et al.* 2005. Postnatal diet-induced obesity in rats upregulates systemic and adipose tissue glucocorticoid metabolism during development and in adulthood: its relationship with the metabolic syndrome. Diabetes **54:** 197–203.

21. DODIC, M., K. MORITZ, I. KOUKOULAS, *et al.* 2002. Programmed hypertension: kidney, brain or both? Trends Endocrinol. Metab. **13:** 403–408.

22. NYIRENDA, M.J., R.S. LINDSAY, C.J. KENYON, *et al.* 1998. Glucocorticoid exposure in late gestation permanently programs rat hepatic phosphoenolpyruvate carboxykinase and glucocorticoid receptor expression and causes glucose intolerance in adult offspring. J. Clin. Invest. **101:** 2174–2181.

23. CLARKE, A.S., D.J. WITTWER, D.H. ABBOTT, *et al.* 1994. Long-term effects of prenatal stress on HPA axis activity in juvenile rhesus monkeys. Dev. Psychobiol. **27:** 257–269.

24. ECONOMIDES, D.L., K.H. NICOLAIDES, E.A. LINTON, *et al.* 1988. Plasma cortisol and adrenocorticotropin in appropriate and small for gestational age fetuses. Fetal Ther. **3:** 158–164.

25. KAJANTIE, E., D.I. PHILLIPS, S. ANDERSSON, *et al.* 2002. Size at birth, gestational age and cortisol secretion in adult life: fetal programming of both hyper- and hypocortisolism? Clin. Endocrinol. (Oxf.) **57:** 635–641.

26. PHILLIPS, D.I., B.R. WALKER, R.M. REYNOLDS, *et al.* 2000. Low birth weight predicts elevated plasma cortisol concentrations in adults from 3 populations. Hypertension **35:** 1301–1306.

27. WARD, A.M., V.M. MOORE, A. STEPTOE, *et al.* 2004. Size at birth and cardiovascular responses to psychological stressors: evidence for prenatal programming in women. J. Hypertens. **22:** 2295–2301.

28. LEVITT, N.S., E.V. LAMBERT, D. WOODS, *et al.* 2000. Impaired glucose tolerance and elevated blood pressure in low birth weight, nonobese, young South African adults: early programming of cortisol axis. J. Clin. Endocrinol. Metab. **85:** 4611–4618.

29. MCINTIRE, D.D., S.L. BLOOM, B.M. CASEY, *et al.* 1999. Birthweight in relation to morbidity and mortality among newborn infants. N. Engl. J. Med. **340:** 1234–1238.

30. TAYLOR, D.J. & P.W. HOWIE. 1989. Fetal growth achievement and neurodevelopmental disability. BJOG **96:** 789–794.

31. BARKER, D.J. 1997. The long-term outcome of retarded fetal growth. Clin. Obstet. Gynecol. **40:** 853–863.

32. PERVANIDOU, P., C. KANAKA-GANTENBEIN & G.P. CHROUSOS. 2006. Assessment of metabolic profile in a clinical setting. Curr. Opin. Clin. Nutr. Metab. Care **9:** 589–595.

33. SNIJDERS, R.J.M., C. SHERROD, C.M. GOSDEN, *et al.* 1993. Fetal growth retardation: associated malformations and chromosome abnormalities. Am. J. Obstet. Gynecol. **168:** 547–555.
34. HECHER, K., S. CAMPBELL, P. DOYLE, *et al.* 1995. Assessment of fetal compromise by Doppler ultrasound investigation of the fetal circulation. Arterial, intracardiac, and venous blood flow velocity studies. Circulation **91:** 129–138.
35. BILARDO, C., K.H. NICOLAIDES & S. CAMPBELL. 1990. Doppler measurements of fetal and uteroplacental circulations: relationship with umbilical venous blood gases measured at cordocentesis. Am. J. Obstet. Gynecol. **162:** 115–120.
36. HECHER, K., R. SNIJDERS, S. CAMPBELL, *et al.* 1995. Fetal venous, intracardiac and arterial blood flow measurements in intrauterine growth retardation: relationship with fetal blood gases. Am. J. Obstet. Gynecol. **173:** 10–15.
37. VISSER, G.H., G. SADOVSKY & K.H. NICOLAIDES. 1990. Antepartum heart rate patterns in small-for-gestational-age third-trimester fetuses: correlations with blood gas values obtained at cordocentesis. Am. J. Obstet. Gynecol. **162:** 698–703.
38. MANNING, F.A., R. SNIJDERS, C.R. HARMAN, *et al.* 1993. Fetal biophysical profile score. Correlation with antepartum umbilical venous fetal pH. Am. J. Obstet. Gynecol. **169:** 755–763.
39. RIBBERT, L.S., R.J. SNIJDERS, K.H. NICOLAIDES, *et al.* 1990. Relationship of fetal biophysical profile and blood gas values at cordocentesis in severely growth-retarded fetuses. Am. J. Obstet. Gynecol. **163:** 569–571.
40. BASCHAT, A., U. GEMBRUCH & C. HARMAN. 2001. The sequence of changes in Doppler and biophysical parameters as severe fetal growth restriction worsens. Ultrasound Obstet. Gynecol. **18:** 571–577.
41. NICOLAIDES, K.H., D.L. ECONOMIDES & P.W. SOOTHILL. 1989. Blood gases, pH, and lactate in appropriate- and small-for-gestational-age fetuses. Am. J. Obstet. Gynecol. **61:** 996–1001.
42. ECONOMIDES, D.L., K.H. NICOLAIDES, W.A. GAHL, *et al.* 1989. Plasma amino acids in appropriate- and small-for-gestational-age fetuses. Am. J. Obstet. Gynecol. **161:** 1219–1227.
43. SOOTHILL, P.W., K.H. NICOLAIDES & S. CAMPBELL. 1987. Prenatal asphyxia, hyperlacticaemia, hypoglycaemia, and erythroblastosis in growth retarded fetuses. Br. Med. J. **25:** 1051–1053.
44. NICOLINI, U., C. HUBINONT, J. SANTOLAYA, *et al.* 1990. Effects of fetal intravenous glucose challenge in normal and growth retarded fetuses. Horm. Metab. Res. **22:** 426–430.
45. ECONOMIDES, D.L., K.H. NICOLAIDES & S. CAMPBELL. 1991. Metabolic and endocrine findings in appropriate- and small-for-gestational-age fetuses. J. Perinat. Med. **19:** 97–105.
46. THORPE-BEESTON, J.G. & K.H. NICOLAIDES. 1993. Fetal thyroid function. Fetal Diagn. Ther. **8:** 60–72.
47. AROSIO, M., D. CORTELAZZI, L. PERSANI, *et al.* 1995. Circulating levels of growth hormone, insulin-like growth factor-I and prolactin in normal, growth retarded and anencephalic human fetuses. J. Endocrinol. Invest. **18:** 346–353.
48. WI, J.M. & B. BOERSMA. 2002. Catch-up growth: definition, mechanisms, and models. J. Pediatr. Endocrinol. Metab. **15:** 1229–1241.
49. TANNER, J.M. 1994. Growth from birth to two: a critical review. Acta Medica. Auxologica. **26:** 7–45.

50. TANNER, J.M. 1986. Childhood epidemiology. Physical development. Br. Med. Bull. **42:** 131–138.

51. ONG, K.K., M.L. AHMED, P.M. EMMETT, *et al.* 2000. Association between postnatal catch-up growth and obesity in childhood: prospective cohort study. Br. Med. J. **320:** 967–971.

52. KARLBERG, J.P., K. ALBERTSSON-WIKLAND, E.Y. KWAN, *et al.* 1995. The timing of early postnatal catch-up growth in normal, full-term infants born short for gestational age. Horm. Res. **48:** 17–24.

53. ONG, K.K. & D.B. DUNGER. 2001. Developmental aspects in the pathogenesis of type 2 diabetes. Mol. Cell Endocrinol. **185:** 145–149.

54. METCALFE, N.B. & P. MONAGHAN. 2001. Compensation for a bad start: grow now, pay later? Trends Ecol. Evol. **16:** 254–260.

55. VICKERS, M.H., B.H. BREIER, W.S. CUTFIELD, *et al.* 2000. Fetal origins of hyperphagia, obesity and hypertension and its postnatal amplification by hypercaloric nutrition. Am. J. Physiol. **279:** 83–87.

56. PLAGEMANN, A., I. HEIDRICH, F. GOTZ, *et al.* 1992. Obesity and enhanced diabetes and cardiovascular risk in adult rats due to early postnatal overfeeding. Exp. Clin. Endocrinol. **99:** 154–158.

57. DESAI, M., D. GAYLE, J. BABU, *et al.* 2005. Programmed obesity in intrauterine growth-restricted newborns: modulation by newborn nutrition. Am. J. Physiol. Regul. Integr. Comp. Physiol. **288:** 91–96.

58. MASORO, E.J. 2000. Caloric restriction and aging: an update. Exp. Gerontol. **35:** 299–305.

59. TEILLET, L., S. GOURAUD & B. CORMAN. 2004. Does food restriction increase life span in lean rats? J. Nutr. Health Aging **8:** 213–218.

60. DAVIS, T.A., C.W. BALES & R.E. BEAUCHENE. 1983. Differential effects of dietary caloric and protein restriction in the aging rat. Exp. Gerontol. **18:** 427–435.

61. ROTH, G.S., D.K. INGRAM, A. BLACK, *et al.* 2000. Effect of reduced energy intake on the biology of ageing: the primate model. Eur. J. Clin. Nutr. **54:** 15–20.

62. RAVELLI, A.C., J.H. VAN DER MEULEN, C. OSMOND, *et al.* 1999. Obesity at the age of 50 years in men and women exposed to famine prenatally. Am. J. Clin. Nutr. **70:** 811–816.

63. ERIKSSON, J.G., T. FORSEN, J. TUOMILEHTO, *et al.* 1999. Catch-up growth in childhood and death from coronary heart disease: longitudinal study. Br. Med. J. **318:** 427–431.

64. BAVDEKAR, A., C.S. YAJNIK, C.H. FALL, *et al.* 1999. Insulin resistance syndrome in 8-year-old Indian children: small at birth, big at 8 years, or both? Diabetes **48:** 2422–2429.

65. CROWTHER, N.J., N. CAMERON, J. TRUSLER, *et al.* 1998. Association between poor glucose tolerance and rapid post natal weight gain in seven-year-old children. Diabetologia **41:** 1163–1167.

66. SINGHAL, A., T.J. COLE, M. FEWTRELL, *et al.* 2004. Is slower early growth beneficial for long-term cardiovascular health? Circulation **109:** 1108–1113.

67. SINGHAL, A., M. FEWTRELL, T.J. COLE, *et al.* 2003. Low nutrient intake and early growth for later insulin resistance in adolescents born preterm. Lancet **361:** 1089–1097.

Pitfalls of the WHIs

Women's Health Initiative

GEORGE MASTORAKOS, EVANGELOS GR. SAKKAS,
ANTONIOS M. XYDAKIS, AND GEORGE CREATSAS

*Endocrine Unit, Second Department of Obstetrics and Gynecology, Aretaieion
Hospital, Medical School, University of Athens, Athens, Greece*

ABSTRACT: Recently, the use of hormone replacement therapy (HRT)
at menopause has become a matter of debate. Its utility has been questioned after the publication of the results of the Women's Health Initiative
(WHI) studies. This trial was divided in two arms of which the first examined the use of combined HRT (continuous estrogens plus progestins) and
the second the use of estrogens alone in menopausal women. The first
arm was terminated prematurely at 5.2 years because the number of
cases of coronary heart disease (CHD), strokes, venous thromboembolic
disease, and breast cancer were more in women receiving HRT than in
women receiving placebo, if the nominal confidence intervals (CIs) were
taken into account. However, in the same study the authors made clear
that the adjusted CIs should be taken into account instead of the nominal ones. These latter ones caused the ending of the trial. Moreover,
WHI was criticized for its conclusions as far as cardiovascular disease
is concerned because of serious defects regarding design of the trial. If
the adjusted CIs were taken into account then the increase in adverse
events was significant only for deep vein thrombosis. The second arm
demonstrated that the use of estrogens was not correlated to an increase
of neither breast cancer incidence nor cardiovascular disease. A closer
look at the results of the WHI trial reveals that the use of HRT for 5 years
should not be considered deleterious for the appearance of breast cancer,
cardiovascular diseases, strokes, and pulmonary embolisms. We suggest
that HRT should be given early in menopause. The regimen should be
individualized for each patient. More intense follow-up should be offered to women with a positive family history of breast cancer, diagnosed
coronary disease, and to women with a predisposition to deep venous
thrombosis.

KEYWORDS: HRT; breast cancer; WHI; cardiovascular

Address for correspondence: George Mastorakos, M.D., D.Sc., 3 Neofytou Vamva Street, Kolonaki
106 74 Athens. Voice: 0030-210-3636230; fax: 0030-210-3636229.
e-mail: mastorak@mail.kapatel.gr

Ann. N.Y. Acad. Sci. 1092: 331–340 (2006). © 2006 New York Academy of Sciences.
doi: 10.1196/annals.1365.030

INTRODUCTION

Recently, the use of hormone replacement therapy (HRT) at menopause has become a matter of debate. Its utility has been questioned after the publication of studies that showed a positive correlation between the use of HRT and the appearance of serious adverse events, such as breast cancer.

The target of HRT is women's relief of menopausal symptoms that are immediate (vasomotor symptoms) and long term (osteoporosis, cardiovascular disease). HRT refers to the use of either estrogens or progestins alone or to the combination of estrogens and a progestin aiming at the protection of the endometrium from hyperplasia or cancer.

The Women's Health Initiative (WHI) was a multicenter study that enrolled 27,347 women aged 50–79 years (mean age 63 years) between 1993 and 1998 and it was scheduled to end in 2005. Its average duration was 8.5 years. It was a large-scale, randomized, NIH-sponsored trial with the purpose of assessing the long-term risk–benefit ratio of estrogen replacement therapy (ERT) and combined HRT (continuous conjugated estrogens and medroxyprogesterone) in disease prevention. The trial consisted of two arms of which the first, which included 16,608 nonhysterectomized menopausal women, examined the use of combined HRT[1] and the second, which included 10,739, studied the use of conjugated estrogens alone[2] to hysterectomized menopausal women. Its primary end points were the prevention of cardiovascular disease and breast cancer.

The combined HRT arm was stopped early because the health risks outweighed the benefits after 5.2 years of follow-up according to the global index. Global index was a summary measure of the overall balance of risks and benefits. The number of heart attacks, strokes, breast cancer cases, endometrium cancer cases, colorectal cancer cases, pulmonary embolisms, hip fractures, and deaths from other causes were taken into account for its calculation. Unfortunately, the trial did not include the calculation of separate measures regarding the effect of combined HRT for each of these parameters. Moreover, WHI did not evaluate symptom relief that was not included in the global index. The combined HRT arm showed a statistically significant increase of the nominal risk for cardiovascular diseases, strokes, venous thromboembolisms, and breast cancer cases.

However, WHI had some important limitations. First, the average age of the women studied was 63 years, approximately 11 years older than the average age of menopause (approximately 52 years). It must be noted that in only 17.1% of them less than 5 years had elapsed since menopause while in 42.8% of them more than 15 years had elapsed since menopause. Women had passed the age at which HRT is usually prescribed in current clinical practice. Moreover, there were relatively high rates of discontinuation in the HRT group (42%) and crossover to HRT treatment in the placebo group (10.7%). Furthermore, 87.3% of the women did not have any vasomotor symptoms, which puts in doubt the necessity of HRT. Finally, attention should be paid at the conclusions drawn from the results. According to the authors "nominal 95% confidence intervals (CIs) describe the variability in the estimates that would arise from a simple trial for a simple outcome. Although traditional, these CIs do not account for the multiple statistical testing issues (across time and across outcome categories) that occurred in this trial, so the probability is greater than 0.05 that at least one of these CIs will exclude unity under an overall null hypothesis. The adjusted 95% CIs presented herein use group sequential methods to correct for multiple analysis over time. The adjusted CIs are closely related to the monitoring procedures and, as such, represent a conservative assessment of the evidence."[1] Surprisingly, the authors chose to focus "primarily on results using the unadjusted statistics."[1]

Breast Cancer

Until now, the majority of the trials were either observational, retrospective, or meta-analyses. A meta-analysis reviewed all the studies published from 1975 to 2000[3] examining the relation between breast cancer and HRT. As far as HRT administration is concerned, 20 studies were reported, 80% of which reported relative risk (RR) estimates not significantly different from 1.0, 10% significantly higher than 1.0, and 10% significantly lower than 1.0. As far as ERT administration is concerned, 45 studies were reported, 82% of which reported RR estimates not significantly different from 1.0. RR equal to 1.0 is the risk for breast cancer for a woman who does not receive HRT. Only 13% of these studies reported RR estimates significantly higher than 1.0 but none higher than 2.0 and 5% of them showed a statistically significant reduction of the RR.

In 1995[4] within the scope of The Nurses' Study, which analyzed retrospectively from 1976 the records of 121,700 nurses aged 30–55 years, Colditz *et al.* showed that the RR for breast cancer for nurses receiving HRT was 1.46 (95%CI: 0.98–2.17). Since RR equal to 1, that is, the risk for breast cancer for a woman receiving placebo, is included within these CIs one should conclude that there is no statistically significant increase of the RR for breast cancer in women aged 50–54 years who took HRT for 5 years as compared to women of the same age who received the placebo. An elevated RR was observed for women over the age of 55 years (RR: 1.37, 95% CI: 1.07–1.76).

In 1997[5] another meta-analysis reviewed 51 studies coming from 21 countries. This was based on 53,865 postmenopausal women with known age at menopause of which 17,830 (33%) were receiving HRT and showed that the administration of HRT even for 14 years was not related to a statistically significant increase of the RR for breast cancer.

In WHI, the RR for breast cancer for all women who received combined HRT was 1.26 (nominal 95% CIs: 1.00–1.59), which was not statistically significant according to the adjusted CIs (adjusted 95% CIs: 0.83–1.92).[1] Moreover, when women who had previously used hormone therapy (26.2%) were excluded from the statistical evaluation, the nominal RR for breast cancer in women who had never taken HRT in the past was not statistically significant from 1 for 5.2 years of HRT use during the study (RR: 1.06, nominal CIs: 0.81-1.38). On the contrary, the RR for breast cancer for women who had taken hormone therapy in the past for less than 5 years (18%, RR: 2.13, 95% CIs: 1.15–3.94) and for 5 to 10 years (5%, RR: 4.61, 95% CIs: 1.01–21.02) were in both cases statistically significant. However, the RR for breast cancer for women who had taken hormone therapy in the past for more than 10 years was not statistically significant (3%, RR: 1.81, 95% CIs: 0.60–5.43) (TABLE 1).

At this point it should be stressed that even the statistically significant nominal RRs mentioned above are close to the RRs for breast cancer after the use of antibiotics in postmenopausal women. In fact, as recently published, the overall nominal RR for breast cancer for women receiving antibiotics for a total of 1 to 50 days was 1.45 (95%CI: 1.24–1.69).[6] Specifically, the nominal RR for breast cancer for women receiving macrolides was 1.49 (95%CI: 1.24–1.78), for women receiving tetracyclines 1.55 (95%CI: 1.28–1.87), for women receiving penicillins 1.52 (95%CI: 1.29–1.79), for women receiving cefalosporines 1.55 (95%CI: 1.30–1.85), for women receiving sulphonamides 1.50 (95%CI: 1.27–1.77), and for women receiving nitrofurantoins 1.44 (95%CI: 1.13–1.84) for 1 to 50 days of total use.[6]

Interestingly, according to the recently published results of the WHI ERT arm in women who had undergone hysterectomy,[2] administration of ERT was not correlated to an increased RR for breast cancer. The nominal RR was 0.77 (95% adjusted CIs: 0.57–1.06). It was observed that if a new additional case of a woman on placebo was diagnosed with breast cancer during the study, the nominal CIs for women taking ERT for 8.2 years would have become 0.55–0.99, which means that ERT would have a protective effect on the appearance of breast cancer.

As far as the type of cancer is concerned, 199 out of 245 who received combined HRT (81%) presented with invasive breast cancer and the rest of them with *in situ* breast cancer. Consequently, it seems that administration of

TABLE 1. Prior hormone therapy use in the HRT arm of the WHI study and the nominal RRs for breast cancer

Prior hormone therapy use	Percentage of women	Nominal RR for breast cancer	95% CIs
0	74%	1.06	0.81–1.38
<5	18%	2.13	1.15–3.94
5–10	5%	4.61	1.01–21.02
>10	3%	1.81	0.60–5.43

Based on the data from Ref. 1.

estrogens does not favor new cancer cases. More likely, these tumors either existed before or were diagnosed accidentally after randomization. Estrogens rather contribute to the increase of their size. Surprisingly, there was no difference in the estrogen receptors incidence between these two groups. It would be expected that combined HRT would have a predisposition for patients with estrogen receptor-positive breast cancer, something which was not the case.

CARDIOVASCULAR DISEASE

Heart Disease

According to the results published in 2003 by the writing group for the WHI Investigators[7] there was no statistically significant RR for women taking combined HRT either for coronary heart disease (CHD) (including acute myocardial infarction necessitating hospitalization, silent myocardial infarction, or death due to CHD), revascularization, and angina (RR: 1.00, 95% adjusted CIs: 0.82–1.22) or for congestive heart failure (RR: 0.99, 95% adjusted CIs: 0.69–1.42). It should be noted that, in the first arm of WHI regarding combined HRT, at the first year of follow-up the RR for CHD was elevated (RR: 1.81 95% CIs: 1.09–3.01) whereas for the subsequent years (2, 3, 4, 5, and over 6 the RR was not statistically significant (TABLE 2).[7]

The second arm of the WHI trial, which studied the administration of ERT, did not show any statistically significant effect on CHD (RR: 0.91, 95% adjusted CIs: 0.72–1.15), the incidence of deaths due to CHD (RR: 0.94, 95% adjusted CIs: 0.54–1.63), or the incidence of nonfatal myocardial infarctions (RR: 0.89, 95% adjusted CIs: 0.63–1.26).[2]

The presence of women with diagnosed CHD (5% of women enrolled in the trial) probably affected these results. A likely explanation is that hormone therapy initially favors ischemic phenomena in women with lesioned arterial endothelium that are followed by the effect of HRT on the surrogate markers (reduction of cholesterol and LDL, elevation of HDL). Similar were the conclusions of the Heart and Estrogen/progestin Replacement Study (HERS).[8]

TABLE 2. Estrogen plus progestin and the risk of CHD in the HRT arm of WHI, according to the year of follow-up

Year of follow-up	RR	95% CIs
1	1.81	1.09–3.01
2	1.34	0.82–2.18
3	1.27	0.64–2.50
4	1.25	0.74–2.12
5	1.45	0.81–2.59
6	0.70	0.42–1.14

Based on the data from Ref. 7.

The latter was a cohort study in which postmenopausal women with active CHD were studied. HERS, as WHI did, showed that there was a statistically significant increase for coronary heart events in women receiving HRT during the first year of use. On the contrary, there was a statistically significant reduction for events in women receiving HRT in the next 4 years. The same explanation, as in WHI, was also given in this case. This led physicians to avoid prescription of HRT regimens for primary prevention of CHD. The age of initiation of HRT to menopausal women with respect to the quality of the arterial wall seems to be crucial (see the chapter by Rosano *et al.* this volume).

Stroke

The first arm of the WHI[1] trial initially demonstrated that the RR for strokes was increased in women receiving HRT (RR: 1.41, 95% nominal CIs: 1.07–1.85). Particularly, there was an increase in fatal strokes (RR: 1.50, 95% nominal CIs: 1.08–2.08). However, when results were adjusted it was evident that there was no statistically significant RR for strokes (95% adjusted CIs: 0.86–2.31). Similarly, neither the second arm of the WHI[2] trial that examined the use of ERT showed that a statistically significant RR for strokes really existed (RR: 1.39, 95% adjusted CIs: 0.97–1.99).

Venous Thromboembolic Disease

As far as venous thromboembolic disease is concerned, in the first arm of the WHI trial the RR was increased (RR: 2.11, 95% nominal CIs: 1.58–2.82 and after the adjustment: 1.26–3.55).[1] Specifically, the RR for deep vein thrombosis was increased (RR: 2.07, 95% nominal CIs: 1.49–2.87 and after the adjustment: 1.14–3.74) whereas the RR for pulmonary embolism was initially elevated (RR: 2.13, 95% nominal CIs: 1.39–3.25) but after adjustment, it was not found to be statistically significant (95% adjusted CIs: 0.99–4.56).

In the second arm of the WHI trial (ERT), the RR for venous thromboembolic disease was 1.33 (95% adjusted CIs: 0.86–2.08), for deep vein thrombosis 1.47 (95% adjusted CIs: 0.87–2.47), and for pulmonary embolism 1.34 (95% adjusted CIs: 0.70–2.55).[2]

Consequently, the incidence of deep vein thrombosis was increased only in women who received combined HRT and not in those who took ERT. On the contrary, the incidence of pulmonary embolism was not influenced by either combined HRT or ERT.

Risk Factors for Cardiovascular Disease

Women with a free cardiovascular history (95.2%) had a mean body mass index (BMI) of 28.5 (±5.8).[7] It is established that BMI over 24.9 characterizes overweight persons. Moreover, increased BMI is considered an important risk factor for cardiovascular disease.[1] BMI 22 has been correlated to a RR for cardiovascular disease equal to 1, and as BMI increases so does the RR. A BMI of 29 is correlated to a RR equal to 3.5.[1,8] Therefore, these women had a considerable predisposition to cardiovascular disease. Furthermore, 35% of them were suffering hypertension, 50% of them were smokers, 4% were suffering diabetes, and 6.9% were receiving statins. Of course, the placebo group had the same characteristics but it is noteworthy that women who took HRT had greater reductions in the total and LDL cholesterol, glucose levels, and insulin levels, and greater increases in HDL and triglyceride levels than women in the placebo group. Systolic blood pressure at year 1 was 1 mmHg higher among women receiving HRT and ERT than among those receiving placebo (remaining 1 to 2 mmHg higher during follow-up), although diastolic blood pressure was not different between groups.[7]

Age and Risk for Cardiovascular Disease

In WHI, as time from menopause and hot flushes increased, a higher RR for CHD was observed suggesting that for the appearance of CHD, age played a critical role regardless of HRT use. It appears that all recent and randomized studies regarding CHD and HRT have included middle-aged women between 64 and 67 years.[1,9-13] Moreover, these studies did not really study if HRT (either combined or ERT) prevented cardiovascular disease. According to biologists' point of view, prevention from cardiovascular disease is defined as prevention of the formation of the fibrous cap around the plaque. Furthermore, it has been observed that HRT administration reduces oxidation of LDL and causes vasodilatation in women without cardiovascular risk factors.[14] Consequently, atherogenesis is prevented because of LDL reduction and improvement in endothelial function. HRT administration also reduces the accumulation of LDL particles ameliorating blood vessel damage. On the other hand, according to cardiologists' point of view, prevention of cardiovascular disease is defined by prevention of a heart event as a result of a preexisting stenosis of the vessel due to atheromatosis. It has been observed that HRT administration can be potentially harmful on existing atheroma because it increases inflammation and expression of metalloproteinase (MMP), which causes disruption of the stable atheroma plaque.[15] It also promotes neovascularization of the plaque and potentially bleeding into the plaque. Therefore, studies that enrolled women of a younger age, like the Nurses' Study, found that HRT had a protective effect on the appearance of heart events since it is less likely to find plaques in these women. In WHI, 70% of the women studied were 60–79 years old. In this age range it is expected that already formed plaques may exist, whereas only 10% of them were 50–54 years old, ages at which HRT could have played a beneficial role. The fact that in WHI, despite the reduction in LDL, total cholesterol, and glucose, and an increase in HDL levels, no improvement of the incidence of cardiovascular diseases was noted or could be attributed to the age of the women included in the trial. This contradiction perhaps emerges from the fact that the administration of HRT in WHI began in an advanced age when atheromatic disease might have already been established. Consequently, it could be proposed that the formation of the plaque is delayed in women who use HRT early in menopause (around 52 years). On the other hand, HRT has no protective effect on menopausal women who begin the use of HRT late (around 65 years).[16]

Examining the Framingham Study,[17,18] the Nurses' Study[4,19] and the WHI,[1] it appears that the first and the last ones studied women of an advanced age. In the Framingham Study and WHI, women aged 50–83 and 50–79 years were studied, respectively. Moreover, in Framingham, mean BMI was 27 and in WHI it was 28.5 (34.1% of the women studied had BMI over 30), whereas in the Nurses' Study mean BMI was 25.1. However, it is noteworthy that the RR for cardiovascular diseases was found elevated only in the Framingham Study, in which HRT was not administered. As far as the nominal RR for strokes is concerned, it was increased in the Framingham Study and in WHI as well.

CONCLUSIONS

According to the adjusted RRs of the WHI, the use of HRT for 5 years should not be considered deleterious for the appearance of breast cancer, cardiovascular events, strokes, and pulmonary embolism. An increase of the RR should be expected for deep vein thrombosis. Moreover, treatment should be individualized, so attention must be paid to women with a positive family history of breast cancer, diagnosed CHD, or a predisposition to deep vein thrombosis.[20] As far as the administration of ERT is concerned, it is safe for a hysterectomized menopausal woman to receive ERT for 8 years. Finally, it appears that the use of HRT should be offered at an early age to a suitable menopausal woman after an individualized decision plan is drawn.

REFERENCES

1. WRITING GROUP FOR THE WOMEN'S HEALTH INITIATIVE INVESTIGATORS. 2002. Risks and benefits of estrogen plus progestin in healthy postmenopausal women. Principal results from the Women's Health Initiative randomized control trial. JAMA **288:** 321–333.
2. THE WOMEN'S HEALTH INITIATIVE STEERING COMMITTEE. 2004. Effects of conjugated equine estrogen in postmenopausal women with hysterectomy. JAMA **291:** 1701–1712.

3. BUSH, T.L., M. WHITEMAN & J.A. FLAWS. 2001. Hormone replacement therapy and breast cancer: a qualitative review. Obstet. Gynecol. **98:** 498–508.
4. COLDITZ G.A., *et al.* 1995. The use of estrogens and progestins and the risk of breast cancer in postmenopausal women. N. Engl. J. Med. **332:** 1589–1593.
5. COLLABORATIVE GROUP ON HORMONAL FACTORS IN BREAST CANCER. 1997. Breast cancer and hormone replacement therapy: collaborative reanalysis of data from 51 epidemiological studies of 52,705 women with breast cancer and 108,411 women without breast cancer. Lancet **350:** 1047–1059.
6. VELICER, C.M., S. HECKBERT, J. LAMPE, *et al.* 2004. Antibiotic use in relation to the risk of breast cancer. JAMA **291:** 827–835.
7. WRITING GROUP FOR THE WOMEN'S HEALTH INITIATIVE INVESTIGATORS. 2003. Estrogen plus progestin and the risk of coronary heart disease. N. Engl. J. Med. **349:** 523–534.
8. WILLETT, W.C., J.E. MANSON, M.J. STAMPFER, *et al.* 1995. Weight, weight change, and coronary heart disease in women: risk within the "normal" weight range. JAMA **273:** 461–465.
9. HULLEY, S., D. GRADY, T. BUSH, *et al.* 1998. Randomized trial of estrogen plus progestin for secondary prevention of coronary heart disease in postmenopausal women. Heart and Estrogen/progestin replacement study research group. JAMA **280:** 605–613.
10. HERRINGTON, D.M., D.M. REBOUSSIN, K.B. BROSNIHAN, *et al.* 2000. Effects of estrogen replacement on the progression of coronary-artery atherosclerosis. N. Engl. J. Med. **343:** 522–529.
11. HULLEY, S., D. GRADY, T. BUSH, *et al.* for the Heart and Estrogen/progestin Replacement Study (HERS) Research Group. 1998. Randomized trial of estrogen plus progestin for secondary prevention of coronary heart disease in postmenopausal women. JAMA **280:** 605–613.
12. WATERS, D.D., E.L. ALDERMAN, J. HSIA, *et al.* 2002. Effects of hormone replacement therapy and antioxidant vitamin supplements on coronary atherosclerosis in postmenopausal women: the women's angiographic vitamin and estrogen (WAVE) trial. JAMA **288:** 2432–2440.
13. CLARKE, S.C., J. KELLEHER, H. LLOYD-JONES, *et al.* 2002. A study of hormone replacement therapy in postmenopausal women with ischaemic heart disease: the papworth HRT atherosclerosis study. Br. J. Obstet. Gynaecol. **109:** 1056–1062.
14. HERRINGTON, D.M., M.A. ESPELAND, J.R. CROUSE, III, *et al.* 2001. Estrogen replacement and brachial artery flow-mediated vasodilation in older women. Arterioscler. Thromb. Vasc. Biol. **21:** 1955–1961.
15. ZANGER, D., B.K. YANG, J. ARDANS, *et al.* 2000. Divergent effects of hormone therapy on serum markers of inflammation in postmenopausal women with coronary artery disease on appropriate medical management. J. Am. Coll. Cardiol. **36:** 1797–1802.
16. POST, W.S., P.J. GOLDSCHMIDT-CLERMONT, C.C. WILHIDE, *et al.* 1999. Methylation of the estrogen receptor gene is associated with aging and atherosclerosis in the cardiovascular system. Cardiovasc. Res. **43:** 985–991.
17. WILSON, P.W., R.J. GARRISON & W.P. CASTELLI. 1985. Postmenopausal estrogen use, cigarette smoking and cardiovascular morbidity in women over 50. The Framingham Study. N. Engl. J. Med. **313:** 1038–1043.

18. KANNEL, W.B. & M. LARSON. 1993. Long-term epidemiologic prediction of coronary disease. Cardiology **82**: 137–152.
19. GRODSTEIN, F., J.E. MANSON, G.A. COLDITZ, *et al.* 2000. A prospective, observational study of postmenopausal hormone therapy and primary prevention of cardiovascular disease. Ann. Intern. Med. **133:** 933–941.
20. MASTORAKOS, G. & E.GR. SAKKAS. 2004. Hormone replacement therapy on menopause: recent data regarding its effect on cancers of the reproductive system and on cardiovascular diseases. Iatriki **86:** 308–319.

Hormone Replacement Therapy and Cardioprotection

What Is Good and What Is Bad for the Cardiovascular System?

GIUSEPPE M.C. ROSANO, CRISTIANA VITALE, AND MASSIMO FINI

Centre for Clinical and Basic Research, Department of Medical Sciences, IRCCS San Raffaele – Roma, Italy

ABSTRACT: The incidence of cardiovascular diseases (CVDs) increases after menopause and at any age postmenopausal women have a significantly higher incidence of CVD compared to premenopausal women. Several epidemiological findings suggest the causative pathogenetic role of ovarian hormone deficiency in the development of CVD in women. Ovarian hormones have several potential protective effects on the cardiovascular system and despite several observational studies have shown the beneficial effect of estrogens and estrogen/progestin associations on CVD, at the present, after the findings of randomized studies, the effect of hormone replacement therapy (HRT) in the prevention of CVD is still under debate. The randomized studies (Heart and Estrogen/Progestin Replacement Study [HERS] and Women's Health Initiative [WHI]) found largely concordant results with the observational studies except for the divergent findings about coronary heart disease (CHD). The discrepancy between the two arms of the WHI study suggests that two factors, time to initiation of HRT since menopause and estrogen/progestin associations, are of pivotal importance to explain the widely divergent findings on the cardiovascular effects of observational studies and randomized clinical studies. Basic science and animal studies together with clinical investigations and the results of clinical studies are concordant in suggesting that a long time since menopause is associated with a reduced protective effect of estrogens while the unfavorable effects upon coagulation remain unaltered. In early postmenopausal women, like the ones included in the observational studies, ovarian hormone replacement may be cardioprotective because of the responsiveness of the endothelium to estrogens that also buffer the detrimental effects upon coagulation. In late postmenopausal women ovarian hormones have either a null effect or even a detrimental effect because of the predominance of the procoagulant or plaque-destabilizing effects over the vasoprotective effects.

Address for correspondence: Giuseppe M.C. Rosano, M.D., Ph.D., Centre for Clinical and Basic Research, IRCCS San Raffaele Roma Via della Pisana 234, 00163 Rome, Italy. Voice: +39-6-660581; fax +39-6-52244512.

e-mail: giuseppe.rosano@sanraffaele.it

Ann. N.Y. Acad. Sci. 1092: 341–348 (2006). © 2006 New York Academy of Sciences.
doi: 10.1196/annals.1365.031

Therefore, HRT has beneficial cardiovascular effects in younger women
while it may have detrimental effect on coagulative balance and vascular
inflammation and has little effect on cardiovascular functions in older
women.

KEYWORDS: estrogen; prognosis; menopause; cardiovascular

INTRODUCTION

Cardiovascular and cerebrovascular diseases in the past 20 years have become the leading cause of mortality and morbidity in postmenopausal women living in industrialized countries. Of importance, while mortality rates for cardiovascular disease (CVD) have been decreasing in the past decades in men, they are still in constant increase in women.[1] The increased incidence of cardiovascular and cerebrovascular diseases in women is mainly attributable to the growing population of postmenopausal women. In fact, the increasing number of women in menopause has made manifest diseases such as CVD, osteoporosis, and dementia that were rare in women until a few decades ago and are influenced by estrogen deficiency.

It is now clear that estrogen deficiency plays a key pathogenetic role in the development of CVD in women as suggested by several epidemiological findings. The cardiovascular risk increases after menopause and at any age postmenopausal women have a significantly higher incidence of CVD compared to normo-menstruating women.[2,3]

Ovarian hormones have several potential protective effects on the cardiovascular system as shown by the beneficial effect of estrogens and estrogen/progestin combinations on surrogate endpoints of CVD and the beneficial effect on cardiovascular events suggested by several observational studies. However, at present the effect of hormone replacement therapy (HRT) in the prevention of CVD is still under debate mainly because of the findings of randomized studies conducted using a fixed estrogen/progestin combination in populations of predominantly late postmenopausal women.[4–13]

MENOPAUSE AS CARDIOVASCULAR RISK FACTOR

In postmenopausal women the state of ovarian hormones deficiency induces changes in metabolic and physiologic functions that lead to a greater prevalence of hypertension, diabetes, hyperlipidemia, and metabolic syndrome compared to the premenopausal period.[2] Although estrogen deficiency may induce detrimental changes in all cardiovascular risk factors, the changes in cardiovascular risk occurring after menopause must be regarded under a unifying mechanism. In fact, menopause causes changes in body weight, insulin sensitivity, plasma lipids, sympathetic tone, and vascular function. These changes interact with each other amplifying the effect of ovarian hormone deficiency and aging.

Menopause is associated with important changes in weight and in body fat distribution. Postmenopausal women tend to gain weight starting within the first year from menopause and redistribute body fat from a gynoid to an android pattern.[13] The fact that the changes in body weight are associated with the state of estrogen deprivation is suggested by the fact that women taking HRT gain weight at a lesser extent than women not on HRT and they maintain the gynoid pattern of fat distribution.[14] The increases in body mass index (BMI) and in the proportion of visceral fat are strongly correlated with the development of arterial hypertension, insulin resistance, and a range of metabolic risk factors for CVD.[13] The pathogenic link between weight gain, hyperinsulinemia/insulin resistance, and hypertension is evoked by the observation that the weight gain-associated worsening of insulin resistance is related to a greater incidence of hypertension. In addition, the improvement in insulin sensitivity by weight loss or treatment with insulin sensitizers is associated with a decrease in blood pressure values.[14–18]

Menopause is associated with unfavorable changes on lipoprotein profile: increase in plasma triglycerides, total and LDL cholesterol, Lp(a), and a decline in HDL levels.[19] As shown by the PROCAM study,[20] significant changes in lipoprotein profile occur in women after the age of 50 years while in men they tend to occur much earlier in life. However, when considering the effect of menopause on lipid metabolism in women it is important to clarify that, conversely to what occurs in men in whom total and LDL cholesterol are the two most important lipid predictors of cardiovascular events, in women high triglycerides and Lp(a) levels as well as low HDL cholesterol are more important than total and LDL cholesterol in the development of CVD. The relative impact of lipid changes occurring after menopause on the overall cardiovascular risk is still to be determined. All studies evaluating the effect of lipid-lowering therapy for primary prevention of CVD have failed to show any effect of this therapy in the reduction of cardiovascular mortality and morbidity.

Blood pressure changes associated with menopause are difficult to evaluate because menopause is associated with aging, and because both menopause and blood pressure are influenced by common factors such as BMI, socioeconomic status, and smoking. However, following middle age both systolic and diastolic blood pressure increase more in women than in men suggesting that menopause has a negative effect on the development of hypertension on top of the aging process. Staessen *et al.* have shown that hypertension in women is more frequent after menopause. After stratification for age and BMI the odds of having hypertension after menopause is 2.2 greater to that before menopause.[21] Several possible mechanisms may explain the increase in blood pressure following menopause. Besides the unfavorable changes in body weight and insulin resistance, postmenopausal estrogen deficiency may affect the balance between various vasoactive hormones and the proliferation and function of vascular smooth muscle cells.

As shown by the DECODE study hypertension has a greater impact as a risk factor for cardiovascular mortality and morbidity in women than in men and, conversely to what happens with hypolipidemic drugs, all therapeutic strategies aimed at reducing blood pressure levels have always shown a beneficial effect on cardiovascular events both in women and men.[22] Furthermore, it has been suggested that blood pressure reduction is more important in women than in men, that is, in patients with metabolic syndrome an aggressive reduction of blood pressure is more effective in reducing cardiovascular events in women than in men.

HORMONE REPLACEMENT THERAPY AND CARDIOPROTECTION

In the past decades and until the publication of the Women's Health Initiative (WHI), estrogen replacement therapy (ERT) and HRT have been prescribed for the relief of menopausal symptoms. In the United States their use had been extended to several years after menopause with the understanding that both replacement regimens might reduce the occurrence of CVD. This belief was based on findings of observational studies, almost all suggesting a significant reduction in cardiovascular events with ERT and HRT, and on a large body of evidence suggesting a favorable effect on lipid pattern and a protective activity of HRT on vascular functions.[5–10]

The results of the randomized studies were largely concordant with the results of the observational studies except for the divergent findings about coronary heart disease (CHD). Indeed, the Heart and Estrogen/Progestin Replacement Study (HERS) study first and the estrogen/progestin arm of the WHI thereafter suggested that HRT may increase cardiovascular risk in late postmenopausal women.[13–23] However, these results have not been confirmed by the recent report of the estrogen-only arm of the WHI.[24] This latter study has also suggested that in early postmenopausal women—women very similar to those included in the observational studies—ERT may reduce cardiovascular risk by an extent similar to that suggested by the observational studies. It seems clear that two factors, time of initiation to HRT since menopause as well as the type of estrogen/progestin combination, are of pivotal importance to explain the widely divergent findings on the cardiovascular effects between observational studies and randomized control trials.

AGING AND CARDIOVASCULAR RESPONSE TO ESTROGENS

The most important difference between the observational and randomized studies is the women under study. In the observational studies women chose to start taking ovarian hormones because of menopausal symptoms while in the randomized studies the absence of menopausal symptoms was a prerequisite for inclusion in the study. The absence of symptoms indicates a physiological adaptation to ovarian hormone deprivation, because of the slow decline in estrogen levels or because of the long time elapsed from menopause, and therefore a new homeostasis.

Almost all studies have suggested substantial benefits of hormone therapy on intermediate markers of CHD (i.e., improved lipid profile and enhanced endothelium-dependent vasodilation). Although it has been suggested that oral HRT may increase plasma levels of C-reactive protein, there is now evidence that this increase is not inflammatory in the majority of women while it may indicate an altered vascular inflammatory status in older women.[12,25–27] Clinical and experimental evidence suggest that many of the cardioprotective and antiatherogenic effects of ovarian hormones are receptor-mediated and endothelium-dependent. Both estrogen receptors and endothelial function are markedly influenced by time of estrogen deprivation and progression of the atherosclerotic injury. However, estrogen receptor expression in the arterial wall diminishes sharply with age as well as time elapsed from menopause. This is suggested by the significant age-related rise in methylation of the estrogen receptor promoter region and that of estrogen receptors in vascular atherosclerotic areas.[28] Therefore, while estrogens may have a detrimental effect in predisposed women, the beneficial cardiovascular effects of estrogen and/or hormone replacement therapy are reduced by a long term since menopause. In early postmenopausal women, like the ones included in the observational studies, ovarian hormone replacement might have been cardioprotective because of the responsiveness of the endothelium to estrogens that also buffer their detrimental effects upon coagulation. In late postmenopausal women, ovarian hormones have either a null effect or even a detrimental effect because of the predominance of the procoagulant or plaque-destabilizing effects over the vasoprotective effects.

Therefore hormone therapy has beneficial cardiovascular effects in younger women while it has little effect on cardiovascular functions or possibly detrimental effect on coagulative balance in older women.

HORMONE REGIMEN

Because of the different findings between the estrogen-only and the estrogen/progestin arm of the WHI it seems clear that the hormone regimen is an important issue.

However, while it is easy to blame the combination of conjugated estrogens and medroxyprogesterone one has to consider that almost all studies suggesting a cardioprotective effect of HRT had been conducted mainly with these two substances. Probably the unfavorable effect of the estrogen/progestin combination used in the randomized studies is related not to the hormone preparation *per se* but to the use of that hormone regimen in the wrong group of women. It is known that the vascular effects of hormones may differ in women in whom different time has elapsed from menopause as well as in women with different clinical characteristics. The Cardiovascular Health Study found that women with cardiovascular risk factors seem to have a reduced vascular response to estrogens.[29] Women recruited in the randomized studies had a high incidence of uncontrolled risk factors such as arterial hypertension and obesity as compared to women included in the observational studies, thus reducing the effectiveness of the cardioprotective effect of estrogens and increasing the likelihood of potential cerebrovascular side effects related to the mineralcorticoid effect of the progestins and their consequent effect upon blood pressure. The effect of HRT upon blood pressure is very relevant since the changes in systolic blood pressure observed in women randomized to estrogen/progestin therapy included in the WHI study are likely to explain the increase in stroke observed in the study.[13] Furthermore, women included in the WHI had often uncontrolled arterial hypertension and this may have intensified the mineralcorticoid effect of medroxyprogesterone.[30] The mineralcorticoid effect of progestins may be increased by the effect of estrogens on the production of angiotensinogen that in turn leads to increased production of angiotensin and aldosterone. Therefore progestins with antimineralcorticoid and antialdosterone effects should be preferred in the treatment of postmenopausal women, especially if they have family history of arterial hypertension or if they report weight gain or bloating with other estrogen/progestin combinations.

It is well known that increased body weight increases the likelihood of venous thromboembolism. Women included in the WHI studies were mostly overweight and obese. The association of increased body weight and oral HRT may therefore increase the risk of venous thromboembolism. It is clear that the long time elapsed from menopause and the excessive body weight of the women included in the WHI were the most important factors in determining the detrimental effects of the estrogen/progestin therapy. In conclusion, HRT is protective in early postmenopausal women. Obesity, time elapsed from menopause, and increased blood pressure may put women at increased risk for cardiovascular events with HRT. Clinical judgment and choice of the right estrogen/progestin combination are of major importance to maximize the beneficial effect of estrogens and estrogen/progestin therapy especially if given shortly after menopause.

REFERENCES

1. AMERICAN HEART ASSOCIATION. 1999. 2000 Heart and Stroke Statistical Update, AHA. Dallas, Texas.
2. COLDITZ, G.A., W.C. WILLETT, M.J. STAMPFER, *et al.* 1987. Menopause and the risk of coronary heart disease in women. N. Engl. J. Med. **316:** 1105–1110.

3. ROSANO, G.M. & M. FINI. 2002. Postmenopausal women and cardiovascular risk: impact of hormone replacement therapy. Cardiol. Rev. **10:** 51–60.
4. STAMPFER, M.J. & G.A. COLDITZ. 1991. Estrogen replacement therapy and coronary heart disease: a quantitative assessment of the epidemiologic evidence. Prev. Med. **20:** 47–63.
5. GRODSTEIN, F. & M. STAMPFER. 1995. The epidemiology of coronary heart disease and estrogen replacement in postmenopausal women. Prog. Cardiovasc. Dis. **38:** 199–210.
6. GRUCHOW, H.W., A.J. ANDERSON, J.J. BARBORIAK & K.A. SOBOCINSKI. 1988. Postmenopausal use of estrogen and occlusion of coronary arteries. Am. Heart. J. **115:** 954–963.
7. MCFARLAND, K.F., M.E. BONIFACE, C.A. HORNUNG, *et al.* 1989. Risk factors and noncontraceptive estrogen use in women with and without coronary disease. Am. Heart J. **117:** 1209–1214.
8. GRODSTEIN, F., M.J. STAMPFER, G.A. COLDITZ, *et al.* 1997. Postmenopausal hormone therapy and mortality. N. Engl. J. Med. **336:** 1769–1775.
9. HENDERSON, B.E., A. PAGANINI-HILL & R.K. ROSS. 1991. Decreased mortality in users of estrogen replacement therapy. Arch. Intern. Med. **151:** 75–78.
10. BUSH, T.L., E. BARRETT-CONNOR, L.D. COWAN, *et al.* 1987. Cardiovascular mortality and noncontraceptive use of estrogen in women: results from the Lipid Research Clinics Program Follow-up Study. Circulation **75:** 1102–1109.
11. THE WRITING GROUP FOR THE PEPI TRIAL. 1995. Effects of estrogen or estrogen/progestin regimens on heart disease risk factors in postmenopausal women. JAMA **273:** 199–208.
12. MENDELSOHN, M.E. & R.H. KARAS. 1999. The protective effects of estrogen on the cardiovascular system. N. Engl. J. Med. **340:** 1801–1811.
13. WRITING GROUP FOR THE WOMEN'S HEALTH INITIATIVE INVESTIGATORS. 2002. Risks and benefits of estrogen plus progestin in healthy postmenopausal women: principal results from the Women's Health Initiative randomized controlled trial. JAMA. **288:** 321–333.
14. GAMBACCIANI, M., M. CIAPPONI, B. CAPPAGLI, *et al.* 1999. Climacteric modifications in body weight and fat tissue distribution. Climacteric **2:** 37–44.
15. CARR, M.C. 2003. The emergence of the metabolic syndrome with menopause. J. Clin. Endocrinol. Metab. **88:** 2404–2411.
16. ROSANO, G.M., C. VITALE, A. SILVESTRI & M. FINI. 2004. The metabolic syndrome in women: implications for therapy. Int. J. Clin. Pract. (Suppl. 139): 20–25.
17. VITALE, C., G. MERCURO, A. CORNOLDI, *et al.* 2005. Metformin improves endothelial function in patients with metabolic syndrome. J. Intern. Med. **258:** 250–256.
18. TUOMILEHTO, J., J. LINDSTROM, J.G. ERIKSSON, *et al.* 2001. Finnish Diabetes Prevention Study Group. Prevention of type 2 diabetes mellitus by changes in lifestyle among subjects with impaired glucose tolerance. N. Engl. J. Med. **344:** 1343–1350.
19. DE ALOYSIO, D., M. GAMBACCIANI, M. MESCHIA, *et al.* 1999. The effect of menopause on blood lipid and lipoprotein levels. Atherosclerosis **147:** 147–153.
20. ASSMANN, G. & H. SCHULTE. 1992. The importance of triglycerides: results from the Prospective Cardiovascular Munster (PROCAM) Study. Eur. J. Epidemiol. **8**(Suppl. 1): 99–103.
21. STAESSEN, J.A., H. CELIS & R. FAGARD. 1998. The epidemiology of the association between hypertension and menopause. J. Hum. Hypertens. **12:** 587–592.

22. Hu, G. 2003. DECODE Study Group. Gender difference in all-cause and cardiovascular mortality related to hyperglycaemia and newly-diagnosed diabetes. Diabetologia **46:** 608–617.

23. HERRINGTON, D.M., D.M. REBOUSSIN, K.B. BROSNIHAN, *et al.* 2000. Effects of estrogen replacement on the progression of coronary-artery atherosclerosis. N. Engl. J. Med. **343:** 522–529.

24. HSIA, J., R.D. LANGER, J.E. MANSON, *et al.* 2006. Women's Health Initiative Investigators. Conjugated equine estrogens and coronary heart disease: the Women's Health Initiative. Arch. Intern. Med. **166:** 357–365.

25. SILVESTRI, A., O. GEBARA, C. VITALE, *et al.* 2003. Increased levels of C-reactive protein after oral hormone replacement therapy may not be related to an increased inflammatory response. Circulation **107:** 3165–3169.

26. SCARABIN, P.Y., M. ALHENC-GELAS, E. OGER & G. PLU-BUREAU. 1999. Hormone replacement therapy and circulating ICAM-1 in postmenopausal women—a randomised controlled trial. Thromb. Haemost. **81:** 673–675.

27. WALSH, B.W., S. PAUL, R.A. WILD, *et al.* 2000. The effects of hormone replacement therapy and raloxifene on C-reactive protein and homocysteine in healthy postmenopausal women: a randomized, controlled trial. J. Clin. Endocrinol. Metab. **85:** 214–218.

28. POST, W.S., P.J. GOLDSCHMIDT-CLERMONT, C.C. WILHIDE, *et al.* 1999. Methylation of the estrogen receptor gene is associated with aging and atherosclerosis in the cardiovascular system. Cardiovasc. Res. **43:** 985–991.

29. HERRINGTON, D.M., M.A. ESPELAND, J.R. CROUSE, III, *et al.* 2001. Estrogen replacement and brachial artery flow-mediated vasodilation in older women. Arterioscler. Thromb. Vasc. Biol. **21:** 1955–1961.

30. WASSERTHEIL-SMOLLER, S., G. ANDERSON, B.M. PSATY, *et al.* 2000. Hypertension and its treatment in postmenopausal women: baseline data from the Women's Health Initiative. Hypertension **36:** 780–789.

Hormone Replacement Therapy in Breast Cancer Survivors

ANTONIOS M. XYDAKIS, EVANGELOS GR. SAKKAS, AND GEORGE MASTORAKOS

Endocrine Unit, Second Department of Obstetrics and Gynecology, "Aretaieion" Hospital, Medical School, University of Athens, Athens, Greece

ABSTRACT: It is well known that women with breast cancer who undergo therapies beyond the surgical intervention (adjuvant chemotherapy, hormone therapy, or both) often suffer from the lack of estrogen, manifesting as climacteric symptoms in either treated premenopausal or postmenopausal women. Although HRT (hormone replacement therapy) is traditionally viewed as a contraindication in women with a history of breast cancer, more women are willing to receive HRT for symptom relief. No observational or retrospective study in breast cancer survivors (whether in pre- or postmenopausal women) has shown an increased risk of tumor recurrence or increased mortality associated with HRT use. Nevertheless, because these studies are retrospective and different in terms of lymph node status, estrogen receptor (ER) status, and type of HRT used, firm conclusions on potential HRT use cannot be safely drawn. The few prospective studies appear controversial possibly due to differences in the studies' design. A potential scheme for possible HRT use in selected breast cancer survivors with severe climacteric symptoms is suggested. The duration of HRT use is debatable because there is insufficient evidence at present. However, the available data suggest that 3-year and possibly 5-year HRT use may be safe. In summary, while HRT cannot currently be recommended as first-line therapy, it may still be of benefit in the management of selected early stage breast cancer survivors with refractory climacteric symptoms after a well-informed decision and an individualized risk benefit discussion.

KEYWORDS: breast cancer survivors; hormone therapy; menopausal symptoms

INTRODUCTION

Breast cancer incidence is increasing worldwide while its mortality decreases due to early screening, enhanced follow-up, and therapeutic advancements. The National Center of Statistics of the United States reported a 6%

Address for correspondence: George Mastorakos, 3 Neofytou Vamva Street, Kolonaki 106 74 Athens, Greece. Voice: 0030-210-3636230; fax: 0030-210-3636229.
e-mail: mastorak@mail.kapatel.gr

Ann. N.Y. Acad. Sci. 1092: 349–360 (2006). © 2006 New York Academy of Sciences.
doi: 10.1196/annals.1365.032

decrease in breast cancer mortality from 1991 to 1995 and the number of breast cancer survivors is continuously rising.[1] Furthermore, it is well known that women with breast cancer who undergo therapies beyond the surgical intervention (adjuvant chemotherapy, hormone therapy, or both) often suffer from the lack of estrogen, which means that climacteric symptoms may appear in treated premenopausal women and become more severe in postmenopausal women. Hot flushes, night sweats, vaginal atrophy, osteoporosis, and cardiovascular disease are the most important adverse consequences associated with estrogen deficiency. The amelioration of severe menopausal symptoms is currently the primary indication for hormone replacement therapy (HRT) in healthy women.[2] The use of combined (estrogen plus continuous progestogen) HRT did not prove effective for either primary or secondary cardiovascular disease prevention, and alternative therapies for osteoporosis prevention and treatment exist.[3–5] Traditionally, HRT has been viewed as an absolute contraindication in women with a history of breast cancer due to fear of reactivating occult disease. However, a US survey showed that 27% of postmenopausal women with a history of breast cancer consider that they need HRT, although the majority think that this may adversely affect their disease prognosis.[2] Therefore, the increased survival rates of breast cancer survivors and the need for better quality of life present new challenges for the physicians caring for such women.

Before analyzing the available studies regarding the effect of HRT in breast cancer survivors, consideration should be given on the effect of HRT on healthy women. A considerable number of older studies being either observational, retrospective, or meta-analyses have failed to convincingly prove a causal association between HRT and an increased breast cancer risk. More recently, the observational Million Women's Study did find a relative risk of 2.0 for women on combined HRT and 1.5 on estrogen alone (ERT) after an average follow-up of about 2.5 years.[6] This study has been criticized due to the potential inclusion of women with more than average risk and possible missing of cancer cases at baseline due to the known reduced sensitivity of mammography in women on HRT. Moreover, the large, prospective, randomized, and placebo-controlled Women's Health Initiative (WHI) study consisted of two arms of which the first lasted 5.2 years and used a conjugated estrogen plus continuous progestin HRT regimen, while the second lasted 8.5 years and studied the use of ERT in postmenopausal women with hysterectomy.[7] Breast cancer hazard ratios were 1.26 (or 8 more cases per 10,000 women per year) (adjusted 95% confidence interval 0.83–1.92) and 0.77, respectively (adjusted 95% confidence interval CI = 0.57–1.06), but statistical significance was not reached in either. Importantly, whatever the quantified excess risk associated with HRT use might be, it has not been translated into an increase in cancer-specific or all-cause mortality in the vast majority of the studies. In fact, most but not all of the available evidence has associated current or previous HRT use with favorable biological features of breast tumors.[8–10] A noteworthy exception is the combined HRT arm of the WHI, in which breast cancers were similar in grade and histology but larger and more advanced compared to those in the placebo group. It must be pointed out, however, that estrogen and progesterone receptor status was unknown in a significant percentage of women in the placebo group making such comparisons difficult to interpret. Estrogen deficiency symptoms pose a difficult management problem. Although nonhormonal alternative therapies are available, such as selective serotonin reuptake inhibitors, gabapentin, and clonidine, HRT remains the most effective option. Therefore, a reconsideration of the available evidence and a reappraisal of relative versus absolute contraindications for HRT use are needed.

RETROSPECTIVE STUDIES

Most of the studies concerning breast cancer survivors and treatment with HRT are retrospective with their inherent limitations, such as selection, reporting, and publication biases.

This review will focus on the most important retrospective studies during the last decade. One of the first studies by Powles *et al.*[11] identified 35 breast cancer survivors taking HRT. The median ERT duration was 15 months and the median follow-up period was 43 months. Subsequently two studies by DiSaia *et al.* were published, the first of which was a retrospective review of 77 breast cancer survivors with a median age at diagnosis of 50 years (range, 26–88 years) who took HRT without a control group, and the second included 41 of the above patients that were matched to 82 comparison patients who did not receive HRT.[12,13] Whether the participants were pre- or postmenopausal at the time of the diagnosis is not clear, while 36% were already receiving HRT at the time of diagnosis. In this study, therapy was given for a mean period of 27 months and the mean follow-up period was 59 months. Shortly thereafter, Vassilopoulou-Sellin *et al.* published the results of a retrospective study, which included 43 women treated with oral HRT,[14] but there was no control group. The median age at the time of cancer diagnosis was 46 years (range 26–66 years), the median duration of ERT was 31 months (range 24–142 months), and the median follow-up period 144 months after cancer diagnosis (range 46–324 months). In 2001 two retrospective studies were published of which the first by O'Meara *et al.*[15] was randomized and compared 174 HRT users (68% were over 55 years old) after cancer diagnosis to 695 nonusers. The median duration of oral HRT use during follow-up was 15 months and the women were followed for a median of 3.7 years for recurrence and 4.6 years for mortality. The second trial by Beckmann *et al.*[16] was nonrandomized and examined a total of 185 breast survivors of which 64 received HRT after diagnosis and 121 did not. In this study, breast cancer survivors were divided in two groups, the first of which included patients under 50 and the second consisted of patients over 50 years old. For breast cancer patients not on HRT, the overall median follow-up was 42 months (range 3–60 months) while for those on HRT it was

37 months (range 3–60 months). One of the most recent studies was published by Durna et al.[17] This was a retrospective observational study, in which 1,122 postmenopausal women with a diagnosis of breast cancer were followed up for a median of 6.08 years (range 0–36 years) and 286 of women who received HRT were compared to nearly 1,000 women not receiving HRT, although 154 of the initial cohort were lost to follow-up.

Lymph Node and Receptors Status

It is not easy to draw any firm conclusion regarding the relationship between breast cancer recurrence and the lymph node state. In the O'Meara et al.[15] study lymph node state is not reported whereas in the Beckmann's study[16] there is considerable difference between users and nonusers; 69% of the HRT users were node positive whereas only 37% of the nonusers were positive. In the Durna et al. study[17] the majority of those who took therapy (91%) had positive nodes. On the contrary DiSaia et al.[12,13] included 75% patients taking therapy with negative nodes with only 16% being node positive.

As far as the estrogen receptor (ER) status is concerned there are also notable differences among the studies. DiSaia et al.[12,13] included mainly positive ER (ER+) patients, nevertheless there were a lot of patients whose status was unknown. Durna et al.[17] did not report the receptor status and in the O'Meara et al.[15] study such reporting is incomplete. Beckmann's[16] study provides sufficient information regarding the receptor status: 50% of the users were ER+ and the rest were negative, while 40% of the non-HRT users were positive and the rest were negative.

HRT Use Before Diagnosis

In most of the studies a significant percentage of women were receiving HRT before breast cancer diagnosis. Some of these women continued HRT after the diagnosis was made and some subsequently stopped. Specifically in the DiSaia et al.[12,13] trial 36% had been receiving postmenopausal HRT at the time of diagnosis. Similarly, in the Durna et al.[17] study 67% of women in the HRT-treated arm used HRT before cancer diagnosis for a median period of 6.5 years while 19% of the non-HRT-treated arm had taken HRT before cancer diagnosis. The respective numbers in the Beckmann et al.[16] study were 40% of the users and 15% of the nonusers. Finally, in the O'Meara et al.[15] study, 68% of the users were taking HRT before diagnosis (35% of the users were receiving therapy for more than 6 years) and 48% of the nonusers, which could be even higher taking into account that there are missing data for some of the patients.

Type of HRT and Combination with Tamoxifene

The specific HRT regimen and route of delivery also vary considerably among the studies. Moreover, some studies included patients who received estrogens or progestins or both in combination with tamoxifen. The effect of the concurrent use of HRT and tamoxifen on breast cancer incidence is truly unknown although it has been stated that one does not alter the other drug's action.[18,19]

Powles *et al.* included patients who took oral conjugated estrogens with tamoxifen. In the DiSaia *et al.*[12,13] study most of the patients received HRT in the form of conjugated estrogen, and patients used estradiol patches, while 39% of women received concomitant tamoxifen therapy during some interval of HRT use. In the Beckmann *et al.*[16] study the regimen used was estrogen plus progestin. Durna *et al.*[17] included 138 patients (48%) who took estrogen plus progestin, 78 (27%) who took oral progestins alone, 32 (11%) who took vaginal estrogen alone, 21 (7%) who took vaginal estrogen plus oral progestin, and 17 (6%) who took oral or transdermal estrogen alone. Finally, in the O'Meara *et al.*[15] study, 79% of the users took unopposed estrogens and the rest of the subjects combined a progestogen with estrogen in a cyclical manner. Among the users, 41% took oral HRT, 43% received only vaginal HRT, and 16% received both vaginal and oral HRT. Whether the timing of tamoxifen use (prior, concurrent, or later) with respect to HRT alters their respective effects on the breast has not been adequately studied.

Stage of Breast Cancer

One of the few parameters appearing to be common in all retrospective studies is the breast cancer stage. In fact, according to a meta-analysis, which covers all studies performed from 1989 to 2000, the majority of women enrolled had survived from a breast cancer stage I or II.[20] Similarly, in the Durna *et al.*[17] and O'Meara *et al.*[15] studies 53% and 80% of subjects were respectively of stage I or II. However, it is inappropriate to associate the stage with the recurrence and mortality risk because of potential selection bias in these studies. Women with stage I and II breast cancers are generally more likely to use HRT than those with advanced stage III or IV disease.

RESULTS

All of the aforementioned studies provide optimistic results regarding the association between HRT use, breast cancer recurrence, and breast cancer mortality. In the Powles *et al.*[11] study two recurrences and one death were observed. DiSaia *et al.*[12,13] found seven recurrences and three deaths of which

20 women took ERT for 2–5 years, and 6 women took ERT for <2 years. As far as receptor and lymph node status are concerned, 70% in the randomized group and 66% in the nonrandomized group were ER⁻, while 83% of both groups had up to three lymph nodes involved. The study participants were women who had survived from breast cancer stage I or II and had remained disease free for 2 years at least. There was no association between ERT use and time to recurrence of breast cancer whether the analysis was performed for the randomized group only or the entire group combined (overall 3.6% of ERT users and 13.5% nonusers developed new or recurrent disease, respectively).[21]

In 2003 the steering committee of the eagerly awaited HABITS study (Hormonal replacement therapy after breast cancer diagnosis—is it safe?)[22] decided to halt the trial prematurely and recommended that all patients on HRT stop treatment. The HABITS trial started to recruit women in 1997, examining whether a 2-year HRT treatment for menopausal symptoms was safe in women with previously treated breast cancer. This trial was designed as a non-inferiority study and was tailored to exclude a relative hazard (RH) equal or greater than 1.36 comparing HRT with no HRT. Women were eligible if they had previously completed treatment for *in situ* up to stage II breast cancer. The choice of the specific type of HRT was directed by local practice, so estrogen–progestin combinations were used except tibolone. Due to slow recruitment, in 2002 HABITS and a similar parallel trial in Stockholm, agreed to pool safety and final analyses in the future. The joint analysis of the two studies showed that the risk of breast cancer recurrence was significantly associated with menopausal hormone therapy (RH = 1.8, 95% CI = 1.03–3.1). However, there was a statistically significant ($P = 0.02$) heterogeneity between the two studies; in HABITS the RH was 3.3 (95% CI = 1.5–7.4) and in the Stockholm trial it was 0.82 (95% CI = 0.35–1.9). According to HABITS alone, among 345 women (434 women had been initially randomized) who were followed up until 2003, 56% of the users were hormone receptor positive versus 48% of the nonusers, 26% had positive lymph nodes versus 21% of the nonusers, and 52% had received HRT before diagnosis versus 56% of the nonusers. A total of 26 women out of 174 (15%) who were followed up and received HRT were reported to have experienced new breast cancer events contrary to 8 out of 171 (4.5%) who were followed up and did not take HRT. The higher number of women with positive nodes and ER⁺ tumors in the HRT group at baseline, as well as the relatively short time interval until recurrence (potential detection of preexisting tumors at follow-up) have been pointed out as limitations in the HABITS study design and the generalization of its conclusions. Notably, there was a striking difference in recurrent events between ER⁺ and ER⁻ study participants and there were a greater number of deaths in the non-HRT group. More controversy is generated after consideration of the Stockholm randomized trial,[23] a study initially thought to be similar to HABITS that was also stopped prematurely. In a separate brief report of their results, von Schoultz *et al.* found that at a median follow-up of 4.1 years, the risk of breast cancer recurrence was not associated with HRT. In this study, patients were randomly allocated to receive HRT for 5 years ($n = 188$) or to receive no HRT ($n = 190$). These women were postmenopausal breast cancer survivors younger than 70 years who were invited to participate irrespective of time since surgery, stage of primary disease, hormone receptor status, and concomitant adjuvant treatment. In contrast to the HABITS trial, there were much fewer events with positive nodes (16% vs. 26%, respectively) and more women who received adjuvant tamoxifen (52% vs. 21%, respectively). Importantly, the Stockholm trial recommended that patients avoid continuous combined HRT but rather use regimens that incorporated 1 week of no treatment every 1 (cyclically) or 3 (spacing out regimen) months. This recommendation resulted in that 73% of HRT users were on either ERT alone or on the spacing out progestogen regimen (2 weeks every 3 months). Finally, most of the recurrences in both groups were ER$^+$ and occurred in women who had previous HRT exposure.

CONCLUSIONS

An ever increasing number of breast cancer survivors (some in their 30s and 40s) suffer from climacteric symptoms more often and for a longer period than women in the general population. Improved treatment outcomes, disease-free intervals, and survival rates call for a better quality of life for these women. In healthy women, the reassuring WHI ERT alone arm results and the abso-lute low breast cancer risk emerging only after 5 years in the WHI combined HRT arm allow for short-term HRT use for vasomotor symptoms. But does HRT have a place in the physician's armamentarium against climacteric symp-toms in breast cancer patients? Specific evidence-based recommendations have been difficult to formulate. Due to concerns for dormant disease reactivation, women carrying a previous diagnosis of breast carcinoma have been strongly discouraged from using HRT and alternative remedies are offered to them. Ob-jectively, however, no observational or retrospective study performed (whether in pre- or postmenopausal women) has shown an increased risk of tumor re-currence or increased mortality from progressive disease. Moreover, according to a meta-analysis published in 2001, which examined the recurrence rate of breast cancer as it appeared in 11 retrospective studies, all performed from 1993 to 1999, the relative risk among 669 HRT total users was 0.82 (95% CI = 0.58–1.15). Nevertheless, these studies are subject to several limitations with respect to selection, reporting, and publication biases. In addition, there are significant differences between the observational studies with a variable number of patients, age, follow-up period, and HRT duration. Reliable conclu-sions cannot be drawn regarding lymph node status, because in some studies it is not reported and in others there is considerable difference between HRT users and nonusers. As far as receptor status is concerned, only Beckmann *et al.*[16] provided sufficient information. Furthermore, in some studies women were premenopausal when breast cancer was diagnosed while other studies included only postmenopausal women. A significant percentage of women had used HRT before diagnosis, which can also be a confounding factor. The type of HRT used was never the same among the studies (type or dose or route of administration) and in the Powles et al.[11] study women were also receiving tamoxifen.

Regarding the evidence from the few prospective studies, the message is rather controversial at present. The discrepant results between the HABITS on the one hand and the Stockholm as well as Vassilopoulou-Sellin et al.[14] studies on the other are difficult to explain. Differences in the study design, patient population, and HRT regimen used may in part be responsible for the conflicting reports. Recent case–control studies have indicated that continuous progestogen exposure is associated with a significant increase in breast cancer risk in contrast with much less risk in women using ERT alone. The mechanism drawn from basic science studies appears to relate the effects of systemic progestogen to both upregulated cell proliferation and blood vessel growth although contradictory reports have also been published. This hypothesis of the adverse impact of continuous progestogen on breast cancer risk is further supported by the discrepant results between the combined HRT and ERT alone WHI arms and between the HABITS and the Stockholm randomized trial. Should the HABITS investigators' general conclusion that even short-term HRT causes an unacceptably high risk of disease recurrence dictate current practice and preclude HRT use in breast cancer survivors? Although concern that risk may outweigh the benefit should definitely not be disregarded, we believe that most retrospective and prospective data allow for possible HRT use in breast cancer survivors with severe climacteric symptoms who had disease stage I or II, negative nodes and ER$^-$ receptor status with preferably at least 2 years disease-free interval. The duration of HRT use is a matter of ongoing debate because there is insufficient evidence but from the available data, it may be suggested that 3-year and possibly 5-year HRT use may be safe. With regards to breast cancer survivors who have advanced stage III or IV, HRT use should still be viewed as an absolute contraindication. As far as breast cancer survivors with ER$^+$ tumors, there is insufficient data because the majority of the retrospective studies did not report the receptor status or this was incompletely documented. With respect to the type of HRT regimen, there is accumulating evidence that ERT at the lowest effective dose alone or combined with minimal systemic progestogen exposure may interfere less with mechanisms that underlie cancer recurrence. There appears that adjuvant therapy with tamoxifen may also reduce the risk of breast cancer recurrence when used concurrently with ERT. The unique properties of tibolone, a selective ER regulator, suggest that it ameliorates vasomotor symptoms without promoting adverse effects on the breast or the endometrium. Preliminary data from pilot studies are encouraging and the effect of tibolone on recurrence rates in women with a history of breast cancer is currently being assessed in a large double-blind, randomized, placebo-controled, 5-year trial (LIBERATE). In summary, while HRT cannot currently be recommended as first-line therapy, it may still be of benefit in the management of selected early stage breast cancer survivors with refractory climacteric symptoms after a well-informed decision and an individualized risk benefit discussion.

Potential options for breast cancer survivors with climacteric symptoms

	Breast cancer survivors	
↓		↓
Not severe symptoms		Severe symptoms
↓		↓
Do nothing		First option
		↓
	Second option	non-HRT
↓		↓
Negative nodes		Positive nodes
ER$^+$		ER$^-$
Stage III or IV		Stage I or II
HRT not recommended		HRT* recommended
		for up to 5 years

*lowest effective dose.

REFERENCES

1. BIGLIA, N., M. COZZARELLA, F. CACCIARI, *et al.* 2003. Menopause after breast cancer: a survey on breast cancer survivors. Maturitas **45:** 29–38.
2. VASSILOPOULOU-SELLIN, R. & M.J. KLEIN. 1996. Estrogen replacement therapy after treatment for localized breast carcinoma: patients responses and opinions. Cancer **78:**1043–1048.
3. HULLEY, S., D. GRADY, T. BUSH, *et al.* 1998. Randomized trial of oestrogen plus progestin for secondary prevention of coronary heart disease in postmenopausal women. JAMA **280:** 605–613.
4. GRADY, D., D. HERRINGTON, V. BITTNER, *et al.* 2002. Cardiovascular disease outcomes during 6.8 years of hormone therapy. Heart and oestrogen-progestin replacement study follow-up (HERS II). JAMA **288:**49–57.
5. WRITING GROUP FOR THE WOMEN'S HEALTH INITIATIVE INVESTIGATORS. 2002. Risks and benefits of estrogen plus progestin in healthy postmenopausal women. Principal results from the Women's Health Initiative randomized control trial. JAMA **288:** 321–333.
6. BERAL, V. MILLION WOMEN 'S STUDY COLLABORATORS. 2003. Breast cancer and hormone replacement therapy in the Million Women Study. Lancet **362:** 419–427.
7. THE WOMEN'S HEALTH INITIATIVE STEERING COMMITTEE. 2004. Effects of conjugated equine estrogen in postmenopausal women with hysterectomy. JAMA **291:**1701–1712.
8. BIGLIA, N., L. SGRO, E. DEFABIANI, *et al.* 2005. The influence of hormone replacement therapy on the pathology of breast cancer. Eur. J. Surg. Oncol. **31:** 467–472.

9. FLETCHER, A.S., B. ERBAS, A.M. KAVANAGH, *et al.* 2005. Use of hormone replacement therapy (HRT) and survival following breast cancer diagnosis. Breast **14:** 192–200.
10. MARSDEN, J., M. WHITEHEAD, R. A'HERN, *et al.* 2000. Are randomized trials of hormone replacement therapy in symptomatic women with breast cancer feasible? Fertil. Steril. **73:** 292–299.
11. POWLES, T.J., T. HICKISH, S. CASEY, *et al.* 1993. Hormone replacement after breast cancer. Lancet **342:** 60–61.
12. DISAIA, P.J., E.A. GROSEN, F. ODICINO, *et al.* 1995. Replacement therapy for breast cancer survivors. A pilot study. Cancer **76:** 2075–2078.
13. DISAIA, P.J., E.A. GROSEN, T. KUROSAKI, *et al.* 1996. Hormone replacement therapy in breast cancer survivors: a cohort study. Am. J. Obstet. Gynecol. **174:** 1494–1498.
14. VASSILOPOULOU-SELLIN, R., R. THERIAULT & M.J. KLEIN. 1997. Estrogen replacement therapy in women with prior diagnosis and treatment of breast cancer. Gynecol. Oncol. **65:** 89–93.
15. O'MEARA, E.S., A. ROSSING, J.R. DALING, *et al.* 2001. Hormone replacement therapy after a diagnosis of breast cancer in relation to recurrence and mortality. J. Natl. Cancer Inst **93:** 754–762.
16. BECKMANN, M.W., D. JAP, S. DJAHANSOUZI, *et al.* 2001. Hormone replacement therapy after treatment of breast cancer: effects on postmenopausal symptoms, bone mineral density and recurrence rates. Oncology **60:** 199–206.
17. DURNA, E.M., B.G. WREN, G.Z. HELLER, *et al.* 2002. Hormone replacement therapy after a diagnosis of breast cancer: cancer recurrence and mortality. Med. J. Aust. **177:** 347–351.
18. MARSDEN, J. 2002. Hormone-replacement therapy and breast cancer. Lancet Oncol. **3:** 303–311.
19. CHANG, J., T. POWLES, S. ASHLEY, *et al.* 1996. The effect of tamoxifen and hormone replacement therapy on serum cholesterol, bone mineral density and coagulation factors in healthy postmenopausal women participating in a randomised, controlled tamoxifen prevention study. Ann. Oncol. **7:** 671–675.
20. COL, N., L. HIROTA, R. ORR, *et al.* 2001. Hormone replacement therapy after breast cancer: a systematic review and quantitative assessment of risk. J. Clin. Oncol. **19:** 2357–2363.
21. VASSILOPOULOU-SELLIN, R., D.S. COHEN, G.N. HORTOBAGYI, *et al.* 2002. Estrogen replacement therapy for menopausal women with a history of breast carcinoma. Cancer **95:** 1817–1826.
22. STEERING COMMITTEE AND DMC OF HABITS. 2004. HABITS (hormonal replacement therapy after breast cancer- is it safe?), a randomized comparison: trial stopped. Lancet **363:** 453–455.
23. RUTQVIST, L., D. CEDERMARK, U. GLAS, *et al.* 1987. The Stockholm trial on adjuvant tamoxifen in early breast cancer. Correlation between estrogen receptor level and treatment effect. Breast Cancer Res. Treat. **10:** 255–266.

Potential Biological Functions Emerging from the Different Estrogen Receptors

KAREN D. CARPENTER AND KENNETH S. KORACH

Receptor Biology Section, Laboratory of Reproductive and Developmental Toxicology, National Institute of Environmental Health Sciences, National Institute of Health, Research Triangle Park, North Carolina, USA

ABSTRACT: **Technological advances and new tools have brought about tremendous advances in elucidating the roles of estradiol and the estrogen receptors (ERs) in biological processes, especially within the female reproductive system. Development and analysis of multiple genetic models have provided insight into the particular functions of each of the ERs. This article reviews the insights into ER biology in female reproduction gained from the development and use of new types of experimental models.**

KEYWORDS: **estradiol; estrogen receptor; uterus; ovary**

INTRODUCTION

It is well known that estrogens are essential for successful mammalian reproduction. Estrogens circulate systemically and effect many target tissues via estrogen receptors (ERs). ERs are members of a family of nuclear transcription factors including receptors for sex steroids, thyroid hormone, vitamin D, retinoids, and many orphan receptors for which ligands have not yet been identified.[1] Two distinct ER molecules, ERα and ERβ, have been identified and are expressed at differing levels in many tissues including the hypothalamus, pituitary, uterus, and ovary. The ER isoforms share a similar structure as illustrated in FIGURE 1. Generally, ERs possess a DNA-binding domain (C domain) that contains two zinc-fingers and binds to estrogen response elements (EREs) in target genes, and a ligand-binding domain that binds estrogen and estrogenic compounds. The AF-1 region in the amino terminus and the AF-2 region within the ligand-binding domain are involved in ligand-independent and ligand-dependent transcriptional activation, respectively.

Address for correspondence: Kenneth S. Korach, Receptor Biology Section, Laboratory of Reproductive and Developmental Toxicology, National Institute of Environmental and Health Sciences, 111 TW Alexander Drive, Research Triangle Park, NC 27709, USA. Voice: 919-541-3512; fax: 919-541-0696.

e-mail: Korach@niehs.nih.gov

Ann. N.Y. Acad. Sci. 1092: 361–373 (2006). © 2006 New York Academy of Sciences.
doi: 10.1196/annals.1365.033

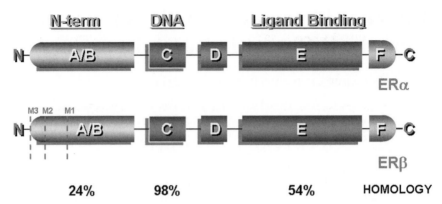

FIGURE 1. Estrogen receptor structure. The domain structures of ERα and ERβ are depicted. Each contains six domains, **A–F**. Three alternative translational start sites, M1, M2, and M3, for ERβ are shown. The degree of homology between the two isoforms is listed below the domains.

In the simplest models of estrogen action, estrogen binds to the ER, which then interacts as dimers with EREs in target genes. The estrogen–ER complex then recruits transcriptional comodulators and consequently regulates transcription of the target genes. The transcriptional coregulators, including members of the steroid receptor complex (SRC)/p160 family and the thyroid receptor-associated protein (TRAP220) complex, mediate interactions between ERs and the transcriptional machinery. Many estrogen-responsive genes lack the canonical ERE sequence and interact with ERs via a tethering mechanism with a combination of ER and SP1 or AP1 transcription factors.[2–4] In addition, very rapid nongenomic or nongenotropic estrogen responses indicate that ERs interact with and activate signaling cascades at the cell membrane.[5,6] Finally, ER-mediated transcription can occur in a ligand-independent manner in response to signaling through growth factor receptors by activators such as insulin-like growth factor I (IGF-I) and epidermal growth factor (EGF).[5] The mechanistic details of ER-directed transcription are more fully described and discussed elsewhere.[7–9]

The development of knockout or transgenic mice with disruptions, mutations, or overexpression of molecules related to reproduction and hormone action has increased our understanding of their relative physiological roles in developmental and biological processes in the mouse. Overt phenotypes are seen in ERα and ERβ and double knockout mice (αERKO, βERKO, and αβERKO) indicating the essential roles of these receptors in certain tissues and biological responses. Briefly, the αERKO and αβERKO females are infertile and βERKO females are subfertile due to distinct ovulatory defects.[10] This article provides an overview of the phenotypes observed in the ERKO models as they apply to the roles of ERs in female reproduction with the potential use for identifying or characterizing clinical conditions which may be a result of compromised activity of the ERs in sexual differentiation and development, where it has been established that AR activity and androgen hormone is required in the male.

ERs IN UTERINE BIOLOGY

Murine models of disrupted ER function suggest that ERα plays a greater role in uterine responsiveness and function than does ERβ. All three lines of ER-null females exhibit uteri that possess the expected tissue compartments (myometrium, endometrial stroma, and epithelium) indicating especially in the αβERKO model that ER signaling is not required for development of the female reproductive tract, which is in contrast to the male. Uteri of αERKO and αβERKO females are hypoplastic and exhibit severely reduced uterine weights relative to wild-type littermates whereas βERKO uteri are grossly normal (FIG. 2).[11,12] The βERKO females are subfertile but are able to carry pregnancies to term indicating adequate uterine function despite the absence of ERβ.[10] Furthermore, the transcriptional response of the βERKO uterus to estrogen is comparable to wild type.[13] These data suggest ERβ is necessary to achieve maximal reproductive performance, but is not required for successful reproduction.

The impact of the loss of ERα is further seen in the adult uterus by the lack of response to exogenous estradiol exposure in the αERKO. The acute treatment of ovariectomized mice with estrogen has long served as a key experimental model

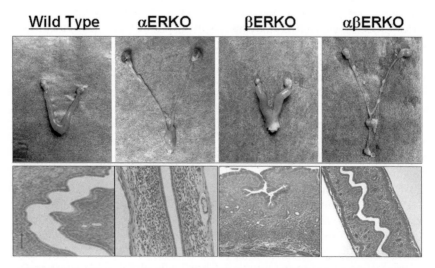

FIGURE 2. Uterine morphology of ERKO mice. Reproductive tracts from wild-type, αERKO, βERKO, and αβERKO mice are shown on the top row. Below, photomicrographs depict the histology of uteri from the wild-type and knockout models.[18,23,39]

in which to study the biochemical mechanisms underlying uterine responses to estradiol. These responses have been described as biphasic as they may be divided into events occurring immediately following estrogen elevation and subsequent responses that follow up to 24 h later.[14] Early events include nuclear ER occupancy, transcription of early phase genes such as *c-fos*, fluid uptake (termed water imbibtion), hyperemia, and infiltration of immune system cells such as macrophages and eosinophils into the uterine tissue.[15,16] Late-phase responses include the transcription of late-phase genes such as *lactoferrin*, increase in uterine wet weight, further accumulation of immune system cells, the development of the epithelial layer into columnar secretory epithelial cells, and subsequent mitosis, which occurs principally in the epithelial layer.[17] In addition, increases in uterine weight after treating ovariectomized mice for 3 days has been used as a bioassay for estrogen sensitivity. Neither of these treatments elicits a response in the αERKO female, and the response in βERKO mice is comparable to that of wild type supporting a role for ERα (FIG. 3).[18]

ERs IN THE OVARIES

The ovary has two major physiological endocrine activities, steroidogenesis and folliculogenesis, and is comprised of many developing follicles that contain oocytes at different stages of maturity embedded in a stromal/interstitial tissue.[19] Layers of granulosa cells that are rich in ERβ surround the oocyte and are the primary location of estrogen biosynthesis. In contrast, the thecal and interstitial cells exclusively express ERα and synthesize androgen and androgen precursors.[10] This compartmentalization of expression has made the ERKO models invaluable in studying specific aspects of the roles of ERs in the ovary and ovulation. In addition, the classical hormone replacement studies to activate ER-mediated responses are not effective for studying the roles of ER in the ovary because it is the source of the hormone of study. Therefore, the ERKO models are a genetic approach to dissecting the roles of the individual receptors in ovarian function.

Adult female mice undergo an estrous cycle every 4–5 days, under the control of the hypothalamic-pituitary-gonadal (HPG) axis. Pulses of gonadotropin-releasing hormone (GnRH) from the hypothalamus regulate the release of the gonadotropins, luteinizing hormone (LH), and follicle-stimulating hormone (FSH), from the pituitary gonadotroph cells. The gondatropins then act on the ovary to direct the maturation of the follicles, which produce estradiol and progesterone prior to and following ovulation, respectively.[20] Estradiol produced by the ovary in response to the gonadotropin signals is also an essential regulator of the HPG axis through ERα. One such action of estradiol suppresses the production of LH in the pituitary. Chronically elevated LH levels in the αERKO suggest a critical role for ERα in this process.[10] These females fail to ovulate and develop cystic and hemorrhagic follicles that eventually become

(A)

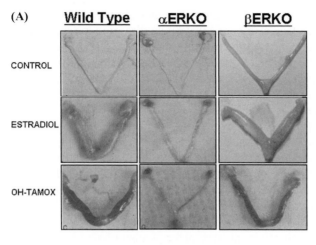

(B)

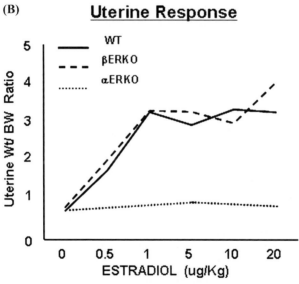

FIGURE 3. (**A**) Uterine response to estradiol esposure. Whole mounts of uteri from wild-type, αERKO, and βERKO mice treated with propylene glycol vehicle, estradiol, or tamoxifen daily for three days are pictured.[18] (**B**) Changes in uterine wet weight in response to estradiol treatment. Changes in uterine wet weight are graphed as a ratio of uterine weight to body weight (y-axis) as compared to increasing doses of estradiol (x-axis) ranging from 0 μg/kg to 20 μg/kg in wild-type, αERKO, and βERKO females.[18]

atretic most likely due to the chronic elevation of circulating LH levels and the lack of an LH surge. Normal preantral and small antral follicles are present, and prepubertal αERKO females are able to respond to exogenous gonadotropins prior to the persistent LH stimulation indicating a normal response to LH and FSH, which was also confirmed by studies of cultured follicles.[12,21] In addition, treatment of prepubertal females with the GnRH antagonist, antide, prevents the rise in LH and the consequent formation of cysts (FIGS. 4A and 4B),[22] thus confirming the cysts are a result of elevated LH due to an absence of ERα, not in the ovary, but rather in the neuroendocrine axis affecting the negative feedback mechanism.

The βERKO females exhibit a less severe phenotype resulting in impaired fertility. A reduction in litter size was consistent in the ERβ-null females; however, the number of litters varied from total infertility to the expected number within a 4-month period.[23] Given the high level of ERβ expression in the granulosa cells of the developing follicle, it is not surprising that the underlying cause of this subfertility is an infrequent and inefficient ovulatory response. While all stages of folliculogenesis can be observed in the βERKO ovary, there is a slight increase in the number of atretic follicles and very few corpora lutea present.[12,23] In fact, there are rarely more than two corpora lutea present per ovary as compared to seven in wild-type females (FIG. 5).[24] The number of oocytes recovered following superovulation of immature βERKO females is significantly reduced as compared to wild-type counterparts (FIGS. 5 and 6).[12,23] Previous studies indicate estradiol acts synergistically with FSH in the differentiation and maturation of follicles.[23,25–31] Two hallmarks of normal granulosa cell differentiation include increases in expression of Cyp19 expression and aromatase activity and acquisition of Lhcgr expression and LH responsiveness.[26–31] These differentiated functions were reduced in the βERKO follicles indicating a deficiency in the response to FSH.[32] In addition, expansion of the cumulus-oocyte complex was reduced in βERKO females as compared to wild-type counterparts following treatment with exogenous gonadotropins.

In superovulation protocols, human chorionic gonadotropin (hCG) is used to simulate the LH surge required for ovulation. Induction of Ptgs2 and Pgr expression, coding for cyclooxygenase-2 and progesterone receptor, respectively, in the granulosa cells by hCG is required for this response.[33,34] Expression of these genes is not sufficiently increased in the βERKO follicles.[32] Administration of an ovulatory dose of hCG also elicits a remarkable decrease in the expression of Cyp19 resulting in a decline in plasma estradiol levels.[35–37] In βERKO mice, Cyp19 expression was increased following treatment with hCG possibly due to the lack of induction of Ptgs2 expression.[32] This resulted in a significant rise in circulating estradiol levels that is uncharacteristic of this point in the estrous cycle when progesterone should be the predominate steroid.[32] The reduced level of LH receptor in the granulosa cells of βERKO females is apparently insufficient to elicit the appropriate response to ovulatory levels of hCG. The resulting increase in Cyp19 gene expression and subsequent elevation of circulating estradiol more closely resembles that seen

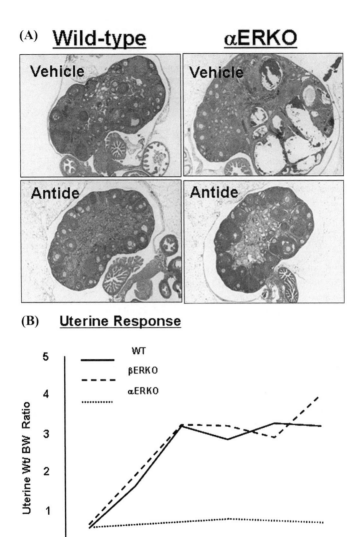

FIGURE 4. (**A**) Prevention of the αERKO ovarian phenotype. Wild-type and αERKO females were treated from age 28 days to 53 days with a GnRH antagonist, antide, or vehicle control every 48 h. Photomicrographs picture cross-sections from the ovaries collected at 53 days of age.[22] (**B**) Prevention of the rise in circulating LH levels in the αERKO. Shown is the average LH (ng/mL) ($\pm$ SEM) for wild-type and αERKO females at 53 days of age following treatment every 48 h with the indicated dose of antide for 24 days. ***$P < 0.001$ when genotypes are compared within the same treatment group.[22]

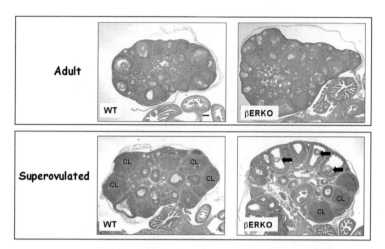

FIGURE 5. Phenotype of βERKO ovary and response to superovulation protocol. Histology of adult wild-type and βERKO ovaries are pictured at the top. Below are cross-sections of ovaries from immature wild-type and βERKO females following superovulation. Arrows indicate unruptured preovulatory follicles in the superovulated βERKO ovary. CL = corpus luteum.[23]

after FSH treatment. The cause of this aberrant expression in βERKO follicles is unclear at this time. These data suggest ERβ is required for proper granulosa cell differentiation and subsequent responses to FSH and LH required for ovulation. In the βERKO females, the end result is impaired ovulation leading to a decrease in fertility, persistent estrous, and a paucity of corpora lutea in the ovary.[12]

Mice in which both ERα and ERβ are absent display a phenotype similar to that observed in the αERKO in that these females are infertile and do not spontaneously ovulate.[23,38,39] While follicles of every developmental stage are present in the αβERKO ovary, the preovulatory follicles display an underdeveloped antrum, reduced granulosa cell number, and a thin, poorly structured thecal layer (FIG. 7).[38,39] The general lack of hemorrhagic and cystic follicles indicated a role for ERβ in the development of this pathology in the αERKO females.[38,39] Subsequent studies using a cross of LH transgenic and βERKO mice showed no cystic development in LH transgenic mice that lacked ERβ.[40] A unique and remarkable feature of the αβERKO ovary is the presence of follicular structures that contain Sertoli-like cells.[38,39] These structures also possess an intact basal lamina, some granulosa cells, and a degenerating oocyte.[39] Interestingly, formation of the structures occurs postpubertally as they are not present in the ovaries of 10-day-old αβERKO females.[39] It is unknown if the Sertoli-like cells originate from precursor cells within the follicle or are the result of granulosa cell transdifferentiation. They express many testis specific factors including *Sox9*.[39] SOX9 is a transcription factor that is critical to normal Sertoli cell differentiation during testis development.[41,42] Expression of

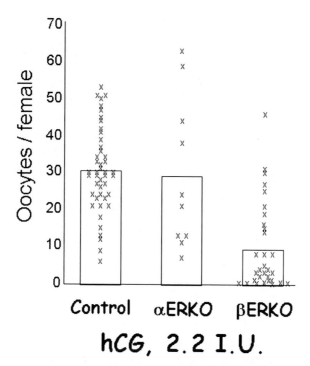

FIGURE 6. Oocyte yield following induced ovulation in immature ERKO mice. Results after treatment with doses of gonadotropin optimum for induced ovulation. Each dot represents the oocyte yield of an individual animal within their respective genotype; vertical bars represent the average oocyte yield within each group.[32]

the *Sox9* gene in the αβERKO ovary is restricted to the atretic follicles and precedes the appearance of Sertoli-like cells.[43] Other testis specific factors expressed in the αβERKO ovary include Müllerian-inhibiting substance (MIS) and sulfated glycoprotein-2.[12] Similar phenotypes are reported in other mouse models including fetal ovaries transplanted to adult hosts,[44,45] *in vitro* exposure of fetal rat, rabbit, or ovine ovaries to purified MIS,[46] overexpression of MIS,[47] overexpression of *Sox9*, or targeted disruption of *Wnt4*;[48] however, the αβERKO female is the first description of this sex reversal occurring in adult tissues. The gonadotropin profile of αβERKO females is similar to that observed in the αERKO with even greater elevations of plasma LH levels.[49] Notably, the increase in ovarian aromatase and estradiol synthesis is not present in the αβERKO females.[49] This finding further supports the hypothesis that elevated LH levels increases substrates for estradiol synthesis, which is enhanced by the actions of ERβ in the αERKO but is disrupted in the αβERKO. In addition, the degeneration of αβERKO germ cells may also impact this system as oocyte-derived factors have been shown to positively influence steroidogenesis.[50]

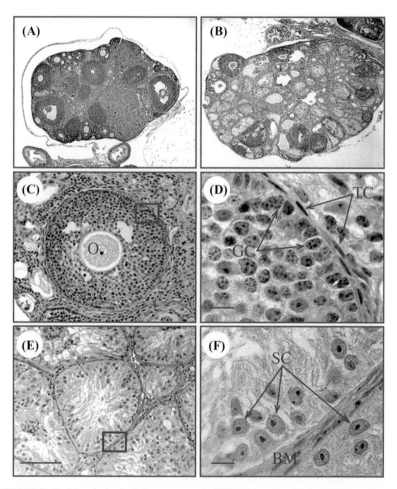

FIGURE 7. Morphological phenotypes of αβERKO ovaries. Representative photomicrographs of cross-sections from αβERKO ovaries (**A** and **B**). Higher magnification (C X66, D X330) of a healthy follicle which contains a single oocyte (O), several layers of granulosa cells (GC), and an intact basal lamina and thecum (TC). The sex-reversed follicle (E X66, FX330) shows that the oocyte has degenerated and the somatic cells have undergone redifferentiation to a sertoli cell (SC) phenotype. The basal membrane (BM) remains intact as it would to provide structure to the cords of the testis. Scale bars in (**C**) and (**E**) equal 100 μm, and in (**D**) and (**F**) 10 μm.[39]

SUMMARY

In this article, a review of data collected regarding the functions of the ER isoforms from genetically engineered mice has been presented. The knowledge gained from these knockout models elucidates many aspects of the roles of the specific ER receptors in reproduction. Specifically, ERα is the primary ER regulating negative feedback of trophic hormones and uterotropic response, and actions of ERβ are crucial for proper differentiation and function of granulosa cells in follicles. It also has been noted how perturbing homeostasis reveals mechanisms of many components both directly related to ER function and other components important to maximal fertility. With more knowledge, more questions arise. Advancements in techniques and technologies hold much promise for furthering our understanding of this critical biological system and the development of therapeutic agents.

REFERENCES

1. MANGELSDORF, D.J. et al. 1995. The nuclear receptor superfamily: the second decade. Cell **83**: 835–839.
2. KUSHNER, P.J. et al. 2000. Estrogen receptor pathways to AP-1. J. Steroid Biochem. Mol. Biol. **74**: 311–317.
3. SAFE, S. 2001. Transcriptional activation of genes by 17 beta-estradiol through estrogen receptor-Sp1 interactions. Vitam. Horm. **62**: 231–252.
4. JAKACKA, M. et al. 2001. Estrogen receptor binding to DNA is not required for its activity through the nonclassical AP1 pathway. J. Biol. Chem. **276**: 13615–13621.
5. COLEMAN, K.M. & C.L. SMITH. 2001. Intracellular signaling pathways: nongenomic actions of estrogens and ligand-independent activation of estrogen receptors. Front. Biosci. **6**: D1379–D1391.
6. CATO, A.C. et al. 2002. Rapid actions of steroid receptors in cellular signaling pathways. Sci. STKE **138**: RE9.
7. SMITH, C.L. & B.W. O'MALLEY. 2004. Coregulator function: a key to understanding tissue specificity of selective receptor modulators. Endocr. Rev. **25**: 45–71.
8. GLASS, C.K. & M.G. ROSENFELD. 2000. The coregulator exchange in transcriptional functions of nuclear receptors. Genes Dev. **14**: 121–141.
9. HERMANSON, O. et al. 2002. Nuclear receptor coregulators: multiple modes of modification. Trends Endocrinol. Metab. **13**: 55–60.
10. COUSE, J.F. & K.S. KORACH. 1999. Estrogen receptor null mice: what have we learned and where will they lead us? Endocr. Rev. **20**: 358–417.
11. HEWITT, S.C. et al. 2005. Lessons in estrogen biology from knockout and transgenic animals. Annu. Rev. Physiol. **67**: 285–308.
12. COUSE, J.F. et al. 2006. Steroid receptors in the ovary and uterus. In The Physiology of Reproduction. J.D. Neill, Ed.: 593–678. Raven. New York, NY.
13. HEWITT, S.C. et al. 2003. Estrogen receptor-dependent genomic responses in the uterus mirror the biphasic physiological response to estrogen. Mol. Endocrinol. **17**: 2070–2083.
14. KATZENELLENBOGEN, B.S. et al. 1979. Estrogen and antiestrogen action in reproductive tissues and tumors. Recent Prog. Horm. Res. **35**: 259–300.
15. PEREZ, M.C. et al. 1996. Role of eosinophils in uterine responses to estrogen. Biol. Reprod. **54**: 249–254.
16. GRIFFITH, J.S. et al. 1997. Evidence for the genetic control of estradiol-regulated responses. Implications for variation in normal and pathological hormone-dependent phenotypes. Am. J. Pathol. **150**: 2223–2230.

17. POLLARD, J.W. *et al.* 1987. Estrogens and cell death in murine uterine luminal epithelium. Cell Tissue Res. **249:** 533–540.
18. LUBAHN, D.B. *et al.* 1993. Alteration of reproductive function but not prenatal sexual development after insertional disruption of the mouse estrogen receptor gene. Proc. Natl. Acad. Sci. USA **90:** 11162–11166.
19. GREENWALD, G.S. & S.K. ROY. 1994. Follicular development and control. *In* The Physiology of Reproduction. E. Knobil & J.D. Neill, Eds.: 629–724. Raven. New York, NY.
20. GHARIB, S.D. *et al.* 1990. Molecular biology of the pituitary gonadotropins. Endocr. Rev. **11:** 177–199.
21. EMMEN, J.M. *et al.* 2005. In vitro growth and ovulation of follicles from ovaries of estrogen receptor (ER){alpha} and ER{beta} null mice indicate a role for ER{beta} in follicular maturation. Endocrinology **146:** 2817–2826.
22. COUSE, J.F. *et al.* 1999. Prevention of the polycystic ovarian phenotype and characterization of ovulatory capacity in the estrogen receptor-alpha knockout mouse. Endocrinology **140:** 5855–5865.
23. KREGE, J.H. *et al.* 1998. Generation and reproductive phenotypes of mice lacking estrogen receptor beta. Proc.N. Y. Acad. Sci. USA **95:** 15677–15682.
24. CHENG, G. *et al.* 2002. A role for the androgen receptor in follicular atresia of estrogen receptor beta knockout mouse ovary. Biol. Reprod. **66:** 77–84.
25. GOLDENBERG, R.L. *et al.* 1972. Estrogen and follicle stimulation hormone interactions on follicle growth in rats. Endocrinology **90:** 1492–1498.
26. FITZPATRICK, S.L. & J.S. RICHARDS. 1991. Regulation of cytochrome P450 aromatase messenger ribonucleic acid and activity by steroids and gonadotropins in rat granulosa cells. Endocrinology **129:** 1452–1462.
27. ZHUANG, L.Z. *et al.* 1982. Direct enhancement of gonadotropin-stimulated ovarian estrogen biosynthesis by estrogen and clomiphene citrate. Endocrinology **110:** 2219–2221.
28. ADASHI, E.Y. & A.J. HSUEH. 1982. Estrogens augment the stimulation of ovarian aromatase activity by follicle-stimulating hormone in cultured rat granulosa cells. J. Biol. Chem. **257:** 6077–6083.
29. KNECHT, M. *et al.* 1984. Estrogens enhance the adenosine $3',5'$-monophosphate-mediated induction of follicle-stimulating hormone and luteinizing hormone receptors in rat granulosa cells. Endocrinology **115:** 41–49.
30. KNECHT, M. *et al.* 1985. Aromatase inhibitors prevent granulosa cell differentiation: an obligatory role for estrogens in luteinizing hormone receptor expression. Endocrinology **117:** 1156–1161.
31. KNECHT, M. *et al.* 1985. Estrogen dependence of luteinizing hormone receptor expression in cultured rat granulosa cells. Inhibition of granulosa cell development by the antiestrogens tamoxifen and keoxifene. Endocrinology **116:** 1771–1777.
32. COUSE, J.F. *et al.* 2005. Estrogen receptor-beta is critical to granulosa cell differentiation and the ovulatory response to gonadotropins. Endocrinology **146:** 3247–3262.
33. DAVIS, B.J. *et al.* 1999. Anovulation in cyclooxygenase-2-deficient mice is restored by prostaglandin E2 and interleukin-1beta. Endocrinology **140:** 2685–2695.
34. STERNECK, E. *et al.* 1997. An essential role for C/EBPbeta in female reproduction. Genes. Dev. **11:** 2153–2162.
35. FITZPATRICK, S.L. *et al.* 1997. Expression of aromatase in the ovary: down-regulation of mRNA by the ovulatory luteinizing hormone surge. Steroids **62:** 197–206.

36. HICKEY, G.J. *et al*. 1988. Hormonal regulation, tissue distribution, and content of aromatase cytochrome P450 messenger ribonucleic acid and enzyme in rat ovarian follicles and corpora lutea: relationship to estradiol biosynthesis. Endocrinology **122:** 1426–1436.

37. HICKEY, G.J. *et al*. 1990. Aromatase cytochrome P450 in rat ovarian granulosa cells before and after luteinization: adenosine $3',5'$-monophosphate-dependent and independent regulation. Cloning and sequencing of rat aromatase cDNA and $5'$ genomic DNA. Mol. Endocrinol. **4:** 3–12.

38. DUPONT, S. *et al*. 2000. Effect of single and compound knockouts of estrogen receptors alpha (ERalpha) and beta (ERbeta) on mouse reproductive phenotypes. Development **127:** 4277–4291.

39. COUSE, J.F. *et al*. 1999. Postnatal sex reversal of the ovaries in mice lacking estrogen receptors alpha and beta. Science **286:** 2328–2331.

40. COUSE, J.F. *et al*. 2004. Formation of cystic ovarian follicles associated with elevated luteinizing hormone requires estrogen receptor-beta. Endocrinology **145:** 4693–4702.

41. MORAIS DA SILVA, S. *et al*. 1996. Sox9 expression during gonadal development implies a conserved role for the gene in testis differentiation in mammals and birds. Nat. Genet. **14:** 62–68.

42. KANAI, Y. & P. KOOPMAN. 1999. Structural and functional characterization of the mouse Sox9 promoter: implications for campomelic dysplasia. Hum. Mol. Genet. **8:** 691–696.

43. DUPONT, S. *et al*. 2003. Expression of Sox9 in granulosa cells lacking the estrogen receptors, ERalpha and ERbeta. Dev. Dyn. **226:** 103–106.

44. TAKETO-HOSOTANI, T. 1987. Factors involved in the testicular development from fetal mouse ovaries following transplantation. J. Exp. Zool. **241:** 95–100.

45. WHITWORTH, D.J. *et al*. 1996. Gonadal sex reversal of the developing marsupial ovary in vivo and in vitro. Development **122:** 4057–4063.

46. VIGIER, B. *et al*. 1989. Anti-Mullerian hormone produces endocrine sex reversal of fetal ovaries. Proc. Natl. Acad. Sci. USA **86:** 3684–3688.

47. BEHRINGER, R.R. *et al*. 1990. Abnormal sexual development in transgenic mice chronically expressing mullerian-inhibiting substance. Nature **345:** 167–170.

48. VAINIO, S. *et al*. 1999. Female development in mammals is regulated by Wnt-4 signalling. Nature **397:** 405–409.

49. COUSE, J.F. *et al*. 2003. Characterization of the hypothalamic-pituitary-gonadal axis in estrogen receptor (ER) null mice reveals hypergonadism and endocrine sex reversal in females lacking ERalpha but not ERbeta. Mol. Endocrinol. **17:** 1039–1053.

50. MAGOFFIN, D.A. 2002. The ovarian androgen-producing cells: a 2001 perspective. Rev. Endocr. Metab. Disord. **3:** 47–53.

The Cardiovascular Effects of Selective Estrogen Receptor Modulators

G.E. CHRISTODOULAKOS, I.V. LAMBRINOUDAKI, AND D.C. BOTSIS

Second Department of Obstetrics and Gynecology, Aretaieion Hospital, University of Athens, Athens, Greece

ABSTRACT: Coronary artery disease (CAD) is the main contributor of mortality among postmenopausal women. Menopause-associated estrogen deficiency has both metabolic and vascular consequences that increase the risk for CAD. Hormone therapy (HT) has been reported to have a beneficial effect on metabolic and vascular factors influencing the incidence of CAD. Although observational studies have reported that HT reduces significantly the risk for CAD, randomized clinical trials (WHI, HERS, ERA) have questioned the efficacy of HT in primary and secondary CAD prevention despite confirming the lipid-lowering effect of HT. In the aftermath of the WHI, increased interest has been given to the action of selective estrogen receptor modulators (SERMs) and their effect on the cardiovascular system. The chemical structure of SERMs, either triphenylethilyn (tamoxifen) or benzothiophene (raloxifene) derivatives, differs from that of estrogens. SERMs are nonsteroidal molecules that bind, with high affinity, to the ER. SERMs induce conformational changes to the ligand-binding domain of the ER that modulate the ability of the ER to interact with coregulator proteins. The relative balance of coregulators within a cell determines the transcriptional activity of the receptor–ligand complex. SERMs therefore may express an estrogen-agonist or estrogen-antagonist effect depending on the tissue targeted. SERMs express variable effects on the metabolic and vascular factors influencing the incidence of CAD. SERMs have been reported to modulate favorably the lipid–lipoprotein profile. Toremifene expresses the most beneficial effect followed by tamoxifene and raloxifene, while ospexifene and HMR-3339 have the least effect and may even increase triglycerides. Raloxifene and tamoxifene decrease serum homocysteine levels and C-reactive proteins (CRP), which are both markers of CAD risk. Raloxifene has been reported to increase the nitric oxide (NO)–endothelin (ET)-1 ratio and, thus, contribute to proper endothelial function and vasodilation. Toremifene has no effect on the NO–ET-1 ratio. Finally, raloxifene decreases the vascular cell adhesion molecules and the inflammatory cytokines TNF-α and IL-6. Of the SERMs, raloxifene has had the most extensive evaluation regarding the effect on the vascular wall of endothelium. Although not confirmed by large clinical trials, raloxifene

Address for correspondence: Irene Lambrinoudaki, 27, Themistokleous St., Dionysos, GR-14578, Athens, Greece. Voice and fax: 0030-210-6410325.
    e-mail: ilambrinoudaki@hotmail.com

Ann. N.Y. Acad. Sci. 1092: 374–384 (2006). © 2006 New York Academy of Sciences.
doi: 10.1196/annals.1365.034

has been reported to have an effect on the cohesion of the intercellular junction (VE-cadherin) and the synthesis—degradation of extracellular matrix (MMP-2). The Multiple Outcomes Raloxifene Evaluation (MORE) study has reported that raloxifene may have a cardioprotective effect when administered to postmenopausal women at high risk for CAD disease.

KEYWORDS: coronary artery disease (CAD); hormone therapy (HT); raloxifene; selective estrogen receptor modulators (SERMs); tamoxifen

INTRODUCTION

Postmenopausal estrogen deficiency has both metabolic and vascular consequences that increase the risk for cardiovascular disease (CVD). CVD is the main contributor of mortality among postmenopausal women.[1-3] Although hormone therapy (HT) has been reported to have a beneficial effect on the metabolic and vascular factors, which define the incidence of CVD, and although observational studies[3,4] have reported that HT significantly reduces CVD risk, randomized clinical trials (RCTs) evaluating the effect of HT in primary (WHI)[5] and secondary (HERS)[6] CVD prevention have questioned the efficacy of HT despite confirming the lipid-lowering effect of estrogens. Furthermore, the WHI trial confirmed that prolonged (> 4 years) exposure to HT increased significantly the risk for breast cancer.

In the aftermath of WHI, research and clinical interest have shifted to different estrogen–progestin regimens of lower dose and administered via different routes and to alternative therapies. Selective estrogen receptor modulators (SERMs) may be alternatives to HT and in particular for the asymptomatic osteopenic–osteoporotic postmenopausal women in need of prolonged therapy.

SERMs differ in their chemical structure. Both benzothiophene and triphenylethylene derivatives are nonsteroidal ligands, which bind with high affinity to the ER.[7] The pharmacological action of SERMs depends on:

a. The concentration of ER and the ratio of Era–ERb on the target cell.
b. The conformational changes induced by the SERM on the ligand-binding domains of the receptor and the ability of the receptor to interact with coregulator proteins either co-activators or co-repressors.
c. The relative balance of co-activators–co-repressors, which modulates the transcriptional activity of the receptor–ligand complex.
d. The cellular signaling that influences the activity of coregulatory proteins.

The above mechanisms play a key role in determining the estrogen (E) agonist versus antagonist activity of the SERM depending on the cell targeted.[8,9] Tamoxifen and raloxifene express an E-agonist, albeit of variable efficacy, effect on bone metabolism. The effect of tamoxifen on bone mineral density (BMD) is minor and transient.[10] Tamoxifen is a potent E-antagonist on breast tissue and is accredited for the prevention of breast cancer.[11] However, its E-agonist action on the endometrium and the resultant increased risk for hyperplasia–cancer do not qualify this molecule as an alternative to HT for prolonged administration.[12] Toremifene is an FDA-approved SERM for the treatment of advanced breast cancer. However, its effect on the endometrium is unknown and it has no effect on postmenopausal bone loss.[8] Raloxifene is the only FDA-approved SERM that prevents bone loss and decreases significantly the risk of vertebral fracture.[13,14] Observational and RCT evidence suggests that raloxifene does not stimulate the endometrium[15–17] and that it may decrease significantly the risk for breast cancer.[18,19]

SERMs have been reported to express a variable but in general E-agonist effect on CV risk factors, such as the lipid profile, homocysteine (Hcy), and factors associated with the vascular wall and endothelium. The cardiovascular effects of SERMs in association with their effect on bone metabolism and breast and endometrium will determine the candidacy of a SERM to function as an alternative to HT.[20–24] The purpose of this presentation is to review the effect of SERMs on the CV system.

Lipids–Lipoproteins

Following menopause the beneficial effect of endogenous estrogens on lipid metabolism is lost[25] and a proatherogenic lipid profile is established, which has been considered to contribute to the postmenopausal increase in CVD risk.[26,27] With the exception of an increase in triglycerides (TG), HT induces beneficial changes on the lipid profile.[28]

Although endothelial and vascular wall factors are now accepted as mainly responsible in defining the incidence of CVD among postmenopausal women, a prominent role is still attributed to lipids–lipoproteins in the genesis of atherosclerosis.[29–31] Toremifene expresses the best action profile on lipids–lipoproteins.[22] However, the significance of this effect is limited because lipid profile modulations may account for only 30% of the total cardiovascular benefit.[29] With the exception of ospemifene,[32,33] tamoxifen,[20] toremifene,[22] raloxifene,[21] droloxifene,[34] and the SERM HMR3339[35] decreased low-density lipoprotein (LDL)-C. Toremifene is the only SERM that increases high-density lipoprotein (HDL)-C[22] while the other SERMs have no effect. Raloxifene, however, increases the HDL2-C subfraction considered as mainly responsible for atheroprotection.[21] Of particular importance is the effect of SERMs on TG. TG have acquired prominence among lipid profile parameters and their levels are now considered as playing a key role in cardiovascular risk particularly among postmenopausal women and particularly when associated with HDL-C < 40 mg/dL.[36–38] TGs are regulators of lipoprotein interactions, are associated with the diameter and density of LDL particles and, in essence, reflect the presence of the highly atherogenic VLDL and sdLDL.[39–41] Both toremifene[22] and raloxifene[21] show a trend to decrease TG, while ospemifene[32,33] and HMR3339[35] may even increase them.

Homocysteine (Hcy)

Homocysteine (Hcy) is a sulfur-containing amino acid, which is an independent risk factor for vascular damage. Complex mechanisms account for the association of even moderate hyperhomocysteinemia to atherosclerosis and the resultant increase in cardio-cerebro-peripheral vascular disease and recurrent arterial–venous thrombosis.[42] Hyperhomocysteinemia results in excess H_2O_2 that promotes the conversion of nitric oxide (NO) to peroxynitrate (ONOO-). Consumption of NO leads to endothelial dysfunction, whereas ONOO- is highly toxic to the endothelium.[43,44] Furthermore, hyperhomocysteinemia associates with decreased glutathione concentrations and, hence, decreased free radical scavenging.[45]

Sex steroids have been reported to modulate Hcy metabolism and decrease Hcy levels.[46] The ability of certain SERMs to express an E-agonist effect and decrease Hcy levels may represent a mechanism of cardioprotection. Tamoxifen[47] and HMR3339[35] decrease Hcy levels. Observational[48] and RCTs[23–49] have reported that raloxifene decreased significantly Hcy. In fact, the effect of raloxifene may be greater compared to that of estrogen and estrogen–progestin regimens.[48]

Nitric Oxide (NO)

Nitric oxide (NO) and endothelin-1 (ET-1) are vasoactive factors expressing a vasodilatory and vasoconstrictive effect, respectively. NO and ET-1 interact and their ratio determines vessel patency. NO exhibits antiatherogenic action via such mechanisms as vasodilation, blood flow modulation in coronary and peripheral vessels, inhibition of LDL-C oxidation, and leukocyte adhesion to the vessel wall. In contrast, ET-1 causes potent vasoconstriction and promotes leukocyte adhesion and smooth muscle cell proliferation.[50–52] NO synthesis is dependent on endothelium NO synthase formation and is regulated by an ER-mediated mechanism.[53] Of the SERMs, although tamoxifen and toremifene did not influence serum NO levels significantly, the NO–ET-1 ratio increased.[54] Raloxifene enhanced the release of NO in the rat aorta[55] and triggered a rapid dose-dependent release of NO from cultured endothelial cells.[53] *In vivo*, raloxifene augmented NO-induced coronary artery dilatation.[56] In postmenopausal women droloxifene has been reported to increase endothelium-dependent vasodilation[34] while raloxifene increases NO and decreases ET-1 levels.[57] This effect of raloxifene and droloxifene may represent a cardioprotective mechanism.

Vascular Cell Adhesion Molecules (VCAMs)

Following activation endothelial cells increase the expression of VCAMs, such as VCAM-1, intercellular adhesion molecule-1 (ICAM-1), and E-selectin.[58] VCAMs mediate adherence at the site of injury of monocytes and T-lymphocytes, which in turn migrate across the endothelium and aggregate in the subendothelial space. Within the intima monocytes differentiate into macrophages, which ingest lipids to become foam cells and initiate the fatty streak.[59,60]

Raloxifene, in contrast to tamoxifen, has been reported to decrease the expression of VCAM-1[61] as well as ICAM-1 and E-selectin.[62] Droloxifene is associated with a significant reduction in E-selectin but also with an unwanted increase in VCAM-1 and has no effect on ICAM-1.[63] The beneficial modulation of adhesion molecules following raloxifene administration may indicate a possible cardioprotective profile.

C-Reactive Protein (CRP) and Interleukin-6 (IL-6)

Inflammation is considered as playing a key role in the genesis and progression of atherosclerosis. The significant increase in C-Reactive Protein (CRP), a global inflammatory marker, reported in the WHI trial was initially implicated as the cause of the early increase in cardiac events.[58] Interleukin-6 (IL-6) is an inflammatory cytokine influencing CRP expression activation.[64] The involvement of CRP in cardiovascular risk is still unresolved. HT-induced elevation of CRP is seen following oral but not transdermal administration of therapy.[65] It is still unknown whether CRP increase is the result of overexpression of proinflammatory cytokines or of increased hepatic synthesis.[64] The effect of droloxifene and raloxifene on CRP and IL-6 differs from that of HT. Droloxifene is associated with a nonsignificant increase in IL-6 and had no effect on CRP.[63] Raloxifene is reported to leave both CRP and IL-6 unchanged and to decrease or have no effect on IL-6 expression.[66]

Venous Thromboembolic Events (VTE)

Treatment with SERMs upsets hemostatic balance and enhances blood clotting. Raloxifene, droloxifene, toremifene, and tamoxifen associate with an increased (twofold) VTE risk similar to that of HT.[13,14,75]

Further Effects of Raloxifene

Raloxifene is a benzothiophene derivative, which expresses an E-antagonist effect on the breast and endometrium.[67] The Multiple Outcomes Raloxifene

Evaluation (MORE)[19] and Continuing Outcomes Raloxifene Evaluation (CORE)[18] trials have reported that raloxifene decreases significantly the risk for breast cancer whereas in a recent 5-year follow-up study[17] raloxifene is associated with the least effect on endometrial thickness and unscheduled vaginal bleeding compared to HT and tibolone. These properties allow the administration of raloxifene for the prolonged period required to exert an osteoprotective effect.[14,15,67] It is probably for these reasons that raloxifene has been most consistently evaluated among postmenopausal women for its effect on CV risk factors. The MORE trial has investigated cerebrovascular and coronary events as a secondary end point and has reported that raloxifene does not increase early cardiac events and, in a subset of high-risk women, decreases significantly both cerebrovascular and coronary events.[19] Although the effect of raloxifene on the vessel wall and endothelium is still not fully established by RCTs,[68] recent studies have further suggested that it may have a role in preventing/delaying the initiation/progression of atherosclerosis.

Matrix Metalloproteinases (MMPs)

Matrix metalloproteinases (MMPs) are Zn- and Ca-dependent endopeptidases that control vascular extracellular matrix metabolism and homeostasis with their tissue-specific inhibitors[24,69] via regulated deposition–degradation of its components. MMPs influence the progression of atherosclerosis and plaque stability.[25,70] In healthy postmenopausal women raloxifene significantly increased serum total MMP-2 as well as its active fraction.[71] Administered when the lesion is at an early stage raloxifene may retard its progression.

Vascular Endothelial Cadherin (VE-cad)

Human vascular endothelial cadherin (VE-cad) is an endothelium-specific Ca-dependent transmembrane glycoprotein responsible for the organization and maintenance of interendothelial junctions. VE-cad interacts with cytoskeleton proteins known as catenins to provide cohesion to the endothelial cell–cell junction. As a result VE-cad influences endothelial permeability. Cleavage of the cadherin–catenin complex and shedding of VE-cad increases its serum levels. Increased VE-cad may represent loss of junction integrity and may promote transendothelial migration of immunoinflammatory elements and lipids resulting in plaque progression.[72,73] Raloxifene has been reported to decrease significantly soluble VE-cad in healthy postmenopausal women.[74] Although it is unknown whether the decrease represents a direct effect of raloxifene in inhibiting cleavage of the cadherin–catenin complex, it may nevertheless suggest a mechanism influencing the progression of atherosclerosis.

CONCLUSIONS

SERMs express variable effects on the metabolic and vascular factors that influence cardiovascular disease risk. There is as yet no RCT that has investigated the impact of SERMs on cardiovascular events as a primary end point. The Raloxifene Use in The Heart (RUTH) trial has concluded the investigation of the effect of raloxifene on coronary events among high-risk postmenopausal women as a primary end point but the results have not yet been presented.

REFERENCES

1. STAMPFER, M.J., G.A. COLDITZ & W.C. WILETT. 1990. Menopause and heart disease. Ann. N.Y. Acad. Sci. **592:** 193–203.
2. HU, F.B. & F. GRODSTEIN. 2002. Postmenopausal hormone therapy and the risk of cardiovascular disease: the epidemiologic evidence. Am. J. Cardiol. **90:** 26F–29F.
3. BARRETT-CONNOR, E. & D. GRADY. 1998. Hormone replacement therapy, heart disease and other considerations. Annu. Rev. Public Health **19:** 55–72.
4. GRODSTEIN, F., M.J. STAMPFER, J.E. MANSON, et al. 1996. Postmenopausal estrogen and progestin use and the risk of cardiovascular disease. N. Engl. J. Med. **335:** 453–461.
5. THE WRITING GROUP FOR THE WOMEN'S HEALTH INITIATIVE INVESTIGATORS. 2002. Risks and benefits of estrogen plus progestin in healthy postmenopausal women. JAMA **288:** 321–333.
6. HULLEY, S., D. GRADY, T. BUSH, et al. FOR THE HERS RESEARCH GROUP. 1998. Randomized trial of estrogen plus progestin for secondary prevention of coronary heart disease in postmenopausal women: Heart and Estrogen/Progestin Replacement Study (HERS) Research Group. JAMA **280:** 605–613.
7. BURGER, H.G. 2000. Selective estrogen receptor modulators. Horm. Res. **53:** 25–29.
8. RIGGS, B.L. & C.L. HARTMANN. 2003. Selective estrogen receptor modulators—mechanisms of action and application to clinical practice. N. Engl. J. Med. **348:** 618–629.
9. SMITH, C.L. & B.W. O'MALLEY. 2004. Co-regulator function: a key to understanding tissue specificity of selective receptor modulators. Endocr. Rev. **25:** 45–71.
10. LOVE, R.R., H.S. BARDEN, R.B. MAZESS, et al. 1994. Effect of tamoxifen on lumbar spine bone mineral density in postmenopausal women after 5 years. Arch. Intern. Med. **154:** 2585–2588.
11. EARLY BREAST CANCER TRIALISTS' COLLABORATIVE GROUP. 1998. Tamoxifen for early breast cancer: an overview of the randomized trials. Lancet **351:** 1451–1467.
12. GARUTI, G., F. CELLANI, G. CENTINAIO, et al. 2006. Histopathologic behavior of endometrial hyperplasia during tamoxifen therapy for breast cancer. Gynecol. Oncol. **101**(2): 269–273.
13. DELMAS, P.D., K.E. ENSRUD, J.D. ADASHI, et al. 2002. Efficacy of raloxifene on vertebral fracture risk reduction in postmenopausal women with osteoporosis: 4-year results from a randomized clinical trial. J. Clin. Endocrinol. Metab. **87:** 3609–3617.

14. ETTINGER, B., D.M. BLACK, B.H. MITLAK, *et al*. 1999. Reduction of vertebral fracture risk in postmenopausal women with osteoporosis treated with raloxifene: results from a 3-year randomized clinical trial. JAMA **282:** 637–645.

15. DELMAS, P.D., N.H. BJARNASON, B.H. MITLAK, *et al*. 1997. Effects of raloxifene on bone mineral density, serum cholesterol concentrations, and uterine endometrium in postmenopausal women. N. Engl. J. Med. **337:** 1641–1647.

16. JOLLY, E.E., N.H. BJARNASON, P. NEVEN, *et al*. 2003. Prevention of osteoporosis and uterine effects in postmenopausal women taking raloxifene for 5 years. Menopause **10:** 337–344.

17. CHRISTODOULAKOS, G.E., D.S. BOTSIS, I.V. LAMBRINOUDAKI, *et al*. 2006. A 5-year study on the effect of hormone therapy, tibolone and raloxifene on vaginal bleeding and endometrial thickness. Maturitas. **53(4):** 413–423.

18. MARTINO, S., J.A. CAULEY, E. BARRETT-CONNOR, *et al*. 2004. Continuing outcomes relevant to Evista: breast cancer incidence in postmenopausal osteoporotic women in a randomized trial of raloxifene. J. Natl. Cancer Instit. **96:** 1751–1761.

19. CAULEY, J.A., L. NORTON, M.E. LIPPMAN, *et al*. 2001. Continued breast cancer risk reduction in postmenopausal women treated with raloxifene: 4-year results from the MORE trial. Breast Cancer Res. Treat. **65:** 125–134.

20. LOVE, R.R., D.A. WIEBE, P.A. NEWCOMB, *et al*. 1991. Effects of tamoxifen on cardiovascular risk factors in postmenopausal women. Ann. Intern. Med. **115:** 860–864.

21. WALSH, B.W., L.H. KULLER, R.A. WILD, *et al*. 1998. Effects of raloxifene on serum lipids and coagulation factors in healthy postmenopausal women. JAMA **279:** 1445–1451.

22. SAARTO, T., C. BLOMQVIST, C. EHNHOLM, *et al*. 1996. Antiatherogenic effects of adjuvant antiestrogens: a randomized trial comparing the effects of tamoxifen and toremifene on plasma lipid levels in postmenopausal women with node-positive breast cancer. J. Clin. Oncol. **14:** 429–433.

23. WALSH, B.W., S. PAUL, R.A. WILD, *et al*. 2000. The effects of hormone replacement therapy and raloxifene on C-reactive protein and homocysteine in healthy postmenopausal women: a randomized, controlled trial. J. Clin. Endocrinol. Metab. **85:** 214–218.

24. CHRISTODOULAKOS, G.E., I.V. LAMBRINOUDAKI, E.V. ECONOMOU, *et al*. 2006. Circulating chemoattractants RANTES, negatively related to endogenous androgens, and MCP-1 are differentially suppressed by hormone therapy and raloxifene. Atherosclerosis. In press.

25. STEVENSON, J.C., D. CROOK & I.F. GODSLAND. 1993. Influence of age and menopause on serum lipids and lipoproteins in healthy women. Atherosclerosis **98:** 83–90.

26. GODSLAND, I.F. 2001. Effects of postmenopausal hormone replacement therapy on lipid, lipoprotein, and apolipoprotein A concentrations: analysis of studies published from 1974–2000. Fertil. Steril. **75:** 898–915.

27. DIAS, A.R., R.N. MELO, O.C.E. GEBARA, *et al*. 2005. Effect of conjugated equine estrogens or raloxifene on lipid profile, coagulation and fibrinolysis factors in postmenopausal women. Climacteric **8:** 63–70.

28. LOBO, R.A. 1990. Cardiovascular implications of estrogen replacement therapy. Obstet. Gynecol. **75:** 18S–25S.

29. NAZR, A. & M. BRECKWOLDT. 1998. Estrogen replacement therapy and cardiovascular protection: lipid mechanisms are the tip of the iceberg. Gynecol. Endocrinol. **12:** 43–59.

30. MENDELSOHN, M.E. & R.H. KARAS. 1999. The protective effects of estrogen on the cardiovascular system. N. Engl. J. Med. **340:** 1801–1811.
31. GODSLAND, I.F. 2004. Biology: risk factor modification by OCs and HRT lipids and lipoproteins. Maturitas **47:** 299–303.
32. KOMI, J., K.S. LANKINEN, P. HARKONEN, et al. 2005. Effects of ospemifene and raloxifene on hormonal status, lipids, genital tract, and tolerability in post-menopausal women. Menopause **12:** 202–209.
33. YLIKORKALA, O., B. CACCIATORE, K. HALONEN, et al. 2003. Effects of ospemifene, a novel SERM, on vascular markers and function in healthy, postmenopausal women. Menopause **10:** 440–447.
34. HERRINGTON, D.M., B.E. PUSSER, W.A. RILEY, et al. 2000. Cardiovascular effects of droloxifene, a new selective estrogen receptor modulator, in healthy postmenopausal women. Arterioscler. Thromb. Vasc. Biol. **20:** 1606–1612.
35. VOGELVANG, T.E., V. MIJATOVIC, P. KENEMANS, et al. 2004. HMR 3339, a novel selective estrogen receptor modulator, reduces total cholesterol, low-density lipoprotein cholesterol, and homocysteine in healthy postmenopausal women. Fertil. Steril. **82:** 1540–1549.
36. DOBIASOVA, M. & J. FROHLICH. 2001. The plasma parameter log (TG/HDL-C) as an atherogenic index: correlation with lipoprotein particle size and esterification rate in ApoB-lipoprotein-depleted plasma (FER_{HDL}). Clin. Biochem. **34:** 583–589.
37. D'AGOSTINO, R.B., M.W. RUSSEL, D.M. HUSE, et al. 2000. Primary and subsequent coronary risk appraisal: new results from the Framingham study. Am. Heart J. **139:** 272–281.
38. KNOPP, R.H., X. ZHU & B. BONET. 1994. Effects of estrogen on lipoprotein metabolism and cardiovascular disease in women. Atherosclerosis **110**(Suppl): S83–S91.
39. TAN, M.H., D. JOHNS & B.N. GLAZER. 2004. Pioglitazone reduces atherogenic index of plasma in patients with type 2 diabetes. Clin. Chem. **50:** 1184–1188.
40. MAAS, A., Y. VAN DER SCHOUW & D. GROBBEE, et al. 2004. "Rise and fall" of hormone therapy in postmenopausal women with cardiovascular disease. Menopause **11:** 228–235.
41. SANADA, M., M. TSUDA, I. KODAMA, et al. 2004. Substitution of transdermal estradiol during oral estrogen–progestin therapy in postmenopausal women. Effects of hypertriglyceridemia. Menopause **11:** 331–336.
42. JACOBSEN, D.W. 1998. Homocysteine and vitamins in cardiovascular disease. Clin. Chem. **44:** 1833–1843.
43. DIMITROVA, K.R., K. DEGROOT & Y.D. KIM. 2002. Estrogen and homocysteine. Cardiovasc. Res. **53:** 577–588.
44. SMOLDERS, R.G., M.J. VAN DER MOOREN, T. TEERLINK, et al. 2003. A randomized placebo-controlled study of the effect of transdermal vs. oral estradiol with or without gestodene on homocysteine levels. Fertil. Steril. **79:** 261–267.
45. MOSHAROV, E., M. CRANFORD & R. BANERJEE. 2000. The quantitatively important relationship between homocysteine metabolism and glutathione synthesis by the transsulfuration pathway and its regulation by redox changes. Biochemistry **39:** 13005–13011.
46. HAK, A.E., K.H. POLDERMAN, I.C. WESTENDORP, et al. 2000. Increased plasma homocysteine after menopause. Atherosclerosis **149:** 163–168.

47. DE LEO, V., A. LA MARCA, G. MORGANTE, *et al.* 2004. Menopause, the cardiovascular risk factor homocysteine, and the effects of treatment. Review. Treat. Endocrinol. **3:** 393–400.
48. CHRISTODOULAKOS, G., I. LAMBRINOUDAKI, C. PANOULIS, *et al.* 2003. Effect of raloxifene, estrogen, and hormone replacement therapy on serum homocysteine levels in postmenopausal women. Fertil. Steril. **79:** 455–456.
49. DE LEO, V., A. LA MARCA, G. MORGANTE, *et al.* 2001. Randomized controlled study on the effects of raloxifene on serum lipids and homocysteine in older women. Am. J. Obstet. Gynecol. **184:** 350–353.
50. BEST, P.J.M., P.B. BERGER, V.M. MILLER, *et al.* 1998. The effect of estrogen replacement therapy on serum nitric oxide and endothelin-1 levels in postmenopausal women. Ann. Intern. Med. **128:** 285–288.
51. WILCOX, J.G., I.E. HATCH, E. GENTZCHEIN, *et al.* 1997. Endothelin levels decrease after oral and non oral estrogen in postmenopausal women with increased cardiovascular risk factors. Fertil. Steril. **67:** 273–277.
52. VOGEL, R.A. & M.C. CORRETI. 1998. Estrogens, progestins and heart disease. Can endothelial function divine the benefit? Circulation **97:** 1223–1236.
53. SIMONCINI, T. & A.R. GENAZZANI. 2000. Raloxifene acutely stimulates nitric oxide release from human endothelial cells via an activation of endothelial nitric oxide synthase. J. Clin. Endocrinol. Metab. **85:** 2966–2969.
54. MARTTUNEN, M.B., P. HIETANEN, A. TIITINEN, *et al.* 2000. Antiestrogens reduce plasma levels of endothelin-1 without affecting nitrate levels in breast cancer patients. Gynecol. Endocrinol. **14:** 55–59.
55. RAHIMIAN, R., I. LAHER, G. DUBE & C. VAN BREEMEN. 1997. Estrogen and selective estrogen receptor modulator LY117018 enhance release of nitric oxide in rat aorta. J. Pharmacol. Exp. Ther. **283:** 116–122.
56. PAVO, I., F. LASZLO, E. MORSCHL, *et al.* 2000. Raloxifene, an oestrogen-receptor modulator, prevents decreased constitutive nitric oxide and vasoconstriction in ovariectomized rats. Eur. J. Pharmacol. **410:** 101–104.
57. SAITTA, A., D. ALTAVILLA, D. CUCINOTTA, *et al.* 2001. Randomized, double-blind, placebo-controlled study on effects of raloxifene and hormone replacement therapy on plasma no concentrations, endothelin-1 levels, and endothelium-dependent vasodilation in postmenopausal women. Arterioscler. Thromb. Vasc. Biol. **21:** 1512–1519.
58. PRADHAN, S. & B.E. SUMPIO. 2004. Do estrogen effects on blood vessels translate into clinically significant atheroprotection? J. Am. Coll. Surg. **198:** 462–474.
59. ROLLINS, B.J., T. YOSHIMURA & E.J. LEONARD. 1990. Cytokine-activated human endothelial cells synthesize and secrete a monocyte chemoattractant, MCP-1/JE. Am. J. Pathol. **136:** 1229–1233.
60. REAPE, T.J. & P.H.E. GROOT. 1999. Chemokines and atherosclerosis. Atherosclerosis **147:** 213–225.
61. SIMONCINI, T., R. DE CATERINA & A.R. GENAZZANI. 1999. Selective estrogen receptor modulators: different actions on vascular cell adhesion molecule-1 (VCAM-1) expression in human endothelial cells. J. Clin. Endocrinol. Metab. **84:** 815–818.
62. COLACURCI, N., D. MANZELLA, F. FORNARO, *et al.* 2003. Endothelial function and menopause: effects of raloxifene administration. J. Clin. Endocrinol. Metab. **88:** 2135–2140.
63. HERRINGTON, D.M., K.B. BROSNIHAN, B.E. PUSSER, *et al.* 2001. Differential effects of E and droloxifene on C-reactive protein and other markers of inflammation in healthy postmenopausal women. J. Clin. Endocrinol. Metab. **86:** 4216–4222.

64. LAKOSKI, S.G. & D.M. HERRINGTON. 2005. Effects of hormone therapy on C-reactive protein and IL-6 in postmenopausal women: a review article. Climacteric **8:** 317–326.
65. CUSHMAN, M., E.N. MEILAHN, B.M. PSATY, *et al.* 1999. Hormone replacement therapy, inflammation, and hemostasis in elderly women. Arterioscler. Thromb. Vasc. Biol **19:** 893–899.
66. WALSH, B.W., D.A. COX, A. SASHEGYI, *et al.* 2001. Role of tumor necrosis factor-alpha and interleukin-6 in the effects of hormone replacement therapy and raloxifene on C-reactive protein in postmenopausal women. Am. J. Cardiol. **88:** 825–828.
67. BRYANT, H.U. & W.H. DERE. 1998. Selective estrogen receptor modulators: an alternative to hormone replacement therapy. Soc. Exp. Biol. Med. **217:** 45–52.
68. KEARNEY, L.E. & D.W. PURDIE. 1998. Selective estrogen receptor modulators. Climacterice **1:** 143–147.
69. NAGASE, H. & J.F. WOESSNER. 1999. Matrix metalloproteinases. J. Biol. Chem. **274:** 21491–21494.
70. GALIS, Z.S. & J.J. KHTZI. 2002. Matrix metalloproteinases in vascular remodeling and atherogenesis: the good, the bad and the ugly. Circ. Res. **90:** 251–262.
71. CHRISTODOULAKOS, G.E., C.P. PANOULIS, I.V. LAMBRINOUDAKI, *et al.* 2004. The effect of hormone therapy and raloxifene on serum matrix metalloproteinase-2 and -9 in postmenopausal women. Menopause **11:** 299–305.
72. BOBRYSHEV, Y.V., S.M. CHERIAN, S.J. INDER & R.S.A. LORD. 1999. Neovascular expression of VE-cadherin in human atherosclerotic arteries and its relation to intimal inflammation. Cardiovasc. Res. **43:** 1003–1017.
73. HOFMANN, S., H. GRASBERGER, P. JUNG, *et al.* 2002. The tumor necrosis factor-a induced vascular permeability is associated with the induction of VE-cadherin expression. Eur. J. Med. Res. **7:** 171–176.
74. CHRISTODOULAKOS, G., I. LAMBRINOUDAKI, C. PANOULIS, *et al.* 2004. Effect of hormone therapy and raloxifene on serum VE-cadherin in postmenopausal women. Menopause **11:** 299–305.
75. MARTTUNEN, M.B., B. CACCIATORE, P. HIETANEN, *et al.* 2001. Prospective study on gynaecological effects of two antioestrogens tamoxifen and toremifene in postmenopausal women. Br. J. Cancer **84:** 897–902.

Bone Remodeling

DIMITRIOS J. HADJIDAKIS AND IOANNIS I. ANDROULAKIS

Second Department of Internal Medicine, Propaedeutic, and Research Institute, Athens University, Attikon University General Hospital, Athens, Greece

ABSTRACT: The skeleton is a metabolically active organ that undergoes continuous remodeling throughout life. Bone remodeling involves the removal of mineralized bone by osteoclasts followed by the formation of bone matrix through the osteoblasts that subsequently become mineralized. The remodeling cycle consists of three consecutive phases: resorption, during which osteoclasts digest old bone; reversal, when mononuclear cells appear on the bone surface; and formation, when osteoblasts lay down new bone until the resorbed bone is completely replaced. Bone remodeling serves to adjust bone architecture to meet changing mechanical needs and it helps to repair microdamages in bone matrix preventing the accumulation of old bone. It also plays an important role in maintaining plasma calcium homeostasis. The regulation of bone remodeling is both systemic and local. The major systemic regulators include parathyroid hormone (PTH), calcitriol, and other hormones such as growth hormone, glucocorticoids, thyroid hormones, and sex hormones. Factors such as insulin-like growth factors (IGFs), prostaglandins, tumor growth factor-beta (TGF-β), bone morphogenetic proteins (BMP), and cytokines are involved as well. As far as local regulation of bone remodeling is concerned, a large number of cytokines and growth factors that affect bone cell functions have been recently identified. Furthermore, through the RANK/ receptor activator of NF-kappa B ligand (RANKL)/osteoprotegerin (OPG) system the processes of bone resorption and formation are tightly coupled allowing a wave of bone formation to follow each cycle of bone resorption, thus maintaining skeletal integrity.

KEYWORDS: bone remodeling; osteoblast; osteoclast; cytokines

INTRODUCTION

The remarkable increase in the research of bone biology over the last two decades has not only enhanced our understanding of the regulation of bone remodeling but also enabled us to address some of the major unanswered

Address for correspondence: Dimitrios J. Hadjidakis, M.D., Second Department of Internal Medicine, Propaedeutic and Research Institute, Athens University, Attikon University Hospital, Rimini 1, Haidari 124 62, Greece. Voice: +30-210-5831153; fax: +30-210-6756-133.
e-mail: dhadjida@med.uoa.gr

Ann. N.Y. Acad. Sci. 1092: 385–396 (2006). © 2006 New York Academy of Sciences.
doi: 10.1196/annals.1365.035

questions. Bone remodeling, a complex process by which old bone is continuously replaced by new tissue, requires interaction between different cell phenotypes and is regulated by a variety of biochemical and mechanical factors. This review outlines our current understanding of bone remodeling and its regulation.

Bone and cartilage constitute the skeletal system, which serves two main functions. The first, a structural function, consists of support and protection of vital internal organs and bone marrow as well as the muscle attachment for locomotion. Second, the skeleton has an essential metabolic function serving as a reserve of calcium and phosphate needed for the maintenance of serum homeostasis by contributing to buffering changes in hydrogen ion concentration. Remodeling is the process by which bone is being turned over, allowing the maintenance of the shape, quality, and size of the skeleton. This is accomplished through the repairing of microfractures and the modification of structure in response to stress and other biomechanical forces. This process is characterized by the coordinated actions of osteoclasts and osteoblasts, organized in bone multicellular units (BMU) that follow an activation-resorption-formation sequence of events.

SKELETAL DEVELOPMENT—BONE ORGANIZATION

Bone is a porous mineralized structure made up of cells, vessels, and crystals of calcium compounds (hydroxyapatite). Their proportion varies according to bone types and regions. The processes of cellular differentiation that give rise to the skeleton are regulated by genes, which first establish the pattern of skeletal structure in the form of cartilage and mesenchyme and then replace them with bone through the differentiation of osteoblasts.[1]

The structural components of bone consist of extracellular matrix (largely mineralized), collagen, and cells. Two types of bone are observed in the normal, mature human skeleton: cortical and trabecular.[2] Although macroscopically and microscopically different, the two forms are identical in their chemical composition. *Cortical bone*, which comprises 80% of the skeleton, is dense and compact, has a slow turnover rate and a high resistance to bending and torsion, and constitutes the outer part of all skeletal structures. The major part of the cortical bone is calcified and its function is to provide mechanical strength and protection, but it can also participate in metabolic responses, particularly when there is severe or prolonged mineral deficit. *Trabecular bone* represents 20% of the skeletal mass but 80% of the bone surface is found inside the long bones throughout the bodies of the vertebrae, and in the inner portions of the pelvis and other large flat bones. Trabecular bone is less dense, more elastic, and has a higher turnover rate than cortical bone exhibiting a major metabolic function. Trabecular bone contributes to mechanical support, particularly in bones such as the vertebrae, and provides the initial supplies of mineral in acute deficiency states.

Bone Matrix

Bone matrix mainly consists of type I collagen fibers (consisting of two a1 chains and one a2 chain) and noncollagenous proteins, and represents approximately 90% of the organic composition of the whole bone tissue. Within lamellar bone, the fibers form arches that allow the highest density of collagen per unit volume of tissue. The lamellae can run parallel to each other (trabecular bone and periosteum), or be concentric surrounding a channel centered on a blood vessel (cortical bone Haversian system). Crystals of hydroxyapatite [3Ca3(PO4)2·(OH)2] are found on the collagen fibers, within them, and in the matrix, and tend to be oriented in the same direction as the collagen fibers.

The role of numerous noncollagenous proteins present in bone matrix has not been fully explained. The major noncollagenous protein produced is osteocalcin (Gla protein), which plays a role in calcium binding, stabilization of hydroxyapatite in the matrix, and regulation of bone formation.[3] Gla protein is a negative regulator of bone formation, which appears to inhibit premature or inappropriate mineralization.[4] In contrast, biglycan, a proteoglycan, is expressed in the bone matrix and positively regulates bone formation.[5]

Osteocytes

Osteoblasts that have been trapped in the osteoid are called osteocytes. Even though the metabolic activity of the osteoblast decreases once it is fully encased in bone matrix, these cells still produce matrix proteins. Osteocytes have numerous long cell processes rich in microfilaments that are organized during the formation of the matrix and before its calcification. They form a network of thin canaliculi permeating the entire bone matrix.

Osteocyte functional activity and morphology varies according to cell age. A young osteocyte has most of the structural characteristics of the osteoblast but decreased cell volume and capacity of protein synthesis. An older osteocyte, located deeper within the calcified bone, presents with a further decrease in cell volume and an accumulation of glycogen in the cytoplasm. The osteocytes are finally phagocytosed and digested during osteoclastic bone resorption.[6]

Despite the complex organization of the osteocytic network, the exact function of these cells remains obscure. It is likely that osteocytes respond to bone tissue strain and enhance bone remodeling activity by recruiting osteoclasts to sites where bone remodeling is required.[7] However, so far there is no direct evidence for osteocytes signaling to cells on the bone surface in response to bone strain or microdamage.

Osteoblast—Bone Formation

The osteoblast is responsible for the production of the bone matrix constituents. Osteoblasts do not function individually but are found in clusters along the bone surface, lining on the layer of bone matrix that they are producing. They originate from multipotent mesenchymal stem cells, which have the capacity to differentiate into osteoblasts, adipocytes, chondrocytes, myoblasts, or fibroblasts.[8] Recent gene deletion studies have shown that absence of runt-related transcription factor 2 (Runx2) or of a downstream factor, osterix, is critical for osteoblast differentiation.[9] Toward the end of the matrix-secreting period, 15% of mature osteoblasts are entrapped in the new bone matrix and differentiate into osteocytes. On the contrary, some cells remain on the bone surface, becoming flat lining cells.

Bone formation occurs in three successive phases: the production and the maturation of osteoid matrix, followed by mineralization of the matrix. In normal adult bone, these processes occur at the same rate so that the balance between matrix production and mineralization is equal. Initially, osteoblasts produce osteoid by rapidly depositing collagen. This is followed by an increase in the mineralization rate to equal that of collagen synthesis. In the final stage the rate of collagen synthesis decreases and mineralization continues until the osteoid becomes fully mineralized.

Osteoblasts produce a range of growth factors under a variety of stimuli including the insulin-like growth factors (IGF),[10] platelet-derived growth factor (PDGF),[11] basic fibroblast growth factor (bFGF),[12] transforming growth factor-beta (TGF-β),[13] and the bone morphogenetic proteins (BMP).[14] Osteoblast activity is regulated in an autocrine and paracrine manner by these growth factors, whose receptors have been found on osteoblasts. Receptors for classical hormones such as parathyroid hormone, parathyroid hormone-related protein, thyroid hormone,[15] growth hormone,[16] insulin,[17] progesterone,[18] and prolactin[19] are located in osteoblasts as well. Osteoblastic nuclear steroid hormone receptors include receptors for estrogens,[20] androgens,[21] vitamin D3,[22] and retinoids.[23]

Osteoclast–Bone Resorption

The osteoclast, a giant multinucleated cell up to 100 mm in diameter, derives from hematopoietic cells of the mononuclear lineage[24] and is the bone lining cell responsible for bone resorption. It is usually found in contact with a calcified bone surface and within a lacuna (Howship's lacunae) as a result of its own resorptive activity.

Osteoclasts have abundant Golgi complexes, mitochondria, and transport vesicles loaded with lysosomal enzymes. They present deep foldings of the plasma membrane in the area facing the bone matrix (called ruffled border) and the surrounding zone of attachment (called sealing zone). Lysosomal enzymes such as tartrate-resistant acid phosphatase and cathepsin K are actively synthesized by the osteoclast and are secreted via the ruffled border into the bone-resorbing compartment.[25]

The process of the osteoclast attachment to the bone surface involves binding of integrins expressed in osteoclasts with specific amino acid sequences within proteins at the surface of the bone matrix.[26] After osteoclast adhesion to the bone matrix, avb3 integrin binding activates cytoskeletal reorganization within the osteoclast.[27] Attachment usually occurs via dynamic structures called podosomes. Through their continual assembly and disassembly they allow osteoclast movement across the bone surface during which bone resorption proceeds. Integrin signaling and subsequent podosome formation is dependent on a number of adhesion kinases including the proto-oncogene src.[28]

Osteoclasts resorb bone by acidification and proteolysis of the bone matrix and of the hydroxyapatite crystals encapsulated within the sealing zone. The first process during bone matrix resorption is mobilization of the hydroxyapatite crystals by digestion of their link to collagen. Then the residual collagen fibers are digested by either cathepsins or activated collagenases and the residues from this digestion are either internalized or transported across the cell and released at the basolateral domain. Osteoclast function is regulated both by locally acting cytokines and by systemic hormones. Osteoclastic receptors for calcitonin,[29] androgens,[30] thyroid hormone,[31] insulin,[32] PTH,[33] IGF-1,[34] interleukin (IL)-1,[35] CSF-1,[36] and PDGF[37] have been demonstrated.

BONE REMODELING

Bone is a living organ that undergoes remodeling throughout life. Remodeling results from the action of osteoblasts and osteoclasts, and defects such as microfractures are repaired by their coupling. In a homeostatic equilibrium resorption and formation are balanced so that old bone is continuously replaced by new tissue so that it adapts to mechanical load and strain. In 1990 Frost defined this phenomenon as bone remodeling.[38]

Osteoclasts and osteoblasts closely collaborate in the remodeling process in what is called a basic multicellular unit (BMU). The organization of the BMUs in cortical and trabecular bone differs, but these differences are mainly morphological rather than biological. In cortical bone the BMU forms a cylindrical canal about 2,000 μm long and 150–200 μm wide and gradually burrows through the bone with a speed of 20–40 μm/day. During a cycle 10 osteoclasts dig a circular tunnel in the dominant loading direction[39] and then they are followed by several thousands of osteoblasts that fill the tunnel.[40] In this manner, between 2% and 5% of cortical bone is being remodeled each year. The trabecular bone is more actively remodeled than cortical bone due to the much larger surface to volume ratio. Osteoclasts travel across the trabecular surface with a speed of approximately 25 μm/day, digging a trench with a depth of 40–60 μm.

The remodeling cycle consists of three consecutive phases: resorption, reversal, and formation. Resorption begins with the migration of partially differentiated mononuclear preosteoclasts to the bone surface where they form multinucleated osteoclasts. After the completion of osteoclastic resorption, there is a reversal phase when mononuclear cells appear on the bone surface. These cells prepare the surface for new osteoblasts to begin bone formation and provide signals for osteoblast differentiation and migration. The formation phase follows with osteoblasts laying down bone until the resorbed bone is completely replaced by new. When this phase is complete, the surface is covered with flattened lining cells and a prolonged resting period begins until a new remodeling cycle is initiated. The stages of the remodeling cycle have different lengths. Resorption probably continues for about 2 weeks, the reversal phase may last up to 4 or 5 weeks, while formation can continue for 4 months until the new bone structural unit is completely created.

The assumption that a coupling mechanism must exist between bone formation and resorption was first reported in 1964.[41] However, the exact molecular mechanism that describes the interaction between cells of the osteoblastic and osteoclastic lineages was only recently identified.[42] The bone remodeling cycle begins with activation mediated by cells of the osteoblast lineage. Activation may involve the osteocytes, the lining cells, and the preosteoblasts in the marrow. The exact cells of the osteoblast lineage responsible have not been fully defined. These cells undergo changes in their shape, they secrete enzymes that digest proteins on the bone surface and express a 317 amino acid peptide, member of the tumor necrosis factor (TNF) superfamily, called receptor activator of NF-kappa B ligand (RANKL). RANKL interacts with a receptor on osteoclast precursors called RANK. The RANKL/RANK interaction results in activation, differentiation, and fusion of hematopoietic cells of the osteoclast lineage so that they begin the process of resorption. Furthermore, it also prolongs osteoclast survival by suppressing apoptosis.[43] This interaction indicates that bone resorption and bone formation are coupled among others through RANKL.

The effects of RANKL are blocked by osteoprotegerin (OPG), a secretory dimeric glycoprotein belonging to the TNF receptor family with a molecular weight of 120 kDa. OPG acts as a decoy receptor (a soluble receptor acting as antagonist) for RANKL and it is mainly produced by cells of the osteoblast lineage, but it can also be produced by the other cells in the bone marrow.[44,45] OPG regulates bone resorption by inhibiting the final differentiation and activation of osteoclasts and by inducing their apoptosis. OPG is not incorporated into bone matrix and its effects on bone resorption are therefore fully reversible.

REGULATION OF BONE REMODELING

The overall integrity of bone appears to be controlled by hormones and many other proteins secreted by both hemopoietic bone marrow cells and bone cells. There is both systemic and local regulation of bone cell function.

Systemic Regulation

Parathyroid hormone is the most important regulator of calcium homeostasis. It maintains serum calcium concentrations by stimulating bone resorption, increasing renal tubular calcium reabsorption and renal calcitriol production. PTH stimulates bone formation when given intermittently and bone resorption when secreted continuously.[46] *Calcitriol* is essential in enhancing intestinal calcium and phosphorus absorption, and in this way it promotes bone mineralization. In addition, vitamin D3 possesses important anabolic effects on bone, thus exerting a dual effect on bone turnover.[47] *Calcitonin*, in pharmacologic doses, mediates loss of the ruffled border, cessation of osteoclast motility, and inhibition of the secretion of proteolytic enzymes through its receptor on osteoclasts. This effect, however, is dose limited and its physiologic role is minimal in the adult skeleton. The growth hormone (GH)/IGF-1 system and IGF-2 are important for skeletal growth, especially at the cartilaginous end plates and during endochondreal bone formation. They are among the major determinants of adult bone mass through their effect on regulation of both bone formation and resorption.[48] *Glucocorticoids* exert both stimulatory and inhibitory effects on bone cells. They are essential for osteoblast maturation by promoting their differentiation from mesenchymal progenitors but they decrease osteoblast activity. Furthermore, glucocorticoids sensitize bone cells to regulators of bone remodeling and they augment osteoclast recruitment.[49] *Thyroid hormones* stimulate both bone resorption and formation. Thus, bone turnover is increased in hyperthyroidism and therefore bone loss can occur.[50] *Estrogens* decrease the responsiveness of the osteoclast progenitor cells to RANKL, thereby preventing osteoclast formation.[51] Furthermore, besides reducing osteoclast life span,[52] estrogens stimulate osteoblast proliferation and decrease their apoptosis. They affect gene coding for enzymes, bone matrix proteins, hormone receptors, transcription factors, and they also upregulate the local production of OPG, IGF I, IGF II, and TGF-β.[53] *Androgens* are essential for skeletal growth and maintenance via their effect on androgen receptor, which is present in all types of bone cells.[54]

Local Regulation

As far as the local regulation of bone cell function is concerned, after the recent discovery of the OPG/RANKL/RANK system, there is a clearer picture regarding the control of osteoclastogenesis and bone remodeling in general. RANKL, expressed on the surface of preosteoblastic/stromal cells binds to RANK on the osteoclastic precursor cells and is critical for the differentiation, fusion into multinucleated cells, activation, and survival of osteoclastic cells.[43] OPG inhibits the entire system by blocking the effects of RANKL.[45] Macrophage colony-stimulating factor (M-CSF), which binds to its receptor, c-Fms, on preosteoclastic cells, appears to be necessary for osteoclast development because it is the primary determinant of the pool of these precursor cells.[55]

The opposite phenotypes of OPG overexpression or with RANKL deletion mice (osteopetrosis) and OPG-deficient or with RANKL overexpression (osteoporosis) have led to the hypothesis that OPG and RANKL can be the mediators for the stimulatory or inhibitory effects of a variety of systemic hormones, growth factors, and cytokines on osteoclastogenesis. This is recently referred to as "the convergence hypothesis" in that the activity of the resorptive and antiresorptive agents "converges" at the level of these two mediators, whose final ratio controls the degree of osteoclast differentiation, activation, and apoptosis.[56]

A number of cytokines such as TNF-α and IL-10 modulate this system primarily by stimulating M-CSF production and by directly increasing RANKL expression.[57] In addition, a number of other cytokines and hormones exert their effects on osteoclastogenesis by regulating cell production of OPG and RANKL (see TABLE 1). Furthermore, IL-6, a pleiotropic cytokine secreted by osteoblasts, osteoclasts, and stromal cells, appears to be an important regulator of bone remodeling by stimulating osteoclastic bone resorption[65] but also by promoting osteoblast generation in conditions of high bone turnover.[66] Recent studies have also suggested that osteoblast-derived PTHrP promotes the recruitment of osteogenic cells and prevents the apoptotic death of osteoblasts, thus being an important regulator of bone cell function.[67]

Abnormalities of bone remodeling can produce a variety of skeletal disorders. The recent advances concerning systemic and local regulation of bone remodeling have led to new approaches in the diagnosis and treatment of

TABLE 1. Effects of cytokines and hormones on bone remodeling through RANKL and OPG secretion

	RANKL	OPG
Transforming growth factor-β[58]	–	↑
Parathyroid hormone[59]	↑	↓
1,25(OH)$_2$ vitamin D$_3$[60]	↑	–
Glucocorticoids[61]	↑	↓
Estrogen[62]	–	↑
Basic fibroblast growth factor 2[63]	↑	↓
Prostaglandin E$_2$[64]	↓	↑

skeletal disorders. In particular, the newer methods in molecular and cellular biology aid to define the abnormalities in cells of the osteoblastic and osteoclastic lineages that lead to bone disease and to develop new therapeutic approaches based on a better understanding of the pathogenetic mechanisms. These involve production of recombinant molecules of cytokines and their soluble receptors, development of inhibitory peptides, and specific inhibition of key signaling pathways.

REFERENCES

1. WELLIK, D.M. & M.R. CAPECCHI. 2003. Hox10 and Hox11 genes are required to lobally pattern the mammalian skeleton. Science **301**: 363–367.
2. ADLER, C.P. 2000. Bones and bone tissue; normal anatomy and histology. *In* Bone Diseases. 1–30. Springer-Verlag. New York.
3. DUCY, P., C. DESBOIS, B. BOYCE, *et al.* 1996. Increased bone formation in osteocalcin-deficient mice. Nature **382**: 448–452.
4. LUO, G., P. DUCY, M.D. MCKEE, *et al.* 1997. Spontaneous calcification of arteries and cartilage in mice lacking matrix GLA protein. Nature **386**: 78–81.
5. XU, T., P. BIANCO, L.W. FISHER, *et al.* 1998. Targeted disruption of the biglycan gene leads to an osteoporosis-like phenotype in mice. Nat. Genet. **20**: 78–82.
6. ELMARDI, A.S., M.V. KATCHBURIAN & E. KATCHBURIAN. 1990. Electron microscopy of developing calvaria reveals images that suggest that osteoclasts engulf and destroy osteocytes during bone resorption. Calcif. Tissue Int. **46**: 239–245.
7. LANYON, L.E. 1993. Osteocytes, strain detection, bone modeling and remodelling. Calcif. Tissue Int. **53**(Suppl 1): S102–S106.
8. BIANCO, P., M. RIMINUCCI, S. GRONTHOS, *et al.* 2001. Bone marrow stromal stem cells: nature, biology, and potential applications. Stem Cells **19**: 180–192.
9. DUCY, P., R. ZHANG, V. GEOFFROY, *et al.* 1997. Osf2/Cbfa1: a transcriptional activator of osteoblast differentiation. Cell **89**: 747–754.
10. CANALIS, E., J. PASH, B. GABBITAS, *et al.* 1993. Growth factors regulate the synthesis of insulin-like growth factor-I in bone cell cultures. Endocrinology **133**: 33–38.
11. RYDZIEL, S., S. SHAIKH & E. CANALIS. 1994. Platelet-derived growth factor-AA and -BB (PDGF-AA and -BB) enhance the synthesis of PDGF-AA in bone cell cultures. Endocrinology **134**: 2541–2546.
12. GLOBUS, R.K., J. PLOUET & D. GOSPODAROWICZ. 1989. Cultured bovine bone cells synthesize basic fibroblast growth factor and store it in their extracellular matrix. Endocrinology **124**: 1539–1547.
13. CANALIS, E., J. PASH & S. VARGHESE. 1993. Skeletal growth factors. Crit. Rev. Eukaryot. Gene Expr. **3**: 155–166.
14. CHEN, D., M. ZHAO & G.R. MUNDY. 2004. Bone morphogenetic proteins. Growth Factors **22**: 233–241.
15. RIZZOLI, R., J. POSER & U. BURGI. 1986. Nuclear thyroid hormone receptors in cultured bone cells. Metabolism **35**: 71–74.
16. BARNARD, R., K.W. NG, T.J. MARTIN, *et al.* 1991. Growth hormone (GH) receptors in clonal osteoblast-like cells mediate a mitogenic response to GH. Endocrinology **128**: 1459–1464.

17. LEVY, J.R., E. MURRAY, S. MANOLAGAS, *et al.* 1986. Demonstration of insulin receptors and modulation of alkaline phosphatase activity by insulin in rat osteoblastic cells. Endocrinology **119:** 1786–1792.

18. WEI, L.L., M.W. LEACH, R.S. MINER, *et al.* 1993. Evidence for progesterone receptors in human osteoblast-like cells. Biochem. Biophys. Res. Commun. **195:** 525–532.

19. CLEMENT-LACROIX, P., C. ORMANDY, L. LEPESCHEUX, *et al.* 1999. Osteoblasts are a new target for prolactin: analysis of bone formation in prolactin receptor knockout mice. Endocrinology **140:** 96–105.

20. ERIKSEN, E.F., D.S. COLVARD, N.J. BERG, *et al.* 1988. Evidence of estrogen receptors in normal human osteoblast-like cells. Science **241:** 84–86.

21. COLVARD, D.S., E.F. ERIKSEN, P.E. KEETING, *et al.* 1989. Identification of androgen receptors in normal human osteoblast-like cells. Proc. Natl. Acad. Sci. USA **86:** 854–857.

22. DARWISH, H.M. & H.F. DELUCA. 1996. Recent advances in the molecular biology of vitamin D action. Prog. Nucleic Acid Res. Mol. Biol. **53:** 321–344.

23. KINDMARK, A., H. TORMA, A. JOHANSSON, *et al.* 1993. Reverse transcription-polymerase chain reaction assay demonstrates that the 9-cis retinoic acid receptor alpha is expressed in human osteoblasts. Biochem. Biophys. Res. Commun. **192:** 1367–1372.

24. TEITELBAUM, S.L. 2000. Bone resorption by osteoclasts. Science **289:** 1504–1508.

25. VAANANEN, H.K., H. ZHAO, M. MULARI, *et al.* 2000. The cell biology of osteoclast function. J. Cell Sci. **113**(Pt 3): 377–381.

26. DAVIES, J., J. WARWICK, N. TOTTY, *et al.* 1989. The osteoclast functional antigen, implicated in the regulation of bone resorption, is biochemically related to the vitronectin receptor. J. Cell Biol. **109:** 1817–1826.

27. REINHOLT, F.P., K. HULTENBY, A. OLDBERG, *et al.* 1990. Osteopontin—a possible anchor of osteoclasts to bone. Proc. Natl. Acad. Sci. USA **87:** 4473–4475.

28. SORIANO, P., C. MONTGOMERY, R. GESKE, *et al.* 1991. Targeted disruption of the c-src proto-oncogene leads to osteopetrosis in mice. Cell **64:** 693–702.

29. WARSHAWSKY, H., D. GOLTZMAN, M.F. ROULEAU, *et al.* 1980. Direct *in vivo* demonstration by radioautography of specific binding sites for calcitonin in skeletal and renal tissues of the rat. J. Cell Biol. **85:** 682–694.

30. MIZUNO, Y., T. HOSOI, S. INOUE, *et al.* 1994. Immunocytochemical identification of androgen receptor in mouse osteoclast-like multinucleated cells. Calcif. Tissue Int. **54:** 325–326.

31. ABU, E.O., S. BORD, A. HORNER, *et al.* 1997. The expression of thyroid hormone receptors in human bone. Bone **21:** 137–142.

32. THOMAS, D.M., N. UDAGAWA, D.K. HARDS, *et al.* 1998. Insulin receptor expression in primary and cultured osteoclast-like cells. Bone **23:** 181–186.

33. TETI, A., R. RIZZOLI & Z.A. ZAMBONIN. 1991. Parathyroid hormone binding to cultured avian osteoclasts. Biochem. Biophys. Res. Commun. **174:** 1217–1222.

34. HOU, P., T. SATO, W. HOFSTETTER, *et al.* 1997. Identification and characterization of the insulin-like growth factor I receptor in mature rabbit osteoclasts. J. Bone Miner. Res. **12:** 534–540.

35. XU, L.X., T. KUKITA, Y. NAKANO, *et al.* 1996. Osteoclasts in normal and adjuvant arthritis bone tissues express the mRNA for both type I and II interleukin-1 receptors. Lab. Invest. **75:** 677–687.

36. HOFSTETTER, W., A. WETTERWALD, M.C. CECCHINI, *et al.* 1992. Detection of transcripts for the receptor for macrophage colony-stimulating factor, c-fms, in murine osteoclasts. Proc. Natl. Acad. Sci. USA **89:** 9637–9641.

37. ZHANG, Z., J. CHEN & D. JIN. 1998. Platelet-derived growth factor (PDGF)-BB stimulates osteoclastic bone resorption directly: the role of receptor beta. Biochem. Biophys. Res. Commun. **251:** 190–194.

38. FROST, H.M. 1990. Skeletal structural adaptations to mechanical usage (SATMU): 2. Redefining Wolff's law: the remodeling problem. Anat. Rec. **226:** 414–422.

39. PETRTYL, M., J. HERT & P. FIALA. 1996. Spatial organization of the haversian bone in man. J. Biomech. **29:** 161–169.

40. PARFITT, A.M. 1994. Osteonal and hemi-osteonal remodeling: the spatial and temporal framework for signal traffic in adult human bone. J. Cell Biochem. **55:** 273–286.

41. FROST, H.M. 1996. Dynamics of bone remodeling. *In* Bone Biodynamics. H.M. Frost, Ed.: 315–333. Littel Brown. Boston, MA.

42. SUDA, T., N. TAKAHASHI, N. UDAGAWA, *et al.* 1999. Modulation of osteoclast differentiation and function by the new members of the tumor necrosis factor receptor and ligand families. Endocr. Rev. **20:** 345–357.

43. HSU, H., D.L. LACEY, C.R. DUNSTAN, *et al.* 1999. Tumor necrosis factor receptor family member RANK mediates osteoclast differentiation and activation induced by osteoprotegerin ligand. Proc. Natl. Acad. Sci. USA **96:** 3540–3545.

44. HOFBAUER, L.C. & M. SCHOPPET. 2004. Clinical implications of the osteoprotegerin/RANKL/RANK system for bone and vascular diseases. JAMA **292:** 490–495.

45. SIMONET, W.S., D.L. LACEY, C.R. DUNSTAN, *et al.* 1997. Osteoprotegerin: a novel secreted protein involved in the regulation of bone density. Cell **89:** 309–319.

46. KIM, C.H., E. TAKAI, H. ZHOU, *et al.* 2003. Trabecular bone response to mechanical and parathyroid hormone stimulation: the role of mechanical microenvironment. J. Bone Miner. Res. **18:** 2116–2125.

47. CHAPUY, M.C., M.E. ARLOT, F. DUBOEUF, *et al.* 1992. Vitamin D3 and calcium to prevent hip fractures in the elderly women. N. Engl. J. Med. **327:** 1637–1642.

48. WANG, J., J. ZHOU, C.M. CHENG, *et al.* 2004. Evidence supporting dual, IGF-I-independent and IGF-I-dependent, roles for GH in promoting longitudinal bone growth. J. Endocrinol. **180:** 247–255.

49. WEINSTEIN, R.S., R.L. JILKA, A.M. PARFITT, *et al.* 1998. Inhibition of osteoblastogenesis and promotion of apoptosis of osteoblasts and osteocytes by glucocorticoids. Potential mechanisms of their deleterious effects on bone. J. Clin. Invest. **102:** 274–282.

50. BRITTO, J.M., A.J. FENTON, W.R. HOLLOWAY, *et al.* 1994. Osteoblasts mediate thyroid hormone stimulation of osteoclastic bone resorption. Endocrinology **134:** 169–176.

51. SRIVASTAVA, S., G. TORALDO, M.N. WEITZMANN, *et al.* 2001. Estrogen decreases osteoclast formation by down-regulating receptor activator of NF-kappa B ligand (RANKL)-induced JNK activation. J. Biol. Chem. **276:** 8836–8840.

52. KAMEDA, T., H. MANO, T. YUASA, *et al.* 1997. Estrogen inhibits bone resorption by directly inducing apoptosis of the bone-resorbing osteoclasts. J. Exp. Med. **186:** 489–495.

53. MANOLAGAS, S.C. 2000. Birth and death of bone cells: basic regulatory mechanisms and implications for the pathogenesis and treatment of osteoporosis. Endocr. Rev. **21:** 115–137.

54. SATO, T., H. KAWANO, S. KATO, *et al.* 2002. Study of androgen action in bone by analysis of androgen-receptor deficient mice. J. Bone Miner. Metab. **20:** 326–330.

55. UDAGAWA, N., N. TAKAHASHI, T. AKATSU, *et al.* 1990. Origin of osteoclasts: mature monocytes and macrophages are capable of differentiating into osteoclasts under a suitable microenvironment prepared by bone marrow-derived stromal cells. Proc. Natl. Acad. Sci. USA **87:** 7260–7264.

56. HOFBAUER, L.C., S. KHOSLA, C.R. DUNSTAN, *et al.* 2000. The roles of osteoprotegerin and osteoprotegerin ligand in the paracrine regulation of bone resorption. J. Bone Miner. Res. **15:** 2–12.

57. HOFBAUER, L.C., D.L. LACEY, C.R. DUNSTAN, *et al.* 1999. Interleukin-1beta and tumor necrosis factor-alpha, but not interleukin-6, stimulate osteoprotegerin ligand gene expression in human osteoblastic cells. Bone **25:** 255–259.

58. THIRUNAVUKKARASU, K., R.R. MILES, D.L. HALLADAY, *et al.* 2001. Stimulation of osteoprotegerin (OPG) gene expression by transforming growth factor-beta (TGF-beta). Mapping of the OPG promoter region that mediates TGF-beta effects. J. Biol. Chem. **276:** 36241–36250.

59. MA, Y.L., R.L. CAIN, D.L. HALLADAY, *et al.* 2001. Catabolic effects of continuous human PTH (1–38) *in vivo* is associated with sustained stimulation of RANKL and inhibition of osteoprotegerin and gene-associated bone formation. Endocrinology **142:** 4047–4054.

60. KITAZAWA, R., S. KITAZAWA & S. MAEDA. 1999. Promoter structure of mouse RANKL/TRANCE/OPGL/ODF gene. Biochim. Biophys. Acta **1445:** 134–141.

61. HOFBAUER, L.C., F. GORI, B.L. RIGGS, *et al.* 1999. Stimulation of osteoprotegerin ligand and inhibition of osteoprotegerin production by glucocorticoids in human osteoblastic lineage cells: potential paracrine mechanisms of glucocorticoid-induced osteoporosis. Endocrinology **140:** 4382–4389.

62. SAIKA, M., D. INOUE, S. KIDO, *et al.* 2001. 17beta-estradiol stimulates expression of osteoprotegerin by a mouse stromal cell line, ST-2, via estrogen receptor-alpha. Endocrinology **142:** 2205–2212.

63. YANO, K., N. NAKAGAWA, H. YASUDA, *et al.* 2001. Synovial cells from a patient with rheumatoid arthritis produce osteoclastogenesis inhibitor factor/osteoprotegerin: reciprocal regulation of the production by inflammatory cytokines and basic fibroblast growth factor. J. Bone Miner. Metab. **6:** 365–372.

64. LIU, X.H., A. KIRSCHENBAUM, S. YAO, *et al.* 2005. Cross-talk between the interleukin-6 and prostaglandin E(2) signaling systems results in enhancement of osteoclastogenesis through effects on the osteoprotegerin/receptor activator of nuclear factor-{kappa}B (RANK) ligand/RANK system. Endocrinology **146:** 1991–1998.

65. MOONGA, B.S., O.A. ADEBANJO, H.J. WANG, *et al.* 2002. Differential effects of interleukin-6 receptor activation on intracellular signaling and bone resorption by isolated rat osteoclasts. J. Endocrinol. **173:** 395–405.

66. SIMS, N.A., B.J. JENKINS, J.M. QUINN, *et al.* 2004. Gp130 regulates bone turnover and bone size by distinct downstream signaling pathways. J. Clin. Invest. **113:** 379–389.

67. MIAO, D., B. HE, Y. JIANG, *et al.* 2005. Osteoblast-derived PTHrP is a potent endogenous bone anabolic agent that modifies the therapeutic efficacy of administered PTH 1–34. J. Clin. Invest. **115:** 2402–2411.

Bisphosphonates

IRENE LAMBRINOUDAKI, GEORGE CHRISTODOULAKOS,
AND DIMITRIOS BOTSIS

*Second Department of Obstetrics and Gynecology, University of Athens,
Artetaieio Hospital, Athens, Greece*

ABSTRACT: Bisphosphonates belong to a class of compounds similar to pyrophosphate. In these compounds the oxygen atom of the pyrophosphate is replaced by a carbon atom resulting in a P-C-P bond. They exert a potent inhibitory effect on osteoclasts and are therefore potent antiresorptive agents. They reduce bone turnover, increase bone mineral density, and decrease fracture risk both at the lumbar spine and the hip. Bisphosphonates have a high affinity for bone surfaces, where they accumulate, mainly at sites of bone remodeling. Due to their selectivity in action, they are usually not associated with systemic side effects. Their main unwanted effect is upper gastrointestinal irritation. Alendronate and risedronate are the two most widely used compounds in the treatment of postmenopausal osteoporosis. They are administered orally either daily or once weekly. Ibandronate is a highly potent newer third-generation bisphosphonate administered once monthly with similar efficacy with respect to bone mineral density and fracture risk. Zoledronate, another potent third-generation bisphosphonate, currently approved for the treatment of malignancy-associated hypercalcemia, is currently undergoing phase III trials for the treatment of postmenopausal osteoporosis as an intravenous (i.v.) infusion once annually.

KEYWORDS: bisphosphonate; osteoporosis; risedronate; alendronate; ibandronate; zoledronate

MECHANISM OF ACTION

Bisphosphonates are phyrophosphate analogues. The central oxygen atom in the bisphosphonate molecule is replaced by a carbon atom, which results in a P-C-P bond. The existence of this bond enables the binding of the molecule to the hydroxyapatite. The structure of the two side chains (R1 and R2) determines the potency of the particular bisphosphonate. The presence of nitrogen in the R2 chain, as is the case in the second-generation bisphosphonates, increases the potency of the drug.

Address for correspondence: Irene Lambrinoudaki, Second Department of Obstetrics and Gynecology, University of Athens, 27, Themistokleous St., Dionysos, GR-14578, Athens, Greece. Voice and fax: 0030-210-6410325.
e-mail:ilambrinoudaki@hotmail.com

Ann. N.Y. Acad. Sci. 1092: 397–402 (2006). © 2006 New York Academy of Sciences.
doi: 10.1196/annals.1365.036

Once bisphosphonates enter the circulation, they preferentially concentrate on exposed bone surfaces in active areas of bone remodeling. The intracellular uptake of bisphosphonates by osteoclasts during bone resorption results in the loss of resorptive function and finally in the apoptosis of the osteoclasts. This is mediated through disruption of cytoskeleton, loss of ruffled border, inhibition of lysosomal enzymes, and protein tyrosine phosphatases. Beyond their primary action on the osteoclast activity and life span, bisphosphonates also reduce the number of active osteoclasts by inhibiting their recruitment and finally they inhibit the osteoclast-stimulating activity by osteoblasts.[1]

PHARMACOKINETICS

Gastrointestinal absorption of bisphosphonates is very poor and it diminishes further with food, so patients should be advised to take their medication on an empty stomach. Depending on the type of bisphosphonate, gastrointestinal absorption ranges between 0.5% and 10%. Once in the bloodstream, bisphosphonates are incorporated up to 80% in bone surfaces within 6–10 h, where they remain for long periods of time and are slowly released over weeks or months. This is the rationale for the intermittent dosaging of bisphosphonates. They are not metabolized in liver, they are not secreted in the bile, and they are eliminated unaltered in the urine.[2]

ALENDRONATE

Alendronate is a second-generation nitrogen containing bisphosphonate. Along with risedronate it is widely used in the prevention and treatment of postmenopausal osteoporosis. It can be used as a daily oral regimen of 5 mg and 10 mg for the prevention and treatment of postmenopausal osteoporosis, respectively. The most popular regimen, however, is the weekly administration of 70 mg. The efficacy of alendronate in reducing osteoporotic fracture risk is documented in the Fracture Intervention Trial (FIT).[3] About 994 women with postmenopausal osteoporosis were treated either with placebo or alendronate (5 or 10 mg daily for 3 years, or 20 mg for 2 years followed by 5 mg for 1 year). Both groups received supplemental calcium. Treatment with alendronate was associated with a 48% reduction of new vertebral fractures (3.2%, vs. 6.2% in the placebo group; $P = 0.03$), a decreased progression of vertebral deformities (33%, vs. 41% in the placebo group; $P = 0.028$), and a reduced loss of height ($P = 0.005$). Alendronate is also capable of reducing hip fractures by 53% as demonstrated by FIT. This effect is apparent as early as the first year of treatment.[4]

Alendronate therapy significantly increases bone mineral density (BMD) at the spine (8.8%) and the femoral neck (5.9%) after 3 years of treatment.[3]

Recently, the 10-year extension of the FIT demonstrated that daily alendronate in the 10 mg dose is associated with continuing increase in BMD at the spine (13.7%) and the femoral neck (6.7%). Women in the active treatment group who stopped their medication at 3 years maintained a stable BMD over the remaining 7 years, an observation implying that alendronate continues to have an effect many years after cessation of therapy.[5] Finally, alendronate improves trabecular connectivity and does not derange the mineralization process.[6]

RISEDRONATE

Risedronate is a potent aminobisphosphonate that is widely prescribed for the prevention and treatment of postmenopausal osteoporosis. It can be administered either daily in the dose of 5 mg or once weekly in the dose of 35 mg. The antifracture efficacy of risedronate is documented in the VERT trial (vertebral efficacy with risedronate therapy). The study enrolled 2,558 osteoporotic postmenopausal women with prevalent vertebral fractures who were randomized to receive daily either risedronate 5 mg or placebo. At the end of the 3 years, women in the active treatment arm had 41% lower incidence of new vertebral fractures (CI 18–58%) and 39% lower incidence of nonvertebral fractures (CI: 6–61%). The antifracture efficacy was most prominent during the first year of treatment.[7] Furthermore, BMD increased significantly in the risedronate group compared to placebo in the lumbar spine (5.4% vs. 1.1%) and femoral neck (1.6% vs. 1.2%). Risedronate preserves bone microarchitecture and restores bone turnover to the premenopausal state.[8]

IBANDRONATE

Ibandronate is a new oral aminobisphosphonate initially approved as a daily oral formulation of 2.5 mg for the prevention and treatment of postmenopausal osteoporosis. Recently, the monthly formulation of 150 mg was approved and marketed. The efficacy of the daily formulation with respect to vertebral fractures was proven in the BONE trial (oral ibandronate osteoporosis vertebral fracture trial in North America and Europe). This study enrolled 2,946 postmenopausal women with low BMD and at least one prevalent vertebral fracture. After 3 years women in the daily ibandronate group had 62% lower incidence of radiologically diagnosed new vertebral fractures and 49% lower incidence of new clinical vertebral fractures compared to women in the placebo group. No difference in the incidence of nonvertebral fractures was recorded in this trial between the active treatment and the placebo group. The trial, however, was not sufficiently powered to detect antifracture efficacy in peripheral skeleton.[9] Significant and progressive increases in lumbar spine (6.5% and 1.3% for daily ibandronate and placebo, respectively at 3 years) and hip BMD (3.4% and

0.7% for daily ibandronate and placebo, respectively at 3 years) were observed in the same trial.

The approval of the monthly formulation was based in the MOBILE trial (monthly oral ibandronate therapy in postmenopausal osteoporosis). This trial compared the monthly formulation of 150 mg to the daily dose of 2.5 mg in women with postmenopausal osteoporosis. At the end of 1 year lumbar spine BMD increased by 3.9% and 4.9% in the 2.5 and 150 mg arms, respectively. Similarly, bone markers decreased by 76% in the monthly ibandronate group compared to 67% decrease in the daily ibandronate group.[10]

ZOLEDRONATE

Zoledronate is a potent nitrogen-containing bisphosphonate approved as an intravenous (i.v.) infusion for the treatment of malignancy-associated hypercalcemia. Currently, it is undergoing a phase III clinical trial for the treatment of postmenopausal osteoporosis as an i.v. infusion once annually. The Health Outcomes and Reduced Incidence with Zoledronic acid Once yearly (HORIZON) Recurrent Fracture trial comprises 1,714 osteoporotic postmenopausal women who have recently (3 months) undergone surgical repair of law trauma hip fracture. These women are randomized either to 5 mg i.v. infusion once annually or to placebo. The primary end point is the occurrence of subsequent skeletal fractures and secondary end points are delayed hip fracture healing, changes in BMD, and the degree of health resource utilization. The trial will stop when 211 primary end points are accrued.[11]

An interim analysis encompassing 99% of the data from the now-completed three-year HORIZON Pivotal Fracture Trial evaluating incident fractures in postmenopausal women with low bone mineral density and/or prevalent fractures showed that patients treated with 5 mg zoledronate once annually experienced a 70% risk reduction in new spine fractures ($P < 0.0001$) and a 40% risk reduction in hip fractures ($P = 0.0032$) over three years compared to placebo.[12]

ADVERSE EFFECTS

Adverse effects are similar with all bisphosphonates and include mainly upper gastrointestinal irritation, which may be manifested with heartburn, esophagitis, abdominal pain, or diarrhea. To avoid gastrointestinal symptoms patients are advised to take their medication with at least one glass of water, not to chew or allow the pill to dissolve in the mouth, and to stay in the upright position for 30 min after the intake of the drug without eating or drinking. Rarer adverse effects include bone, joint, and muscle pain that subsides after the drug is discontinued, osteonecrosis of the jaw, which occurs mainly with the i.v. preparations and ocular inflammation manifesting as scleritis, uveitis, or conjunctivitis.

CONCLUSIONS

Bisphosphonates are the mainstay in the treatment of osteoporosis. They have documented efficacy in reducing fracture risk both at the spine and at the peripheral skeleton. Due to their extremely long half-life in bone they can be administered intermittently, currently either weekly or monthly, and possibly in the future annually. Moreover, they may exert antifracture activity even after the drug is discontinued. The safety profile is favorable with upper gastrointestinal irritation being the principal adverse effect.

REFERENCES

1. MILLER, P.D. 2005. Optimizing the management of postmenopausal osteoporosis with bisphosphonates: the emerging role of intermittent therapy. Clin. Ther. **27:** 361–376.
2. RUSSELL, R.G., *et al.* 1999. The pharmacology of bisphosphonates and new insights into their mechanisms of action. J. Bone Miner Res. **14**(Suppl 2): 53–65.
3. LIBERMAN, U.A., *et al.* 1995. Effect of oral alendronate on bone mineral density and the incidence of fractures in postmenopausal osteoporosis. The Alendronate Phase III Osteoporosis Treatment Study Group. N. Engl. J. Med. **333:** 1437–1443.
4. BLACK, D.M., *et al.* 2000. Fracture risk reduction with alendronate in women with osteoporosis: the Fracture Intervention Trial. FIT Research Group. J. Clin. Endocrinol. Metab. **85:** 4118–4124.
5. BONE, H.G., *et al.* 2004. Ten years' experience with alendronate for osteoporosis in postmenopausal women. N. Engl. J. Med. **350:** 1189–1199.
6. BONE, H.G., *et al.* 2000. Alendronate and estrogen effects in postmenopausal women with low bone mineral density. Alendronate/Estrogen Study Group. J. Clin. Endocrinol. Metab. **85:** 720–726.
7. HARRIS, S.T., *et al.* 1999. Effects of risedronate treatment on vertebral and non-vertebral fractures in women with postmenopausal osteoporosis: a randomized controlled trial. Vertebral Efficacy With Risedronate Therapy (VERT) Study Group. JAMA **282:** 1344–1352.
8. BORAH, B., *et al.* 2006. Long-term risedronate treatment normalizes mineralization and continues to preserve trabecular architecture: sequential triple biopsy studies with micro-computed tomography. Bone **39:** 345–352.
9. CHESNUT, I.C., *et al.* 2004. Effects of oral ibandronate administered daily or intermittently on fracture risk in postmenopausal osteoporosis. J. Bone Miner Res. **19:** 1241–1249.
10. MILLER, P.D., *et al.* 2005. Monthly oral ibandronate therapy in postmenopausal osteoporosis: 1-year results from the MOBILE study. J. Bone Miner Res. **20:** 1315–1322.

11. COLON-EMERIC, C.S., *et al.* 2004. The HORIZON Recurrent Fracture Trial: design of a clinical trial in the prevention of subsequent fractures after low trauma hip fracture repair. Curr. Med. Res. Opin. **20:** 903–910.
12. BLACK, D.M., *et al.* 2006. Effect of once-yearly infusion of Zoledronic Acid 5 mg on spine and hip fracture reduction in postmenopausal women with osteoporosis: the HORIZON pivotal fracture trial. Presented at 28th annual meeting of the American Society for Bone and Mineral Research (ASBMR), 15–19 September. Philadelphia, PA.

Strontium Ranelate

A Novel Treatment in Postmenopausal Osteoporosis

S. TOURNIS, D. ECONOMOPOULOS, AND G.P. LYRITIS

Laboratory for Research of Muskuloskeletal System, University of Athens, Athens, Greece

ABSTRACT: Strontium ranelate (SR) is a novel antiosteoporotic agent, electively concentrated in positions of active bone formation, and especially onto the crystal surface that allows permanent exchanges with extracellular fluid. Although the mechanism(s) of action is still under rigorous research, SR appears to reduce bone resorption by decreasing osteoclast differentiation and activity and to stimulate bone formation by increasing replication of preosteoblast cells, leading to increased matrix synthesis. In the placebo-controlled, phase III trial spinal osteoporosis therapeutic intervention (SOTI) (no = 1442; mean age 69 years), there was a 41% decrease over 3 years in the number of patients with new vertebral fractures in the SR (2 g/day) group versus placebo ($P < 0.001$), already detected after 12 months (49% lower risk, $P < 0.001$). The phase III treatment of peripheral osteoporosis (TROPOS) study assessed the efficacy of SR (2 g/day) in preventing nonvertebral fractures in postmenopausal osteoporosis (no = 4932; mean age 77 years). SR reduced nonvertebral fracture risk by 16% versus placebo ($P = 0.04$) and hip fracture risk by 36% ($P = 0.031$) in osteoporotic patients older than 74 years. Thus SR is an effective and safe treatment for vertebral and hip osteoporosis with a unique mode of action.

KEYWORDS: strontium ranelate; spinal osteoporosis therapeutic intervention; treatment of peripheral osteoporosis

INTRODUCTION

Strontium (Sr) was first used for the treatment of osteoporosis in the 1950s.[1] Because of its tendency to oxidate, it is not found in its free form. The main natural sources of strontium are vegetables and cereals, with its concentration

Address for correspondence: Symeon Tournis, M.D., Laboratory for Research of Musculoskeletal System "Th. Garofalidis," University of Athens, KAT Hospital, 10 Athinas Str., Kifissia, PC: 14561, Athens, Greece. Voice: +30-2108018123; fax: +30-2108018122.
e-mail: stournis@med.uoa.gr

Ann. N.Y. Acad. Sci. 1092: 403–407 (2006). © 2006 New York Academy of Sciences.
doi: 10.1196/annals.1365.037

varying between 0.001 and 39 mg/L in soil and <1 mg/L in water. Strontium daily intake is 2 to 4 mg, while the ratio of ingested Sr to Ca is 8/1,000. Plasma Sr levels vary from 0.11 μmol/L to 0.31 μmol/L. When 1.9 mg of Sr is consumed daily, 0.34 mg is excreted in the urine, 1.5 mg in feces, 0.02 mg in sweat, and $0.2 \, 10^{-3}$ mg in growing hair. About 25–30% of the administered dosage of Sr is absorbed by the jejunum, with active transport. Substances like vitamin D, lactose, and generally all carbohydrates have a positive impact on Sr absorption in contrast to chelating agents Ca and P. The Sr/Ca absorption ratio is 0.6–0.7 and after coadministration of Sr and Ca it declines to 0.45–0.5.

The renal clearance of Sr is three times higher compared to calcium. The mechanism of tubular reabsorption is similar for both Sr and Ca. However, since the atom of Sr is larger, its tubular reabsorption is significantly lower than that of Ca. After intravenous Sr administration, serum iPTH levels, serum Ca and renal Ca reabsorption decline, whereas serum P levels increase and 1a-hydroxylase activity is suppressed thus decreasing calcitriol levels.

About 50–80% of the absorbed dosage is concentrated electively in positions of active bone formation.[1,2] The heterogeneous distribution of Sr in the skeleton depends on its plasma concentration, time of exposure, sex, skeletal site (trabecular or cortical), and the age of bone, with newly formed bone showing higher Sr concentration than that of older bone. The majority of strontium is adsorbed onto the crystal surface that allows permanent exchanges with extracellular field; at most 1 atom of calcium out of 10 is replaced by strontium at high doses (monkey-52 weeks treatment).

STRONTIUM RANELATE

Strontium ranelate (SR), which consists of two atoms of stable strontium and an organic acid, ranelate, is a new orally administered drug for the treatment of postmenopausal osteoporosis.[3] Its effects on bone mass and architecture have been thoroughly studied in models of normal and osteopenic animals as well as on bone cells *in vitro*. The effects of SR seem to be mediated through activation of the calcium-sensing receptor on osteoblasts or another functionally different cation-sensing receptor on the same cells.[1] SR administration in intact female rats (225–900 mg/kg/day) dose-dependently increased bone mass of the vertebra body and midshaft femur, while indices of microarchitecture such as trabecular and cortical bone volume as well as trabecular number and thickness improved, thereby increasing bone strength.[4] In animal models with predominant bone remodeling (*Macaca fashicularis*), SR (0.39–2.91 mmol/kg/day for 6 months) dose-dependently decreased bone resorption and increased the extent of mineralizing surfaces.[5] These findings indicate that SR has a unique uncoupling action on bone, increasing bone formation and decreasing bone resorption. In animal models of osteopenia such as ovariectomized rats and after limb immobilization, SR decreased bone resorption while bone formation, contrary to the classic antiresorptive compounds, was maintained or increased.[6,7] *In vitro* studies indicate that the favorable effect on bone formation is mediated by amplification of preosteoblastic cells replication and by secondary or primary increase synthesis of bone matrix.[8] Furthermore, by monitoring the expression of carbonic anhydrase and fibronectin receptor, it was concluded that the osteoclast differentiation is decreased by SR leading to suppression of bone resorption.[9] The suppressing activity of strontium is also established in cell cultures,[9,10] where a decrease of the resorption surface has been observed.

Collectively, opposite to other drugs employed in the treatment of osteoporosis, which act by either increasing bone formation or decreasing bone resorption, SR does both simultaneously. As a result, it increases bone density and bone strength in intact rats, while improving the architecture of the cortical and trabecular bone in normal and ovariectomized experimental animals. Its distinctive impact on bone metabolism results in the formation of a new bone with higher bone strength.

But is there any connection between the formation of a new and stronger bone and the decrease of risk fracture? The answer is given by two multicenter, randomized, double-blind, controlled trials concerning women with postmenopausal osteoporosis. In the Spinal Osteoporosis Therapeutic Intervention study (SOTI),[11] 1,649 postmenopausal women with low lumbar spine bone mineral density (BMD) (<0.840 g/m^2) and at least one vertebral fracture were randomly assigned to receive 2 g/day SR or placebo, both groups being supplemented with calcium and vitamin D according to their needs. Over 1 and 3 years there was a significant decrease in the relative risk of new vertebral fractures of 49% and 41%, respectively, with 9 patients requiring treatment for 3 years to prevent one vertebral fracture. Furthermore, there was a significant relative risk reduction at 1 (52%) and 3 (38%) years in new clinical vertebral fractures. Height loss more than 1 cm was less in the treatment group (30.1% vs. 37.3%, $P = 0.003$), while new or worsening back pain tended to be lower (17.7% vs. 21.3%, $P = 0.07$). Over a period of 3 years, BMD in the SR group increased from baseline by 12.7% at the lumbar spine, 7.2% at the femoral neck, and 8.6% at the total hip ($P < 0.001$ for all three comparisons with baseline values), corresponding to differences between the placebo and the treatment groups at 3 years of 14.4%, 8.3%, and 9.8%, respectively. At 3 years, the BMD at the lumbar spine, adjusted for Sr content, showed an increase over the baseline value of 6.8% in the SR group and a decrease of 1.3% in the placebo group ($P < 0.001$); these changes correspond to a treatment-related increase of 8.1%. Regarding indices of bone turnover there was a significant increase of bone-specific alkaline phosphatase, while C-telopeptide cross-links decreased during the first year and subsequently increased remaining at all times significantly lower compared with controls. The tolerability profile of SR was good. There was no evidence of osteomalacia in a small group of patients on whom bone biopsy was performed, while there was a slight transient increase in the incidence of diarrhea in the active group during the first 3 months of treatment.

The Treatment of Peripheral Osteoporosis study (TROPOS)[12] randomized 5,091 osteoporotic (T-score $_{FN}$ < −2.5) women (≥ 74 years or 70–73 years with at least one risk factor for fracture—previous fracture, frequent falls, living in retirement home, or family history of osteoporotic fracture) to receive either 2 g/day SR or placebo, both groups being supplemented with calcium and vitamin D according to their needs. Over 3 years there was a 16% decrease in the relative risk of nonvertebral fracture (RR = 0.84; 95% CI [0.702; 0.995], 19% relative risk reduction of major nonvertebral osteoporotic fractures (RR = 0.81; 95%CI [0.66; 0.98], while risk of hip fracture was significantly decreased by 36% in a high-risk subgroup (femoral neck BMD t-score ≤ −3 and age ≥ 74 years) (RR = 0.64; 95%CI [0.412; 0.997]. Concerning vertebral fractures there was 45% and 39% relative risk reduction of new vertebral fractures over 1 and 3 years (RR = 0.55; 95%CI [0.39; 0.77], RR = 0.61; 95%CI [0.51; 0.73], respectively). This favorable effect was evident in patients with (RR = 0.68; 95%CI [0.53; 0.85]) and without (RR = 0.55; 95%CI [0.42; 0.72]) previous prevalent vertebral fractures. BMD at the femoral neck and total hip increased significantly in the active treatment group by 8.2% (95%CI [7.7; 8.7] and 9.8% (95%CI [9.3; 10.4] at 3 years compared to placebo. The safety profile was good as it was shown in the Spinal Osteoporosis Therapeutic Intervention (SOTI) trial.

In summary, SR 2 g orally, once daily reduces the risk of vertebral, nonvertebral, and hip fractures and has a good tolerability profile. It is obvious that SR dual activity in bone metabolism is a breakthrough for the treatment of postmenopausal osteoporosis.

REFERENCES

1. PORS NIELSEN, S. 2004. The biological role of strontium. Bone **35:** 583–588.
2. BROWN, E.M. 2003. Is the calcium receptor a molecular target for the actions of strontium on bone? Osteoporos. Int. **14**(Suppl 3): S25–S34.
3. MARIE, P.J. 2003. Optimizing bone metabolism in osteoporosis: insight into the pharmacologic profile of strontium ranelate. Osteoporos. Int. **14**(Suppl 3): S9–S12.
4. AMMANN, P., V. SHEN, B. ROBIN, *et al.* 2004. Strontium ranelate improves bone resistance by increasing bone mass and improving architecture in intact female rats. J. Bone Miner. Res. **19:** 2012–2020.
5. BUEHLER, J., P. CHAPPUIS, J.L. SAFFAR, *et al.* 2001. Strontium ranelate inhibits bone resorption while maintaining bone formation in alveolar bone in monkeys (*Macaca fascicularis*). Bone **29:** 176–179.
6. MARIE, P.J., M. HOTT, D. MODROWSKI, *et al.* 1993. An uncoupling agent containing strontium prevents bone loss by depressing bone resorption and maintaining bone formation in estrogen deficient rats. J. Bone Miner. Res. **8:** 607–615.

7. HOTT, M., P. DELOFFRE, Y. TSOUDEROS & P.J. MARIE. 2003. S12911-2 reduces bone loss induced by short-term immobilization in rats. Bone **33:** 115–123.

8. CANALIS, E., M. HOTT, P. DELOFFRE, *et al.* 1996. The divalent strontium salt S12911 enhances bone cell replication and bone formation in vitro. Bone **18:** 517–523.

9. BARON, R. & Y. TSOUDEROS. 2002. *In vitro* effects of S12911-2 on osteoclast function and bone marrow macrophage differentiation. Eur. J. Pharmacol. **450:** 11–17

10. TAKAHASHI, N., T. SASAKI, Y. TSOUDEROS & T. SUDA. 2003. S12911-2 inhibits osteoclastic bone resorption *in vitro*. J. Bone Miner. **18:** 1082–1087.

11. MEUNIER, P.J., C. ROUX, E. SEEMAN, *et al.* 2004. The effects of strontium ranelate on the risk of vertebral fracture in women with postmenopausal osteoporosis. N. Engl. J. Med. **350:** 459–468.

12. REGINSTER, J.Y., E. SEEMAN, E.M. DE VERNEJOUL, *et al.* 2005. Strontium ranelate reduces the risk of nonvertebral fractures in postmenopausal women with osteoporosis: Treatment of Peripheral Osteoporosis (TROPOS) study. J. Clin. Endocrinol. Metab. **90:** 2816–2822.

Myomectomy during Cesarean Section

A Safe Procedure?

D. HASSIAKOS, P. CHRISTOPOULOS, N. VITORATOS,
E. XARCHOULAKOU, G. VAGGOS, AND K. PAPADIAS

Second Department of Obstetrics and Gynecology, Medical School, University of Athens, Aretaieion Hospital, Athens, Greece

ABSTRACT: A patient's frequent request is the simultaneous surgical removal of a previously diagnosed myoma during cesarean section. The aim of this study was to evaluate the safety and efficacy of myomectomy during cesarean section. From January 1995 until December 2004, 47 pregnant women with coexisting uterine myomas underwent cesarean section and simultaneous myomectomy. All cesarean sections were performed by residents while myomectomies were conducted by the senior staff. Intraoperative and postoperative complications such as blood loss were estimated and compared with 94 women with uterine myomas who underwent surgical delivery without removal of the fibroids. Furthermore, the length of hospitalization was compared between the two groups. Myomectomy added a mean time of 15 min to the operative time of cesarean section. No hysterectomy was performed at the time of the cesarean section. No complications were developed during the puerperium. The difference between the preoperative and postoperative hemoglobin mean value was statistically significant ($P = 0.001$) but did not differ between isolated cesarean and myomectomy-combined cesarean groups. None of the patients received blood transfusion. The length of hospitalization was comparable between the two groups. Despite controversial literature data, we suggest that myomectomy during cesarean section could be generally recommended. Depending on size and location of myomas, the associated risks are similar to those of isolated cesarean section.

KEYWORDS: cesarean section; fibroids; myomectomy; uterine myomas

INTRODUCTION

Uterine myomas are the most common pelvic tumors over the age of 30 years.[1] Given the fact that their growth is related to their exposure to circulating estrogens, fibroids obtain their maximum dimensions during the reproductive period.[2]

Address for correspondence: Panagiotis Christopoulos, 1 Hariton Str., Kifissia, 14564 Athens, Greece. Voice: 2107217835, 2107286353; fax: 2107233330, 2107286282.
e-mail: dr_christopoulos@yahoo.gr

Ann. N.Y. Acad. Sci. 1092: 408–413 (2006). © 2006 New York Academy of Sciences.
doi: 10.1196/annals.1365.038

TABLE 1. Patient characteristics

	Myomectomy ($n = 47$) (mean $\pm$ S.D.)	(Controls ($n = 94$) mean $\pm$ S.D.)	P value
Maternal age (years)	32.1 ± 4.5	30.9 ± 3.3	NS
Parity (n)	0.8 ± 1.2	1.1 ± 1.1	NS
Gestational age (weeks)	37.7 ± 2.5	37.6 ± 1.4	NS
Myoma diameter (cm)	7.9 ± 4.2	5.9 ± 2.9	<0.05

NS = not statistically significant

Nowadays they are encountered more frequently during gestation as many women are delaying childbearing. Adverse events concerning delivery of the embryo or suturing of the uterine incision, caused by the presence of myomas, may require and finally lead to their removal during cesarean section. A patient's frequent request is the simultaneous surgical removal of a previously diagnosed myoma during cesarean section.

In practice though, many surgeons are hesitant regarding the combined procedure because of the potential complications. Several authors report that it would be better to avoid myomectomy during cesarean section with the exception of small, pedunculated fibroids.[3–5] Caesarean-combined myomectomy is usually avoided because of the high risk of uterus atony and severe hemorrhage that can often lead to hysterectomy and subsequent impairment of fertility.[6–8] This is why most obstetricians are trained to avoid myomectomy during cesarean delivery.

In contrast to these opinions, the strategy of avoiding cesarean-combined myomectomy is gradually changing. Some authors suggest myomectomy at cesarean section in selected patients.[6,9,10] Several reports have shown that by taking into consideration certain factors such as uterine contractility, anatomic location, number and size of myomas, and proximity to large vessels, the cesarean-combined myomectomy could be considered a safe procedure. However, multiple fibroids are unfavorable for myomectomy.[3,5,6,8,9,11–16]

In this study, our aim was to evaluate the outcome of myomectomy during cesarean section and to compare it with a control group.

TABLE 2. Location of removed myomas

Type	N (%)
Pedunculated	10.0
Subserosal	38.5
Intramural	24.5
Submucosal	5.0
Multiple sites	22.0

TABLE 3. Outcomes of cesarean myomectomy patients compared with controls

	Myomectomy ($n = 47$)	Controls ($n = 94$)	P value
Preoperative haemoglobin values (g/dl) (mean ± S.D.)	11.6 ± 0.8	11.2 ± 1.6	NS
Postoperative hemoglobin values (g/dl) (mean ± S.D.)	10.6 ± 1.1	10.4 ± 1.2	NS
Mean change in hemoglobin values (g/dl)	1.0 ± 0.3	0.8 ± 0.4	NS
Incidence of hemorrhage	10.6%	9.6%	NS
Frequency of blood transfusion	0%	0%	NS
Frequency of postoperative fever	5.5%	7.5%	NS
Duration of operation (minutes) (mean ± S.D.)	63.2 ± 16.4	48.5 ± 5.6	<0.05
Length of hospital stay (days) (mean ± S.D.)	3.7 ± 0.6	3.3 ± 0.8	<0.05

NS = not statistically significant

MATERIALS AND METHODS

In this retrospective case-control study conducted at Aretaieion Hospital, Second Department of Obstetrics and Gynecology, Medical School, University of Athens, Greece, 141 women with myomas who underwent cesarean delivery between January 1995 and December 2004 were recruited.

The inclusion criteria were: (1) documented myoma during the index pregnancy by antepartum ultrasound or by intraoperative findings; (2) no evidence of antenatal bleeding; (3) no other procedures at the time of cesarean section besides myomectomy; (4) no comorbid conditions with evidence of coagulopathy.

The surgical deliveries were carried out between the 35th and 40th weeks of pregnancy. The study group composing group A consisted of 47 patients who underwent myomectomy at the time of cesarean delivery after delivery of the neonate. Control subjects ($n = 94$), composing group B, were selected in a 2:1 control subject/study subject ratio among patients with myomas who underwent isolated cesarean delivery without removal of fibroids. Characteristics such as age, parity, gestational age at delivery, and number, size, and location of the myomas were recorded and completely matched between study group A and control group B.

The main outcomes were preoperative and postoperative hemoglobin values and the difference between them, hemorrhage (defined as decrease in hematocrit of 10 points from the preoperative value), the need for intraoperative or postoperative blood transfusion, postoperative fever (defined as temperature greater than or equal to 38.0 °C), duration of operation (calculated from skin incision to skin closure), and length of postoperative hospital stay. Prophylactic antibiotic therapy was used for all patients.

RESULTS

The mean $\pm$ SD age of groups A and B was 32.1 ± 4.5 and 30.9 ± 3.3 years, respectively. The mean size of fibroids removed in groups A and B was 7.9 ± 4.2 cm (range: 3–15.5 cm) and 5.9 ± 2.9 cm (range: 2–21 cm), respectively (TABLE 1). Twenty-two percent of the fibroids were located in multiple sites while the majority of them (38.5%) were subserosal (TABLE 2).

In group A, patients had larger myomas and more than 24% of the removed fibroids were intramural. There was no difference in the incidence of hemorrhage between groups A (10.6%) and B (9.6%). The difference between the preoperative (11.6 ± 0.8 mg/dL) and postoperative (10.6 ± 1.1mg/dL) hemoglobin mean value was statistically significant ($P = 0.001$) but did not differ between groups A and B. None of the patients received blood transfusion.

Despite the high rate of large myomas, no hysterectomy or other procedures to control bleeding were performed in any case. The mean operative time was significantly longer for group A (63.2 ± 16.4 min) as compared to control group B (48.5 ± 5.6 min) ($P < 0.05$). Myomectomy added an average 15 min to the operation time of cesarean section. Compared to the related literature this is a prolonged procedure, but this is due to the fact that approximately 93% of all obstetrical operations in our institution are performed by trainees, while myomectomies are conducted by the senior staff. No complications were developed during puerperium. The average length of hospitalization was 0.4 days longer for group A (3.7 ± 0.6 days) as compared to control group B (3.3 ± 0.8 days).

There was no difference in the incidence of postoperative fever between groups A and B (TABLE 3).

DISCUSSION

The adequate management of fibroids, previously known or surprisingly met during cesarean delivery, is controversial. Additional benefits of surgical management of uterine fibroid during cesarean section include reduction of the risk of anesthesia as well as of the cost.[13]

In this study, results indicate that in selected patients and in experienced hands, myomectomy during cesarean delivery is generally a safe procedure. The decision whether to interve depends mainly on the location of the fibroid and the surgeon's experience. If the myoma is located in the area of the uterine incision, it can be safely removed with an easy and bloodless procedure. There is no doubt that large, fundal, intramural fibroids in the vicinity of the tubes should be avoided. Intramural fibroids in general should be excised with caution. Although no available literature exists, it seems that fibroids located at the cornual region of the uterus should not be removed as this may affect subsequent fertility.[13]

Kwawukume removed from one solitary fibroid nodule to six nodules with an average diameter of 6 cm. Eighty-five percent of the fibroids were intramural within the body of the uterus. There were no significant complications during puerperium. In addition, there was no significant difference in intraoperative and postoperative morbidity and blood loss in performing cesarean section alone and cesarean section with myomectomy when a tourniquet was applied.[17]

Kaymak et al. found no significant difference over any studied parameters between the study and control groups, although 60% of the myomas measured more than 6 cm and more than 30% were intramural.[18]

Uterine tourniquet,[17] electrocautery,[19] bilateral uterine artery ligation,[20] or other intraoperative techniques[21] can minimize blood loss during the surgery. In our study, none of them was employed because they were not necessary. Similarly to others,[21,22] oxytocin infusion was continued for 12 to 24 h while antibiotic treatment was administrated in all patients to avoid infection and possible dehiscence of suture. In accordance with almost all the above studies, we also believe that adequate experience at routine myomectomy and the use of high-dose oxytocin infusion during the intra- and postoperative period will curtail severe hemorrhage.

Our results indicate that removing accessible subserosal or pedunculated fibroid is a safe procedure. The case in which the myomas are located elsewhere but are asymptomatic, to our knowledge and experience despite the controversial literature data, myomectomy during cesarean section could be generally recommended and it can be safely performed without any serious or life-threatening complications by experienced hands. Depending on size and location of the myomas, a detailed discussion should be carried out with the patients regarding the associated risks, which, in general, are equal to those of an isolated cesarean section.

REFERENCES

1. Novak, E.R. & J.D. Woodruff. 1979. Myoma and other benign tumours of the uterus. Novak's gynecologic and obstetric pathology with clinical and endocrine relations. 260. W.B. Saunders. Philadelphia.
2. Wallach, E.E. 1992. Myomectomy. In Te Linde's operative gynecology. Seventh edition. J.D. Thompson & J.A. Rock, Eds.: 647–662. Lippincott. Philadelphia PA.
3. Davis, J.L., S. Ray-Mazumder, C.J. Hobel, et al. 1990. Uterine leimyomas in pregnancy: a prospective study. Obstet. Gynecol. 75: 41–44.
4. Hasan, F., K. Arumugam & V. Sivanesaratnam. 1990. Uterine leimyomata in pregnancy. Int. J. Gynecol. Obstet. 34: 45–48.
5. Ortaç, F., M. Güngör & M. Sönmezer. 1999. Myomectomy during cesarean section. Int. J. Gynecol. Obstet. 67: 189–190.
6. Burton, C.A., D.A. Grimes & C.M. March. 1989. Surgical management of leiomyoma during pregnancy. Obstet. Gynecol. 74: 707–709.

7. EXACOUSTOS, C. & P. ROSATI. 1993. Ultrasonographic diagnosis of uterine leiomyomas and complications in pregnancy. Obstet. Gynecol. **82:** 97–101.
8. LOIS, D., K. ZIKOPOULOS & E. PARASKEVAIDIS. 1994. Surgical management of leiomyomata during pregnancy. Int. J. Obstet. Gynecol. **44:** 71–72.
9. KWAWUKUME, E.Y. 2002. Myomectomy during cesarean section. Int. J. Gynecol. Obstet. **76:** 183–184.
10. ROMAN, A.S. & K.M.A. TABSH. 2004. Myomectomy at time of cesarean delivery: a retrospective cohort study. BMC Pregnancy Childbirth **4:** 14–17.
11. EHIGIEGBA, A.E., A.B. ANDE & S.I. OJOBO. 2001. Myomectomy during cesarean section. Int. J. Gynecol. Obstet. **75:** 21–25.
12. ACIEN, P. & F. QUERADA 1996. Abdominal myomectomy: results of a simple operative technique. Fertil. Steril. **65:** 41–51.
13. FEBO, G., M. TESSAROLO, L. LEO, *et al.* 1997. Surgical management of leiomyomata in pregnancy. Clin. Exp. Obstet. Gynecol. **24:** 76–78.
14. GLAVIND, K., D.H.B. PALVI & J.G. LAURISTEN 1990. Uterine myoma in pregnancy. Acta Obstet. Gynecol. Scand. **69:** 617–619.
15. BROWN, D. & M. MYRIE. 1997. Caesarean myomectomy—a safe procedure. West Ind. Med. J. **46**(Suppl 2): 45–49.
16. EHIGIEGBA, A.E. & C.E. EVBUOMWAN. 1998. Inevitable caesarean myomectomy. Trop. J. Obstet. Gynaecol. **5:** 62–63.
17. KWAWUKUME, E.Y. 2002. Caesarean myomectomy. Afr. J. Reprod. Health **6:** 38–43.
18. KAYMAK, O., E. USTUNYURT, R.E. OKYAY, *et al.* 2005. Myomectomy during cesarean section. Int. J. Gynecol. Obstet. **89:** 90–93.
19. COBELLIS, L., P. FLORIO, L. STRADELLA, *et al.* 2002. Electro-cautery of myomas during caesarean section—two case reports. Eur. J. Obst. Gynecol. Reprod. Biol. **102:** 98–99.
20. SAPMAZ, E., H. CELIK & A. ALTUNGUL. 2003. Bilateral ascending uterine artery ligation vs. tourniquet use for hemostasis in cesarean myomectomy. A comparison. J. Reprod. Med. **48:** 950–954.
21. COBELLIS, L., E. PECORI & G. COBELLIS. 2002. Hemostatic technique for myomectomy during cesarean section. Int. J. Gynecol. Obstet. **79:** 261–262.
22. ANDE, A.B., A.E. EHIGIEGBA & O.U.J. UMEORA. 2004. Repeat myomectomy at caesarean section. Arch. Gynecol. Obstet. **270:** 296–298.

Maternal Age and the Duration of the Second Stage of Labor

K. PAPADIAS, P. CHRISTOPOULOS, E. DELIGEOROGLOU,
N. VITORATOS, E. MAKRAKIS, P. KALTAPANIDOU, A. TSOUKAS,
AND G. CREATSAS

*Second Department of Obstetrics and Gynecology, Medical School,
University of Athens, Aretaieion Hospital, Greece*

ABSTRACT: The purpose of this study was to investigate the relationship
between parity, maternal age at delivery, gestational age, and duration
of the second stage of labor. In this article a retrospective analysis of
deliveries during the period from 2000 to 2005 in our Institution was
made. We recorded 208 pregnant women under the age of 20 years , 6,115
between 20 and 40 years, and 188 over the age of 40 years considering
parity, duration of second stage of labor, birth weight, and gestation
age. The correlation of the above parameters was statistically analyzed.
In primigravidas, under the age of 20 years, the second stage of labor
was significantly shorter compared to women aged over 40 years, and
significantly shorter compared to women between the age of 20 and 40
years. Gestational age at delivery was significantly shorter in women
aged over 40 years compared to those under the age of 20 years as well as
to those between 20 and 40 years of age. Age was positively correlated to
the duration of the second stage of labor and negatively correlated to the
gestation age at delivery. In multigravidas, age was negatively correlated
to the gestational age at delivery. In primigravidas, maternal age was
positively correlated with the duration of the second stage of labor. On
the contrary, gestational age at delivery was negatively correlated with
maternal age. In multigravidas, a negative correlation between maternal
age and gestational age at delivery was statistically significant.

KEYWORDS: maternal age; second stage of labor; duration

INTRODUCTION

The ideal management of the second stage of labor should maximize the
probability of vaginal delivery with the least risk of maternal and neonatal
morbidity and mortality.[1-3] Prolonged second stage of labor is associated with
increased perinatal mortality.[4] Prolonged labor can have deleterious effects on

Address for correspondence: Panagiotis Christopoulos, 1 Hariton Str., Kifissia, 14564 Athens,
Greece. Voice: 2107217835; fax: 2107233330.
e-mail: dr_christopoulos@yahoo.gr

Ann. N.Y. Acad. Sci. 1092: 414–417 (2006). © 2006 New York Academy of Sciences.
doi: 10.1196/annals.1365.039

both fetus and mother, such as uterine atony with possible hemorrhage, trauma, infection, fetal asphyxia, or finally cerebral fetal damage because of prolonged head pressure.

Unfortunately, there is little knowledge on the impact of various obstetrical parameters influencing the duration of the second stage of labor. Maternal age at delivery, gestational age, and parity are considered to be factors determining the duration of labor stages, but are poorly understood.

The purpose of our study was to evaluate the duration of the second stage of labor and to investigate the impact of a variety of obstetrical parameters, such as maternal age, parity, birth weight, and gestational age at delivery, on the duration of the second stage of labor.

MATERIALS AND METHODS

We retrospectively investigated 6,511 consecutive deliveries that took place during the period from 2000 to 2005 at the Second Department of Obstetrics and Gynaecology of Aretaieion Hospital (Athens University Medical School). Inclusion criteria were gestational age of at least 35 weeks, singleton pregnancies, and cephalic presentation. Induced labors, as well as those ending in cesarean section, or instrumental delivery, were excluded.

Women had vaginal examinations at least every 60 min, and/or when progress to full dilatation was suspected. The second stage of labor was defined as the time period from dilatation of the cervix until the moment of delivery. Cardiotocography, with continuous electronic fetal heart rate and uterine contraction registration, was applied in all women. The whole management of each labor and delivery was undertaken by the physician on duty. We registered parameters, such as duration of the second stage of labor, maternal age, parity, birth weight, and gestational age at delivery. Statistical analysis was performed with the use of Spearman's correlation.

RESULTS

Mean maternal age was 31 years (range 16–46, SD 5.5). In 3.2% of the studied subjects ($n = 208$) maternal age was <20 years (mean age 18.38), in 93.9% ($n = 6,115$) it was between 20 and 40 years (mean 27.87), and in 2.9% ($n = 188$) maternal age was >40 years (mean 41.11). The mean parity was 1.3 (range 1–5). Of the studied subjects 55.6% ($n = 3,623$) were primagravidas and 44.4% ($n = 2,888$) were multiparous.

The second stage of labor, in primigravidas under the age of 20 years (mean $31.83 \pm$ SD 21.59 min), was significantly shorter compared to women aged over 40 years (mean $45.83 \pm$ SD 29.06 min), ($P = 0.03$) and significantly shorter compared to women between 20 and 40 years of age (mean

TABLE 1. Duration of the second stage of labor (in minutes) in relation to maternal age

Age (years)	Duration of the second stage (mean ± SD)	P-value
< 20	31.83 ± 21.59	
20–40	41.71 ± 36.02	0.05
> 40	45.83 ± 29.06	0.03

41.71 ± SD 36.02 min), ($P = 0.05$) (TABLE 1). Maternal age was positively correlated to the duration of the second stage of labor (correlation coefficient 0.11, $P = 0.02$).

Gestational age at delivery was significantly shorter in women aged over 40 years (mean 37.5 ± SD 2.6 weeks), compared to those under the age of 20 years (mean 38.8 ± SD 1.2 weeks), ($P < 0.001$) and to those between 20 and 40 years of age (mean 40.9 ± SD 2.7 weeks) ($P < 0.001$) (TABLE 2). Maternal age was negatively correlated to the gestation age at delivery (correlation coefficient –0.15, $P < 0.001$). Maternal age was not significantly correlated to the fetal birth weight.

In multigravidas, the stages of labor were not significantly different between all age subgroups. Age was negatively correlated to the gestation age at delivery (correlation coefficient –0.119, $P = 0.005$). Maternal age was not significantly correlated to the fetal birth weight.

DISCUSSION

Maternal age is often discussed as a factor influencing the second stage of labor. Nowadays there is a trend toward delaying childbearing, most likely because of women's interest in further education and success in a professional career. In addition, assisted reproduction techniques give women the chance to conceive in more advanced ages. Albers reported that when maternal age was over 30 years, the second stage was found to be prolonged.[5] Also, Paterson et al. reported a positive association between maternal age and the second stage of labor.[6] According to our results, in primigravidas, maternal age was correlated with the duration of the second stage of labor: as maternal age was advancing, the duration of the second stage of labor was lasting longer. It is important to mention that there is a constant increase in the duration of second

TABLE 2. Gestational age at delivery (in weeks) in relation to maternal age

Age (years)	Gestational age at delivery (mean ± SD)	P-value
< 20	38.8 ± 1.2	
20–40	40.9 ± 2.7	$P < 0.001$
> 40	37.5 ± 2.6	$P < 0.001$

stage along with maternal age without the existence of a certain cutoff point. This finding is in accordance with the pattern suggested in earlier studies by Friedman and Sachtleben,[7] Cohen *et al.*,[8] and Adashek.[9] According to their theory, there is a gradual decrease in myometrial function with increasing age. On the contrary, gestation age at delivery was decreasing as the maternal age was advancing.

In multigravidas, only a negative correlation between maternal age and gestation age at delivery was statistically significant. In favor of this study is the great number of carefully selected and analyzed pregnant women. Unfortunately, it remained quite difficult to evaluate the interactive effect of epidural anesthesia.

In conclusion, our results are in agreement with other investigators.[10] Maternal age turns out to be one of the most influential maternal characteristics on the duration of the second stage of labor. It seems that the myometrium is affected by aging as are the rest of the muscles. As a result, the uterine muscle weakens along with the advancing age and this may explain the prolongation of the second stage of labor.

REFERENCES

1. SCHIESSL, B., W. JANNI, K. JUNDT, *et al.* 2005. Obstetrical parameters influencing the duration of the second stage of labor. Eur. J. Obstet. Gynecol. Repr. Biol. **118:** 17–20.
2. SAUNDERS, N.S., C.M. PATERSON & J. WADSWORTH. 1992. Neonatal and maternal morbidity in relation to the length of the second stage of labor. Br. J. Obstet. Gynaecol. **5:** 381–385.
3. CHENG, Y.W., L.M. HOPKINS & A.B. CAUGHEY. 2004. How long is too long: does a prolonged second stage of labor in nulliparous women affect maternal and neonatal outcomes? Am. J. Obstet. Gynecol. **191:** 933–938.
4. PIPER, J.M., D.R. BOLLING & E.R. NEWTON. 1991. The second stage of labor: factors influencing duration. Am. J. Obstet. Gynecol. **165:** 976–979.
5. ALBERS, L.L. 1999. The duration of labor in healthy women. J. Perinatol. **19:** 114–119.
6. PATERSON, C.M., N.S. SAUNDERS & J. WADSWORTH. 1992. The characteristics of the second stage of labor in 25,069 singleton deliveries in the North West Thames Health Region, 1988. Br. J. Obstet. Gynaecol. **99:** 377–380.
7. FRIEDMAN, E.A. & M.R. SACHTLEBEN. 1965. Relation of maternal age to the course of labor. Am. J. Obstet. Gynecol. **91:** 915–924.
8. COHEN, W.R., L. NEWMAN & E.A. FRIEDMAN. 1980. Risk of labor abnormalities with advancing maternal age. Obstet. Gynecol. **55:** 414–416.
9. ADASHEK, J.A., A.M. PEACEMAN, J.A. LOPEZ-ZENO, *et al.* 1993. Factors contributing to the increased cesarean birth rate in older parturient women. Am. J. Obstet. Gynecol. **169:** 936–940.
10. RASMUSSEN, S., L. BUNGUM & K. HOIE. 1994. Maternal age and duration of labor. Acta Obstet. Gynecol. Scand. **73:** 231–234.

Poor Responders in IVF

Cancellation of a First Cycle Is Not Predictive of a Subsequent Failure

STAVROULA BAKA, EVANGELOS MAKRAKIS, DESPOINA
TZANAKAKI, SOCRATES KONIDARIS, DIMITRIS HASSIAKOS,
THEODOROS MOUSTAKARIAS, AND GEORGE CREATSAS

*IVF Unit, Second Department of Obstetrics and Gynecology, Aretaieion
Hospital, University of Athens, Athens, Greece*

ABSTRACT: Management of women with a poor response to controlled
ovarian hyperstimulation during IVF remains a frustrating challenge.
The present study included 96 cycles from an equal number of women
with a poor ovarian response and successful oocyte retrieval. Poor response was defined by the presence of at least one of the following characteristics: three or fewer oocytes on retrieval, serum estradiol level less
than 500 pg/mL on the day of hCG administration, and serum FSH levels less than 20 IU/L. The same patients had a previous cycle cancelled
because of a poor ovarian response whereas in the second cycle they preferred to continue the treatment despite the poor prognosis. We obtained
241 oocytes in the 96 IVF cycles. The fertilization rate was 60.2%. Three
oocytes per cycle were retrieved in 56 cycles (58.3%), two oocytes per
cycle in 33 cycles (34.4%), and one oocyte per cycle in 7 cycles (7.3%). In
19 cycles (19.8%) no fertilization was achieved. An embryo transfer was
finally performed in 74 out of 96 cycles. Pregnancy rate was 12.5% per
cycle and 16.2% per transfer. Among the 12 pregnancies achieved, 7 were
in the 3-oocyte cycles and 5 in the 2-oocyte cycles. No pregnancies were
achieved in the 1-oocyte cycles. Our data demonstrate that continuation
of therapy in poor responders undergoing IVF can be an option despite
the low pregnancy rates. The prognosis of these patients is not affected
by a poor response in the first cycle and for some of them the outcome
can be favorable.

KEYWORDS: poor responders; IVF; ovarian stimulation; pregnancy rate

Address for correspondence: Stavroula Baka, M.D., IVF Unit, Second Department of Obstetrics
and Gynecology, Aretaieion Hospital, University of Athens, 76 Vas. Sofias Ave., GR-11528 Athens,
Greece. Voice: +30-210-6517467; fax: +30-210-7233330.
 e-mail: ivf@aretaieio.uoa.gr

Ann. N.Y. Acad. Sci. 1092: 418–425 (2006). © 2006 New York Academy of Sciences.
doi: 10.1196/annals.1365.040

INTRODUCTION

Assisted reproduction outcomes are strongly dependent on the ovarian response after controlled ovarian hyperstimulation (COH). The major goal of COH is to provide a higher number of good quality oocytes that can lead to good quality embryos for transfer and, if available, cryopreservation of excess embryos to improve the total reproductive potential.[1]

Poor response in patients with diminished ovarian reserve after a standard stimulation protocol is not unusual.[2] In this group of infertility patients an insufficient number of oocytes are obtained resulting in a low number of embryos, if any, for transfer and poor pregnancy outcome.[1] The first description of a poor response after a standard ovarian stimulation with human menopausal gonadotropins (hMG) comes from Garcia *et al.*[3] whereas the prevalence of poor responders can vary anywhere from 9% to 24% of IVF patients.[4] Most of assisted reproduction technologies (ART) specialists agree that a poor ovarian response is characterized by the production of less than three to four oocytes after intense COH, low E2 levels (500–1,000 pg/mL) on the day of human chorionic gonadotropin (hCG) administration, and high baseline (cycle day 2) serum FSH levels.[1,2,5]

Treating poor responders remains a challenge for all specialists involved in ART. Different ovarian stimulation regimens have been tested.[1,5–7] Nevertheless, most of the time, the results have been disappointing, probably because one has to deal with a nonhomogeneous population of patients.[1,2,5,6] In general, a poor response usually means a longer duration of the medication prescribed associated with a higher cost[8] whereas cancellation rates are increased.[5]

It has been suggested that cycles with a large number of recruited follicles and high estrogen levels are associated with biochemical[9] and morphological[10] endometrial alterations, which can lead to low implantation rates.[11] Therefore, in contrast, patients with a reduced number of follicles might present a better endometrium that can lead to a better implantation rate.[12]

It is already known that a diminished ovarian response declines with age and has been associated with ovarian aging.[13,14] Many poor responders can be found in the 40 and older age group.[15] Often, these patients are not treated with IVF because of poor results. The same can be the case in younger patients too[16] where cancellation rate can be as high as >15%.[17] The purpose of this study was to examine pregnancy rates in poor responders presenting for a second IVF cycle and who preferred to cancel their first cycle.

MATERIALS AND METHODS

The study included a total of 96 patients with primary "unexplained" infertility undergoing IVF–ET in the IVF Unit, Second Department of Obstetrics and Gynecology, University of Athens, with a documented poor response to

COH and successful oocyte retrieval, and who had presented a poor ovarian response in a previous IVF cycle, too. The criterion for inclusion in the study was the presence of at least one of the following characteristics: three or fewer oocytes upon retrieval, serum estradiol levels less than 500 pg/mL on the day of hCG administration, or serum FSH baseline levels less than 20 IU/L.

After being informed by the clinicians about their treatment options (to continue treatment, to have intrauterine insemination, whenever indicated, or to be cancelled), all the study subjects opted for the continuation of treatment.

All the study subjects underwent controlled ovarian hyperstimulation (COH) with a short protocol (from cycle day 2: daily administration of GnRH agonist, and from cycle day 3: daily administration of 300 IU recombinant FSH and 150 IU human menopausal gonadotropin), followed by transvaginal ultrasound-guided oocyte retrieval 35 h after the administration of 10,000 IU of human chorionic gonadotropin. IVF or ICSI was performed with the respective husband's spermatozoa, and all embryo transfers were performed on day 3 with a Wallace catheter under ultrasound guidance. Statistical analysis was performed using the Fisher's exact test. A P-value < 0.05 was considered as significant.

RESULTS

The mean age of the study subjects was 36 years (range 32–41). From the 96 oocyte retrieval procedures, 241 oocytes were recovered (TABLE 1) as follows: in 56 (58.3%) cycles 3 oocytes per cycle were retrieved, in 33 (34.4%) cycles 2 oocytes per cycle, and 1 oocyte per cycle was retrieved in 7 (7.3%) cycles (TABLE 2).

All gametes were treated by conventional IVF. In 96 oocytes no fertilization or abnormal fertilization was observed. Normal fertilization occurred in 145 oocytes (60.2%) from 77 cycles (TABLE 1). Embryo transfer was performed in 74 patients (77.1%) and a clinical (detected by ultrasonography) pregnancy was achieved in 12 patients (12.5% per cycle and 16.2% per transfer). Out of the 12 pregnancies achieved, 7 were in the 3-oocyte cycles while the remaining 5 in the 2-oocyte cycles. No pregnancies were achieved in the 1-oocyte cycles. The Fisher's exact test did not detect any significant differences between 3-oocyte versus 2-oocyte cycles ($P = 0.47$), 2-oocyte versus 1-oocyte cycles ($P = 0.36$), or 3-oocyte versus 1-oocyte cycles ($P = 0.41$) (TABLE 2).

DISCUSSION

The aim of COH for IVF treatment is to obtain as many oocytes as possible in every cycle to achieve high implantation and pregnancy rates. Unfortunately, some women are more prone than others to develop a poor response following COH.

TABLE 1. Outcomes of IVF cycles in the study population

Number of cycles	96
Collected oocytes	241
Fertilized oocytes	145
Cycles with fertilization	77
Transfer cycles	74
Pregnancies	12

Problems with poor responders in IVF arise from the difficulty of specialists to uniformly characterize this specific population,[2,18] which in fact, seems to be a heterogeneous group with various causes in different patients.[19] A poor response is often associated with ovarian reserve depletion or with older age.[20–22]

Different approaches in the treatment of poor responders have been developed[2,5] for a better outcome with no impressive or clear results: various ovulation induction protocols[6,18,23–27] with or without adjuvant therapy to COH, include growth hormone,[28,29] glucocorticoids,[30,31] oral contraceptives,[24,32] nitric oxide donors,[33] IUI,[34] natural cycle,[35–38] transfer at blastocyst stage,[39] assisted hatching,[40] intracytoplasmic sperm injection,[41] as well as other forms of special treatment like co-culture,[42] cytoplasm, and nuclear transfer,[43,44] and *in vitro* maturation of immature oocytes.[45,46]

Different classifications have been suggested for a better management of poor responders[47,48] with no significant improvement in their response to ovarian hyperstimulation protocols.[27] Actually, a poor response is a retrospective diagnosis being confirmed only after failing to respond properly to a standard protocol.[2]

The prediction of a poor response before starting therapy is difficult and challenging since no test is as accurate as the ovarian response itself to exogenous stimulation. Previous cycle cancellation and high FSH baseline levels are usually used as predictors.[2,18]

Even if cancellation can be an option,[17] patients are always given the opportunity to continue therapy with some success.[12,49] It has been shown that results can be improved by continuing the treatment despite the poor response in their first cycle.[21] In this respect, even if statistical significance could not be achieved, our results are in agreement with the previous study.[21]

TABLE 2. Categorization of achieved pregnancies in the study population regarding the collected oocytes per cycle

	Number of collected oocytes per cycle		
	3 oocytes	2 oocytes	1 oocyte
No cycles	56	33	7
No pregnancies	7	5	0

Our study group preferred continuation of therapy in their second cycle despite the repeated poor response. Pregnancy rates were not very high but obviously 12 out of our 96 patients became pregnant, a number that cannot be ignored.

In conclusion, there is a need for continuous evaluation of the methods employed to improve pregnancy rates in poor responders. We believe that, whenever possible, the continuation of therapy in poor responders can be justified even by low pregnancy rates as those in our study.

REFERENCES

1. ARSLAN, M., S. BOCCA, S. MIRKIN, *et al.* 2005. Controlled ovarian hyperstimulation protocols for *in vitro* fertilization: two decades of experience after the birth of Elizabeth Carr. Fertil.Steril. **84:** 555–569.
2. TARLATZIS, B.C., L. ZEPIRIDIS, G. GRIMBIZIS, *et al.* 2003. Clinical management of low ovarian response to stimulation for IVF: a systematic review. Hum. Reprod. Update **9:** 61–76.
3. GARCIA, J., G.S. JONES, A.A. ACOSTA, *et al.* 1983. Human menopausal gonadotropin/human chorionic gonadotropin follicular maturation for oocyte aspiration: phase II, 1981. Fertil. Steril. **39:** 174–179.
4. KEAY, S.D., N.H. LIVERSEDGE, R.S. MATHUR, *et al.* 1997. Assisted conception following poor ovarian response to gonadotrophin stimulation. Br. J. Obstet. Gynecol. **104:** 521–527.
5. FASOULIOTIS, S.J., A. SIMON & N. LAUFER. 2000. Evaluation and treatment of low responders in assisted reproductive technology: a challenge to meet. J. Assist. Reprod. Genet. **17:** 357–373.
6. MOHAMED, K.A., W.A. DAVIES, J. ALLSOPP, *et al.* 2005. Agonist "flare-up" versus antagonist in the management of poor responders undergoing *in vitro* fertilization treatment. Fertil. Steril. **83:** 331–335.
7. CHUNG, K., L. KREY, J. KATZ, *et al.* 2005. Evaluating the role of exogenous luteinizing hormone in poor responders undergoing *in vitro* fertilization with gonadotropin-releasing hormone antagonists. Fertil. Steril. **84:** 313–318.
8. LOK, I.H., S.K. YIP, L.P. CHEUNG, *et al.* 2004. Adjuvant low-dose aspirin therapy in poor responders undergoing *in vitro* fertilization: a prospective, randomized, double-blind, placebo-controlled trial. Fertil. Steril. **81:** 556–561.
9. SIMON, C., A. MERCADER, A. FRANCES, *et al.* 1996. Hormonal regulation of serum and endometrial IL-1 alpha, IL-1 beta and IL-1ra: IL-1 endometrial microenvironment of the human embryo at the apposition phase under physiological and supraphysiological steroid level conditions. J. Reprod. Immunol. **31:** 165–184.
10. KOLB, B.A., S. NAJMABADI & R.J. PAULSON. 1997. Ultrastructural characteristics of the luteal phase endometrium in patients undergoing controlled ovarian hyperstimulation. Fertil. Steril. **67:** 625–630.
11. SIMON, C., J.J. GARCIA VELASCO, D. VALBUENA, *et al.* 1998. Increasing uterine receptivity by decreasing estradiol levels during the preimplantation period in high responders with the use of a follicle-stimulating hormone step-down regimen. Fertil. Steril. **70:** 234–239.

12. BILJAN, M.M., W.M. BUCKETT, N. DEAN, *et al.* 2000. The outcome of IVF-embryo transfer treatment in patients who develop three follicles or less. Hum. Reprod. **15:** 2140–2144.

13. BECKERS, N.G.M., N.S. MACKLON, M.J.C. EIJKEMANS, *et al.* 2002. Women with regular menstrual cycles and a poor response to ovarian hyperstimulation for *in vitro* fertilization exhibit follicular phase characteristics suggestive of ovarian aging. Fertil. Steril. **78:** 291–297.

14. NIKOLAOU, D., S. LAVERY, C. TURNER, *et al.* 2002. Is there a link between an extremely poor response to ovarian hyperstimulation and early ovarian failure? Hum. Reprod. **17:** 1106–1111.

15. MUASHER, S.J. 1993. Treatment of low responders. J. Assist. Reprod. Genet. **10:** 112–114.

16. JACOBS, S.L., D.A. METZGER, W.C. DODSON, *et al.* 1990. Effect of age on response to human menopausal gonadotropin stimulation. J. Clin. Endocrinol. Metab. **71:** 1525–1530.

17. TANBO, T., P.O. DALE, T. ABYHOLM, *et al.* 1989. Follicle-stimulating hormone as a prognostic indicator in clomiphene citrate/human menopausal gonadotrophin-stimulated cycles for in-vitro fertilization. Hum. Reprod. **4:** 647–650.

18. SURREY, E.S. & W.B. SCHOOLCRAFT. 2000. Evaluating strategies for improving ovarian response of the poor responder undergoing assisted reproductive techniques. Fertil. Steril. **73:** 667–676.

19. LOUTRADIS, D., P. DRAKAKIS, S. MILINGOS, *et al.* 2003. Alternative approaches in the management of poor response in controlled ovarian hyperstimulation (COH). Ann. N.Y. Acad. Sci. **997:** 112–119.

20. FADDY, M.J., R.G. GOSDEN, A. GOUGEON, *et al.* 1992. Accelerated disappearance of ovarian follicles in mid-life: implications for forecasting menopause. Hum. Reprod. **7:** 1342–1346.

21. KLINKERT, E.R., F.J.M. BROEKMANS, C.W.N. LOOMAN, *et al.* 2004. A poor response in the first *in vitro* fertilization cycle is not necessarily related to a poor prognosis in subsequent cycles. Fertil. Steril. **81:** 1247–1253.

22. GALEY-FONTAINE, J., I. CEDRIN-DURNERIN, R. CHAIBI, *et al.* 2005. Age and ovarian reserve are distinct predictive factors of cycle outcome in low responders. Reprod. Biomed. Online **10:** 94–99.

23. BENADIVA, C.A., O. DAVIS, I. KLIGMAN, *et al.* 1995. Clomiphene citrate and hMG: an alternative stimulation protocol for selected failed *in vitro* fertilization patients. J. Assist. Reprod. Genet. **12:** 8–12.

24. SCOTT, R.T. & D. NAVOT. 1994. Enhancement of ovarian responsiveness with microdoses of gonadotropin-releasing hormone agonist during ovulation induction for *in vitro* fertilization. Fertil. Steril. **61:** 880–885.

25. LAND, J.A., M.I. YARMOLINSKAYA, J.C.M. DUMOULIN, *et al.* 1996. High-dose human menopausal gonadotropin stimulation in poor responders does not improve *in vitro* fertilization outcome. Fertil. Steril. **65:** 961–965.

26. FABER, B.M., J. MAYER, B. COX, *et al.* 1998. Cessation of gonadotropin-releasing hormone agonist therapy combined with high-dose gonadotropin stimulation yields favorable pregnancy results in low responders. Fertil. Steril. **69:** 826–830.

27. WANG, P.T., R.K. LEE, J.T. SU, *et al.* 2002. Cessation of low dose gonadotropin releasing hormone agonist therapy followed by high-dose gonadotropin stimulation yields a favorable ovarian response in poor responders. J. Assist. Reprod. Genet. **19:** 1–6.

28. SUIKKARI, A.M., V. MACLACHLAN, R. KOISTINEN, *et al.* 1996. Double-blind placebo controlled study: human biosynthetic growth hormone for assisted reproductive technology. Fertil. Steril. **65:** 800–805.

29. KOTARBA, D., J. KOTARBA & E. HUGHES. 2002. Growth hormone for *in vitro* fertilization (Cochrane Review). *In* The Cochrane Library, Vol. 1. Update Software. Oxford.

30. BIDER, D., J. BLANKSTEIN, J. LEVRON, *et al.* 1997. Gonadotropins and glucocorticoid therapy for "low responders"—A controlled study. J. Assist. Reprod. Genet. **14:** 328–331.

31. KEAY, S.D., E.A. LENTON, I.D. COOKE, *et al.* 2001. Low-dose dexamethasone augments the ovarian response to exogenous gonadotrophins leading to a reduction in cycle cancellation rate in a standard IVF programme. Hum. Reprod. **16:** 1861–1865.

32. LINDHEIM, S.R., D.H. BARAD, B. WITT, *et al.* 1996. Short-term gonadotropin suppression with oral contraceptives benefits poor responders prior to controlled ovarian hyperstimulation. J. Assist. Reprod. Genet. **13:** 745–747.

33. BATTAGLIA, C., M. SALVATORI, N. MAXIA, *et al.* 1999. Adjuvant L-arginine treatment for *in vitro* fertilization in poor responder patients. Hum. Reprod. **14:** 1690–1697.

34. WOOD, S., R. RAHIM, T. SEARLE, *et al.* 2003. Optimal treatment for poor responders to ovarian stimulation: does *in vitro* insemination offer any advantages to intrauterine insemination? Hum. Fertil. (Camb) **6:** 13–18.

35. BASSIL, S., P.A. GODIN & J. DONNEZ. 1999. Outcome of IVF through natural cycles in poor responders. Hum. Reprod. **14:** 1262–1265.

36. MORGIA, F., M. SBRACIA, M. SCHIMBERNI, *et al.* 2004. A controlled trial of natural cycle versus microdose gonadotropin-releasing hormone analog flare cycles in poor responders undergoing *in vitro* fertilization. Fertil. Steril. **81:** 1542–1547.

37. UBALDI, F.M., L. RIENZI, S. FERRERO, *et al.* 2005. Management of poor responders in IVF. Reprod. Biomed. Online **10:** 235–246.

38. KOLIBIANAKIS, E., K. ZIKOPOULOS, M. CAMUS, *et al.* 2004. Modified natural cycle for IVF does not offer a realistic chance of parenthood in poor responders with high day 3 FSH levels, as a last resort prior to oocyte donation. Hum. Reprod. **19:** 2545–2549.

39. GARDNER, D.K., P. VELLA, M. LANE, *et al.* 1998. Culture and transfer of human blastocysts increases implantation rates and reduces the need for multiple embryo transfers. Fertil. Steril. **69:** 84–88.

40. SCHOOLCRAFT, W.B., T. SCHLENKER, M. GEE, *et al.* 1994. Assisted hatching in the treatment of poor prognosis *in vitro* fertilization candidates. Fertil. Steril. **62:** 551–554.

41. MORENO, C., A. RUIZ, C. SIMON, *et al.* 1998. Intracytoplasmic sperm injection as a routine indication in low responder patients. Hum. Reprod. **13:** 2126–2129.

42. WIEMER, K.E., J. COHEN, M.J. TUCKER, *et al.* 1998. The application of co-culture in assisted reproduction: 10 years of experience with human embryos. Hum. Reprod. **13:** 226–238.

43. KEEFE, D.L., T. NIVEN-FAIRCHILD, S. POWELL, *et al.* 1995. Mitochondrial deoxyribonucleic acid deletions in oocytes and reproductive aging in women. Fertil. Steril. **64:** 577–583.

44. COHEN, J., R. SCOTT, M. ALIKANI, *et al.* 1998. Ooplasmic transfer in mature human oocytes. Mol. Hum. Reprod. **4:** 269–280.

45. RUSSELL, J.B. 1998. Immature oocyte retrieval combined with *in vitro* oocyte maturation. Hum. Reprod. **13:** 63–70.
46. LIU, J., G. LU, Y. QIAN, *et al.* 2003. Pregnancies and births achieved from *in vitro* matured oocytes retrieved from poor responders undergoing stimulation in *in vitro* fertilization cycles. Fertil. Steril. **80:** 447–449.
47. BARRI, P.N., F. MARTINEZ, B. COROLEU, *et al.* 1998. Managing non-responders. Fertility and Reproductive Medicine. Proceedings of XVI World Congress on Fertility and Sterility. 127–137.
48. GORGY, A. & M. TARAMISSI. 2001. Defining and predicting the poor responder. Fertil. Steril. **75:** 226–227.
49. LASHEN, H., W. LEDGER, A. LOPEZ-BERNAL, *et al.* 1999. Poor responders to ovulation induction: is proceeding to *in vitro* fertilization worthwhile? Hum. Reprod. **14:** 964–969.

The Varying Patterns of Neurotrophin Changes in the Perinatal Period

K.E. NIKOLAOU, A. MALAMITSI-PUCHNER, T. BOUTSIKOU,
E. ECONOMOU, M. BOUTSIKOU, K-P. PUCHNER, S. BAKA,
AND D. HASSIAKOS

*Neonatal Division, Second Department of Obstetrics and Gynecology,
University of Athens, Athens, Greece*

ABSTRACT: Neurotrophins (NTs), nerve growth factor (NGF), brain-derived neurotrophic factor (BDNF), NT-3, and NT-4 are of major importance in prenatal and postnatal brain development, due to their neuroprotective action. Developmental changes alter the neuronal responsiveness to certain NTs, which subsequently are variously expressed, to properly balance their action. The following study aimed at examining the pattern of perinatal changes of the four NTs—NGF, BDNF, NT-3, and NT-4 in 30 appropriate for gestational age (AGA) full-term fetuses and neonates by determining their circulating levels at characteristic time points. This study show a gradual decrease of circulating levels of the NTs, NT-3 and NT-4 from umbilical cord (UC) to neonates day 4 (N4), while circulating levels of NGF and BDNF present the opposite pattern: an increase from UC to N4. These patterns of perinatal changes differ according to their impact on the process of neuronal development and their reaction to perinatal stress. NT3 and NT4 have been documented to act at early stages of neuronal development and to decrease after hypoxia-ischemia, while NGF and BDNF to increase. Further studies should investigate these patterns in premature or full-term infants, presenting various pathological conditions in the perinatal period.

KEYWORDS: neurotrophins; NT-3; BDNF; NT-4; NGF; fetus; neonate; neuronal development

INTRODUCTION

In humans, four structurally related molecules: nerve growth factor (NGF), brain-derived neurotrophic factor (BDNF), neurotrophin-3 (NT-3) and neurotrophin-4 (NT-4) comprise the NT family,[1] a group of substances rendering neuroprotection, by reducing apoptosis and promoting survival and

Address for correspondence: A. Malamitsi-Puchner, M.D., Neonatal Division, Second Department of Obstetrics and Gynecology, University of Athens, 19, Soultani Street, GR-10682 Athens, Greece. Voice: +30-6944-443815; fax: +30-210-7233330.
e-mail: malamitsi@aias.gr

Ann. N.Y. Acad. Sci. 1092: 426–433 (2006). © 2006 New York Academy of Sciences.
doi: 10.1196/annals.1365.041

maintenance of neurons in the peripheral and central nervous system.[2–5] Therefore, NTs are of major importance in prenatal and postnatal brain development.[6]

Previous studies have shown that developmental changes alter the neuronal responsiveness to certain NTs, which subsequently are variously expressed, to properly balance their action.[7,8]

The following study aimed at examining the pattern of perinatal changes of the four NTs—NGF, BDNF, NT-3, and NT-4 in appropriate for gestational age (AGA) full-term fetuses and neonates by determining their circulating levels at characteristic time points.

MATERIAL AND METHODS

The study was approved by the Ethics Committee of our teaching hospital and informed consent was acquired from mothers of participating infants.

The study comprised 30 AGA full-term fetuses-neonates. For the characterization of a fetus-neonate as AGA customized centiles were calculated according to the principles of the gestation-related optimal weight (GROW) program.[9,10] This computer-generated antenatal chart takes into consideration determinants of birth weight (gestational age, neonatal gender, maternal weight at the beginning of pregnancy, maternal height, ethnic group, and parity), which adjust the normal birth weight centile limits.[9]

Mothers of included neonates were healthy and had uncomplicated pregnancy and delivery, either vaginally or by elective cesarean section. Neonates, included in the study, were single and presented neither intrauterine infection nor genetic syndromes. One and five minute Apgar scores were in all infants ≥ 7 and ≥ 8, respectively. Placentas were in all cases normal in appearance and weight. Demographic data of participating infants are given in TABLE 1.

Blood was drawn from the doubly clamped umbilical cord (UC), reflecting fetal state and from the neonates on day 1 (N1) and 4 (N4), characteristic for transition and stabilization to extrauterine life, respectively.

Collected blood was centrifuged and supernatant plasma was kept frozen at $-80°C$ until assayed. The determination of all NTs was performed by enzyme

TABLE 1. Demographic data of AGA infants and their mothers

	Mean (m)	Standard deviation (SD)
Centile	37.2	18.84
Gestational age (weeks)	38.42	1.12
Placental weight (grams)	603.79	153.19
Birth weight (grams)	3080.5	328.28
Maternal age (years)	31.1	4.38
Maternal height (cm)	165.97	6.2
Maternal weight (kilograms)	60.67	8.68

immunoassays (human β-NGF, Catalog Number DY256; human BDNF, Catalog Number DY248; human NT-3, Catalog Number DY267; human NT-4, Catalog Number DY268; R&D Systems, Inc., Minneapolis, MN). The minimum detectable concentration, intra- and interassay coefficients of variation were for: β-NGF 31.3 pg/mL, 8.9% and 12.7%, BDNF 20 pg/mL, 7.5% and 11.3%, NT-3 40.3 pg/mL, 8.2% and 11.9%, NT-4 25.8 pg/mL, 10.5%, and 15%, respectively.

STATISTICAL ANALYSIS

Shapiro Wilk normality test was applied and proved that NT-3, NT-4, and NGF levels were not normally distributed. Therefore, nonparametric procedures were used in the analysis. Wilcoxon sum rank test was used to indicate differences in NT-3, NT-4, NGF levels in plasma from the UC and the infant on the first (N1) and fourth day (N4) after birth. Spearman Rank correlation was applied to determine positive or negative relationships between the three groups in NT-3, NT-4, NGF plasma levels. In contrast to data of the previous NTs, BDNF data followed normal distribution in UC, N1, and N4. Thus, in this case, parametric procedures were applied. Paired sample t-test was performed to detect differences in BDNF levels between the groups, while Pearson correlation coefficient was applied to determine positive or negative relationships. P values <0.05 were considered significant.

RESULTS

Data on UC, N1, and N4, of NT-3, NT-4, NGF, and BDNF levels in AGA neonates are presented in FIGURES 1–4, respectively.

NT-3 levels appear to decrease gradually with time. UC NT-3 levels were found to be significantly elevated compared to N1 NT-3 levels ($P = 0.022$). Significant positive correlations were observed between UC NT-3 and N1 NT-3 ($r = 0.810$, $P < 0.001$) as well as between UC NT-3 and N4 NT-3 ($r = 0.797$, $P < 0.001$). Finally a significant positive correlation was evident between N1 NT-3 and N4 NT-3 ($r = 0.869$, $P < 0.001$).

NT4 levels followed the same pattern. UC NT-4 levels were found to be elevated compared to N1 NT-4 as well as N4 NT-4 levels, and these differences were statistically significant ($P = 0.04$ and $P < 0.001$, respectively). UC NT-4 was positively correlated to N1 NT-4 ($r = 0.966$, $P < 0.001$) and N4 NT-4 ($r = 0.957$, $P < 0.001$). A significant positive correlation was evident between N1 NT-4 and N4 NT-4 ($r = 0.978$, $P < 0.001$) as well.

NGF levels presented initially a decrease from UC to N1 and afterward an increase to N4. N4 NGF levels were significantly elevated compared to UC NGF levels ($P = 0.03$) and N1 NGF ($P = 0.019$) levels. Significant positive

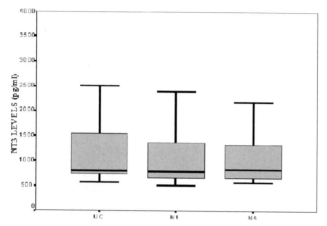

FIGURE 1. Box and whiskers plots of the concentration of NT-3 in fetal (UC), neonatal day 1 (N1) and day 4 (N4) serum samples from AGA neonates. Each box represents the median concentration with the interquartile range (25th and 75th percentiles). The upper and lower whiskers represent the range.

correlations were observed between UC NGF and N1 NGF ($r = 0.806$, $P < 0.001$) as well as N4 NGF ($r = 0.561$, $P = 0.001$). In addition, a significant positive correlation was evident between N1 NGF and N4 NGF ($r = 0.766$, $P < 0.001$).

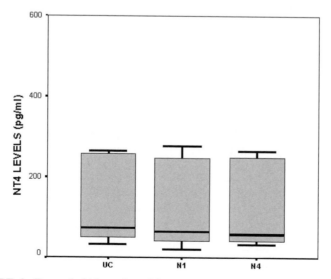

FIGURE 2. Box and whiskers plots of the concentration of NT-4 in fetal (UC), neonatal day 1 (N1) and day 4 (N4) serum samples from AGA neonates. Each box represents the median concentration with the interquartile range (25th and 75th percentiles). The upper and lower whiskers represent the range.

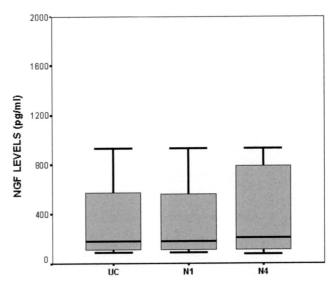

FIGURE 3. Box and whiskers plots of the concentration of NGF in fetal (UC), neonatal day 1 (N1) and day 4 (N4) serum samples from AGA neonates. Each box represents the median concentration with the interquartile range (25th and 75th percentiles). The upper and lower whiskers represent the range.

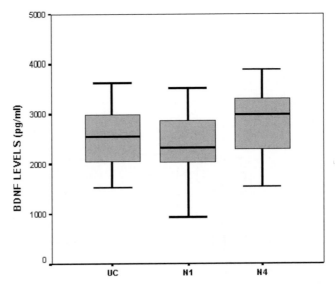

FIGURE 4. Box and whiskers plots of the concentration of BDNF in fetal (UC), neonatal day 1 (N1) and day 4 (N4) serum samples from AGA neonates. Each box represents the median concentration with the interquartile range (25th and 75th percentiles). The upper and lower whiskers represent the range.

BDNF levels appear to follow the same pattern with NGF. Testing the equality of BDNF levels between UC, N1, N4 statistical significant differences were observed between UC, N1, and N4 levels. N4 BDNF levels were elevated compared to N1 BDNF ($P = 0.001$) and UC BDNF ($P = 0.03$) levels. A significant positive correlation was observed between UC BDNF and N1 BDNF levels ($r = 0.534$, $P = 0.002$).

DISCUSSION

The results of this study show a gradual decrease of circulating levels of the NTs NT-3 and NT-4 from UC to N4. However, circulating levels of NGF and BDNF present the opposite pattern: an increase from UC to N4. These findings could be explained taking into consideration previous studies.

During the perinatal period the blood-brain barrier is immature and thus, circulating levels of NTs may represent respective central nervous system (CNS) levels.[11] After a brain injury many recovery developmental cellular mechanisms are reused in order to limit the amount of cell death and to promote plasticity, neurogenesis, and subsequent functional recovery.[12] NTs are therefore strongly upregulated following brain injury in the adult, in what can be called the brain's "endogenous neuroprotective system."[12] In particular, BDNF and NGF have been shown to be upregulated following hypoxic/ischemic (HI) type insults[12] and following insulin induced hypoglycemia.[13] NGF, BDNF, and their receptors proved to be upregulated in neurons, which are generally resistant to brain-injury-mediated cell death; this resistance may therefore be due to their NT content.[14] In contrast, NT-3 has been shown to be downregulated following HI injury.[15,16]

Treatment studies, using the NTs BDNF and NGF have shown both these factors to offer significant neuroprotection against delayed (apoptotic) neuronal death when administered centrally or systemically following brain injury in the adult[17–19] as well as in the neonate.[20,21] In agreement with its opposite response to brain injury, NT-3 was shown not to be protective against MPPt (1-methyl-4-phenylpyridinium ion)-mediated oxidative stress *in vivo*.[21] Although in our cases there were no obvious HI insults, stress and hypoxia are present in all forms of delivery.[22] Our results may imply that the increase of BDNF and NGF possibly reflect the neuroprotection against perinatal stress and hypoxia. The decrease in NT-3 levels is in agreement with the previously published data showing its downregulation after hypoxia. The decrease in NT-4 might imply similar reaction with that of NT-3.

In conclusion, circulating NTs in healthy full-term fetuses and neonates present different patterns of perinatal changes, according to their impact on the process of neuronal development and their reaction to perinatal stress. Thus, NT-3 and NT-4 levels present a gradual drop, from intra- to extrauterine life, and oppositely NGF and BDNF present an increase in their levels. Further studies should investigate these patterns in premature or full-term infants, presenting various pathological conditions in the perinatal period.

REFERENCES

1. BARDE, Y.A. 1990. The nerve growth factor family. Prog. Growth Factor Res. **2:** 237–248.
2. LEWIN, G. & Y.A. BARDE. 1996. Physiology of the Neurotrophins. Annu. Rev. Neurosci. **19:** 289–317.
3. HEFTI, F. 1986. Nerve growth factor promotes survival of septal cholinergic neurons after fimbrial transections. J. Neurosci. **6:** 2155–2162.
4. HYMAN, C., M. HOFER, Y.A. BARDE, et al. 1991. BDNF is a neurotrophic factor for dopaminergic neurons of the substantia nigra. Nature **350:** 230–232.
5. ARENAS, E. & H. PERSSON. 1994. Neurotrophin-3 prevents the death of adult central noradrenergic neurons in vivo. Nature **367:** 368–371.
6. CHOUTHAI, N.S., J. SAMPERS, N. DESAI, et al. 2003. Changes in neurotrophin levels in umbilical cord blood from infants with different gestational ages and clinical conditions. Pediatr. Res. **53:** 965–969.
7. CICCOLINI, F. & C.N. SVENDSEN. 2001. Neurotrophin responsiveness is differentially regulated in neurons and precursors isolated from the developing striatum. J. Mol. Neurosci. **17:** 25–33.
8. OPPENHEIM, R.W. 1996. The concept of uptake and retrograde transport of neurotrophic molecules during development: history and present status. Neurochem. Res. **21:** 769–777.
9. GARDOSI, J., A. CHANG, B. KALYAN, et al. 1992. Customised antenatal growth charts. Lancet **339:** 283–287.
10. GARDOSI, J., M. MONGELLI, M. WILCOX, et al. 1995. An adjustable fetal weight standard. Ultrasound Obstet. Gynecol. **6:** 168–174.
11. POLIN, R.A. & W.W. FOX. 1998. Fetal and Neonatal Physiology. WB Saunders. Philadelphia, PA.
12. HASHIMOTO, Y. & H. KAWATSURA, et al. 1992. Significance of nerve growth factor content levels after transient forebrain ischemia in gerbils. Neurosci. Lett. **139:** 45–46.
13. LINDVALL, O., P. ERNFORS, et al. 1992. Differential regulation of mRNAs for nerve growth factor, brain-derived neurotrophic factor, and neurotrophin 3 in the adult rat brain following cerebral ischemia and hypoglycemic coma. Proc. Natl. Acad. Sci. USA **89:** 648–652.
14. LEE, T.H., H. KATO, et al. 1996. Temporal profile of nerve growth factor-like immunoreactivity after transient focal cerebral ischemia in rats. Brain Res. **713:** 199–210.
15. HICKS, R.R., S. NUMAN, et al. 1997. Alterations in BDNF and NT-3 mRNAs in rat hippocampus after experimental brain trauma. Brain Res. Mol. Brain Res. **48:** 401–406.
16. LINDVALL, O., Z. KOKAIA, et al. 1994. Neurotrophins and brain insults. Trends Neurosci. **17:** 490–496.
17. CHENG, Y., J.M. GIDDAY, et al. 1997. Marked age-dependent neuroprotection by brain-derived neurotrophic factor against neonatal hypoxic-ischemic brain injury. Ann. Neurol. **41:** 521–529.

18. EBADI, M., R.M. BASHIR, *et al.* 1997. Neurotrophins and their receptors in nerve injury and repair. Neurochem. Int. **30**: 347–374.
19. SCHABITZ, W.R., S. SCHWAB, *et al.* 1997. Intraventricular brain-derived neurotrophic factor reduces infarct size after focal cerebral ischemia in rats. J. Cereb. Blood Flow Metab. **17**: 500–506.
20. ALMLI, C.R., T.J. LEVY, *et al.* 2000. BDNF protects against spatial memory deficits following neonatal hypoxia-ischemia. Exp. Neurol. **166**: 99–114.
21. KIRSCHNER, P.B., B.G. JENKINS, *et al.* 1996. NGF, BDNF and NT-5, but not NT-3 protect against MPP+ toxicity and oxidative stress in neonatal animals. Brain Res. **713**: 178–185.
22. NIKISCHIN, W., D. WEISNER & H.D. OLDIGS. 1990. Perinatal glucose metabolism as an indicator for stress and hypoxia during different forms of delivery. J. Perinat. Med. **18**: 209–213.

Insulin-Like Growth Factor–1 Isoform mRNA Expression in Women with Endometriosis

Eutopic Endometrium Versus Endometriotic Cyst

DIMITRIOS MILINGOS,[a,b] HARALAMPOS KATOPODIS,[b]
SPYROS MILINGOS,[a] ATHANASIOS PROTOPAPAS,[a]
GEORGE CREATSAS,[c] STELIOS MICHALAS,[a] ARIS ANTSAKLIS,[a]
AND MICHAEL KOUTSILIERIS[b]

[a]First Department of Obstetrics and Gynecology, Medical School, University of Athens, Greece

[b]Department of Experimental Physiology, Medical School, University of Athens, Greece

[c]Second Department of Obstetrics and Gynecology, Medical School, University of Athens, Greece

ABSTRACT: Pathogenesis of endometriosis involves growth factors, which are synthesized locally. Insulin-like growth factor-1 (IGF-1) prevents apoptosis and has mitogenic action on endometrial cells. The IGF-1 gene undergoes alternative splicing and results in three isoforms (IGF-1Ea, IGF-1Eb, and IGF-1Ec or MGF). We analyzed the mRNA expression of IGF-1 isoforms in tissue samples of eutopic endometrium and endometriotic cyst obtained during laparoscopy from women with endometriosis. We documented that all three IGF-1 isoforms are expressed in both eutopic endometrium and ovarian endometrioma. Furthermore, we documented a significant decrease in all IGF-1 isoform expression in endometriotic cyst compared to endometrium of women with endometriosis. The reduction may correlate with the disease status and presence of fibrotic inactive tissue found in late stages of the disease.

KEYWORDS: endometriosis; IGFs; IGF-1Ea; IGF-1Eb; MGF

Address for correspondence: Michael Koutsilieris, M.D., Department of Experimental Physiology, Medical School, University of Athens, 75 Micras Asias, Goudi, Athens, 115 27, Greece. Voice: 0030210-7462507; fax: 0030210-7462571.
e-mail: mkouts@medscape.com

Ann. N.Y. Acad. Sci. 1092: 434–439 (2006). © 2006 New York Academy of Sciences.
doi: 10.1196/annals.1365.042

INTRODUCTION

Endometriosis is a benign gynecologic disease that affects women of reproductive age and is defined as the presence of endometrial glandular and stromal cells outside the uterine cavity, such as the pelvic peritoneum, the ovary, the Douglas pouch, the uterosacral ligaments, the urinary bladder, and the sigmoid colon.

It is a very common condition with almost 10% prevalence in women of reproductive age and approximately 30% in women with infertility.[1] Regarding the pathogenesis of endometriosis, numerous theories have been proposed, and although the etiology still remains enigmatic there is evidence that retrograde menstruation is the primary factor for the development of the disease.[2] It is assumed that one or more mechanisms exist that enable ectopic endometrial cells to survive in the peritoneal cavity[3] and recently, there are studies investigating the role of immunological and growth factors, which are synthesized locally in the peritoneal cavity, and enhance the establishment and maintenance of endometriotic lesions.

It has been documented that ectopic endometrial cells undergo reduced spontaneous apoptosis as compared to eutopic endometrium.[4] Insulin-like growth factor-1 (IGF-1) has been shown to be one of the factors that prevents apoptosis[5] and acts mitogenically on endometrial cells, thus promoting their growth in the peritoneal cavity.[6] Furthermore, in the peritoneal fluid of women with endometriosis there are increased levels of IGF-1 compared to healthy women.[7]

The IGF-1 gene contains six exons, which undergo alternative splicing at the 3′ end and give rise to different mRNAs. The resulting peptides have a common 16 amino acid N-terminal sequence and alternative C-terminal sequence.[8] Until now, three isoforms of IGF-1 (IGF-1Ea, IGF-1Eb, and IGF-1Ec) have been identified, all of which are expressed in human tissue. They probably have different actions and bind to different receptors.[9,10] However, the physiological and molecular mechanisms that regulate their expression and their exact physiological function are still unclear.

The first isoform, IGF-1Ea, is similar to the hepatic endocrine type of IGF-1. It is the most abundant isoform in liver and contributes to growth hormone-dependent and growth hormone-independent secretion of IGF-1 into the circulation.[8,9] IGF-1Eb isoform has not been much studied but it is thought to be predominantly expressed in the liver.[11,12] The third isoform IGF-1Ec has been investigated in skeletal muscle and has been termed *mechano growth factor* (MGF) because it is increased after muscle tissue has been subjected to damage (mechanosensitive response).[10]

The purpose of our study was to evaluate the expression of IGF-1 isoforms (IGF-1Ea, IGF-1Eb, MGF) in eutopic endometrium and endometriotic cyst of women with endometriosis. In addition, we analyzed comparatively the mRNA expression of IGF-1 isoforms in tissue samples obtained from ovarian endometriotic cysts of women with endometriosis and normal endometrium of the same women.

MATERIALS AND METHODS

Tissue Sampling

Endometriotic tissue samples were collected from ovarian endometriotic cysts, from women with stage III–IV endometriosis, undergoing laparoscopy during the proliferative phase of the menstrual cycle. From the same women normal endometrium was aspirated using the Cornier device (Laboratoire C.C.D., France).

RNA Isolation and Quantitative PCR

RNA was extracted from tissue biopsies using Tri-Reagent TR (MRI Cat. TR-118) and quantified spectrophotometrically. To detect changes in gene expression between eutopic and endometriotic tissue, we performed relative quantitative reverse transcription (rqRT-PCR) analysis of total RNA extracted from tissue using the Quantum RNA 18S Internal Standards Kit (Ambion, Austin, TX, USA Cat 1716). The reverse transcriptase reaction was carried out using Superscript II RNase H' as suggested by the manufacturer (Invitrogen Corp., Cat. 18064-014, Carlsbad, CA, USA). Briefly, 2 μg of total RNA was mixed in thin walled tubes with 0.5 mM dNTPs, 5 μM random hexamer primers, and filled to 12 μL with depc-treated ddH2O. The reaction was then heated to 65 °C for 5 min and quickly chilled on ice water. The RT buffer containing 200 U/μL of superscript reverse transcriptase was then added and mixed. The reactants were incubated at 42°C for 50 min. The PCR mix for the amplification of IGF-1 isoforms consisted of 0.05 units of Taq Polymerase (Invitrogen Corp. Cat pri 10342-020), 1 × PCR Buffer, 200 μM of each dNTP, 1.6 mM MgCl2 and 4 μL of primer: Competimers mix per 100 μL of PCR mix at a ratio of 2:8, and 2 μL of RT reaction per 100 μL of PCR mix. The oligonucleotide sequence of the primer used in the PCR amplification of IGF-1Ea was: forward: 5'-GCCTGCTCACCTTCACCAGC-3' and reverse: 5'-TCAAATGTACTTCCTTCTGGGTCTTG-3'.[8] The primer sequence for PCR amplification of MGF was: forward: 5'-ACCAACAAGAACACGAAGTC-3' and reverse: 5'- CAAGGTGCAAATCACTCCTA-3'.[13] The primer sequence for PCR amplification of IGF-1Eb was selected using the Primerfinder Program based on sequences obtained from the gene bank and the specificity of the resulting primers was examined by a BLAST search.

The cycle parameters for the PCR of IGF-1Ea target fragments were: one cycle 95°C: 3 min, followed by 30 cycles at 95°C: 1 min, 54 °C: 45 sec, 72°C

45 sec, and a final cycle at 72°C for 6 min. The cycle parameters for the PCR of the IGF-1Eb fragments were: one cycle 94 °C for 4 min, followed by 32 cycles at 94°C: 45 sec, 54°C: 45 sec, 72°C: 45 sec, and a final cycle at 72°C: 4 min. The cycle parameters for MGF were: 95 °C: 3 min followed by 32 cycles at 95°C: 1 min, 58°C: 45 sec, 72 °C: 30 sec, and a final cycle at 72°C for 6 min.

The level of IGF-1 expressed in tissue biopsies was quantified using the Quantum 18S RNA Internal Standards Kit (Ambion Cat 1617). The RT-PCR products were then analyzed using the Kodak EDAS 290 Electrophoresis Documentation & Analysis System Software.

Statistical Analysis

Differences of group means were assessed for statistical significance using the one-tailed multiple comparison procedure of the Dunnett test only when treatments were compared with control values. When single comparisons were made, the Student's *t*-test was used.

RESULTS

We documented that all isoforms: IGF-1Ea, IGF-1Eb, and MGF were expressed in both eutopic endometrium and ovarian endometriotic cysts of women with endometriosis (FIG. 1).

We assessed quantitatively the mRNA expression of IGF-1 isoforms in eutopic endometrium compared to endometriotic cyst. The samples of endometrium and cyst were collected from the same women, at the same time. When we analyzed the results, we detected in all cases a decrease in the expression of IGF-1 isoforms in endometriotic cyst compared to eutopic endometrium. The IGF-1Ea expression was reduced by fourfold in endometriotic cysts, while the expression of IGF-1Eb and MGF was about half the expression in normal endometrium (FIG. 2).

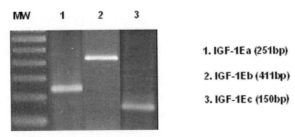

1. IGF-1Ea (251bp)

2. IGF-1Eb (411bp)

3. IGF-1Ec (150bp)

FIGURE 1. Detection of IGF-1 isoforms mRNA expression in eutopic endometrium.

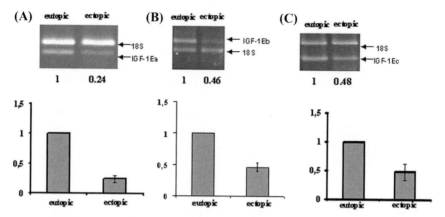

FIGURE 2. An example of the analysis of the relative expression of (**A**) IGF-1Ea, (**B**) IGF-1Eb, (**C**) IGF-1Ec mRNA as depicted by the relative quantitative-PCR normalized to 18S. There was a significant decrease in endometriotic cysts as compared to eutopic endometrium in all IGF-1 isoforms.

DISCUSSION

The role of growth factors synthesized locally in the peritoneal cavity and acting in a paracrine/autocrine way, is increasingly studied as potential factors involved in the pathogenesis of endometriosis. Levels of insulin-like growth factor have been found elevated in the peritoneal fluid of women with endometriosis, and shown to have antiapoptotic and mitogenic activity on endometriotic cells.[5-7] Therefore, IGF-1 has been implicated in the mechanism that enhances the establishment and maintenance of endometriotic cells, which reach the peritoneal cavity with retrograde menstruation. The IGF-1 gene undergoes alternative splicing, resulting in three isoforms (IGF-1Ea, IGF-1Eb, and MGF) with so far unknown physiological function.

In our study, in addition, we documented that eutopic endomerium and endometriotic cyst obtained from women with endometriosis, express all IGF-1 isoforms. The detection of MGF mRNA expression was particularly important because until now, MGF had been investigated in muscle tissue and related to features of muscle repairing mechanisms.[10]

Furthermore, we compared quantitatively the expression of IGF-1 isoforms between eutopic endometrium and ovarian endometrioma. Since endometriomas represent late stages of endometriosis, the reduction in the expression of IGF-1 isoforms in cysts correlates with the disease status. The natural history of the disease is progressive, and active endometriotic tissue is substituted by fibrotic tissue, accounting for the increase of scarring and adhesion formation met in late stages of the disease.[14] This is consistent with the results of our previous studies, where we documented increased expression of other components (uPA/IGFBP-3) of the IGF bioregulatory system, in endometriotic peritoneal lesions of women with endometriosis.[15] Thus, low IGF-1 expression represents a state of late disease, where endometrioma cells show low levels of expression.

REFERENCES

1. GIUDICE, L.C., S.I. TAZUKE & L. SWIERSZ. 1998. Status of current research on endometriosis. J. Reprod. Med. **43:** 252–262.
2. SAMPSON, J.A. 1927. Peritoneal endometriosis due to the menstrual dissemination of endometrial tissue into the peritoneal cavity. Am. J. Obstet. Gynecol. **14:** 422–469.
3. SELI, E., M. BERKKANOGLOU & A. ARICI. 2003. Pathogenesis of endometriosis. Obstet. Gynecol. Clin. N. A. **30:** 41–61.
4. GEBEL, H.M., D.P. BRAUN, A. TAMBUR, *et al.* 1998. Spontaneous apoptosis of endometrial tissue is impaired in women with endometriosis. Fertil. Steril. **69:** 1042–1047.
5. KOUTSILIERIS, M., G. MASTROGAMVRAKIS, P. LEMBESSIS, *et al.* 2001. Increased insulin-like growth factor −1 activity can rescue KLE endometrial like cells from apoptosis. Mol. Med. **7:** 20–26.
6. KOUTSILIERIS, M., E. LAVERGNE & A. LEMAY. 1997. Association of protease activity against IGFBP-3 with peritoneal fluid mitogens: possible implications for the ectopic growth of endometrial cells in women with endometriosis. Anticancer Res. **17:** 1239–1244.
7. KIM, J.G., C.S. SUH, S.H. KIM, *et al.* 2000. Insulin-like growth factors (IGFs), IGF-binding proteins (IGFBPs), and IGFBP-3 protease activity in the peritoneal fluid of women with and without endometriosis. Fertil. Steril. **73:** 996–1000.
8. HAMEED, M., R.W. ORELL, M. COBBOLD, *et al.* 2003. Expression of IGF-1 splice variants in young and old human skeletal muscle after high resistance exercise. J. Physiol. **547:** 247–254.
9. YAKAR, S., Y. WU, J. SETSER & C.J. ROSEN. 2002. The role of circulating IGF-1. Endocrine **19:** 239–248.
10. HILL, M. & G. GOLDSPINK. 2003. Expression and splicing of the insulin-like growth factor gene in rodents is associated with muscle satellite (stem) cell activation following local tissue damage. J. Physiol. **549:** 409–418.
11. HAMEED, M., K.H.W. LANGE, J.L. ANDERSEN, *et al.* 2003. The effect of recombinant human growth hormone and resistance training on IGF-1 mRNA expression in the muscles of elderly men. J. Physiol. **555:** 231–240.
12. ROTWEIN, P. 1986. Two insulin-like growth factor 1 messenger RNAs are expressed in human liver. Proc. Natl. Acad. Sci. USA **83:** 77–81.
13. BICKEL, C.S., J.M. SLADE, F. HADDAD, *et al.* 2003. Acute molecular responses of skeletal muscle to resistance exercise in able-bodied and spinal cord-injured subjects. J. Appl. Physiol. **94:** 2255–2262.
14. NISSOLE, M. & J. DONNEZ. 1997. Peritoneal endometriosis, ovarian endometriosis, and adenomyotic nodules of the rectovaginal septum are three different entities. Fertil. Steril. **68:** 585–596.
15. LEMBESSIS, P., S. MILINGOS, S. MICHALAS, *et al.* 2003. Urokinase-type plasminogen activator and insulin-like growth factor-binding protein 3 mRNA expression in endometriotic lesions and eutopic endometrium. Ann. N.Y. Acad. Sci. **997:** 223–228.

Possible Early Prediction of Preterm Birth by Determination of Novel Proinflammatory Factors in Midtrimester Amniotic Fluid

ARIADNE MALAMITSI-PUCHNER,[a] NIKOLAOS VRACHNIS,[a]
EVI SAMOLI,[b] STAVROULA BAKA,[a] ZOE ILIODROMITI,[a]
KARL-PHILIPP PUCHNER, PANTELIS MALLIGIANIS,[c]
AND DIMITRIOS HASSIAKOS[a]

[a]Second Department of Obstetrics and Gynecology, University of Athens, Athens, Greece

[b]Department of Hygiene and Epidemiology, University of Athens, Athens, Greece

[c]Iaso Maternity Hospital, Athens, Greece

ABSTRACT: Interferon-γ-inducible T cell-α chemoattractant (ITAC) is a chemokine, directing activated T lymphocytes toward sites of inflammation. ADAM-8 (A disintegrin and metalloprotease-8) is a glycoprotein expressed in cells promoting inflammation. Elastase, a protease targeting at the degradation of intra- or extracellular proteins, is inhibited by secretory leukocyte proteinase inhibitor (SLPI), which protects against microbial invasion. Adhesion molecules (soluble intercellular adhesion molecule—sICAM-1 and soluble vascular cell adhesion molecule—sVCAM-1) serve as markers of inflammation or tissue damage. We hypothesized that elevated midtrimester amniotic fluid concentrations of above substances, and decreased levels of SLPI could possibly be useful predictors of asymptomatic intra-amniotic inflammation and/or infection, eventually resulting in preterm labor and delivery. The study involved 312 women undergoing midtrimester amniocentesis. Thirteen cases, progressing to preterm delivery (<37 weeks), were matched with 21 controls (delivering >37 weeks) for age, parity, and gestational age at amniocentesis. Amniotic fluid levels of the above substances were measured by enzyme-linked immunosorbent assay (ELISA). Only amniotic fluid ITAC and ADAM-8 levels were significantly higher ($P = 0.005$ and $P < 0.02$, respectively) in women delivering at <37 weeks than at >37 weeks. SLPI concentrations significantly increased in women going into labor without ruptured membranes irrespective of pre- or term delivery ($P < 0.007$, $P < 0.001$, respectively) and

Address for correspondence: Ariadne Malamitsi-Puchner, M.D., Second Department of Obstetrics and Gynecology, University of Athens, 19, Soultani Str., GR-10682 Athens, Greece. Voice: +30-6944-443815; fax: +30-210-7233330, +30-210-3303110.
e-mail: malamitsi@aias.gr

Ann. N.Y. Acad. Sci. 1092: 440–449 (2006). © 2006 New York Academy of Sciences.
doi: 10.1196/annals.1365.043

correlated with elastase ($r = 0.508$, $P < 0.002$). In conclusion, elevated midtrimester amniotic fluid levels of ITAC and ADAM-8 could predict occult infections/inflammations, possibly resulting in preterm birth.

KEYWORDS: ITAC; ADAM-8; elastase; SLPI; adhesion molecules; midtrimester amniotic fluid; preterm birth; amniocentesis; inflammation; infection

INTRODUCTION

Intra-amniotic inflammation characterized by amniotic cavity invasion of neutrophils and secretion of cytokines and enzymes participating in the inflammatory process[1] is considered a main factor for preterm delivery.[2–5] Several studies have shown that preterm birth could result from a preexisting, occasionally asymptomatic intrauterine infection occurring relatively early in pregnancy.[6–8] In this respect, amniotic fluid microbial invasion[7,9,10] and elevated levels of the proinflammatory cytokines and chemokines[11,12] have been documented.

Interferon-γ-inducible T cell-α chemoattractant (ITAC/CXCL11), a member of the α chemokine family, is an interferon-γ-inducible protein, structurally characterized by the presence of a single amino acid, separating the first two cysteine residues of the sequence.[13–15] The main function of ITAC is to direct the migration of leukocytes, particularly activated T lymphocytes, in basal states from the bone marrow toward sites of inflammation following injury.[16] The relatively low basal ITAC expression is generally regulated by inflammation.[17,18]

ADAM-8 (A disintegrin and metalloprotease-8), naturally occurring as a membrane-bound and a soluble form,[19,20] is a glycoprotein, expressed in cells promoting inflammation, such as macrophages, granulocytes, monocytes, and B cells (also known as cell-surface antigen CD156 and MS2).[21,22] ADAM-8 is capable of cleaving a variety of peptide substrates, based on the cleavage sites of membrane-bound cytokines, growth factors, and receptors that are known to be processed by metalloproteases.[23] Furthermore, ADAM-8 may mediate extravasation of leukocytes.[24]

Elastase, a protease produced by neutrophils, histiocytes, and macrophages, is secreted during cell activation. It targets the degradation of intra- or extracellular proteins, among which elastin, collagen, and fibronectin[25,26] are included. Main inhibitor of elastase is the secretory leukocyte proteinase inhibitor (SLPI), present in the secretions of the respiratory and genital system.[27–29] SLPI limits the proinflammatory cascades ongoing during parturition, protects against microbial invasion and the response to infection,[30] and inhibits the proinflammatory action of bacterial products.[31,32] Increased elastase concentrations have been documented at the site of ruptured membranes in cases of preterm delivery.[33] The ratio of elastase to SPLI concentrations is important for the evolution of a normal delivery, as SPLI seems to protect both fetal membranes and cervical tissue.[34]

Adhesion molecules (ICAM-1 and VCAM-1), are expressed on hematopoietic and nonhematopoietic cell surfaces, particularly on endothelial cells[35] and are induced or upregulated by proinflammatory cytokines (e.g., interleukin (IL)-1, tumor necrosis factor (TNF)-α, interferon-γ).[36,37] As they mediate the adhesion of lymphocytes, monocytes, and eosinophils on activated endothelium they enable circulating white cells to enter inflamed tissues[38,39] and thus, they are used as markers of inflammation or tissue damage.[40] Both molecules exist in transmembrane and soluble (s) forms.[41,42]

The following studies[43–45] were based on the hypothesis that elevated amniotic fluid concentrations of all the above substances and decreased levels of SLPI could possibly serve as useful predictors of asymptomatic intra-amniotic inflammation and/or infection, eventually resulting in preterm labor and delivery. Therefore, we aimed to determine amniotic fluid concentrations of the above substances in women undergoing second trimester amniocentesis and subsequently delivering pre- or full-term infants.

MATERIALS AND METHODS

During the second trimester of pregnancy and under aseptic conditions, ultrasound-guided transabdominal amniocentesis was performed in 312 women for several reasons (advanced maternal age, nuchal translucency of the fetus, family history of congenital anomalies, and parental hemoglobinopathies). Out of the total 312 women, 13 progressed to spontaneous preterm delivery before 37 weeks of gestation. These women were subsequently matched for maternal age, parity, and gestational age at amniocentesis (within 2 weeks) with 21 controls (out of the initial 312 women), who delivered at or after 37 weeks of gestation healthy, appropriate for gestational age neonates (all with birth weights between the 30th and 70th customized centile, controlling for maternal height, booking weight, ethnic group, parity, gestational age, birth weight, and neonatal gender.[46] Women with multiple pregnancies, cervical dilatation (>1 cm) or ruptured membranes at the time of amniocentesis, abnormal fetal karyotype, or major fetal anomalies were excluded. All included cases and controls in this study were nonsmokers and did not report previous preterm deliveries, clinical signs of chorioamnionitis (temperature $\geq 37.8°C$, uterine tenderness, malodorous vaginal discharge, fetal tachycardia >160 beats/min, maternal tachycardia >100 beats/min, and maternal leukocytosis $>15,000$ cells/mm^3), or bleeding during the current pregnancy. Demographic data of the participating women are shown in TABLE 1. The study was approved by the Ethical Committee of our teaching hospital and included subjects who gave written informed consent.

TABLE 1. Demographic data of women participating in the study and delivering at <37 weeks of gestation (cases) or at term (≥37 weeks of gestation controls)

	Cases ($n = 13$)	Controls ($n = 21$)	P-values
Age	38.0 (±1.1)	37.1 (±0.7)	0.50
Gestational week at amnioncentesis	18.5 (±0.6)	17.4 (±0.3)	0.07
BMI	25.5 (±1.8)	22.5 (±0.9)	0.12
Gender of offspring			0.64
Male	5 (45.5%)	13 (61.9%)	
Female	6 (54.5%)	8 (38.1%)	

Amniotic fluid was drawn, centrifuged, and stored in polypropylene tubes at –80°C until assay. Levels of the substances were determined by commercially available enzyme-linked immunosorbent assays (ELISA) (R&D Systems, Minneapolis, MN 55413, USA and Immundiagnostik AG D-64625, Bensheim for elastase). Sensitivity, intra- and interassay coefficients of variation were: 13.9 pg/mL, 5.9% and 7.4% for ITAC, 16.9 pg/mL, 3.1% and 4.8% for ADAM-8, <0.12 ng/mL, 7.5% and 8.4% for elastase, <25 pg/mL, 4.5% and 6.2% for SPLI, 0.35 ng/mL, 3.5% and 5.9% for sICAM-1 and 2 ng/mL, 6.3% and 8.2% for sVCAM-1, respectively.

After applying the Kolmogorow–Smirnov test, data concerning ITAC were not normally distributed. Thus, nonparametric tests (Mann-Whitney U test and Spearman correlation coefficient) were applied in the statistical analysis. Data concerning all other parameters presented normal distribution, therefore t-test was applied in the statistical analysis. $P < 0.05$ was considered statistically significant. A receiver operating characteristic (ROC) curve was used for each variable to identify its cutoff concentrations in amniotic fluid for spontaneous preterm delivery after midtrimester amniocentesis.

RESULTS

Concentrations of amniotic fluid concentrations of all examined factors in the two groups with term or preterm delivery are demonstrated in TABLE 2. ITAC values were significantly higher ($P = 0.005$) in the amniotic fluid of women delivering before 37 weeks than after 37 weeks. Also, women with spontaneous preterm delivery after midtrimester amniocentesis had significantly higher mean amniotic fluid ADAM-8 concentrations than women in

TABLE 2. Mean value, standard error (SE), and ranges for each determined substance

	Cases ($n = 13$)			Controls ($n = 21$)			
	Mean	SE	Ranges	Mean	SE	Ranges	P
ITAC (pg/mL)	92.5	35.5	13.8–454	27.6	8.0	13.8–126	0.005
ADAM-8 (pg/mL)	1213.9	96.7	780–1,854	937.2	50.3	486–1,508	< 0.02

the control group ($P < 0.02$). Elastase, sICAM-1, and sVCAM-1 levels were higher and SLPI levels were lower in second trimester amniotic fluid of mothers, delivering preterm as compared to mothers delivering at term, however, these findings did not reach statistical significance. In contrast, SLPI levels in second trimester amniotic fluid were significantly higher in the group of women who delivered either preterm ($P < 0.007$) or at term ($P < 0.001$) with the absence of ruptured membranes prior to delivery. Furthermore, a statistical significant correlation existed between elastase and SLPI ($r = 0.508$, $P < 0.002$).

DISCUSSION

The results of the studies indicate, on the one hand, the presence of examined substances in midtrimester amniotic fluid, and on the other, that increased concentrations of ITAC and ADAM-8 may reflect intrauterine inflammation, possibly due to an occult amniotic infection responsible for preterm delivery.[7,47] Furthermore, we have shown that even from the early second trimester of pregnancy, in preterm or full-term deliveries, preceded by rupture of membranes, levels of SLPI are significantly decreased, possibly implying influence of the latter on membrane integrity.

Evidence for intrauterine infection is difficult to be uncovered since detection of microbes in the amniotic fluid is successful in only 3–48% of cases,[7,10,11] despite application of modern techniques (polymerase chain reaction). During amniocentesis, bacteria from the maternal skin can contaminate the amniotic culture[48] and lastly, more than one microorganism can be isolated from the amniotic fluid.[10,12,48]

In contrast to the diagnosis of infection, intrauterine inflammation can be easily detected by laboratory tests determining cytokines.[8] Elevated levels of several amniotic fluid cytokines (IL-1, IL-6, IL-8, and TNF-α)[49,50] have been associated with preterm prelabor rupture of membranes and preterm birth. Particularly, elevated intra-amniotic IL-6 and IL-8 concentrations are excellent predictors of preterm delivery[12,48] and of preterm prelabor rupture of membranes.[48] In this respect, the elevated amniotic fluid levels of ITAC, which is also an α-chemokine, can be explained.

In our study as much as 61.5% of preterm deliveries (<37 weeks) were associated with an elevated ADAM-8 level and thus, with assumed intra-amniotic inflammation. On the other hand, it is noteworthy that only 14% (3/21) of women who delivered at term had elevated midtrimester ADAM-8 levels, implying that an inflammation present around that time may have subsequently resolved. Analogous explanations have been given concerning IL-6 and MMP-8.[2,51]

It is known that bacterial proteases may cause fetal membrane weakening and rupture, as they decrease their strength and elasticity.[52,53] Elastase demonstrates adverse effects on the growth and properties of elastic tissue in the amnion of rabbits[54] and immunohistochemical studies of fetal ruptured membranes have shown accumulation of elastase at the ruptured site both in full- and preterm deliveries.[55,56] Nevertheless, in our study the determination of amniotic fluid elastase both in pre- and full-term deliveries could imply the participation of this substance in the common metabolic pathway of labor and therefore, its concentrations did not change significantly in both groups of the study.

On the other hand, amniotic fluid protease inhibitors (alpha 1-protease inhibitor—α1-PI-, urinary trypsine inhibitor, and SLPI) control elastase activity.[34,57–59] Thus, Zhang *et al.*[60] reported that SLPI functions as a potent anti-inflammatory agent by interfering with the signal transduction pathway leading to production of monocyte matrix metalloproteinases, which are also implicated in membrane rupture. A possible explanation for the lower SLPI concentrations in cases of ruptured membranes could be its consumption early in pregnancy during repeated inflammatory processes.

Increased circulating sICAM-1 levels in midtrimester amniotic fluid have been related to a shortened length of gestation at delivery,[61] while determination of sICAM-1, expressed on fetal membranes and mononuclear cells of amniotic fluid, has been considered a valuable biomarker for early detection of acute chorioamnionitis and the possibility of premature rupture of membranes.[62] Nevertheless, another study could not show amniotic fluid sICAM-1 concentrations significantly different between patients with and without intra-amniotic infection,[63] a finding being in accordance with our result, referring to the incidence of preterm delivery. As for midtrimester amniotic fluid sVCAM-1 concentrations no relevant studies exist in the international literature.

In conclusion, our data indicate that two novel proinflammatory substances, ITAC and ADAM-8, demonstrate elevated midtrimester amniotic fluid concentrations in women who subsequently deliver before 37 weeks of gestation as compared to women who deliver at term. Additionally, second trimester amniotic fluid SLPI levels are significantly decreased in cases where pre- or full-term delivery is preceded by membrane rupture. Therefore, determination of ITAC, ADAM-8, and SLPI, either alone or in combination with other cytokines, in transabdominally acquired amniotic fluid, during second trimester amniocentesis, could be a helpful tool for timely detection and treatment of occult infections/inflammations, as well as prediction of rupture of membranes either in the second or in the third trimester.

REFERENCES

1. SCHETTLER, A., H. THORN, B.M. JOCKUSCH, *et al.* 1991. Release of proteinases from stimulated polymorphonuclear leukocytes. Evidence for subclasses of the main granule types and their association with cytoskeletal components. Eur. J. Biochem. **197:** 197–202.

2. ROMERO, R., H. MUNOZ, R. GOMEZ, *et al.* 1995. Two thirds of spontaneous abortion/fetal deaths after amniocentesis are the results of a pre-existing subclinical inflammatory process of the amniotic cavity [abstract No. 24]. Am. J. Obstet. Gynecol. **172:** 261.

3. WENSTROM, K.D., W.W. ANDREWS, T. TAMURA, *et al.* 1996. Elevated amniotic fluid interleukin-6 levels at genetic amniocentesis predict subsequent pregnancy loss. Am. J. Obstet. Gynecol. **175:** 830–833.

4. SPONG, C.Y., A. GHIDINI, D.M. SHERER, *et al.* 1997. Angiogenin: a marker for preterm delivery in midtrimester amniotic fluid. Am. J. Obstet. Gynecol. **176:** 415–418.

5. WENSTROM, K.D., ANDREWS, W.W., HAUTH, J.C. *et al.* 1998. Elevated mid-trimester amniotic fluid interleukin-6 levels predict preterm delivery. Am. J. Obstet. Gynecol. **178:** 546–550.

6. WENSTROM, K.D., W.W. ANDREWS, N.E. BOWLES, *et al.* 1998. Intrauterine viral infection at the time of second trimester genetic amniocentesis. Obstet. Gynecol. **92:** 420–424.

7. GOLDENBERG, R.L., J.C. HAUTH & W.W. ANDREWS. 2000. Intrauterine infection and preterm delivery. N. Engl. J. Med. **342:** 1500–1507.

8. YOON, B.H., R. ROMERO, J.B. MOON, *et al.* 2001. Clinical significance of intra-amniotic inflammation in patients with preterm labor and intact membranes. Am. J. Obstet. Gynecol. **185:** 1130–1136.

9. CARROLL, S.G., S. PAPAIOANNOU, I.L. NTUMAZAH, *et al.* 1996. Lower genital tract swabs in the prediction of intrauterine infection in preterm prelabour rupture of the membranes. Br. J. Obstet. Gynaecol. **103:** 54–59.

10. GOMEZ, R., R. ROMERO, S.S. EDWIN, *et al.* 1997. Pathogenesis of preterm labor and preterm premature rupture of membranes associated with intraamniotic infection. Infect. Dis. Clin. North Am. **11:** 135–176.

11. HSU, C.D., E. MEADDOUGH, K. AVERSA, *et al.* 1998. Elevated amniotic fluid levels of leukemia inhibitory factor, interleukin 6 and interleukin 8 in intra-amniotic infection. Am. J. Obstet. Gynecol. **179:** 1267–1270.

12. EL-BASTAWISSI, A.Y., M.A. WILLIAMS, D.E. RILEY, *et al.* 2000. Amniotic fluid interleukin-6 and preterm delivery: a review. Obstet. Gynecol. **95:** 1056–1064.

13. COLE, K.E., C.A. STRICK, T.J. PARADIS, *et al.* 1998. Interferon-inducible T cell alpha chemoattractant (I-TAC); a novel non-ELR CXC chemokine with potent activity on activated T cells through selective high affinity binding to CXCR3. J. Exp. Med. **187:** 2009–2021.

14. BAGGIOLINI, M., B. DEWALD & B. MOSER. 1994. Interleukin 8 and related chemotactic cytokines-CXC and CC chemokines. Adv. Immunol. **55:** 97–179.

15. SOZZANI, S., M. LOCATI, P. ALLAVENA, *et al.* 1996. Chemokines: a superfamily of chemotactic cytokines. Int. J. Clin. Lab. Res. **26:** 69–82.

16. LU, B., A. HUMBLES, D. BOTA, C. GERARD, *et al.* 1999. Structure and function of the murine chemokine receptor CXCR3. Eur. J. Immunol. **29:** 3804–3812.

17. LOETSCHER, P., M. SEITZ, M. BAGGIOLINI, *et al.* 1996. Interleukin-2 regulates CC chemokine receptor expression and chemotactic responsiveness in T lymphocytes. J. Exp. Med. **184:** 569–577.

18. BLUEL, C.C., L. WU, J.A. HOXIE, T.A. SPRINGER, *et al.* 1997. The HIV coreceptors CXCR4 and CCR5 are differentially expressed and regulated on human T lymphocytes. Proc. Natl. Acad. Sci. USA **94:** 1925–1930.

19. CHOI, S.J., J.H. HAN & G.D. ROODMAN. 2001. ADAM-8: a novel osteoclast stimulating factor. J. Bone Miner. Res. **16:** 814–822.

20. PRIMAKOFF, P. & D.G. MYLES. 2000. The ADAM gene family: surface proteins with adhesion and protease activity. Trends Genet. **16:** 83–87.
21. YOSHIYAMA, K., Y. HIGUCHI, M. KATAOKA, *et al.* 1997. CD156 (Human ADAM-8): expression, primary amino acid sequence, and gene location. Genomics **41:** 56–62.
22. YOSHIDA, S., M. SETOGUCHI, Y. HIGUCHI, *et al.* 1990. Molecular cloning of cDNA encoding MS2 antigen, a novel cell surface antigen strongly expressed in murine monocytic lineage. Int. Immunol. **2:** 585–591.
23. AMOUR, A., C.G. KNIGHT, W.R. ENGLISH, *et al.* 2002. The enzymatic activity of ADAM-8 and ADAM9 is not regulated by TIMPs. FEBS Lett. **31:** 154–158.
24. YAMAMOTO, S., Y. HIGUCHI, K. YOSHIYAMA, *et al.* 1999. ADAM family proteins in the immune system. Immunol. Today **20:** 278–284.
25. GADEK, J.E., G.A. FELLS, D.G. WRIGHT, *et al.* 1980. Human neutrophil elastase functions as a type III collagen "collagenase." Biochem. Biophys. Res. Commun. **95:** 1815–1822.
26. MAINARDI, C.L., D.L. HASTY, J.M. SEYER, *et al.* 1980. Specific cleavage of human type III collagen by human polymorphonuclear leukocyte elastase. J. Biol. Chem. **255:** 12006–12010.
27. SALLENAVE, J.M., M. SI TAHAR, G. COX, *et al.* 1997. Secretory leukocyte proteinase inhibitor is a major leukocyte elastase inhibitor in human neutrophils. J. Leukoc. Biol. **61:** 695–702.
28. BERGENFELDT, M., L. AXELSSON & K. OHLSSON. 1992. Release of neutrophil proteinase 4 and leukocyte elastase during phagocytosis and their interaction with proteinase inhibitors. Scand. J. Clin. Lab. Invest. **52:** 823–829.
29. HELMIG, R., N. ULDBJERG & K. OHLSSON. 1995. Secretory leukocyte protease inhibitor in the cervical mucus and in the fetal membranes. Eur. J. Obstet. Gynecol. Reprod. Biol. **59:** 95–101.
30. DENISON, F.C., R.W. KELLY, A.A. CALDER, *et al.* 1999. Secretory leukocyte protease inhibitor concentration increases in amniotic fluid with the onset of labour in women: characterization of sites of release within the uterus. J. Endocrinol. **161:** 299–306.
31. JIN, F.Y., C. NATHAN, D. RADZIOCH, *et al.* 1997. Secretory leukocyte protease inhibitor: a macrophage product induced by and antagonistic to bacterial lipopolysaccharide. Cell **88:** 417–426.
32. DING, A., N. THIEBLEMONT, J. ZHU, *et al.* 1999. Secretory leukocyte protease inhibitor interferes with uptake of lipopolysaccharide by macrophages. Infect. Immun. **67:** 4485–4489.
33. HELMIG, B.R., R. ROMERO, J. ESPINOZA, *et al.* 2002. Neutrophil elastase and secretory leukocyte protease inhibitor in prelabor rupture of membranes, parturition and intra-amniotic infection. J. Matern. Fetal Neonatal Med. **12:** 237–246.
34. HELMIG, R., N. ULDBJERG & K. OHLSSON. 1995. Secretory leukocyte protease inhibitor in the cervical mucus and in the fetal membranes. Eur. J. Obstet. Gynecol. Reprod. Biol. **59:** 95–101.
35. DUSTIN, M.L., R. ROTHLEIN, A.K. BHAN, *et al.* 1986. Induction by IL-1 and interferon-gamma: tissue distribution, biochemistry, and function of a natural adherence molecule (ICAM-1). J. Immunol. **137:** 245–254.
36. ROTHLEIN, R., M. CZAJKOWSKI, M.M. O'NEILL, *et al.* 1988. Induction of intercellular adhesion molecule 1 on primary and continuous cell lines by pro-inflammatory cytokines. Regulation by pharmacologic agents and neutralizing antibodies. J. Immunol. **141:** 1665–1669.

37. MASINOVSKY, B., D. URDAL & W.M. GALLATIN. 1990. IL-4 acts synergistically with IL-1 beta to promote lymphocyte adhesion to microvascular endothelium by induction of vascular cell adhesion molecule-1. J. Immunol. **145:** 2886–2895.

38. YAN, H.C., I. JUHASZ, J. PILEWSKI, et al. 1993. Human/severe combined immunodeficient mouse chimeras. An experimental in vivo model system to study the regulation of human endothelial cell-leukocyte adhesion molecules. J. Clin. Invest. **91:** 986–996.

39. LOBB, R. 1991. Vascular adhesion molecules. In Cellular and Molecular Mechanisms of Inflammation. C.G.Cochrane & M.A. Gimbrone Eds: 151–167 Academic Press. London.

40. ROTHLEIN, R., E.A. MAINOLFI, M. CZAJKOWSKI, et al. 1991. A form of circulating ICAM-1 in human serum. J. Immunol. **147:** 3788–3793.

41. VAN DE STOLPE, A. & P.T. VAN DER SAAG. 1996. Intercellular adhesion molecule-1. J. Mol. Med. **74:** 13–33.

42. TERRY, R.W., L. KWEE, J.F. LEVINE, et al. 1993. Cytokine induction of an alternatively spliced murine vascular cell adhesion molecule (VCAM) mRNA encoding a glycosylphosphatidylinositol-anchored VCAM protein. Proc. Natl. Acad. Sci. USA **90:** 5919–5923.

43. MALAMITSI-PUCHNER, A., N. VRACHNIS, E. SAMOLI, et al. 2006. Elevated second trimester amniotic fluid interferon gamma-inducible T-cell alpha chemoattractant concentrations as a possible predictor of preterm birth. J. Soc. Gynecol. Investig. **13:** 25–29.

44. VRACHNIS, N., A. MALAMITSI-PUCHNER, E. SAMOLI, et al. 2006. Elevated midtrimester amniotic fluid ADAM-8 concentrations as a potential risk factor for preterm delivery. J. Soc. Gynecol. Investig. **13:** 186–190.

45. MALAMITSI-PUCHNER, A., N. VRACHNIS, E. SAMOLI, et al. 2006. Investigation of midtrimester amniotic fluid factors as potential predictors of term and preterm deliveries. Mediators Inflamm. **2006**(4): 1–5.

46. GARDOSI, J., A. CHANG, B. KAYLAN, et al. 1992. Customised antenatal growth charts. Lancet **339:** 283–287.

47. WATTS, D.H., M.A. KROHN, S.L. HILLIER, et al. 1992. The association of occult amniotic fluid infection with gestational age and neonatal outcome among women in preterm labor. Obstet. Gynecol. **79:** 351–357.

48. JACOBSSON, B., I. MATTSBY-BALTZER, B. ANDERSCH, et al. 2003. Microbial invasion and cytokine response in amniotic fluid in a Swedish population of women with preterm prelabor rupture of membranes. Acta Obstet. Gynecol. Scand. **82:** 423–431.

49. ASRAT, T. 2001. Intra-amniotic infection in patients with preterm prelabor rupture of membranes. Pathophysiology, detection and management. Clin. Perinatol. **28:** 735–751.

50. ROMERO, R., B.H. YOON, M. MAZOR, et al. 1993. A comparative study of the diagnostic performance of amniotic fluid glucose, white blood cell count, interleukin-6 and gram stain in the detection of microbial invasion in patients with preterm premature rupture of membranes. Am. J. Obstet. Gynecol. **169:** 839–851.

51. YOON, B.H., S.Y. OH, R. ROMERO, et al. 2001. An elevated amniotic fluid matrix metalloproteinase-8 level at the time of mid-trimester genetic amniocentesis is a risk factor for spontaneous preterm delivery. Am. J. Obstet. Gynecol. **185:** 1162–1167.

52. MCGREGOR, J.A., D. LAWELLIN, A. FRANCO-BUFF, et al. 1986. Protease production by microorganisms associated with reproductive tract infection. Am. J. Obstet. Gynecol. **154:** 109–114.

53. McGregor, J.A., J.I. French, D. Lawellin, *et al.* 1986. *In vitro* study of bacterial protease–induced reduction of chorioamniotic membrane strength and elasticity. Obstet. Gynecol. **69:** 167–174.

54. Chimura, T. & K. Fujimori. 1989. An experimental study on the effects of elastase, bleomycin and infection on the growth and tensile strength of elastic tissue in rabbit fetal membranes. Asia Oceania J. Obstet. Gynaecol. **15:** 307–312.

55. Kanayama, N., T. Terao & K. Horiuchi. 1988. The role of human neutrophil elastase in the premature rupture of membranes. Asia Oceania J. Obstet. Gynaecol. **14:** 389–397.

56. Halaburt, J.T., N. Uldbjerg, R. Helmig, *et al.* 1989. The concentration of collagen and the collagenolytic activity in the amnion and the chorion. Eur. J. Obstet. Gynecol. Reprod. Biol. **31:** 75–82.

57. Denison, F.C., R.W. Kelly, A.A. Calder, *et al.* 1999. Secretory leukocyte protease inhibitor concentration increases in amniotic fluid with the onset of labour in women: characterization of sites of release within the uterus. J. Endocrinol. **161:** 299–306.

58. Kanayama, N., H. Kamijo & T. Terao. 1986. The relationship between trypsin activity in amniotic fluid and premature rupture of membranes. Am. J. Obstet. Gynecol. **155:** 1043–1048.

59. Akutsu, H. & H. Iwama. 2000. Concentrative relationship between polymorphonuclear elastase and urinary trypsin inhibitor in amniotic fluid. Arch. Gynecol. Obstet. **263:** 156–159.

60. Zhang, Y., D.L. DeWitt & T.B. McNeely. 1997. Secretory leukocyte protease inhibitor suppresses the production of monocyte prostaglandin H synthase-2, prostaglandin E2, and matrix metalloproteinases. J. Clin. Invest. **99:** 894–900.

61. Salafia, C.M., G.R. DeVore, E. Mainolfi, *et al.* 1993. Circulating intercellular adhesion molecule-1 in amniotic fluid, maternal serum alpha-fetoprotein levels, and intrauterine growth retardation. Am. J. Obstet. Gynecol. **169:** 830–834.

62. Shaarawy, M., S.Y. El-Mallaah, A.S. El-Dawakhly, *et al.* 1998. The clinical value of assaying maternal serum and amniotic fluid intercellular adhesion molecule-1 (ICAM-1) in cases of premature rupture of membranes. Cytokine. **10:** 989–992.

62. Hsu, C.D., K. Aveersa & E. Meaddough. 2000. The role of amniotic fluid interleukin-6, and cell adhesion molecules, intercellular adhesion molecule-1 and leukocyte adhesion molecule-1, in intra-amniotic infection. Am. J. Reprod. Immunol. **43:** 251–254.

Effect of Prolactin in the Absence of hCG on Maturation, Fertilization, and Embryonic Development of *in Vitro* Matured Mouse Oocytes

ERASMIA KIAPEKOU,[a] EVANGELIA ZAPANTI,[b]
GEORGE MASTORAKOS,[c] PANAGIOTIS BERETSOS,[a] RITSA BLETSA,[a]
PETER DRAKAKIS,[a] DIMITRIS LOUTRADIS,[a]
AND ARISTIDIS ANTSAKLIS[a]

[a]*First Department of Obstetrics and Gynecology, Alexandra Hospital, University of Athens, Athens, Greece*

[b]*First Endocrine Section, Alexandra Hospital, Athens, Greece*

[c]*Endocrine Unit, Second Department of Obstetrics and Gynecology, Aretaieion Hospital, University of Athens, Athens, Greece*

ABSTRACT: Oocyte maturation is a complex process involving both the progression of meiotic cycle and the reprogramming of cytoplasmic events. The aim of this study was to investigate the effects of prolactin (PRL) in the *in vitro* maturation (IVM) of preantral mouse oocytes, in the absence of human chorionic gonadotrophin (hCG). Mouse preantral follicles were collected from female mice without prior hormonal ovarian stimulation and were cultured in the presence of varying concentrations of PRL (20, 100, 200, and 300 ng/mL) for 12 days. A group of *in vitro* matured oocytes were assessed for polar body (PB) formation, while the rest were fertilized and embryonic development was recorded. The maturation of preantral mouse follicles, as well as their fertilization and cleavage rates, observed when the culture medium was supplemented with middle- and high-range doses of PRL was beneficially affected. This effect was considerably high, although the culture media lacked hCG, a hormone extensively used in modern ovulation induction regiments, as well as in IVM media.

KEYWORDS: embryonic development; fertilization; IVM; oocyte maturation; prolactin

Address for correspondence: Erasmia Kiapekou, 25 Karaiskaki Street, 15 772 Athens, Greece. Voice: 0030-697-7252111; fax: 0030-210-7470460.
e-mail: ekiapek@otenet.gr

Ann. N.Y. Acad. Sci. 1092: 450–459 (2006). © 2006 New York Academy of Sciences.
doi: 10.1196/annals.1365.044

INTRODUCTION

Oocyte maturation begins with the migration of primordial germ cells to the genital ridge of a developing female embryo and the release of an ovum that has completed metaphase II in a postpubertal ovary.

Oocyte maturation is a complex process involving both the progression of meiotic cycle and the reprogramming of cytoplasmic events. Meiotic maturation of mammalian oocytes *in vitro* was first described in rabbits by Pincus and Enzmann in 1935.[1] Nevertheless, the developmental potential after *in vitro* maturation (IVM) is disappointingly low even nowadays.

One of the most significant aspects on this field is to establish a culture system to provide the experimental framework for identification of molecular events of oocyte growth and maturation and for resolving the complex interactions of hormones, growth factors, and cell-to-cell communication that will lead to the formation of oocytes fully competent to confer successfully to embryonic development.

However, in the near future, immature oocyte retrieval, combined with IVM, could possibly replace standard stimulated *in vitro* fertilization (IVF). Maturation of oocytes has two aspects: (i) nuclear maturation, leading to the extraction of the first polar body (PB), and (ii) cytoplasmic maturation that permits the protein synthesis required for normal fertilization and early embryonic development to happen.

The growth of preantral follicles renders them more dependent on follicle-stimulating hormone (FSH),[2] the primary factor responsible for ovarian follicular recruitment. In addition, some growth factors, such as epidermal growth factor (EGF) and insulin-like growth factor I (IGF I),[3,4] have been identified to hold a significant role, while several nonsteroid hormones, like growth hormone (GH)[4] and prolactin (PRL),[5] have also been implicated in the process of IVM.

The present study was designed to further investigate the effects of PRL in the maturation of preantral mouse oocytes during the IVM process, particularly in the absence of human chorionic gonadotrophin (hCG), a hormone extensively used in modern ovulation induction regiments, as well as in IVM media.

MATERIALS AND METHODS

Animals

Preantral follicles were obtained from 14-day-old female mice (New Zealand Black [NZB] × New Zealand White [NZW]) (Hellenic Pasteur Institute, Athens, Greece) without prior hormonal ovarian stimulation. The mice were sacrificed by cervical dislocation and their ovaries were removed.

MATERIALS

Dulbecco's phosphate-buffered saline (DPBS), α-minimal essential medium (α-MEM) culture medium, fetal bovine serum (FBS), insulin-transferrin-selenium (ITS), human EGF from Invitrogen Life Technologies (Paisley, UK); bovine serum albumin (BSA) and human PRL from Sigma-Aldrich (Dorset, UK); recombinant human FSH (r-FSH) from Organon (Oss, the Netherlands); culture dishes (Falcon, No. 3037) from Becton Dickinson Co., (New Jersey, NJ).

METHODS

Isolation of Mouse Preantral Follicles

Mouse preantral follicles were released by puncturing the ovaries in Leibovitz L15 medium (with L-Glutamine) supplemented with 10% FBS, penicillin, and streptomycin.[6] The diameter of preantral follicles selected for culture was 100–130 μm. The follicles had at least one granulosa cell layer and the oocyte was centrally located.

IVM of Preantral Follicles

Collected follicles were cultured in α-MEM supplemented with 100 mIU/mL r-FSH, 5% FBS, and ITS in a concentration of 10 mL ITS per medium litre. To investigate the role of PRL on the IVM of mouse preantral follicles, different sets of cultures were set up with varying concentrations of this hormone in the medium. Four concentrations of PRL were employed (20, 100, 200, and 300 ng/mL). Two different sets of control samples were also employed. In particular, both FSH and PRL were omitted for the first set of controls, while only PRL was absent in the second set. A total of 10–20 follicles were placed in the central well of a culture dish with 500 μL of the corresponding culture medium under 500 mL of mineral oil. In addition, 4 mL of culture medium were placed in the surrounding area of the dish to maintain humidity. Culture conditions were adjusted at 37°C, 5% CO_2 concentration, 95% humidity, and pH 7.3–7.4. On day 2 of culture 500 μL of medium were added to each well. Subsequently, half of the medium was replaced by fresh medium every other day. After 12 days of culture, 5 ng/mL of EGF were added to the culture medium, for the improvement of oocyte maturation.[7,8]

A total of 16–18 h after the addition of EGF, the formation of cumulus oocyte complexes (COCs) was assessed and they were collected and mechanically denuded to either assess nuclear maturation or be *in vitro* fertilized.

IVF

IVF of *in vitro* matured oocytes of all groups was performed to evaluate the capacity for fertilization of the oocytes and their capacity for early embryonic development. The *in vitro* matured COCs were transferred into a Falcon culture dish (No. 3037) containing 1 mL drop of Ham's F-10 medium supplemented with 4 mg/mL of BSA, under oil.

Spermatozoa were collected by adult male mice of the same strain as the females. In particular, the mice were sacrificed as described earlier and after the dissection of epididymitis, the vas deferens was cut close to the epididymitis and was placed into 500 μL drop of pregassed Ham's F-10 medium supplemented with 10 mg/mL BSA under oil. Subsequently, the sperm was squeezed out by watchmaker's forceps and was incubated for 1.5 h at 37°C to undergo capacitation. At 16–18 h post-EGF addition 100 μL of sperm (1–2×10^6 spermatozoa/mL) was added to the drops containing mature oocytes and the whole was incubated for 3–4 hours at 37°C. The fertilized oocytes were transferred to the culture medium that contained Ham's F-10 medium supplemented with (4 mg/mL) BSA under oil for 5 days until the blastocyst stage.

Assessment of IVM and Early Embryonic Development of Mouse Preantral Follicles

By employing an inverted microscope (Nikon, Japan) the percentage of nuclear maturation was evaluated as the percentage of oocytes with the first PB to the total number of COCs. In addition, the percentage of GV (germinal vesicle formation) stage oocytes, and the percentage of oocytes that reinitiated meiosis (GV breakdown oocytes, GVBD) to the total number of COCs were evaluated.

Fertilization was assessed by the development of the embryo to the four-cell stage. Embryonic development was assessed by the presence of two-cell embryos, morulae and blastocysts (2nd, 4th, and 5th day after fertilization, respectively). The development rate for each group was calculated as the percentage of fertilized oocytes developed to the corresponding embryonic stage.

Statistical Analysis

The replicate data were converted to the corresponding rates and the results were expressed as mean percentages ± SEM. Analysis was performed using one factor ANOVA of repeated measures. Groups with $P < 0.05$ were considered statistically different.

RESULTS

Evaluation of PRL Effect on IVM of Mouse Oocytes

More than half of the preantral follicles that were cultured in the absence of FSH and/or PRL progressed only to the GV stage of oocyte development (59.8% ± 1.7%), while those that were cultured in the presence of FSH only or FSH supplemented by low doses of PRL (20 ng/mL) were found in their majority to be in the GVBD stage when assessed (55.5% ± 1.1% and 55.2% ± 0.4%, respectively) (FIG. 1). When middle- and high-range doses of PRL (100, 200, 300 ng/mL) were added to the culture medium, the percentage of nuclear maturation of oocytes (PB maturation group) was statistically higher, compared to the control and FSH only samples (FIG. 1). In fact, the maturation rates to PB in those PRL groups varied between 37.5% and 41.5%, compared to 9.1% ± 0.8% and 22.3% ± 1.4% in the control and FSH only groups, respectively ($P < 0.01$). Interestingly, the presence of FSH in the culture medium resulted

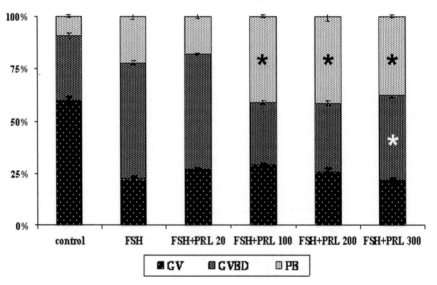

FIGURE 1. Percentage of *in vitro* matured oocytes at the GV, GV breakdown (GVBD), and PB extrusion stages of meiosis, after IVM of different groups of mouse preantral follicles in the presence of varying concentrations of PRL (20, 100, 200, and 300 ng/mL) supplemented by FSH/EGF. Controls (no medium supplementation) and FSH only samples were also included. Each bar represents the total number of mouse preantral follicles used in each condition and consists of three parts that correspond to the percentage of matured oocytes that reached the GV, GVBD, and PB stages of meiosis. Percentages are presented as means (±standard error of means) and groups statistically different from both the control and FSH only samples are noted by an asterisk.

to more oocytes undergoing full nuclear maturation (PB stage) compared to the control sets where no hormones were employed ($P < 0.01$). On the contrary, the supplementation of the culture medium with low doses of PRL (20 ng/mL) did not appear to influence the maturation rate to PB (18% ± 1%) more than the presence of FSH ($P > 0.05$ when compared to the FSH sets and $P < 0.1$ compared to the control sets). Clearly, only a small proportion of preantral follicles had undergone nuclear maturation to the GV stage after culture in the absence of PRL or small doses of PRL.

Evaluation of PRL Effect on IVF of Mouse Oocytes

Fertilization was assessed by the development of mouse embryos to the two-cell stage. The fertilization rate of mouse *in vitro*-matured oocytes in the absence of FSH and/or PRL (control) was significantly low (13.7% ± 2%). The supplementation of the culture medium with FSH did not appear to influence the capacity for fertilization of the *in vitro* matured oocytes (11.5% ± 1.2%, $P > 0.05$) and neither did low doses of PRL (12.7% ± 1.3%, $P > 0.05$) (FIG. 2). Nevertheless, the addition of middle- to high-range doses of PRL (100,

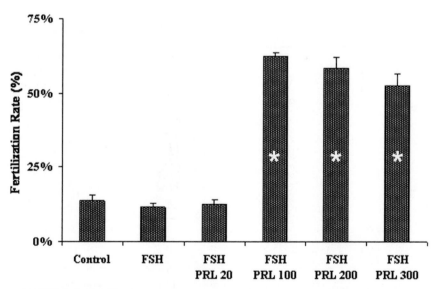

FIGURE 2. Fertilization rate of *in vitro* matured oocytes, after IVM of different groups of mouse preantral follicles in the presence of varying concentrations of PRL (20, 100, 200, and 300 ng/mL) supplemented by FSH/EGF. Controls (no medium supplementation) and FSH only samples were also included. Percentages are presented as means (±standard error of means) and groups statistically different from both the control and FSH only samples are noted by an asterisk.

200, and 300 ng/mL) during the maturation process increased the fertilization of the resulting oocytes about five times (62.5% ± 1.3%, 58.4% ± 3.6%, and 52.7% ± 3.9%, $P < 0.01$ compared to the previous sets). Furthermore, the fertilization rate in those sets did not appear to be affected by the dose of PRL ($P > 0.05$), although a tendency for a higher rate was observed when the medium was supplemented with 100–200 ng/mL of PRL.

Evaluation of PRL Effect on Embryonic Development

As described in the previous section, only about one-tenth of the oocytes matured *in vitro* in the absence of any hormones (control) or in the presence of FSH, supplemented or not by low doses of PRL, reaching the two-cell embryonic stage of development. Nonetheless, none of these progressed to the morula or blastocyst stage (FIG. 3). On the contrary, the maturation of oocytes in the presence of 100, 200, or 300 ng/mL of PRL resulted in a successful fertilization of more than half of them (see above). Of those embryos, less than half progressed to the morula (40.3% ± 2.4%, 37.1% ± 0.7%, and 37.7% ± 2%, respectively) and blastocyst (40.3% ± 2.4%, 34.0% ± 3.4%, and 34.9% ± 0.8%, respectively) stage (FIG. 3). As previously, the dose of PRL did not appear

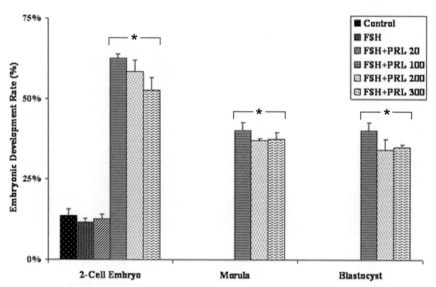

FIGURE 3. Embryonic development (two-cell embryo, morula, and blastocyst) after IVF of *in vitro* matured oocytes, after IVM of different groups of mouse preantral follicles in the presence of varying concentrations of PRL (20, 100, 200, and 300 ng/mL) supplemented by FSH/EGF. Controls (no medium supplementation) and FSH only samples were also included. Percentages are presented as means (±standard error of means) and groups statistically different from both the control and FSH only samples are noted by an asterisk.

to influence the morula or the blastocyst formation rates ($P > 0.05$ in all cases). Even so, both those rates tended to be higher when 100 ng/mL of PRL were employed. Almost all embryos reaching the morula stage progressed to the blastocyst stage ($P > 0.05$ for all sets).

DISCUSSION

The maturation of preantral mouse follicles, as well as their fertilization and cleavage rates, observed when the culture medium was supplemented with middle- and high-range doses of PRL was beneficially affected. Preantral follicles, matured *in vitro* with PRL, FSH, and EGF, showed a high percentage of mature oocytes, even though hCG was not included in the medium. In fact, the absence of hCG did not appreciably influence meiosis, neither fertilization nor early embryonic development. Interestingly, our previous study showed that mouse embryonic development to the morula and blastocyst stages can be significantly higher when oocytes mature with the combination of hCG, PRL, EGF, and FSH, compared to those matured in the absence of hCG.

The beneficial effect of LH on bovine embryonic development has been reported previously.[9] In fact, LH has been shown to enhance maturation of immature oocytes obtained from cattle as reflected by elevated proportions of oocytes that fertilized and reached blastocyst stages *in vitro* after IVF. The action of LH in preantral and small antral follicles was recently reported to be limited.[10] However, granulosa cells express LH/hCG receptors and can be stimulated by both FSH and LH. In the past we have also demonstrated that FSH and LH receptor mRNA is expressed in denuded oocytes as well as in preimplantation embryos of different stages, indicating a physiological role of these hormones in the oocyte maturation process and early embryonic development in both mouse and human.[11,12]

It has been demonstrated that the supplementation of FSH and LH/hCG to the IVM medium of human, murine, and bovine oocytes improves their consequent embryonic development, which underscores the important action of these hormones in the regulation of oocyte maturation and embryonic development.[13]

Furthermore, we have recently demonstrated the beneficial effect of PRL in the IVM of preantral mouse follicles to blastocyst formation (unpublished data).We have also shown that different isoforms of the PRL receptor are present in the various stages of *in vitro* matured mouse follicles.[5] PRL appears to act through its receptor in early preantral follicles, in COCs and in GV stage oocytes resulting in increased nuclear maturation rates. In addition, fertilization and early embryonic development rates were augmented when preantral follicles were cultured in the presence of PRL. PRL in specific concentrations enhances the stimulating effect of FSH in the proliferation of its receptors and in progesterone production in granulose cell cultures.[14]

Consistent with the studies of Cortvrindt *et al.*,[15,16] the addition of rFSH in long-term *in vitro* cultures is essential. Without the addition of r-FSH *in vitro* growth and differentiation of early preantral follicles was compromised and antral cavity formation was never observed. In addition, the maturation rate was higher when hCG and EGF were added to the culture medium on the 12th day of culture. Accordingly, in our study, oocyte nuclear maturation rate increased by the addition of EGF in the culture medium. This observation confirms previous reports.[7,17]

PRL seems to regulate many gonadal functions such as steroidogenesis and corpus luteum formation. Homogenous PRL knock-out mice are sterile, have reduced ovulation and fertilization rates, and their oocytes fail to reinitiate meiosis, while preimplantation development and implantation are altered. In mice, most of these dysfunctions are related to the absence of the long isoform of PRL-R, because this is the major isoform in the cells of reproductive tissues.[18]

As we mentioned previously, PRL, the mRNA receptor of which has been detected in preantral and COCs stages of oocyte development, accelerated the progression of meiosis and fertilization ability, and enhanced the cleavage rate and the rate of blastocyst formation. In addition, hCG has been shown to increase the activity of PRL and hence regulate the nutritional environment of the culture system and consequently oocyte maturation. Therefore, hCG *in vitro* improves embryonic development of embryos when it is combined with PRL. These findings were attributed to an improvement in maturation rate and blastosyst formation when hCG was also present in the culture medium.

In this study, we have shown that the IVM, fertilization, and embryonic development of mouse oocytes from preantral mouse follicles benefits from the supplementation of the culture system with PRL and that the hCG addition seems not to be absolutely necessary for the studied processes. What remains to be clarified is the mechanisms that underlie the interaction of PRL and hCG in this complicated and still not fully elucidated process of IVM.

REFERENCES

1. PINCUS, G. & E.V. ENZMANN. 1935. The comparative behavior of mammalian eggs *in vivo* and *in vitro*: I. The activation of ovarian eggs. J. Exp. Med. **62:** 665–675.
2. GOUGEON, A. & B. LEFEVRE. 1984. Histological evidence of alternating ovulation in women. J. Reprod. Fertil. **70:** 7–13.
3. PAWSHE, C.H., K.B. RAO & S.M. TOTEY. 1998. Effect of insulin-like growth factor I and its interaction with gonadotropins on *in vitro* maturation and embryonic development, cell proliferation, and biosynthetic activity of cumulus-oocyte complexes and granulosa cells in buffalo. Mol. Reprod. Dev. **49:** 277–285.
4. KIAPEKOU, E. *et al.* 2005. Effects of GH and IGF-I on the *in vitro* maturation of mouse oocytes. Hormones (Athens) **4:** 155–160.

5. KIAPEKOU, E. *et al.* 2005. Prolactin receptor mRNA expression in oocytes and preimplantation mouse embryos. Reprod. Biomed. Online **10**: 339–346.
6. CORTVRINDT, R., Y. HU & J. SMITZ. 1998. Recombinant luteinizing hormone as a survival and differentiation factor increases oocyte maturation in recombinant follicle stimulating hormone-supplemented mouse preantral follicle culture. Hum. Reprod. **13**: 1292–1302.
7. DOWNS, S.M. 1989. Specificity of epidermal growth factor action on maturation of the murine oocyte and cumulus oophorus *in vitro*. Biol. Reprod. **41**: 371–379.
8. BEN-YOSEF, D. *et al.* 1992. Rat oocytes induced to mature by epidermal growth factor are successfully fertilized. Mol. Cell Endocrinol. **88**: 135–141.
9. ZUELKE, K.A. & B.G. BRACKETT. 1990. Luteinizing hormone-enhanced *in vitro* maturation of bovine oocytes with and without protein supplementation. Biol. Reprod. **43**: 784–787.
10. FLEMMING, R. *et al.* 2006. Pre-treatment with rhLH: respective effects on antral follicular count and ovarian response to rhFSH. Human Reproduction, Abstracts of the 22nd Annual Meeting of the ESHRE. **21**(Suppl. 1): i54.
11. PATSOULA, E. *et al.* 2001. Expression of mRNA for the LH and FSH receptors in mouse oocytes and preimplantation embryos. Reproduction **121**: 455–461.
12. PATSOULA, E. *et al.* 2003. Messenger RNA expression for the follicle-stimulating hormone receptor and luteinizing hormone receptor in human oocytes and preimplantation-stage embryos. Fertil. Steril. **79**: 1187–1193.
13. ANDERIESZ, C. *et al.* 2000. Effect of recombinant human gonadotrophins on human, bovine and murine oocyte meiosis, fertilization and embryonic development *in vitro*. Hum. Reprod. **15**: 1140–1148.
14. PORTER, M.B., J.R. BRUMSTED & C.K. SITES. 2000. Effect of prolactin on follicle-stimulating hormone receptor binding and progesterone production in cultured porcine granulosa cells. Fertil. Steril. **73**: 99–105.
15. CORTVRINDT, R., J. SMITZ & A.C. VAN STEIRTEGHEM. 1996. In-vitro maturation, fertilization and embryo development of immature oocytes from early preantral follicles from prepuberal mice in a simplified culture system. Hum. Reprod. **11**: 2656–2666.
16. CORTVRINDT, R., J. SMITZ & A.C. VAN STEIRTEGHEM. 1997. Assessment of the need for follicle stimulating hormone in early preantral mouse follicle culture *in vitro*. Hum. Reprod. **12**: 759–768.
17. DOWNS, S.M., S.A. DANIEL & J.J. EPPIG. 1988. Induction of maturation in cumulus cell-enclosed mouse oocytes by follicle-stimulating hormone and epidermal growth factor: evidence for a positive stimulus of somatic cell origin. J. Exp. Zool. **245**: 86–96.
18. ORMANDY, C.J. *et al.* 1997. Null mutation of the prolactin receptor gene produces multiple reproductive defects in the mouse. Genes. Dev. **11**: 167–178.

Greek Experience in the Use of Thermachoice™ for Treating Heavy Menstrual Bleeding

Prospective Study

MINAS PASCHOPOULOS,[a] LAZAROS G. LAVASIDIS,[a]
THOMAS VREKOUSSIS,[a] NIKOLAOS P. POLYZOS,[a]
NIKOLAOS DALKALITSIS,[a] PANAGIOTIS STAMATOPOULOS,[b]
ODYSSEAS GRIGORIOU,[c] GEORGE VLACHOS,[d]
PANAGIOTIS SKOLARIKOS,[e] GEORGE ADONAKIS,[f]
ANASTASIA GOUMENOU,[g] GEORGE LIALIOS,[h] GEORGE MAROULIS,[i]
AND EVANGELOS PARASKEVAIDIS[a]

[a]*Department of Obstetrics and Gynecology, Medical School, University of Ioannina, Greece*

[b]*First Department of Obstetrics and Gynecology, Medical School, University of Thessaloniki, Greece*

[c]*Second Department of Obstetrics and Gynecology, Medical School, University of Athens, Greece*

[d]*First Department of Obstetrics and Gynecology, Medical School, University of Athens, Greece*

[e]*Department of Obstetrics and Gynecology, "Elena Venizelou" Maternity Hospital, Athens, Greece*

[f]*Department of Obstetrics and Gynecology, Medical School, University of Patra, Greece*

[g]*Department of Obstetrics and Gynecology, Medical School, University of Crete, Greece*

[h]*Department of Obstetrics and Gynecology, Medical School, University of Thessaly, Greece*

[i]*Department of Obstetrics and Gynecology, Medical School, University of Thrace, Greece*

ABSTRACT: Heavy menstrual bleeding (HMB) occurs in a considerable percentage of the general population and is one of the main causes due

Address for correspondence: Minas Paschopoulos, M.D., Department of Obstetrics and Gynecology, Medical School and University Hospital, Ioannina 45110, Greece. Voice: +30-26510-99302; fax: +30-26510-99224.
e-mail: mpasxop@cc.uoi.gr

Ann. N.Y. Acad. Sci. 1092: 460–465 (2006). © 2006 New York Academy of Sciences.
doi: 10.1196/annals.1365.045

to which a patient is referred to health services. Despite the efforts for pharmaceutical interventions, the symptom usually persists, therefore operative techniques are needed to control the bleeding. Today, apart from the choice of hysterectomy, other less aggressive techniques have been invented. The first results of the Greek Study Group on Gynecological Endoscopy regarding the use of the Thermachoice™ device are hereby presented. One hundred patients suffering HMB were treated with the Thermachoice™ device following a standard protocol designed by the Study Group. The follow-up meetings with the patients were held at 3, 6, 12, 24, and 36 months. It seems that the overall effectiveness rate (96%) is satisfactory and it is similar to the overall effectiveness rate reported in other relevant studies upon the Thermachoice™ device.

KEYWORDS: heavy menstrual bleeding; second-generation ablation techniques; Thermachoice™

INTRODUCTION

Heavy menstrual bleeding (HMB) is one of the main causes for inpatient care. It is objectively defined as menstrual blood loss of more than 80 mL/cycle, or menstrual bleeding lasting longer than 7 days, over several consecutive cycles.[1] It is reported that 5% of the women admitted to gynecological units in the USA suffer from HMB.[2] Also, recent studies in the UK show that HMB occurs at a rate of 5% in women aged between 30 and 49 years.[2] Excessive bleeding eventually leads to a contact with the Health Services.

Hysterectomy used to be the treatment of choice for HMB because it provides 100% efficacy. It was estimated that around 800,000 hysterectomies were performed for treating HMB during the year 2005 in the USA alone.[2] Nevertheless, the prolonged time of inpatient treatment, the extended time needed for a patient to abstain from everyday activities—leading to higher health and social services expenses—and various complications, have made hysterectomy less appealing than it used to be. Newer techniques—less aggressive but of comparable efficacy—are offered to patients.

The Thermachoice™ device is one of the ablating devices used toward this treatment direction. It was introduced in 1994 and was FDA approved in 1997.[3–5] In this report, the first results from the use of the Thermachoice™ device in Greece for treating HMB are presented.

MATERIALS, PATIENTS, AND METHODS

Protocol Design

The current study was a prospective multicenter study. It was designed by consensus among the participants of the Greek Study Group for Gynecological

Endoscopy and included the first and the second departments of Obstetrics and Gynecology (OB-GYN) of the University of Athens, and the departments of OB-GYN of the "Elena Venizelou" Hospital (Athens), the "Papageorgiou" University Hospital (Thessaloniki), and the University Hospitals of Patra, Heraklion, Alexandroupoli, and Ioannina.

Patients

The present study included 100 patients suffering from dysfunctional uterine bleeding for a period of 3–11 years (median 6.4 years). The median age was 40.7 years (33–49 years). Exclusion criteria for this study were systemic disorders, prior intervention with ablation techniques, and proven gynecological malignancy. Prior to therapy, all patients underwent a transvaginal ultrasound scan to evaluate endometrial thickness and to exclude uterine or ovarian pathology. A Pap test and a histologic evaluation of the endometrium were performed to exclude an underlying malignancy.

Treatment of HMB

All patients were treated with GnRH analogues for 3 months. A transvaginal ultrasound was then performed to reevaluate endometrial thickness. If endometrial thickness was greater than 6 mm, curettage was performed immediately prior to ablation. In cases with endometrium thinner than or equal to 6 mm, endometrial ablation was performed without curettage. Endometrial ablation was performed using the Thermachoice II™ (Gynecare, CA, USA) device according to the manufacturer's protocol. In brief, during the procedure the balloon is inserted in the uterine cavity without direct visualization. While the balloon is situated inside the uterine cavity, it is carefully inflated with 5% dextrose water up to a pressure of 180 mmHg. Once the pressure is stabilized, the heating element and the impeller fan are activated, circulating the fluid and maintaining its temperature at $87°C \pm 5°C$. The duration of the ablating procedure is 8 min and it is electronically monitored. The procedure is electronically cutoff if the pressure falls below 45 mmHg or rises over 210 mmHg. The procedure is also terminated if the temperature exceeds 95°C or falls below 75°C.

Follow-Up

Follow-up was performed at 3, 6, 12, 24, and 36 months after treatment to evaluate the quality of menses.

TABLE 1. Menstruation quality after treatment with Thermachoice™

	3 months	6 months	12 months	24 months	36 months
Amenorrhea (%)	35	19	4	2	2
Hypomenorrhea(%)	55	58	48	45	39
Normal menses (%)	10	23	48	51	55
Menorrhagia (%)	0	0	0	2	4
Overall effectiveness of the method (%)	100	100	100	98	96

RESULTS

The endometrial thickness was between 5 mm and 10 mm (median 7.3). Among the 100 patients no cervical or endometrial malignancy was identified. No cervical high-grade squamus intraepithelial lesion or columnar lesion was found as well. Patients presenting benign or equivocal smear findings were not excluded from the study.

The results of the study (TABLE 1) revealed that amenorrhea, initially caused by endometrial ablation, decreased in a 3-year interval. Although 35% of the cases were diagnosed to have amenorrhea in the first follow-up visit, this symptom persisted only in 2% of the cases 3 years postoperatively. On the contrary, most of the patients experienced menses either frequently (normal menses) or infrequently (hypomenorrhea). Surprisingly, the normal menses' rate gradually increased along the follow-up period. At the end of the study, 55% of the patients declared to have normal menstruation. Also, hypomenorrhea was a common outcome after treatment. However, the rate of hypomenorrhea decreased from 55% to 41% along the follow-up period. No major complications occurred during the procedure, but in two cases temperature elevation was not achieved due to equipment failure. In both cases the silicon balloon was substituted and the procedure continued with no further obstacles.

Four cases out of the 100 presented menorrhagia at 24 months (2 cases) and at 36 months (2 cases) postoperatively. The relative effectiveness of the method was estimated as 96% in 3 years, due to these treatment failures.

DISCUSSION

In this study, the first results of the Greek Study Group on Gynecological Endoscopy are presented. The 3-year follow-up program, as it was designed, is considered satisfactory for efficacy evaluation, although in other studies 5-year programs are also performed.[6] The efficacy of the method in the first year of follow-up seems satisfactory, presenting absolute success in controlling HMB. However, during the second and third year four cases were characterized as failures, since they reported metrorrhagia. These cases, however, were anticipated to fail due to the presence of multiple small submucous myomas. In these cases the GnRH analogue treatment was supposed to minimize the danger of relapse, a thought that was proven to be false. For this reason, after treatment failure, all four cases were treated with modalities other than ablative techniques. In general, however, the efficacy of Thermachoice™ is proven high and is consistent with other reports in the field.[7]

Endometrial thickness over 5 mm does not seem to be an absolute contraindication for endometrial ablation as initially stated within the manufacturer's instructions. On the contrary, administration of GnRH analogues for 3 months, assisted by mild curettage prior to ablation whenever needed, seems to increase the range of treatment success to endometrium up to 10 mm thick. The possibility of relapse in cases presented with thicker endometrium after the 3 years of follow-up is still an issue to be studied in the future.

This study presented as well that the majority of the cases ended up with normal menses or hypomenorrhea, although a substantial proportion reported amenorrhea at the first visit. This can be explained by the proportion of the endometrium that the current method is able to ablate. The balloon inserted in the endometrial cavity cannot extend to the whole endometrial surface. It is extremely difficult for some endometrial regions, especially those proximal to the uterine cornuates, to be totally destroyed. Thus, it is quite possible for menstruation to occur, since the endometrium functions under the influence of estrogens and progesterone still secreted by the ovary. Hypomenorrhea or normal menses may be just different quantity results of the same phenomenon, depending on the extent of the residual endometrium.

The mode of anesthesia is also a matter to comment on. Local or even no anesthesia may be used during this procedure.[8] However, the study group decided to perform the ablation under general anesthesia to avoid possible pain observed in cases of local anesthesia (a fact that could reduce patient compliance in the follow-up program) and to use a uniform protocol, whether curettage was performed or not.

In conclusion, the Thermachoice™ endometrial ablation system seems both efficient and safe in treating HMB. Its efficacy depends on the experience of the performer to avoid complications, as well as on prudent selection of patients for this therapeutic choice. After all, endometrial ablation cannot be considered as the absolute substitute to other operative alternatives, such as hysterectomy or transcervical endometrial resection, but it seems that it is here to stay.

REFERENCES

1. NATIONAL INSTITUTE FOR CLINICAL EXCELLENCE, 2004. Fluid-filled thermal balloon and microwave endometrial ablation techniques for heavy menstrual bleeding: Guidance. NICE Technology Appraisal (TA 078): 1–28.
2. PORKAS, R. & V.G. HUFNAGEL. 1988. Hysterectomy in the United States, 1965–1984. Am. J. Public Health 78: 852–853.

3. AMSO, N.N., S.A. STABINSKY, P. McFAUL, *et al.* 1998. Uterine thermal balloon therapy for the treatment of menorrhagia: the first 300 patients from a multi-centered study. Br. J. Obstet. Gynaecol. **105:** 517–523.
4. MEYER, W.R., B.W. WALSH, D.A. GRAINGER, *et al.* 1998. Thermal balloon and rollerball to treat menorrhagia: a multicenter comparison. Obstet. Gynecol. **92:** 98–103.
5. COOPER, J. & R.J. GIMPELSON. 2004. Summary of safety and effectiveness data from FDA: a valuable source of information on the performance of global endometrial ablation devices. J. Reprod. Med. **49:** 267–273.
6. LOFFER, F.D. & D. GRAINGER. 2002. Five-year follow-up of patients participating in a randomized trial of uterine balloon therapy versus rollerball ablation for treatment of menorrhagia. J. Am. Assoc. Gynecol. Laparosc. **9:** 429–435.
7. OLAH, K.S., J. ALLISTON, J. JONES, *et al.* 2005. Thermal ablation performed in a primary care setting: the South Warwickshire Experience. BJOG **112:** 1117–1120.
8. MARSH, F., J. THEWLIS & S. DUFFY. 2005. Thermachoice endometrial ablation in the outpatient setting, without local anesthesia or intravenous sedation: a prospective cohort study. Fertil. Steril. **83:** 715–720.

Oxytocin Receptor Is Differentially Expressed in Mouse Endometrium and Embryo during Blastocyst Implantation

PANAGIOTIS BERETSOS,[a,b] DIMITRIS LOUTRADIS,[a]
STAUROS KOUSSOULAKOS,[b] LOUKAS H. MARGARITIS,[b]
ERASMIA KIAPEKOU,[a] GEORGE MASTORAKOS,[c]
IRINI PAPASPIROU,[a] NIKOLAOS MAKRIS,[a]
ANTONIS MAKRIGIANNAKIS,[d] AND ARIS ANTSAKLIS[a]

[a]First Department of Obstetrics and Gynecology, Division of Reproductive Medicine, Athens University Medical School, Athens, Greece

[b]Department of Cell Biology and Biophysics, Faculty of Biology, University of Athens, Athens, Greece

[c]Endocrine Unit, Second Department of Obstetrics and Gynecology, Aretaieion Hospital, University of Athens, Athens, Greece

[d]Laboratory of Human Reproduction, Department of Obstetrics and Gynecology, Medical School, University of Crete, Heraklion, Greece

ABSTRACT: The oxytocin (OT)-oxytocin receptor (OTR) system of the mammalian uterus has mainly been studied in relation to its involvement in the onset of labor. The aim of this study was to elucidate the *in vivo* expression and localization pattern of OTR in the mouse endometrium and embryo during implantation, as well as OTR mRNA expression in the *in vitro* developing mouse embryo. The expression of OTR or OT was detected immunohistochemically in uterine tissue sections of 5- to 8-week-old female mice between days 4 and 10 of an established pregnancy. In addition, the expression of OTR mRNA was detected by means of reverse transcription polymerase chain reaction (RT-PCR) in mouse oocytes and embryos up to the blastocyst stage. The mean ratios of normalized expression levels of OTR gene in all samples were also calculated. The recorded increase in OTR mRNA immediately after fertilization could mean a possible role of OT in this process, as OTR mRNA gradually decreased after the four-cell stage of pre-embryonic development. The differential expression of OTR during embryonic apposition and embryonic invasion/placentation in the mouse uterus suggests a potential role of OT in the implantation process of the mouse. It is possible that the interaction of OTR with the hormones included in the ovulation

Address for correspondence: Panagiotis Beretsos, First Department of Obstetrics and Gynecology, Division of Reproductive Medicine, Athens University Medical School, 50 Achaias St., 115 23, Athens, Greece. Voice: 0030-694-6902173; fax: 0030-210-7470460.
e-mail: pberet@biol.uoa.gr

Ann. N.Y. Acad. Sci. 1092: 466–479 (2006). © 2006 New York Academy of Sciences.
doi: 10.1196/annals.1365.046

induction regiments utilized today in *in vitro* fertilization (IVF) could be affecting the receptivity/quality of the implanting endometrium.

KEYWORDS: early development; embryo; implantation; oxytocin; oxytocin receptor

INTRODUCTION

Approximately 50% of all biochemically and clinically recognized pregnancies in humans end in spontaneous abortion before or during the implantation of the pre-embryo into the uterus. The successful implantation of the developing pre-embryo and the establishment of pregnancy is the result of highly orchestrated actions and interactions of many factors, which regulate the maturation of the endometrium, the communication between the conceptus and the uterus, as well as embryonic apposition and invasion.[1-3] A potential modulator of uterine function that has been receiving attention concerning its involvement in the implantation process is oxytocin (OT).

OT is a nine-amino acid peptide produced by the paraventricular and the supraoptic nuclei of the hypothalamus as a large precursor molecule and secreted by the posterior pituitary gland in a spurt or pulsatile fashion.[4] Nevertheless, the expression of OT has also been detected in many other organs, including the uterus,[5,6] of several species. OT is involved to some extent in most of the acute reproductive functions, of which the induction of uterine smooth muscle contraction at birth and the stimulation of milk production are nowadays well established and the most studied.[7] Furthermore, it has been recently documented that OT is able to induce the differentiation of mouse embryonic stem cells[8] and regulate the proliferation of cancer cells[9,10] *in vitro*. Although the controlled pattern of OT release appears to be an important factor in the regulation of the hormonal homeostasis, there is no doubt that the OT receptor (OTR) plays the most crucial role in this operational web. OT receptor is a G protein-coupled receptor with seven transmembrane domains and is expressed in many organs, including the kidneys, ovaries, uterus, testes, as well as in various cancer cell lines.[4] The expression of the receptor undergoes dramatic cell-specific upregulation and downregulation, allowing the circulating OT to switch its target organs and its actions. A variety of factors, including progesterone, estrogen,[11-13] and interleukins,[14,15] are implicated in the control of OTR expression, although the exact mechanisms of this regulation remain largely unknown.

Although the OT/OTR system of the mammalian uterus has mainly been studied in relation to its involvement in the onset of labor, OT and its receptor seem to be dynamically regulated during estrus and early pregnancy, implying further physiological roles in other reproductive functions, too. The receptor, as well as its mRNA, have been detected in the endometrium of various mammals where they are expressed mainly in the endometrial glands of the epithelium.[16–18] Both are downregulated throughout the luteal phase of the reproductive cycle, especially around the implantation window.

In this study, we have investigated the pattern of OTR expression in the mouse endometrium during embryonic apposition and trophoblast invasion, focusing on the peri-implantation area. In addition, the temporospatial expression of OT in the mouse uterus was detected during the phases of embryonic invasion.

MATERIALS AND METHODS

Animals and Cell/Tissue Collection

All operations were performed according to the guidelines of the Federal Animal Welfare Regulations. Adult female crossbred (New Zealand Black [NZB] × New Zealand White [NZW]) mice with normal ovarian cycles were obtained (Hellenic Pasteur Institute, Athens, Greece) and kept under a 12 h light/dark cycle under standardized conditions ($22 \pm 1°C$; $60 \pm 5\%$ humidity) with free access to standard diet and tap water. They were induced to super-ovulate with intra-abdominal injections of 5 IU eCG (Sigma-Aldrich, Dorset, UK) followed after 48 h by similar injections of 5 IU hCG (Sigma-Aldrich).

For the collection of oocytes, mice were sacrificed 15–17 h after hCG administration by cervical dislocation and their ovaries were removed and placed in Dulbecco's phosphate-buffered saline (DPBS; Invitrogen Life Technologies, Paisley, UK), supplemented with bovine serum albumin (BSA) (9:1) (Sigma-Aldrich). Oocytes were collected by puncturing the ovaries, followed by addition of 60 IU/mL hyaluronidase (Sigma-Aldrich) for 2–3 min and removal of the cumulus cells. Hyaluronidase was removed by washing the cumulus-free oocytes in fresh medium and the cells were processed for mRNA extraction.

For the collection of mouse embryos, female mice were allowed to mate with males of the same age and strain overnight. The females were sacrificed by cervical dislocation 15–17 h after hCG administration, their oviducts were removed and washed in DPBS and zygotes were collected by puncturing. A number of the collected zygotes were cultured in modified Ham's culture medium without hypoxanthine[19] (Invitrogen Life Technologies) at 37°C, 95% humidity, 5% CO_2, and pH 7.3. Four-cell embryos, morulae, and blastocysts were collected 42–46 h, 70 h, and 96 h, respectively, after the initiation of culture. The embryos were washed several times in DPBS/BSA prior to mRNA extraction.

Similarly, for the collection of pregnant uteri, females were allowed to mate with males of the same age and strain overnight. The detection of a copulatory plug the following morning designated day 1 of pregnancy. Two mice were sacrificed by cervical dislocation every 24 h and their uteri were removed. Two uteri were obtained from each animal. Each collected uterus was fixed in formalin overnight before being sequentially dehydrated and embedded in paraffin routinely destined to immunohistochemistry.

Immunohistochemistry

Serial sections (4 μm) of the paraffin-embedded uteri were prepared and mounted on Super-Frost Plus® slides (Menzel Gläser, Braunschweig, Germany) to be used for immunological detection of OTR or OT. All sections were incubated overnight at 50°C, dewaxed in xylol three times for 5 min each at 50°C, and 2 min at room temperature, followed by descending concentrations of ethanol. Every fifth section was counterstained by hematoxylin and eosin to study the microscopic anatomy of the uterus. The sections destined to immunological detection were incubated for 15 min (3 × 5 min) in 10 mM citrate buffer, pH 6.0 at 120°C, allowing them to cool over 45 min and were washed twice in PBS.

The immunohistochemical detection of OTR was performed using the Abcam ABC HRP-AEC complex (Abcam, Cambridgeshire, UK) according to the manufacturer's instructions, while for OT an alkaline phosphatase-based assay (Biogenex, San Ramon, CA) was employed. Briefly, a specific, commercially available, primary antibody against OTR (Abcam, Cambridgeshire, UK) or OT (Abcam) was applied (dilution 1:100) to the slides and incubated at 4°C overnight in a moist chamber. After washing with PBS, the secondary antibody was applied to the slides and incubated for 60 min at room temperature. The signal was visualized by incubating the slides in 3-amino-9-ethylcarbazole and H_2O_2 (ABC complex) or Fast Red substrate solution (alkaline phosphatase assay). The slides were counterstained with hematoxylin and mounted with aqueous mounting medium (Abcam).

For the determination of the signal specificity, the primary antibody was omitted in control sections. Depending on the experimental setup, the uterine sections from all animals were examined immunohistochemically together and several times to obtain consistent patterns of staining.

RNA Extraction

Total RNA was extracted from 30 oocytes and groups of 10–20 zygotes, four-cell stage embryos, morulae, and blastocysts. A commercially available kit was used for RNA isolation (RNAeasy micro kit; Qiagen, Valencia, CA), according to the manufacturer's instructions. The RNase-free DNase I and carrier RNA, included in the kit, were utilized to obtain highly purified RNA.

Reverse Transcription-Polymerase Chain Reaction (RT-PCR)

Total RNA from oocytes, zygotes, four-cell stage embryos, morulae and blastocysts was reverse transcribed (RT) to cDNA by using a commercially available kit (Retroscript kit; Ambion, Austin, TX), according to the manufacturer's instructions, in the presence (RT+) or absence (RT−) of reverse transcriptase. Reactions were incubated for 60 min at 42°C, followed by 10 min at 92°C.

The reverse transcription reaction was followed by two separate rounds of PCR for the detection of OTR and rig/S15 mRNAs, respectively. For the detection of OTR mRNA, a commercially available primer set amplifying a 151 bp of the mouse OTR gene was used (SuperArray Bioscience Corp., Frederick, MD). Similarly, a commercially available primer pair was used for the detection of Rig/S15 mRNA (forward: 5–TTCCGCAAGTTCACCTACC, reverse: 5–CGGGCCGGCCATGTTTACG), which is a constitutively expressed "housekeeping" gene encoding for a small ribosomal subunit protein (Retroscript kit; Ambion). The primer pair amplified a 361 bp region of the S15 gene.

For the PCR reactions the ReactionReady™ Hotstart "Sweet" PCR master mix (SuperArray, USA) was used, according to the manufacturer's instructions. Briefly, 1 μL of cDNA and 1 μL of the appropriate primer pair were added to 12.5 μL of ReactionReady™ Hotstart "Sweet" PCR master mix and 10.5 μL of ddH$_2$O. The reaction mixture was incubated at 95°C for 15 min, followed by 25 cycles of denaturation at 94°C for 15 sec, annealing at 55°C for 30 sec and extension at 72°C for 30 sec. A low number of denaturation cycles were used to eliminate the possibility of nonlinear amplification. In each round, a reaction where the cDNA was omitted was also included as a control of contamination from other DNA sources. The products were stored at −20°C.

The amplified products (10 μL) were electrophoresed on a 3% agarose gel containing ethidium bromide (Sigma-Aldrich), in parallel with a 100 bp DNA ladder (Fermentas Life Sciences, Ontario, Canada) and the appropriate negative controls.

Agarose Gel Analysis

An image of the agarose gel was captured with a UV Trans Illuminator using a Gel-Doc Station (Biosure, Athens, Greece), while acquisition and analysis of the obtained data was performed with Gel Analyser v. 1.0 (Biosure). The expression levels of OTR mRNA were normalized by dividing by the background-corrected value for the corresponding S15 control band.[20] The fold-change in the expression of OTR gene between different sample groups was determined by calculating the ratio of its normalized expression levels between those samples. Means of the obtained ratios from all repeats of RT-PCRs and standard errors of mean were calculated with SPSS for Windows v. 13.0 (SPSS, Inc., Chicago, IL).

RESULTS

OT Receptor mRNA Expression in Mouse Oocytes and Early Embryos

The presence of OTR mRNA was investigated by PCR in mouse oocytes (meiosis II) and embryos of various developmental stages (zygotes, four-cell

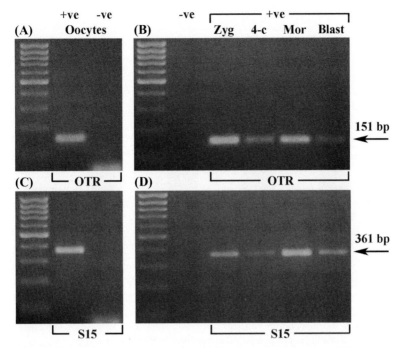

FIGURE 1. Gel electrophoresis of RT-PCR products for OTR and S15 protein (**A** and **C**, respectively) in mouse oocytes, and OTR and S15 protein (**B** and **D**, respectively) in mouse zygotes (Zyg), four-cell stage embryos (4-c), morulae (Mor), and blastocysts (Blast). In each case, a sample where the cDNA was omitted is presented (negative). The detection of S15 mRNA confirmed the integrity of the RNA isolation and the RT-PCR process.

stage embryos, morulae, blastocysts). The receptor mRNA was expressed in all group samples examined, giving rise to the expected 151 bp band during electrophoresis (FIGS. 1A and B). All oocytes (FIG. 1C) and embryos (FIG. 1D) expressed S15 mRNA, while no products were observed in the absence of reverse transcriptase or cDNA. During electrophoresis, variability was observed in the band intensity of the S15 sample products, although this is probably due to the variable number of cells used in the total RNA extraction process. The experiments were performed in triplicate with total RNA extractions from different groups of cells or embryos, yielding statistically identical results.

The mean ratios and standard errors of mean of normalized expression levels of OTR gene in oocytes, zygotes, four-cell stage embryos, morulae, and blastocysts, after acquisition and analysis of data obtained from the corresponding electrophoresed RT-PCR products, were also calculated (FIG. 2). The expression of OTR gene was upregulated after fertilization of the oocytes (mean ratio 0.98 ± 0.05 in zygotes and 0.73 ± 0.11 in oocytes, $P < 0.01$). Nevertheless, embryonic development appeared to be related to the downregulation of OTR

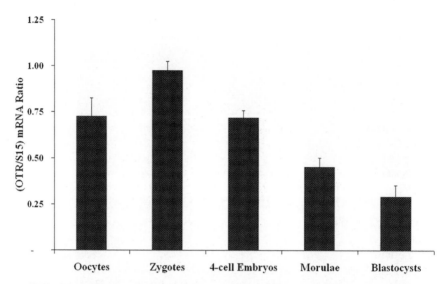

FIGURE 2. Semiquantitative analysis of OTR mRNA expression in mouse oocytes, zygotes, four-cell stage embryos, morulae, and blastocysts. The mean ratios and standard errors of mean of normalized expression levels of OTR gene in oocytes, zygotes, four-cell stage embryos, morulae, and blastocysts were calculated, after acquisition and analysis of data obtained from the corresponding electrophoresed RT-PCR products.

gene expression (mean ratio 0.72 ± 0.04 in four-cell stage embryos, 0.45 ± 0.05 in morulae, and 0.29 ± 0.06 in blastocysts, $P < 0.01$ when compared to stage the zygote stage and to each other), with the ratio of expression decreasing more than threefold at the blastocyst stage compared to OTR gene expression in the zygote.

Early Implantation and Embryonic Apposition

Histological slides from pregnant mice uteri including part of an attaching mouse embryo (days 4–5 of pregnancy) were examined. The presence of OTR in the endometrium was immunohistochemically detected in the form of red granules of minor staining intensity; therefore the receptor was considered to be expressed in low amounts (FIGS. 3A and B). The receptor was predominantly detected in the epithelial cells of the endometrial glands of the uterus, with the intensity of staining varying among the cells that constituted the glands (FIG. 3A). The distribution of OTR on the cytoplasmic membrane of positive cells followed a constant, granulated pattern. The endometrial cells surrounding the implanting embryo did not yield any positive immunoreactivity suggesting lack of OTR expression at this stage (FIG. 3B). On the contrary, OTR appeared to be expressed in the embryonic cells of the implanting embryos.

Positive immunoreactivity was absent when the primary antibody was omitted (FIG. 3G).

Trophoblast Invasion and Establishment of Pregnancy

The expression of OTR was also studied in more progressed stages of implantation, especially during trophoblast invasion and early stages of placentation. As in the case of embryonic apposition, histological sections from various stages (days) of pregnancy were studied to find the suitable samples, focusing on uteri from mice that were on days 7–9 of pregnancy. These samples were characterized by the early stages of placental formation, as well as the development of early embryonic tissues. Immunohistochemical localization revealed the expression of OTR in both the endometrium of the uterus and the embryonic tissues. In fact, endometrial OTR continued to be expressed mainly in the glandular epithelium, showing a higher level of expression compared to the peri-implantation stages. Endometrial OTR expression was also detected at the sites of embryonic implantation (FIGS. 3C and 3D). The immunoreactivity was localized predominantly at the site of conceptus-uterine interaction, namely the cytotrophoblastic and syncytiotrophoblastic tissues. However, the receptor was also detected at low levels in some of the peripheral to the embryo endometrial cells, showing a differential expression pattern. The distribution of embryonic OTR expression during the first stages of embryo development and differentiation appeared to be rather organized compared to the early embryo, as positive immunoreactivity was mainly present at the peripheral embryonic tissues (FIGS. 3C and D). Positive immunoreactivity was absent when the primary antibody was omitted.

Various sites of embryonic invasion were also accessed for the presence of OT. The hormone was found to be present throughout the endometrium of the mouse uterus (FIG. 3E), with the greatest intensity being observed at the endometrial tissues peripherally to the implanting embryo, as well as the embryo itself and the cytotrophoblast (FIG. 3F). Large amounts of OT, compared to the rest of the mouse endometrium, were also detected at the developing syncytiotrophoblastic tissues (FIG. 3F). In the absence of the primary antibody no immunoreactivity was observed (FIG. 3H).

DISCUSSION

Although OT was first discovered by Sir Henry Dale in 1909,[21] who noticed its uterine contractile effect, it is only the last few years that the OT-OTR system has been studied in relation to the establishment of pregnancy. We have recently presented data showing the downregulation of OTR in the cycling mouse endometrium during the peri-implantation period, after the LH surge and the physiological rise of progesterone.[22] Similar findings have been

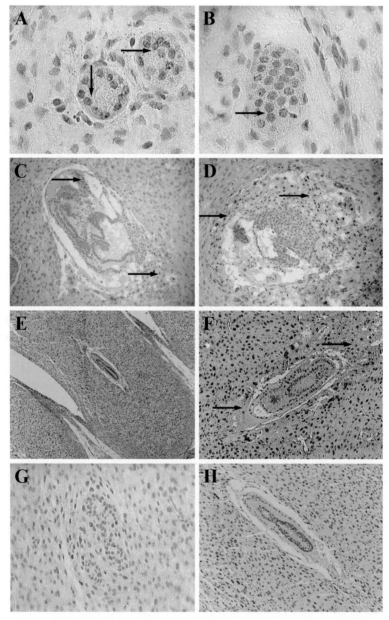

FIGURE 3. Immunohistochemical localization of OTR (**A**, **B**, **C**, and **D**) and OT (**E** and **F**) on sections obtained from the mouse pregnant uterus during embryonic apposition (days 4–5 of pregnancy) (**A**, **B**, and **G**) and embryonic invasion and placental development (days 7–9 of pregnancy) (**C**, **D**, **E**, **F**, and **H**). Positive staining is revealed as red color (red chromogen), whereas the light blue color of hematoxylin stains nonspecifically all cell nuclei. Black arrows point to the sites of OTR (**A**, **B**, **C**, and **D**) or OT (**F**) expression.

rreported by others in the cow,[16] the marmoset monkey,[17] and in humans.[18] In this study, we have demonstrated the localization pattern of OTR expression at the peri-implantation endometrial area of the mouse uterus throughout the early implantation stages, showing the differential expression of OTR during embryonic apposition and embryonic invasion/early placentation. Although previous investigations have shown that the onset of pregnancy in humans[17,23] and cows[16] is accompanied by a downregulation of endometrial OTR expression, this is the first time, to our knowledge, that a differential, localized expression of endometrial OTR at various stages of the implantation processes is presented.

In mammals, it is well established that the LH surge and therefore ovulation is accompanied by an upregulation of progesterone and estrogens. Several studies have shown that both hormones have an effect on OTR expression in a cell-specific manner. In fact, estrogens have been suggested to cause the upregulation of OTR in a variety of tissues in the female rat,[24] including the uterus,[25] although some investigators have questioned the degree of this effect.[26,27] Furthermore, progesterone has been reported to induce a dose-dependent inhibition of specific OT binding to its receptor,[28] as well as to downregulate the receptor itself.[29] In addition, both have recently been shown to have an opposing role in the regulation of uterine peristalsis caused by OT.[30] Actually, estrogens have been reported to stimulate uterine peristalsis, an effect that was antagonized by progesterone, which suppressed uterine contractility. This effect is more clearly presented by our results, where we have seen that OTR is downregulated at the endometrial areas surrounding the attaching embryo, as during embryonic apposition the suppression of uterine contractility may be important for the successful initiation of implantation.[31] However, uterine contractility appears to hold an important role in the successful implantation of the pre-embryo in general,[32] for example during embryonic invasion, which was verified by the upregulation of OTR at the periembryonic endometrial areas, as well as the presence of OT in the uterus, especially at the peri-implantation areas of the endometrium, throughout the later stages of

---

(A) Positive immunoreactivity in the epithelial cells of endometrial glands (magnified 100×); the endometrial glands are round, small, and not very dense, a situation characteristic of the endometrium during the follicular or proliferative phase. (B) Positively stained cells of attaching embryo. No specific staining can be observed in the surrounding endometrial cells. (D) Positively stained cells of an invading embryo and endometrial cells of the peri-implantation area (magnified 60×). (E and F) Positive immunoreactivity in the endometrial cells of the pregnant mouse uterus and invading embryo. Staining was more intense in the peri-implantation areas of the endometrium. [magnified (E) 20× and (F) 40×]. (G and H) Control samples, where the primary antibody was omitted, were also included. No specific staining can be observed in the epithelial cells of endometrial glands (G), the endometrial cells (G and H), or the embryonic cells (H) (magnified 40×).

implantation. Progesterone appears to hold a crucial role in the control of OTR expression and therefore uterine contractility and it has actually been proposed to have beneficiary effects in *in vitro* fertilization (IVF) cycles by supporting early pregnancy.[33,34] Nevertheless, the protocols of progesterone administration that are currently adopted include high dosages of the hormone that may be affecting the subsequent upregulation of OTR observed throughout embryonic invasion and early placentation, resulting therefore to poorer implantation rates. A more sophisticated protocol of progesterone administration, in respect to the dosage and time of administration, could prove beneficial in the outcome of IVF cycles, at least at the level of early pregnancy establishment.

The role of OT during implantation may not be limited strictly in the control of uterine contractility. The last few years, OT has been suggested to be implicated in the proliferation of cancer cells,[9,10] as well as the induction of differentiation of mouse embryonic stem cells to cardiomyocytes.[8] The association of the OT-OTR system with processes of cellular proliferation and differentiation could explain the upregulation of OTR and the accumulation of OT at the peri-implantation endometrial areas we recorded during embryonic invasion and early placentation, which include proliferation and differentiation of the trophoblast, regulation of placental growth and regulation of vascular mimicry. A number of additional factors could be involved in the regulation of OTR expression at this level. A strong candidate is interleukin 6 (IL-6), which is upregulated during the peri-implantation period of pregnancy and remains high throughout the early embryo invasion phase.[35] In fact, the rat and human OTR genes contain several potential interleukin response elements,[36] while IL-6 has been reported to upregulate OTR mRNA expression and binding capacity in cultured human uterine smooth muscle cells.[15] In addition, interferon tau (INF-τ) has been suggested to hold an important role in the control of OTR expression on behalf of the embryo. This characteristic type I interferon is produced by the trophoblast of the developing blastocyst of many species, including the cow[37] and sheep,[38] where it is most studied. This molecule has been related to the downregulation of both OTR and its gene transcripts in cows[39] and sheep,[40] and other ruminants in general.[41] The short time that this molecule is produced by the blastocyst during its presence in the uterus may represent a potential accessory mechanism for the embryo to control the receptivity status of the endometrium and to prevent the development of the endometrial luteolytic mechanism exerted by the OT-OTR system.

The expression of OTR and its mRNA in the cells of the developing embryo has also been presented in the present study. The receptor appears to be expressed as far as the invading embryo, while it is not completely downregulated during embryonic apposition. This, however, does occur in the surrounding endometrial cells, suggesting the existence of alternate, cell-specific mechanisms of OTR expression control between the embryonic cells and the endometrial cells of the uterus. Such a cell-specific type of control in the OTR expression has been suggested by various studies in the past in order to explain the variability in the actions of various molecules, such as estrogens, on OTR expression, as well as the differential pharmacological profiles or immunoreactivity patterns of OT observed.[4,42] The receptor until now has been identified in the cumulus cells of both human[43] and bovine[44] preovulatory follicles, in human trophoblast and choriocarcinoma cell lines,[45] as well as in the developing rat brain.[42] At this study, we have shown that OTR mRNA is constantly expressed during *in vitro* early mouse embryonic development. Although the extent of this expression was assessed in a semiquantitative manner, the level of expression appears to be downregulated from the zygote to the blastocyst stage. In fact, mouse blastocysts showed a more than threefold decrease of OTR expression in comparison to the zygote, while *in vivo* fertilization of the mouse oocytes resulted in a transient upregulation of the OTR mRNA. It remains to investigate further this increase in the OT binding sites during fertilization and examine whether it has a physiological role during this process, considering the fact that OT exerts its actions by activating phospholipase C-β, which results to the release of Ca^{2+} from intracellular stores.[4]

In conclusion, the present study describes a complex mechanism of OTR expression in the mouse endometrium and developing pre-embryo during the implantation process, which in fact is accompanied by certain physiological processes where OT has been suggested to be involved. The utilization of this knowledge in ovulation induction and IVF protocols could be proven beneficial for the patient, although the necessity of the role of OT in those processes remains to be further investigated.

ACKNOWLEDGMENTS

The project is cofinanced within Op. Education by the ESF (European Social Fund) and National Resources. Part of this project has been awarded with the ESHRE Promising Young Scientist Award 2006 at ESHRE 22nd Annual Meeting, Prague, 2006.

REFERENCES

1. BEIER, H.M. & K. BEIER-HELLWIG. 1998. Molecular and cellular aspects of endometrial receptivity. Hum. Reprod. Update **4:** 448–458.
2. MINAS, V., D. LOUTRADIS & A. MAKRIGIANNAKIS. 2005. Factors controlling blastocyst implantation. Reprod. Biomed. Online. **10:** 205–216.
3. MAKRIGIANNAKIS, A. *et al.* 2006. Hormonal and cytokine regulation of early implantation. Trends Endocrinol. Metab. **17:** 178–185.
4. GIMPL, G. & F. FAHRENHOLZ. 2001. The oxytocin receptor system: structure, function, and regulation. Physiol. Rev. **81:** 629–683.
5. STEINWALL, M. *et al.* 2004. Oxytocin mRNA content in the endometrium of nonpregnant women. BJOG **111:** 266–270.

6. BAE, S.E. & E.D. WATSON. 2003. A light microscopic and ultrastructural study on the presence and location of oxytocin in the equine endometrium. Theriogenology **60:** 909–921.
7. ZEEMAN, G.G., F.S. KHAN-DAWOOD & M.Y. DAWOOD. 1997. Oxytocin and its receptor in pregnancy and parturition: current concepts and clinical implications. Obstet. Gynecol. **89:** 873–883.
8. PAQUIN, J. *et al.* 2002. Oxytocin induces differentiation of P19 embryonic stem cells to cardiomyocytes. Proc. Natl. Acad. Sci. USA **99:** 9550–9555.
9. CASSONI, P. *et al.* 2004. Evidence of oxytocin/oxytocin receptor interplay in human prostate gland and carcinomas. Int. J. Oncol. **25:** 899–904.
10. REVERSI, A. *et al.* 2005. The oxytocin receptor antagonist atosiban inhibits cell growth via a "biased agonist" mechanism. J. Biol. Chem. **280:** 16311–16318.
11. AMICO, J.A., P.N. RAUK & H.M. CAI. 2002. Estradiol and progesterone regulate oxytocin receptor binding and expression in human breast cancer cell lines. Endocrine **18:** 79–84.
12. KOMBE, A., J. SIROIS & A.K. GOFF. 2003. Prolonged progesterone treatment of endometrial epithelial cells modifies the effect of estradiol on their sensitivity to oxytocin. Steroids **68:** 651–658.
13. MURATA, T. *et al.* 2000. Oxytocin receptor gene expression in rat uterus: regulation by ovarian steroids. J. Endocrinol. **166:** 45–52.
14. LEUNG, S.T. *et al.* 2001. The effects of lipopolysaccharide and interleukins-1alpha, -2 and -6 on oxytocin receptor expression and prostaglandin production in bovine endometrium. J. Endocrinol. **168:** 497–508.
15. RAUK, P.N. *et al.* 2001. Interleukin-6 up-regulates the oxytocin receptor in cultured uterine smooth muscle cells. Am. J. Reprod. Immunol. **45:** 148–153.
16. ROBINSON, R.S. *et al.* 2001. Expression of oxytocin, oestrogen and progesterone receptors in uterine biopsy samples throughout the oestrous cycle and early pregnancy in cows. Reproduction **122:** 965–979.
17. EINSPANIER, A., A. BIELEFELD & J.H. KOPP. 1998. Expression of the oxytocin receptor in relation to steroid receptors in the uterus of a primate model, the marmoset monkey. Hum. Reprod. Update **4:** 634–646.
18. KIMURA, T. 1998. Regulation of the human oxytocin receptor in the uterus: a molecular approach. Hum. Reprod. Update **4:** 615–624.
19. LOUTRADIS, D. *et al.* 1994. The effect of compounds altering the cAMP level on reversing the 2-cell block induced by hypoxanthine in mouse embryos *in vitro*. Eur. J. Obstet. Gynecol. Reprod. Biol. **57:** 195–199.
20. SAMBROOK, J., T. MANIATIS & E.F. FRITSCH. 1989. Molecular Cloning a Laboratory Manual. Cold Spring Harbor Laboratory Press. New York, NY.
21. DALE, H.H. 1909. The action of extracts of the pituitary body. Biochem. J. **4:** 427–447.
22. BERETSOS, P. *et al.* 2006. The role of oxytocin in early embryo development and implantation of mouse embryos. Hum. Reprod. Abstracts of the 22nd Annual Meeting of the ESHRE. **21**(Suppl. 1): i29.
23. HELMER, H. *et al.* 1998. Oxytocin and vasopressin 1a receptor gene expression in the cycling or pregnant human uterus. Am. J. Obstet. Gynecol. **179:** 1572–1578.
24. QUINONES-JENAB, V. *et al.* 1997. Effects of estrogen on oxytocin receptor messenger ribonucleic acid expression in the uterus, pituitary, and forebrain of the female rat. Neuroendocrinology **65:** 9–17.
25. LARCHER, A. *et al.* 1995. Oxytocin receptor gene expression in the rat uterus during pregnancy and the estrous cycle and in response to gonadal steroid treatment. Endocrinology **136:** 5350–5356.

26. PATISAUL, H.B. *et al.* 2003. Oxytocin, but not oxytocin receptor, is regulated by oestrogen receptor beta in the female mouse hypothalamus. J. Neuroendocrinol. **15:** 787–793.
27. SIEBEL, A.L., H.M. GEHRING & L.J. PARRY. 2004. Steroid-independent regulation of uterine oxytocin receptors. J. Neuroendocrinol. **16:** 398–402.
28. GRAZZINI, E. *et al.* 1998. Inhibition of oxytocin receptor function by direct binding of progesterone. Nature **392:** 509–512.
29. ZHANG, J., P.G. WESTON & J.E. HIXON. 1992. Role of progesterone and oestradiol in the regulation of uterine oxytocin receptors in ewes. J. Reprod. Fertil. **94:** 395–404.
30. MUELLER, A. *et al.* 2006. Role of estrogen and progesterone in the regulation of uterine peristalsis: results from perfused non-pregnant swine uteri. Hum. Reprod. **21:** 1863–1868.
31. FANCHIN, R. *et al.* 2001. Uterine contractility decreases at the time of blastocyst transfers. Hum. Reprod. **16:** 1115–1119.
32. BULLETTI, C. & D. DE ZIEGLER. 2006. Uterine contractility and embryo implantation. Curr. Opin. Obstet. Gynecol. **18:** 473–484.
33. LOUTRADIS, D. *et al.* 2006. Estradiol and progesterone supplementation during luteal phase improved the receptivity of the endometrium in a patient with a history of diethylstilboestrol exposure in-utero. Hormones (Athens) **5:** 147–150.
34. PROCTOR, A. *et al.* 2006. Effect of progesterone supplementation in early pregnancy on the pregnancy outcome after *in vitro* fertilization. Fertil. Steril. **85:** 1550–1552.
35. DE, M., T.R. SANFORD & G.W. WOOD. 1993. Expression of interleukin 1, interleukin 6 and tumour necrosis factor alpha in mouse uterus during the peri-implantation period of pregnancy. J. Reprod. Fertil. **97:** 83–89.
36. KUBOTA, Y. *et al.* 1996. Structure and expression of the mouse oxytocin receptor gene. Mol. Cell Endocrinol. **124:** 25–32.
37. STOJKOVIC, M. *et al.* 1999. Secretion of interferon-tau by bovine embryos in long-term culture: comparison of *in vivo* derived, *in vitro* produced, nuclear transfer and demi-embryos. Anim. Reprod. Sci. **55:** 151–162.
38. LO, W.C. & P.M. SUMMERS. 2002. *In vitro* culture and interferon-tau secretion by ovine blastocysts. Anim. Reprod. Sci. **70:** 191–202.
39. HORN, S. *et al.* 1998. Bovine endometrial epithelial cells as a model system to study oxytocin receptor regulation. Hum. Reprod. Update **4:** 605–614.
40. SPENCER, T.E. & F.W. BAZER. 1996. Ovine interferon tau suppresses transcription of the estrogen receptor and oxytocin receptor genes in the ovine endometrium. Endocrinology **137:** 1144–1147.
41. FLINT, A.P. 1995. Interferon, the oxytocin receptor and the maternal recognition of pregnancy in ruminants and non-ruminants: a comparative approach. Reprod. Fertil. Dev. **7:** 313–318.
42. YOSHIMURA, R. *et al.* 1996. Differential expression of oxytocin receptor mRNA in the developing rat brain. Neurosci. Res. **24:** 291–304.
43. COPLAND, J.A. *et al.* 2002. Oxytocin receptor regulation and action in a human granulosa-lutein cell line. Biol. Reprod. **66:** 1230–1236.
44. JO, M. & J.E. FORTUNE. 2003. Changes in oxytocin receptor in bovine preovulatory follicles between the gonadotropin surge and ovulation. Mol. Cell. Endocrinol. **200:** 31–43.
45. CASSONI, P. *et al.* 2001. Activation of functional oxytocin receptors stimulates cell proliferation in human trophoblast and choriocarcinoma cell lines. Endocrinology **142:** 1130–1136.

Index of Contributors